MW00843510

Clinical Essentials of Contemporary Series
Chinese Medicine

Chinese Herbal Medicine

现代中医临床备要丛书

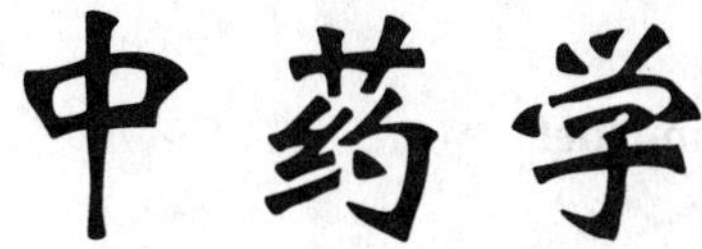

Editors-in-chief ***Lin Gongwang***

Translators-in-chief ***Cao Liya***

Hua Xia Publishing House
华夏出版社

Editor-in-chief

Liu Gongwang

Associate Editor-in-chief

Hyodo Akira　Li Qinghe　Wang Yuxing　Jiao Mao

Editors

Chen Shungbai	Han Yu	Lzimi Takasi
Li Jianyu	Liu Hongchao	Nian Li
Wan Zengzhi	Yu Hong	Zhang Guozhong

Translator-in-chief

Cao Liya

Associate Translator-in-chief

Chu Lirong

Translators

Hu Limin	Li Jie	Liang Chunyu
Liu Weiwei	Liu Wenhong	Liu Yi
Ma Zuoying	Pan Xingfang	Shang Xiukui
Sun Yanming	Wang Wei	Xu Junjuan
Xu Li	Zhang Biao	Zhong Qiangwei

Foreign Translators

Jean Damascene Nsabimana　H. Colin Ohler Anne Troulay

Assistants

Liu Lu　Li Jie　Wu Ming

English Editor

Donald P. Lauda　Jeffrey L. Carnett

Translation Reviser

Shuji Goto　Liu Gongwang

Illustrator

Gong Baoxi

Supervisors

Shuji Goto　Dai Ximeng　Donald P. Lauda

祝「现代中医临床备要」出版发行：

博采精收，衷中参西，

堪称当代中医临床佳作。

吴咸中

九九年十一月

Congratulations on the publication of the book *Clinical Essentials of Contemporary Chinese Medicine*! This book has an extensive collection of TCM essence. It is an integration of Chinese Medicine and Western Medicine and may be rated as a fine clinical piece of modern Chinese Medicine!

Wu Xianzhong

Nov. 1999

(Inscription by Prof. Wu Xianzhong, Acdemician of Academy of Engineering of China, chairman of the Chinses Association of the Integration of Traditional and Western Medicine)

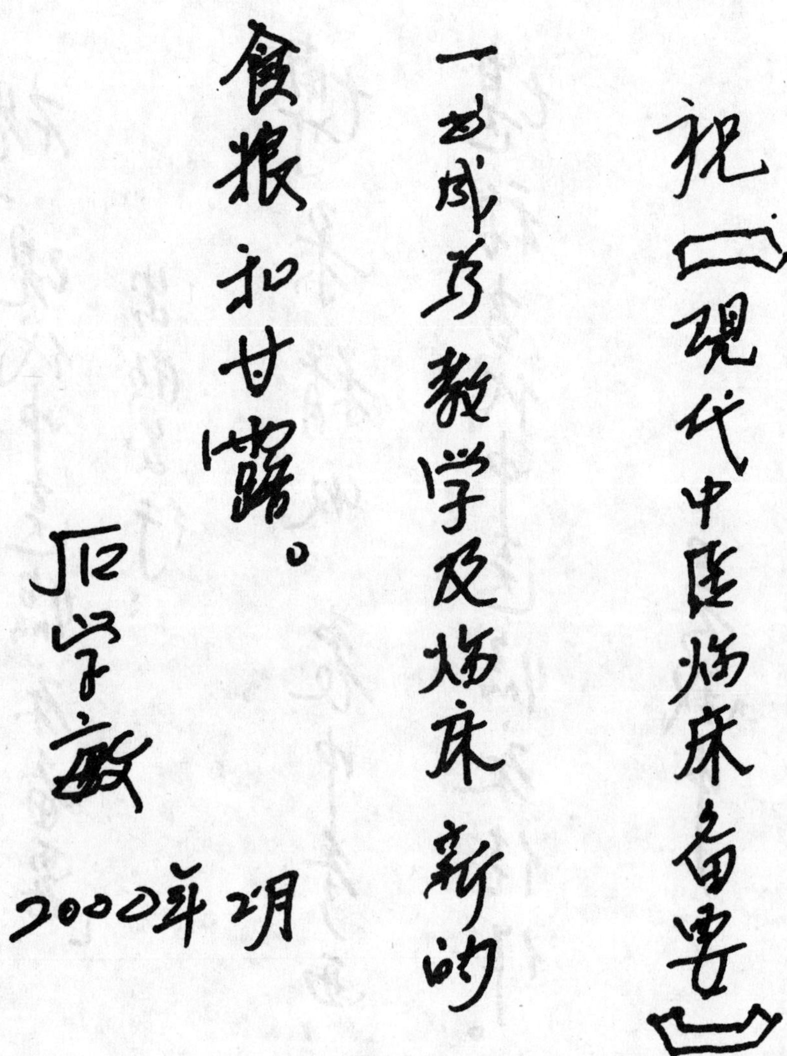

I wish that the book *Clinical Essentials of Contemporary Chinese Medicine* will be a new nourishment and sweet essence for teaching and clinical treatment!

Shi Xuemin
Feb. 2000

(Inscription by Prof. Shi Xuemin, Academician of Academy of Engineering of China, member of the Council of China Acupuncture Association). President of the First Hospital Affiliated to Tianjin College of TCM.)

Preface & Acknowledgement

The material for this book came from my lectures on Chinese Pharmacology prepared for Gero Missoni, an Austrian physician, in 1989. The material was enhanced during the next two years when I lectured at the Toulouse University in France. It became especially valuable when we began to work with the Goto College of Medical Arts and Sciences postgraduate students in a master's degree course in TCM in 1996. It has been continually revised based on my annual lectures in Japan. These efforts resulted in this book, which lists about 500 Chinese herbs and has translated into Japanese and English.

Today, significant progress has been made through research in Chinese pharmacology. This has rendered considerable advancements in clinical application. Conversely, the traditional pharmacological theories such as flavor, tropism, action directions, etc. still serve as major principles in organizing prescriptions. Drugs that are classified in nature as warm, cold, reinforcing or reducing benefit related syndromes such as cold, heat, deficiency and excess respectively. Therefore, the drugs in this book are categorized as reinforcing and reducing, cold and warm, qi and blood, for consciousness, cough and asthma, phlegm and dampness, food retention and external use. Further division depends upon functions of the herbs.

My lectures abroad were given primarily to medical doctors and acupuncturists, including pharmacologists. They emphasized the application of Chinese herbs and their compatibility. This is of critical importance for their application and constitutes a special entry in this book.

Special notations are attached to emphasize similar herbs when they are compared. Precautions are provided particularly on their use in clinical application. In order to give a comprehensive description, the notations cite materials from an extensive list of ancient and modern documents.

Dosage is quite complicated since it varies in different, syndromes, physicians and compatibility. Consequently, routine dosage is only suggested.

Readers will find five references that present a classification of herbs, modern research, and herb selection according to symptoms, syndromes and diseases.

Before publication, parts of this book were used by many practitioners during the last ten years. With the encourage and support from Professor Dai Ximeng, the President of Tianjin College of TCM, and Dr. Shuji Goto, the President of Goto College of Medical Arts and Science, I was determined to have it published in order to share it with more people. Acknowledgment should also be presented to Professor Hiromitsi Yasui and Akira Hyodo from Japan, and Professor Li Qinghe and Professor Wang Yuxing for their concerned assistance and constant hard work. Through their efforts, it became possible to publish the book after the original material had been revised several times.

In the course of translation, help from Dr. Donald P. Lauda and Dr. Jeffrey L. Carnett were sought to ensure the accuracy of the English translation.

During ancient times, the property of herbs was called 'herb character' suggesting that herbs, like people, also have variable characters. How can we understand them when there is a lack of behavior or words to show their characters? The only pathway consists of understanding concerns and clinical practice. Chinese Pharmacology seems to be easy to learn at first glance, but it is difficult to master or understand. I am looking forward to your reactions to my writing and appreciate any advice you can provide to help in improving upon this book.

At the time of publication, I am greatly indebted to Dr. Shuji Goto (Ph. D.), the President of Goto College of Medical Arts and Sciences, Tokyo Japan, for his help in completing this book. It is an exhilarating coincidence that May 1st, 2000 is his 51st birthday. I have the honor to take this opportunity to extend my congratulations to him.

Editor-in-chief

Liu Gongwang

Dec. 2000

CONTENTS

Reference

General Introduction

Chinese drugs generally refer to those grown and produced from the natural world, and they are roughly classified into plant drugs, animal drugs, mineral drugs and their processed materials. As the number of plant drugs increased in ancient times, they were called "Materia Medica". The application of "Materia Medica" is based on the basic theory of Chinese medicine, possessing a unique theoretical system and applicable form. In the late Qing Dynasty after western learning appeared in the east, "Materia Medica" was named "Chinese drugs." These show those Chinese drugs are inherent in Chinese pharmacology.

Chinese pharmacology is a branch of scientific learning, specialized in the basic theory of Chinese drugs and their source, collection, property, effect, and their application. This is thought to be an important component of Chinese medicine.

Differentiation and treatment systems in Chinese medicine aim at a specific syndrome. Treatment is completed with the use of drugs, prescriptions and a certain therapy combined with differentiation theory. Therefore, Chinese pharmacology occupies an important place in the differentiation and treatment system.

Chapter One Initiation from Shennong(神农) Tasting Materia Medica

Chinese pharmacology date back to more than 1,000 years B. C. at the times of Xizhou (1066～771B. C.), when professional "physicians" started "to have medical practice by collection of poison". It is recorded in *Huai Nan Zi* (《淮南子》, Huainanzi) that the founder of Chinese pharmacology was Shennong(神农), who tasted all kinds of herbs, and was poisoned almost 70 times a day. It has been stated that the study of Chinese pharmacology originated from the people's health care and hygiene in the remote antiquity of human history.

The Yellow Emperor's Internal Classic (《黄帝内经》, Huangdineijing), the original work of Chinese medicine, was published during Qin and Han times (221～220 B. C.). It not only established the theoretical system of Chinese medicine, but also summarized such pharmacological theories as "four natures and five tastes." It created a favorable condition for the later development of pharmacology.

By the end of the Eastern Han, the first Chinese monograph on pharmacology *Shengnong's Herbal Classic* (《神农本草经》, Shennongbencaojing) was published. It summarized pharmacological knowledge and the accumulated experience of using drugs before the 2nd century. The complete work is in 3 volumes and lists 365 kinds of drugs and their functions in three grades: superior (top grade), medium (middle grade) and inferior (low grade) according to their functions. It was thought at that time that 120 kinds, which are non-toxic, and used for tonifying and long-term administration, were rated as superior. other 120 kinds in the medium grade, which were toxic or non-toxic, were used for invigorating deficiency; and Another 125 which are toxic and unable to be taken for a long time, were used only in treating diseases as inferior. It was the first time that drugs were classified according to their functions. Most of these drugs recorded in the book proved effective and they have been frequently used ever since. For example, Ginseng(人参, Renshen) can be used to benefit intelligence. Antifebrile Dichroa Root (常山, Changshan) can be used to stop malaria, Coptis Rhizome(黄连, Huanglian) to cure dysentery, Chinese Angelica Root(当归, Danggui) to regulate menstruation, Ass-hide Glue (阿胶, Ejiao) to stop blood and Common Monkshood's Mother Root (乌头, Wutou) to stop pain. Besides, this book gives a brief account of the basic theory of Chinese pharmacology. *Shengnong's Herbal Classic* (《神农本草经》, Shennongbencaojing) lays a foundation for Chinese pharmacology. Consequently, the later physicians could make further supplement based ont his book.

During Liang times, (456～536 A.D.), based on *Shengnong's Herbal Classic* (《神农本草经》, Shennongbencaojing), Tao Hongjing (陶弘景) sorted it out, made notes and added 365 more drugs into the book, thereby, compiling a new book named *Variorum of Shengnong's Herbal Classic* (《神农本草经集注》, Shemnongbencaojingjizhu). It recorded 730 kinds of Chinese drugs altogether and created a new way of classification according to natural properties. Besides, it was the first time to advance such "commonly-used drugs" in this book as Divaricate Saposhnikovia Root(防风, Fangfeng) for treating wind syndrome and Capillary Wormwood Herb(茵陈蒿, Yinchenhao) for treating jaundice.

The two books on Chinese drugs mentioned above may be said to be the classical works on Chinese pharmacology. From then on, the most influential pharmacological monograghs published since the 6th century A.D. can be listed as follows:

The Newly-revised Materia Medica (《新修本草》, Xinxiubencao) was compiled by Li Ji (李勣) and Su Jing(苏敬) etal, as ordered by the Tang Dynasty in the year of 659 A.D. After it was revised and supplemented based on *Variorum of Shengnong's Herbal Classic* (《神农本草经集注》, Shennongbencaojingjizhu). In this book, 850 kinds of drugs are recorded and 120 more kinds were supplemented, among which, many were imported, such as Benzoinum (安息香, Anxixiang) and Pepper(胡椒, Hujiao) etc. Drug pictures and diagrams found in this book are thought to be the initial use of figures. The method of contrasting the essay against figures created a precedent for pharmacological works throughout the world. This book was revised and published in the power of state. It is the first pharmacopoeia of China, and also the earliest one in the world. It was developed 800 years earlier than the pharmacopoeia of Nuruberg in Europe in 1542 A. D. It was introduced to Japan in 731 A.D. It was recorded in *Enkisiki* (《延喜式》, Yanxishi), a Japanese ancient history book, that physicians should read *The*

Newly-revised Materia Medica (《新修本草》, Xinxiubencao). This shows that the book made a great contribution to the development of pharmacology in the world.

During times of 1086～1093 A. D., Tang Shenwei(唐慎微), a well-known physician in Sichuan province(四川) compiled Proved and *Classified Materia Medica* (经史证类备急本草, Jingshizhengleibeijibencao) based on *Illustrated Classic of the Materia Medica of Jiayou Era* (《嘉祐图经本草》, Jiayoutujingbencao) after he extensively collected and proved prescriptions and the materials concerning drugs. It has substantial content and records 1558 kinds of drugs, each of which has a diagram. Besides, it attaches more than 3000 prescriptions. This book is not only practical but also valuable, for it provides a large amount of medical documents describing ancient prescriptions.

Compendium of Materia Medica (《本草纲目》, Bencaogangmu) is a great work of over 2,000,000 words on pharmacology, completed over 27 years by Li Shizhen (李时珍), a famous pharmacologist during the Ming Dynasty. He referred to more than 800 books concerning pharmacology based on *Materia Medica of Zhenghe* (《政和本草》, Zhenghebencao). It records 1892 kinds of drugs and attaches more than 11,000 prescriptions and 1,160 diagrams of drugs. The drugs in the book are classified into 16 classes and 60 categories according to their natural properties. It was the most accurate classification in materia medica at the time. The book selected the refined and corrected the errors made by physicians of the past dynasties and added 374 more kinds of drugs. *Compendium of Materia Medica* 《(本草纲目》, Bencaogangmu) synthesized the knowledge in many fields before the 16th century, such as zoology, botany, mineralogy and metallurgy. Therefore, it is a quite brilliant achievement in the history of Chinese science and technology. Charles Robert Darwin said: " *Compendium of Materia Medica* (《本草纲目》, Bencaogangmu) published in 1596 is an encyclopedia of China".

Supplement to the Compendium of Materia Medica (《本草纲目拾遗》, Bencaogangmushiyi) was completed in the 30th year of Qian Long of the Qing Dynasty (1765 A. D.). Zhao Xuemin(赵学敏)(the author of the book) collected and sorted out folk herbs, recorded 921 kinds of drugs and added 716 kinds of more. The form, function and effect of the drugs found in this book are quite extensive and accurate with practical value. The book also revised errors found in *Compendium of Materia Medica* (《本草纲目》, Bencaogangmu). This book is another summary on pharmacology following Li Shizhen(李时珍). Up to that time, the number of Chinese drugs reached 2,608 kinds.

In addition, the following three books *New Compilation of Materia Medica* (《本草从新》, Bencaocongxin) written by Wu Zuncheng (吴遵程), *Essentials of Materia Medica* (《本草备要》, Bencaobeiyao) by Wang Ang(汪昂) in the early Qing Dynasty, and *Required Reading of Materia Medica* (《本草备读》, Bencaobeidu) by Zhang Bingcheng(张秉成) in the late Qing Dynasty were all completed with the aim of making them brief, practical and easy to learn for beginners. These books play an important role in spreading Chinese pharmacology and are still served as the essential reference books in learning Chinese pharmacology up to the present.

According to historical records, there were 400 kinds of books on Materia Medica from the Han to the Qing Dynasty. These books accumulated substantial theories and experiences, so they deserve to be called treasure of the Chinese civilization. So far, Chinese drugs have come up to more than 5,000 kinds. With the worldwide trend of health care returning to nature, it is predicted that Chinese pharmacology will continue to make significant contributions to the health of mankind.

Chapter Two Medicinal Properties of Traditional Chinese Drugs

Medicinal properties of Chinese drugs are considered a methodological theory based on the nature and function of drugs, and regarded as the theoretical basis in clinical application. In Chinese pharmacology, a variety of properties and functions of drugs, based on the theory of Chinese medicine, can be generalized as having four natures, five kinds of tastes, meridian tropism, ascending, descending, floating and sinking, poisonous and non-poisonous drugs.

In Chinese medicine, under the guidance of theories of yinyang, five elements, zang and fu organs, meridian and collateral, the understanding of medicinal properties of drugs has been gradually deepened and perfected in the long-term medical practice, hereby, forming a unique pharmacological system, namely, the theory of "medicinal properties".

1. Four Natures, Five Kinds of Tastes

Cold, hot, warm and cool are the four different properties of drugs. They were called "four natures" in ancient times. Four natures are generalized according to the reaction of the body after the drugs are administered.

Cold and cool drugs have the actions of relieving or removing heat syndrome and can generally be used for clearing away heat, eliminating pathogenic fire and detoxicating. Warm and hot drugs relieve or remove cold syndrome can generally be used for dispelling cold, warming the interior and invigorating yang. It is said in *Plain Question* (《素问》, Suwen): "Cold syndrome should be treated by warm and hot drugs, whereas heat syndrome by cold and cool drugs." The application of cold and cool drugs or warm and hot drugs is contradicted with the nature of syndrome. (See table 1)

Warm hot and cold cool fall into two different natures. But warm and hot, cold and cool have respective generalities. Cool is the beginning of cold while warm is the beginning of hot.

There are some other drugs whose properties are not obvious, they are mild and called "medium property".

Table. One

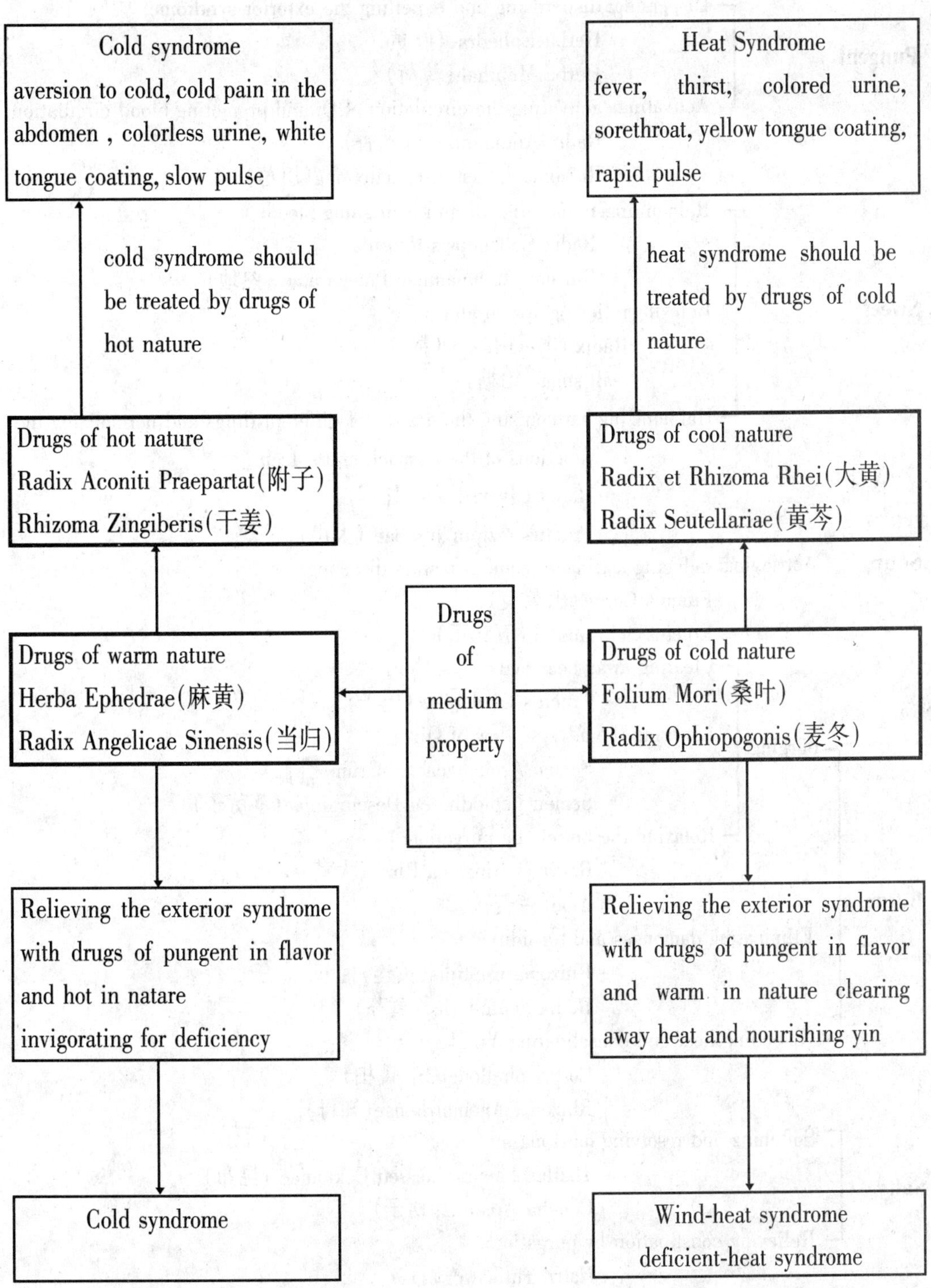

Five tastes of traditional Chinese drugs refer to pungent, sweet, sour, bitter and salty. Besides, some are astringent and tasteless. Five tastes are the indications of actual effects of drugs. Different tastes have different functions, which are listed as follows:

Table. Two

Pungent
- Dispersing: disperesing and expelling the exterior syndrome:
  - Herba Ephedrae(麻黄)
  - Herba Menthae(薄荷)
- Activating: activating the circulation of Qi and promoting blood circulation:
  - Radix Aucklandiae (木香)
  - Rhizoma Ligustici Chuanxiong(川芎)

Sweet
- Reinforcing: reinforcing Qi and nourishing blood:
  - Radix Codonopsis Pilosulae(党参)
  - Rhizoma Rehmanniae Praeparatae (熟地)
- Releving: relieving spasm and pain:
  - Radix Glyeyrrhizae (甘草)
  - malt sugat(饴糖)
- Harmonizing: harmonizing the actions of different drugs and normolizing the functions of the stomach and spleen:
  - Radix Glycyrrhizae(甘草)
  - Fructus Ziziphi Jujubae (大枣)

Sour
- Actringing: inducing astringency and arresting dischange:
  - Fructus Corni (山茱萸)
  - Fructus Schisandrae(五味子)

Bitter
- purging
  - Clearing away heat evils:
    - Fructus Cardeniae (栀子)
  - Lowering the adverse flow of Qi:
    - Semen Armeniacae Amarum(杏仁)
    - Semen Lepiddii seu Descurainiae(葶苈子)
  - Relaxing the bowels by purgation:
    - Radix et Rhizoma Rhei (大黄)
    - Aloe(芦荟)
- Eliminating dampness and turbidity:
  - Rhizoma Coptidis(黄连)
  - Radix Scutellariae(黄芩)
- Dispelling heat and consolidating Yin:
  - Cortex phellodendri(黄柏)
  - Rhizoma Anemarrhenae(知母)

Salty
- Softening and resolving hard mass:
  - Thallus Laminariae seu Eckloniae (昆布)
  - Concha Arcae(瓦楞子)
- Relieving constipation by purgation:
  - Natrii Sulfas(芒硝)
  - Radix Scrophulariae(玄参)

Tasteless
- Eliminating dampness and inducing diuresis:
  - Poria(茯苓)
  - Polyporus Umbellatus(猪苓)

Drugs of astringent taste have similar effects to those of sour taste.

Nature and taste of traditional Chinese drugs demonstrate their effects in different aspects. The actions of all drugs are summarized by nature and taste. For instance, Baikal Skullcap Root(黄芩, Huangqin) is bitter in flavor and cold in nature and used for clearing away heat and eliminating dampness. Buffalo Horn(水牛角, Suiniujiao) is salty in flavor and cold in nature and used for clearing away heat and cooling the blood. Cochinchinese Asparagus Root (天门冬, Tianmendong) is sweet in flavor and cold in nature, so it is used for nourishing yin. Dang-shen Root(党参, Dangshen) is sweet in flavor and warm in nature and used for reinforcing qi. Those drugs with the same nature and taste usually have similar effects. In the same way, drugs with different nature and taste usually have different actions. Drugs with the same nature but different taste or the same taste but different nature may also have different actions.

Table. Three

drugs warm in nature	Herba Ephedrae(麻黄):	diaphoresis with drugs pungent is flavor and warm in nature
	Cortex Maguoliae Officinalis(厚朴):	dispelling dampness with drugs bitter in flavor and warm in nature
	Radix Astragaliseu Hedysari(黄芪):	reinforcing Qi with drugs sweet in flavor and warm in nature
drugs pungent in flavor	Rhizoma Zingiberis Recens(生姜):	dispersing cold with drugs sweet in flavor and warm in nature
	Radix Aconiti Praeparata(附子):	invigorating yang with drugs of pungent taste and hot nature
	Cypsum Fibrosum(石膏):	clearing away heat with drugs of pungent taste and cold nature

Caution should also be taken with those drugs that have the same nature and taste but have different actions. For example, Baikal Skullcap Root(黄芩, Huangqin), Coptis Rhizome(黄连, Huanglian) and Chinese Corktree Bark(黄柏, Huangbai) are all drugs bitter in flavor and cold in nature and have the actions of clearing away heat, eliminating dampness and detoxicating. But Baikal Skullcap Root(黄芩, Huangqin) is used for treating the diseases of the Upper-jiao, Coptis Rhizome (黄连, Huanglian) for those of the Middle-jiao and Chinese Corktree Bark (黄柏, Huangbai) for those of the Lower-jiao.

Besides, in compatibility of drugs, several kinds of tastes may produce compound actions. Officinal Magnolia Bark(厚朴, Houpo) in combination with Coptis Rhizome(黄连, Huanglian) is pungent and bitter in flavor, having the effect of lowering damp-heat.

White Peony Root (白芍药, Baishaoyao) in combination with Licorice Root (甘草, Gancao) is sour and sweet in flavor, having the effect of nourishing yin and relieving spasm.

In a word, we should not only learn about the general rule of the four natures and five tastes, but also know well their therapeutic actions of each kind of drug. Only in this way, can we distinguish better the medicinal properties of drugs, and apply them in accordance with the syndrome.

2. Ascending, Descending, Floating and Sinking

Normal circulation of qi Energy should be in a good state of ascending, descending, going out and coming in. When the circulation of qi Energy becomes abnormal, ascending and descending fails to function, leading to diseases. For example, stomach-qi being unable to descend normally causes adverse flow of qi and it is manifested as vomiting. Impairment of purifying and descending function of the lung causes asthma and cough. Collapse of qi leads to prolapse of the anus. Comparatively speaking, those drugs, which can relieve and cure these syndromes respectively, have the actions of ascending, descending, floating and sinking. So we say, ascending, descending, floating and sinking refer to the functional trend of drugs in the human body.

Ascending refers to upward rising or lifting. Drugs with lifting effect are used to treat the diseases in a worsened condition. Descending means lowering the adverse flow of qi. Drugs with lowering effect are used to treat diseases characterized by adverse flow of qi. Floating means superficial and the exterior, drugs with floating effect are used to treat the diseases in the exterior. Sinking refers to descending drugs and is used to treat the diseases in the interior. In general, drugs of ascending and floating effects have the action of invigorating yang qi, relieving the exterior, expelling wind and cold, inducing vomiting and resuscitation. These drugs can act on the upper part and the exterior of the body. Drugs with sinking and descending effects have the actions of lowering adversed flow of qi and arresting vomiting, promoting diuresis to eliminate dampness, relieving constipation by purgation, tranquilizing the mind, calming down the floating yang to arrest wind, relieving cough and asthma, clearing away heat and reducing fire, promoting digestion and removing stagnated food. These drugs can act on the lower part and the interior of the body. But, such drugs as Ephedra (麻黄, Mahuang), Apricot Seed (杏仁, Xingren), Szechwan Lovage Rhizome (川芎, Chuanxiong), Buffalo Horn (水牛角, Suiniujiao) and Cow-bezoar (牛黄, Niuhuang) have two-way properties.

Ascending, descending, floating and sinking of drugs have a close relation with their own property, taste and quality. Drugs with flower or leaf and light in quality generally have ascending and floating effects and can be used to treat the diseases in the upper part and the exterior of the body, such as Mulberry Leaf (桑叶, Sangye), Chrysanthemum Flower (菊花, Juhua) and Wild Mint (薄荷, Bohe). Drugs like fruit, mineral and shell usually have sinking and descending effects and can be used to treat the diseases in the lower part and the interior of the body, such as Immature Bitter Orange (枳实, Zhishi), Hematite (代赭石, Daizheshi) and Abalone Shell(石决明,Shijueming).

Besides, the properties of ascending, descending, floating and sinking of drugs, are probably affected by processing drugs or compatibility, thereby changing the original effect. For instance, Rhubarb(大黄, Dahuang) is of sinking and descending in nature. But after it is prepared with vine or compatible with Shunk Bugbane Rhizome(升麻, Shengma), it can be used to clear away heat evil in the Upper-jiao.

3. Meridian Tropism

Meridian tropism refers to a theory, which relates the therapeutic action of drugs to the viscera and meridians so as to explain their specific selective actions on the body.

Examples are listed as follows:

Table. Four

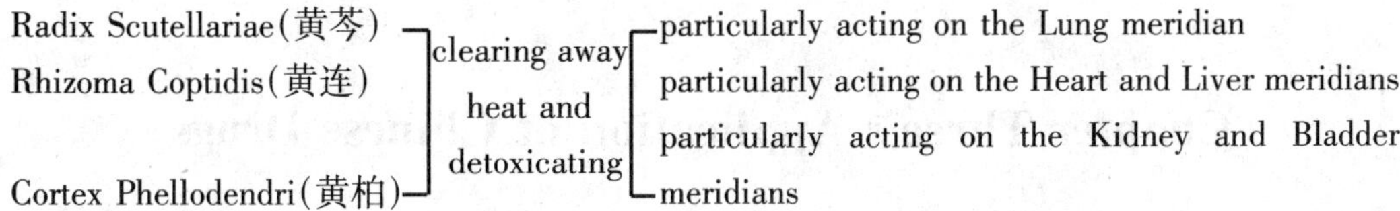

Drug	Action	Meridian
Radix Scutellariae(黄芩)	clearing away heat and detoxicating	particularly acting on the Lung meridian
Rhizoma Coptidis(黄连)		particularly acting on the Heart and Liver meridians
Cortex Phellodendri(黄柏)		particularly acting on the Kidney and Bladder meridians

Taking the taste and color of drugs as a guide, meridian tropism is determined in combination with the therapeutic actions of drugs. Also, it is summarized in the practice according to upon which organ or which part of the body the drugs act. But, even if the meridian tropism is the same, its therapeutic action is not necessarily the same. For example:

Table. Five

Drug	Meridian	Action
Rasiz Scutellariae(黄芩)	acting on the Lung meridian	clearing away lung heat→cough and asthma due to phlegm-heat
Rhizoma Zingiberis(干姜)		warming lung cold→profuse saliva due to cold phlegm
Bulbus Lilii(百合)		tonifying lung deficiency→hemoptysis due to yin deficiency
Semen Lepididii seu Descurainiae (葶苈子)		eliminating the excess from the lung→asthma due to fluid retention in the chest and hypochondrium

Meridian tropism, the theory of pharmacology, must be applied in combination with the nature, taste, ascending, descending, floating and sinking of drugs to show the use of Chinese drugs. Then we can achieve the desired therapeutic effect.

4. Poisonous and Non-poisonous Drugs

"Toxicants" in ancient times had a different implication from that of today. "Drugs are all poison" is considered as a guiding ideology. So-called "toxicants" refer to the general term of drugs. Drugs have their own particularities, which refer to "poison". "Severe poison" and "mild poison" called by the later generations refer to poisonous property and side effect. Such as Pinellia Rhizome (半夏, Banxia) and Common Monkshood's Mother Root (乌头, Wutou).

When the poisonous drugs are applied, dosage should be strictly limited. Try to relieve or eliminate the poison and side effects by way of processing, compatibility and preparation in order to assure the safety when administering. Besides, the law of "combat poison with poison" can be taken as grounds to treat some difficult and complicated diseases or critically ill patients.

Chapter Three Application of Chinese Drugs

The Application of Chinese Drugs includes compatibility and incompatibility of drugs, dosage and administration, etc.

1. Compatibility

When Chinese drugs are applied in clinical treatment, one drug prescribed is called a single prescription, several kinds of drugs combined in use is called compound prescription. Since diseases in the human body are complicated and changeable, several diseases may accompany another, or diseases occurring either in the exterior and interior, or in the state of both deficiency and excess, or alternatively cold and heat. Many diseases are difficult to be cured with a single drug. Under the guidance of differentiation, treatment and pharmacological method, more than two kinds of drugs are selectively used in combination according to the actual condition of the diseases and the properties of drugs. Only in this way, can we achieve the desired effect.

Physicians in ancient times, after they accumulated experiences on compatibility, classified the Chinese drugs into six types: mutual reinforcement, mutual assistance, mutual restraint, mutual detoxication, mutual inhibition and antagonism, When adding the application of a single drug (going alone), they are called the seven prescriptions.

(1) Going alone: one of the seven prescriptions, by using a single drug to achieve the desired therapeutic effect, such as Decoction of Ginseng (独参汤, Dushen Tang). Strictly speaking, going alone doesn't belong to compatibility.

(2) Mutual reinforcement: one of the seven

different effects in compatibility of Chinese drugs. Two or more kinds of drugs with similar properties and functions are used in combination to strengthen their effects. For example: the application of Ephedra (麻黄, Mahuang) in combination with Cassia Twig (桂枝, Guizhi) can strengthen the effectiveness of relieving the exterior syndrome by diaphoresis. Gypsum (石膏, Shigao) in combination with Common Anemarrhea Rhizome (知母, Zhimu) can enhance the function of clearing away heat, dispelling pathogenic fire and replenishing body fluid.

(3) Mutual assistance: The effect of a major drug may be enhanced by subsidiary drug when two drugs with the same properties are used together. For example: Membranous Milkvetch Root (黄芪, Huangqi) for reinforcing qi and promoting diuresis and Poria (茯苓, Fuling) for invigorating the spleen to promote diuresis are used together, the effect of Poria (茯苓, Fuling) can assist Membranous Milkvetch Root (黄芪, Huangqi) to improve the therapeutic effect of reinforcing qi and promoting diuresis.

(4) Mutual restraint: When two kinds of drugs are used in combination, the toxicity or side effects of one drug can be reduced or eliminated by the other. For example: toxicity of Pinellia Rhizome (半夏, Banxia) can be reduced or eliminated by Fresh Ginger (生姜, Shengjiang)

(5) Mutual detoxication: When two kinds of drugs are used in combination, one drug can lessen or remove the toxicity or side effects of the other. For example: Fresh Ginger (生姜, Shengjiang) can lessen or remove the toxicity of Pinellia Rhizome (生半夏, Shengbanxia).

(6) Mutual inhibition: When two kinds of drugs are used together, one drug can damage or reduce the effects of the other. For example: The effect of Ginseng (人参, Renshen) inhibits that of Radish Seed (莱菔子, Laifuzi) and Radish Seed (莱菔子, Laifuzi) may reduce the action of reinforcing qi of Ginseng (人参, Renshen).

(7) Antagonism: When two drugs are used in combination, toxicity or side effects may be produced. This leads to the incompatibility of drugs in a prescription. Toxicity of Lilac Daphne Flower-bud (芫花, Yuanhua) may be increased if it is used with Licorice Root (甘草, Gancao)

(See details in "Incompatibility of Drugs")

Compatibility of drugs can be summarized as follows:

(1) Cooperative function: When two or more than two drugs are used together, they can strengthen the effects, such as "mutual reinforcement" and "mutual assistance".

(2) Antagonistically function: when two or more drugs are used together, they may reduce or counteract the drug effects, such as "mutual inhibition".

(3) Application of toxic drugs or severe poisons can lessen or remove the toxicity or side effects of one drug after compatibility, such as, "mutual restraint" and "mutual detoxication".

(4) Incompatibility of drugs refers to the combined application of certain drugs in a prescription, which will give rise to toxic reactions or side effects, or increase their original toxic and side effects, such as "antagonism".

The compatibility of drugs in a prescription is the major application of drugs in Chinese medicine, which is scientific and reasonable. By way of compatibility, effects of drugs can be enhanced, toxicity of drugs can be reduced, and their therapeutic effects can be increased.

Drugs should be applied in accordance with the disease and for the prevention of drug poisoning.

2. Contraindication of Drugs

Traditional contraindication includes incompatibility of Chinese drugs, contraindication of drugs in pregnancy and contraindication of food during the period when medicine is being taken.

(1) Incompatibility of Drugs

To ensure the compatibility of compound prescription, some drugs should be avoided in combination to prevent the increase or occurrence of poisonous effect or other serious side effects. The early generations identified the drugs that are not advisable for use as "incompatibility among eighteen medicaments" and "Mutual antagonism among nineteen medicaments".

(A) Incompatibility among eighteen medicaments: Common Monkshood's Mother Root (乌头, Wutou) is incompatible with Pinellia Rhizome(半夏, Banxia), Snakegourd Fruit(瓜蒌, Gualou), Tendrilleaf Fritillary Bulb(贝母, Beimu), Japanese Ampelopsis Root (白蔹, Bailian) and Bletilla Rhiozome (白及, Baiji). Licorice Root(甘草, Gancao) compatible with Peking Euphorbia Root (大戟, Daji), Lilac Daphne Flower-bud(芫花, Yuanhua), Kansui Root (甘遂, Gansui) and Seaweed (海藻, Haizao). Black Falsehellebore Root And Rhizome(藜芦, Lilu) incompatible with Ginseng (人参, Renshen), Dang-shen Root(党参, Dangshen), Dan-shen Root(丹参, Danshen), Figwort Root(玄参, Xuanshen), Fourleaf Ladybell Root(沙参, Shashen), Lightyellow Sophora Root(苦参, Kushen), Manchurian Wildginger Herb(细辛, Xixin) and White Peony Root (白芍药, Baishaoyao).

(B) Mutual Antagonism among nineteen medicaments: Sulfur (硫黄, Liuhuang) is antagonistic to Mirabilite(芒硝, Mangxiao), Sulfur(硫黄, liuhuang) to Mirabilite(朴硝, Puxiao). Mercury(水银, Shuiyin) to Arsenolite Ore (砒霜, Pishuang). Chinese Stellera Root (狼毒, Langdu) to Litharge(密陀僧, Mituoseng). Croton Seed (巴豆, Badou) to Pharbitis Seed (牵牛子, Qianniuzi). Clove Flower-bud (丁香, Dingxiang) to Turmeric Root-tuber(郁金, Yujin). Mirabilite (芒硝, Mangxiao) to Common Burreed Rhizome(三棱, Sanleng). Common Monkshood'sMother Root(川乌, Chuanwu), Kusnezoff Monkshood Root (草乌, Caowu) to Asiatic Rhinoceros Horn(犀角, Xijiao). Ginseng(人参, Renshen) to Trogopterus Dung(五灵脂, Wulingzhi) and Cassia Bark(官桂 Guangui) to Red Halloysite (赤石脂, Chishizi).

Incompatibilities among eighteen medicaments and mutual antagonism among nineteen medicaments are both serve to identify the incompatibility of drugs in clinical application. In ancient times or in previous centuries, there were some prescriptions, in which those drugs recorded in incompatibility among eighteen medicaments and mutual antagonisms among nineteen medicaments were used in combination. For example, decoction of Kansui Root (甘遂, Gansui), and Pinellia Rhizome(半夏, Banxia) that is Licorice Root (甘草, Gancao) set in combination. With Kansui Root(甘遂, Gansui), decoction of Sargassum Yuhu, that is Licorice Root(甘草, Gancao) with Seaweed(海藻, Haizao). Ganying Pills, that is Croton Seed

(巴豆, Badou) with Pharbitis Seed(牵牛子, Qianniuzi) Shixiang Fanhun Powder, that is Clove Flower-bud (丁香, Dingxiang) With Turmeric Root-tuber (郁金, Yujin) etc. Indeed, these drugs can cause a poisonous reaction and severe side effects when they are used in combination. For example, if Manchurian Wildginger Herb(细辛, Xixin) is used in combination with Black Falsehellebore Root And Rhizome(藜芦, Lilu) it may lead to death of the experimental animal due to poisoning. There is still much to be tested and verified concerning incompatibility among eighteen medicaments and mutual antagonism among nineteen medicaments through scientific research. Do not neglect this and try to avoid blind compatibility.

(2) Contraindication of drugs in pregnancy

Some drugs may impair parent substance and the embryo (original qi of the fetus) and affect the normal development of the fetus. Some may even have the danger of causing criminal abortion. Therefore, these drugs should be taken as contraindications during women's pregnancy so as to prevent abortion, premature delivery, or fetal malformation, etc. Generally, extremely toxic drugs, purgatives, drugs for removing blood stasis, drugs of hot nature and drugs of fragrant in taste and migratory in nature fall into contraindication of drugs in pregnancy.

According to toxicity (either severe or mild) and actions of drugs (either strong or weak) and the effect of parent substance on the fetus, traditional contraindication of drugs is classified as contraindicated or cautiously used drugs in application. Contraindicated drugs are all severe poisons, such as Mercury (水银, Shuiyin), Arsenolite Ore (砒霜, Pishuang), Red Orpiment (雄黄, Xionghuang), Mercuros Chloride(轻粉, Qingfen), Large Blister Beetle (斑蝥, Banmao), Toad Skin Secretion Cake (蟾酥, Chansu), Nux Vomica (马钱子, Maqianzi), Blue Vitriol(胆矾, Danfan), Malachite Ore(皂矾, Zaofan), Black Falsehellebore Root And Rhizome(藜芦, Lilu), Muskmelon Fruit Pedicel (瓜蒂, Guadi), Resina Toxicodendri (干漆, Ganqi), Centipede (蜈蚣, Wugong), Mush (麝香, Shexiang), Kansui Root (甘遂, Gansui), Peking Euphorbia Root (大戟, Daji), Lilac Daphne Flower-bud (芫花, Yuanhua), Croton Seed (巴豆, Baduo), Caper Euphorbia Herb(千金子, Qianjinzi), Pokeberry Root(商陆, Shanglu), Common Monkshood Root(川乌, Chuanwu), Kusnezoff Monkshood Root (草乌, Caowu), Gadfly (虻虫, Mengchong), Leech (水蛭, Shuizhi), Mirabilite (芒硝, Mangxiao), Senna Leaf (番泻叶, Fanxieye), Aloes (芦荟, Luhui), Common Burreed Rhizome (三棱, Sanleng), Zedoray (莪术, Ezhu) etc. Cautiously-used drugs include those for dredging meridians to remove blood stasis, promoting qi circulation to remove blood stasis and those pungent in taste and hot in nature, such as Cassia Bark(肉桂, Rougui), Tree Peony Bark(牡丹皮, Mudanpi), Rhubarb(大黄, Dahuang), Akebia Stem(木通, Mutong), Trogopterus Dung(五灵脂, Wulingzhi), Cowherb Seed(王不留行, Wangbuliuxing), Immature Bitter Orange (枳实, Zhishi), Bitter Orange (枳壳, Zhike), Prepared Daughter Root Of Common Monkshood (附子, Fuzi), Cluster Mallow Root(冬葵子, Dongkuizi) etc.

Modern pharmacological research has proved that: (a) some drugs have the effect of contraction on the uterus, especially on the uterus in pregnancy, such as, Safflower (红花, Honghua), Twotooth Achyranthes Root (牛膝, Niuxi), Turmeric Rhizome (姜黄, Jianghuang), Cicada Slough(蝉蜕, Chantui),

Szechwan Lovage Rhizome(川芎, Chuanxiong)etc. (b) Some drugs have the actions of stopping pregnancy, inducing labor and resisting early pregnancy, such as, Snakegourd Root (天花粉, Tianhuafen) Turmeric Rhizome(姜黄, Jianghuang), Szechwan Lovage Rhizome (川芎, Chuanxiong), Japanese Pagodatree Flower(槐角, Huaijiao) etc. (c) Some drugs contains certain active mass which may cause fetal malformation, such as, Peach Seed(桃仁, Taoren), Bushcherry Seed(郁李仁, Yuliren), Rhubarb(大黄, Dahuang), Giant Knotweed Rhizome(虎杖, Huzhang), Cassia seed(决明子, Juemingzi), Senna Leaf(番泻叶, Fanxieye), Tuber Fleeceflower Root(何首乌, Heshouwu)Herba Capsellae(荠菜, jiecai), Spreading Hedyotis Herb(白花蛇舌草, Baihuashecao), Tonkin Sophora Root(山豆根, Shandougen), Lily Bulb(百合, Baihe), White Mustard Seed(白芥子, Baijiezi) etc. The abovementioned drugs all fall into contraindication of drugs in pregnancy.

(3) Contraindication of diet in the period of medicine is being taken

Contraindication of diet is commonly referred to "avoid certain food". It means that when medicine is being taken, certain kinds of food, which may affect the treatment of disease, should be avoided. Moderate in eating and drinking is advised. Those food which are not easy to digest, such as, uncooked, cold, sticky, greasy, fishy, food with the smell of mutton and other irritating food should be avoided according to the actual condition.

It was recorded in ancient medical documents that with Antifebrile Dichroa Root(常山, Changshan) avoid onion, with Prepared Rhizome Of Adhesive Rehmannia(地黄, Dihuang)and Tuber Fleeceflower Root(何首乌, Heshouwu) avoids onion, garlic and Turtle Carapace(鳖甲, Biejia) avoids Amaranth(苋菜, Jiancai). Wild Mint(薄荷, Bohe) avoids Turtles.(鳖鱼, Bieyu), Licorice Root(甘草, Gancao) avoids Silver Carp Meat(鲢鱼, Lianyu), Tuckahoe(茯苓, Fuling) avoids vinegar, Chinese Clematis Root(威灵仙, Weilingxian), Glabrous Greenbrier Rhizome(土茯苓, Tufuling) and Rangooncreeper Fruit(使君子, Shijunzi) avoid tea water and Honey(蜂蜜, Fengmi) avoids fresh onion, etc. Besides, we should also pay attention to the contraindication of diet in diseased condition. For example: it is not advisable to have uncooked and cold food in the case of cold syndrome, pungent and greasy food in the case of heat syndrome, pungent and heat food in the case of hyperactivity of liver-yang. Patients with skin disease should avoid such fishy and irritative food as fish, shrimp and crab. Patients with indigestion should avoid fried, sticky and greasy food. Those patients who have frequent headache, insomnia and who are short-tempered should avoid pepper, chili, alcohol and tea. Patients with exogenous and exterior syndrome should avoid oily and greasy food, etc.

3. Dosage

Dosage means the amount of drugs applied to the patients. It refers to the doses of one kind of dry drug an adult needs in decoction for one day. It includes the following 3 aspects:

(1) Dosage of a single drug that an adult needs in decoction(the dosage of all kinds of drugs marked in this book refers to the daily

dosage for internal use of crude drugs after being dried.).

(2) Relative dosage of all drugs in a prescription.

(3) Actual dosage of the preparation.

As the dosage of Chinese drugs directly affects the clinical therapeutic effect, the compatibility between the nature of drugs, condition of the diseases, types of prescription, the age and physical constitution of patients should all be taken into consideration.

Determine the dosage according to compatibility and type of prescription: Non-poisonous drugs are usually prescribed in a large dose if they are used alone and in a small dose in a compound prescription.. Major drugs can be prescribed in a large dose, supplementary drugs in a small dose. In a prescription with many kinds of drugs, going alone should be prescribed in a small dose, and in a prescription with fewer kinds of drugs, going alone should be prescribed in a large dose. The dosage in the decoction is usually larger than that in the pills and powder.

Determine the dosage according to the properties of drugs: Drugs with severe poison should be used in a small dose, being strictly controlled for safety. Drugs like flower and leaf which are light in quality and easy to dissolve are usually used in a small dose, whereas drugs like mineral and shell which are heavy in quality and difficult to dissolve are usually used in a large dose.

Determine the dosage according to the condition of disease, physical constitution and age of patients: Generally speaking, drugs for treating severe and acute diseases are used in a large dose, and mild and chronic diseases in a small dose. Drugs applied to people with a strong constitution are usually given a large dose, while those who are old and weak are usually given a small dose. Babies who are under the age of 1 year take 1/4 dose, those who are 1～5 years old take 1/3 dose, those who are 6～15 years old take 1/2 dose of adults and those who are above 16 years old take an adults' dose.

The normal dose of Chinese drugs for internal use (effective dose) is 6～9g except drugs with severe poison and some refined preparations. There are other drugs, whose normal dose is 15～30g.

4. Decoction and Administration

Decoction and administration include methods of decocting drugs and the recommended time to take drugs.

Administration (method of taking medicine): This depends on the application of drugs. It is advisable to take decoction warm. Drugs for dispelling wind and cold may be taken hot. Drugs for arresting vomiting should be taken in a small amount from time to time. As far as the therapy is concerned, drugs in hot nature can be taken cold, whereas drugs in cool nature can be taken hot. Patients unconsciousness, or with trismus, should be given drugs by nasal feeding. Pill and power are usually taken with warm water that has been boiled. Common diseases should be treated with one dose a day. The dosage can be divided and taken 2～3 times a day if needed. Drugs for serious and acute diseases should be taken every four hours. Some drugs can be taken, according to the patient' condition, several times even at night so as to consolidate the medicinal effect to control the disease.

Time for Taking Medicine: the patients' condition and property of the drugs determine the time. Generally, drugs for tonifying may be taken before meals. Drugs for expelling intestinal parasites and purgation are usually taken when the stomach is empty. Drugs for invigorating the stomach and those that may greatly stimulate the stomach and intestine may well be taken after meals. Drugs for treating malaria should be taken 1～2 hours before an attack. Drugs for tranquilizing the mind are taken before going to bed. Drugs for treating acute diseases are usually taken without a fixed time and those for treating chronic diseases should be taken regularly. Drugs for treating other diseases are also taken after meals. There should have an interval between taking drugs and meals(either before or after meals)so that the therapeutic effect can be ensured.

Methods of decocting drugs: Methods of decocting drugs can directly affect the medicinal effect. The utensils for decocting drugs should be in good quality and should not negatively affect the quality of the decoction. Nowadays, sand pots are usually used or sometimes enamel pots. It is advisable to use clear and purified well water and running water for decocting drugs. One dose should be decocted at least twice. Heat control should be determined according to the property and action of the drugs. For example: drugs of fragrant taste with flower and leaf are generally decocted with high heat, That can not be decocted for a long time or the medicinal effect may be completely lost. Drugs that are greasy and heavy and whose root and stem do not easily give off juice by heating are usually decocted for a longer time with gentle fire.

Otherwise, these drugs cannot be decocted thoroughly and the therapeutic effect will be affected. The Time for decocting drugs cannot last longer or shorter than the fixed time, so this may affect the medicinal effect. Those drugs, which should be decocted in a specific way, are listed as follows:

Mineral drugs and drugs with shells decocted before other drugs are: Tortoise Shell and Plastron(龟板, Guiban), Turtle Carapace(鳖甲, Biejia), Abalone Shell(石决明, Shijueming), Hematite(代赭石, Daizheshi), Drangon's Bone(龙骨, Longgu), Oyster Shell(牡蛎, Muli), Magnetite(磁石, Cishi), Gypsum(石膏, Shigao). These drugs are hard in quality, their effective compositions are difficult to be given off by decocting. So they should be broken into pieces before being decocted. Put other drugs into the decoction after these drugs are decocted for 10～20 minutes.

Drugs which are fragrant in taste and achieve the effect with the help of volatile oil should be decocted after the other drugs: Wild Mint(薄荷, Bohe), Common Aucklandia Root (木香, Muxiang), Villous Amomum Fruit(砂仁, Sharen), Round Cardamom Seed(白豆蔻, Baidoukou), Chinese Eaglewood Wood(沉香, Chenxiang), Sweet Wormwood(青蒿, Qinghao), Rhubarb(大黄, Dahuang), Gambirplant Hooked Stem And Branch(钩藤, Gouteng) etc. These drugs should be decocted after the other drugs are decocted for 4～5 minutes, so that the effective compositions may not volatilize.

Drugs like pollen, seeds and broken mineral powder should be decocted after they are put into a small sack. Inula Flower(旋覆花, Xuanfuhua), Talc(滑石, Huashi), Plantain Seed(车前子, Cheqianzi) and Japanese Climbing Fern Spores(海金沙, Haijinsha) etc. should be put into a small sack made of gauze, placed into a sand pot and decoct it. By doing this, it may prevent the decoction from being turbid and relieve the stimulation caused by the drugs acting on the throat and digestive tract.

Drugs which are costly should be decocted alone: Ginseng (人参, Renshen), American Ginseng Root (西洋参, Xiyangshen), Hairy Antler(鹿茸, Lurong) should be cut into a small slice, put into a pot and decocted for 2～3 hours. Then mix them with the decoction made with the other drugs before taking. The purpose of doing this is to preserve the effective compositions of these drugs and avoid having them absorbed by the other drugs.

Drugs of gluey quality and easy to get melt are: Ass-hide Glue(阿胶, Ejiao), Antler Glue (鹿角胶, Lujiaojiao) and Mirabilite (芒硝, Mangxiao)etc. These drugs should be put into the decoction and stirred, or they can melt alone before being put into the decoction. The purpose of doing this is to prevent the drugs from sticking to the pot or to the other drugs while decocting them.

Drugs which are costly, can not stand high heat, or are difficult to dissolve in water should be taken by mixing them with water, such as, Sanchi Root (三七, Sanqi), Amber (琥珀, Hupo), Cinnabar(朱砂, Zhusha), Cow-bezoar (牛黄, Niuhuang) and Mush(麝香, Shexiang) etc. These drugs should be ground into powder and then mixed with the decoction or boiling water before they are taken.

PART Ⅰ
Purgatives and Tonifying Drugs

In syndrome differentiation there are deficiency syndrome and excess syndrome.

For that reason the treatment will be divided into two parts: reinforcing method and reducing method. In clinic the reinforcing method will be applied to deficiency syndrome and the reducing method will be applied to excess syndrome.

In *The Yellow Emperor's Internal Classic* (《黄帝内经》, Huangdineijing) it is said: excess syndrome refers to pathogenic factors in excess and deficiency syndrome refers to essence qi deficiency. Pathogenic factors refers to body attacked by six abnormal excess factors and also includes pathogenic products such as qi stagnation, blood stasis, phlegm, fluid retention, food retention.

The key point of the treatment is to eliminate pathogenic factors by purgatives.

If the pathogenic factor is in the superficial part of the body, the drugs to relieve the exterior by sweating can be used.

If the factor is in the chest and upper part of the epigastric region, the drugs to induce vomiting can be used.

If the pathogenic factor is retained in stomach or intestines, downward draining drugs (purgatives) can be used.

Ancient physicians summarized that to eliminate pathogenic factors must involve these three methods: sweating, vomiting, and purgation.

As the vomiting therapy has many side effects it is not advised to be used. It can be substituted by a new therapy. Sweating and purgation are still used for treating excessive syndromes.

Deficiency syndrome refers to insufficiency of essence qi. Essence -qi means qi, blood, yin and yang.

The key point of treating deficiency is using tonifying drugs to reinforce body resistance and to enhance the immunity and reduce or eliminate the power of pathogenic factor.

Before tonifying, the type of deficiency must be differentiated if it is qi, blood, yin or yang defective.

if it is qi deficiency, tonify qi; if it is blood deficiency, just tonify blood; If it is yin deficiency, reinforce yin; if it is yang deficiency, just warm yang.

The deficiency syndrome has many complications and different manifestations such as deficiency with excess syndrome; transformation of excess in deficiency, the body resistance fails to eliminate the pathogenic factor or the pathogenic factor is strong enough to consume essence qi. So the treatment will include tonification and purgation. It is very important to differentiate excess from deficiency and to decide which one is the cause and which one is appeared secondary. It will guide to choose the methods of treatment: purgation or tonification therapy.

That is why we introduce the purgatives and tonifying drugs at the beginning of this book.

Chapter 1
Drugs for Relieving the Exterior Syndromes

Definition: These drugs refer to those that have the function of dispersing the exterior pathogenic factors and relieving the exterior syndrome.

Functions: Most of these drugs are pungent in taste and have a dispersing action. The main function of these drugs is relieving the exterior syndrome through diaphoresis and dispersing the pathogenic wind. Furthermore, some of them can relieve asthma, promote diuresis, promote eruptions, remove pathogenic dampness and alleviate itching pain, etc.

Indications: The drugs are used to treat the exterior syndrome including the Taiyang syndrome of exogenous febrile diseases and Wei stage syndrome of epidemic febrile diseases, especially those syndromes caused by the invasion of exterior pathogenic wind-cold or wind-heat, manifested as aversion to cold, fever, headache, body pain, superficial pulse, etc. Some of these drugs can be used for edema, cough, asthma and incomplete eruptions. Some can cure pain of the limbs due to pathogenic wind-cold, and dampness by removing pathogenic dampness. Furthermore the drugs may be used in the early stage of various febrile diseases and skin and external diseases complicated by exterior syndrome by dispersing pathogenic factors and reducing heat.

Classification: The drugs may be classified into two categories. One is the pungent and warm drugs for relieving exterior syndrome used for the exterior syndrome due to wind-cold. The other is the pungent and cool drugs for relieving exterior syndrome used for the exterior syndrome due to wind-heat.

Notes: 1. The drugs which have the function of dispersing wind-cold or dispersing wind-heat should be used correctly according to different exterior syndromes, which may be caused by exterior wind-cold or wind-heat.

2. For those with healthy qi deficiency, the drugs for invigorating yang, benefiting qi and nourishing yin must be used first and simultaneously in order to protect healthy qi and remove pathogenic factors.

3. The drugs with a strong action of diaphoresis should be used cautiously, for profuse sweating may cause deficiency of yang-qi and body fluid.

4. These drugs can not be applied in the case of profuse sweating and the later stage of epidemic febrile diseases with body fluid deficiency. They should be used cautiously for chronic skin and external diseases, stranguria syndrome and loss of blood with exterior syndrome.

Section 1
Drugs of Pungent Taste and Warm Nature for Relieving the Exterior Syndromes

1.麻黄,Mahuang

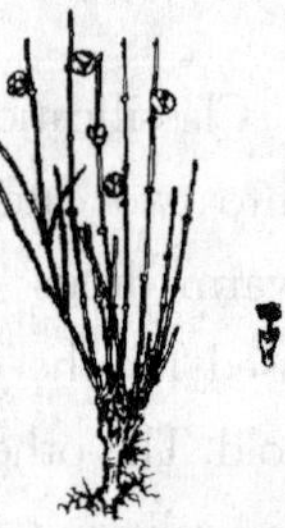
麻 黄

English name: Ephedra

Pharmaceutical name: Herba Ephedrae

Botanical name: Ephedra sinica Stapf. or E. Equistesting Bge

Properties and tastes: pungent, slightly bitter and warm.

Meridian tropism: lung and urinary bladder

Functions: 1. induce diaphoresis and disperse cold

2. control asthma

3. promote urination to reduce edema

4. relieve chronic cellulitis

5. stop pain due to arthralgia

6. inhibit excite virus of influenza

7. excite center

8. contract blood vessels and elevate blood pressure

9. excite the heart

10. mydriasis

Indications: 1. wind cold for aversion to cold, fever without sweating, headache and pain all over the body, nasal obstruction, a floating and tense pulse.

2. cough and asthma for major used is for excessive syndrome of cough and asthma, but after combination, it can be used in all kinds of cough and asthma.

3. edema for manifested in the first stage as instincted facial edema, accompanied by with aversion to cold, fever and anhidrosis (wind-edema syndrome).

4. chronic cellulitis (osteomyelitis, bone tubeculosis)

5. the early stage of rheumatic arthritis

6. acute urticaria

Dosage: 1.5～9g for decoction. When used to relieve exterior, the herb is used fresh. When used to control asthma, the herb is fried with honey.

Contraindication: This herb may cause profuse sweating, so do not use for spontaneous sweating due to qi deficiency, night sweating due to yin deficiency, cough and asthma due to failure of the kidney in receiving qi. Use cautiously in patients with hypertension or tachycardia.

Combinations: 1. add Gypsum (石膏, Shigao)——cough and asthma due to lung heat

2. add Cassia Twig(桂枝, Guizhi)——wind cold exterior excess patterns which are manifested as sweating

3. add Common Ducksmeat Herb (浮萍, Fuping)——wind-edema syndrome, fever and aversion to wind, facial edema, urine retention or rubella itching

4. add Apricot Seed(杏仁, Xingren)——invasion of the lung by wind cold, cough, reversed upward flow of qi

5. add Dried Ginger(干姜, Ganjiang)——asthma and cough due to cold water retention

6. add Prepared Daughter Root of Common Monkshood(附子, Fuzi)——arthralgia syn-

drome due to wind-cold and exopathic disease due to yang deficiency

7. add Largehead Atractylodes Rhizome(白术,Baizhu)——wind-edema syndrome

8. add Coix Seed(薏苡仁, Yiyiren)——arthralgia due to dampness, pain and swelling in the joints

9. add Cassia Bark(肉桂,Rougui),Prepared Rhizome of Adhesive Rehmannia(熟地黄, Shoudihuang)——chronic cellulitis

10. add Fineleaf Schizomepeta Herb(荆芥, Jingjie),Cicada Slough(蝉蜕,Chantui)——acute urticaria

11. add Ginkgo Seed(白果, Baiguo)——used for dispersing and arresting cough and asthma without consuming qi

Prescription: 1. Ephedra Decoction(麻黄汤, Mahuang Tang)

2. Decoction of Ephedra, Aconite and Asarum(麻黄附子细辛汤, Mahuang Fuzi Xixin Tang)

3. Decoction of Ephedra, Apricot, Gypsum and Licorice(麻杏石甘汤, Maxingshigan Tang)

4. Small Blue Dragon Decoction(小青龙汤, Xiaoqinglong Tang)

Notes: Ephedra(麻黄, Mahuang) has bidirectional action which refers to its upward or downward tendency. It can promote the dispersing function of the lung, open the pores and cause sweating, and also promote the descending function of the lung to relieve asthma and promote diuresis. Therefore Ephedra(麻黄, Mahuang) is a key drug for treating diaphoresis, relieving asthma and promoting diuresis.

Ephedra(麻黄, Mahuang), which can inhibit influenza virus, has a strong action for diaphoresis and dispersing cold. Thus it can be used for influenza due to wind-cold, especially those manifested as severe aversion to cold, slight fever, no sweating and superficial and tense pulse. It is said in *Mystery of Herbology* (《本草通玄》, Bencaotongxuan): "Ephedra(麻黄, Mahuang) with light mass can cure excessive exterior syndrome. It is the principal drug used for dispersing exterior pathogenic factors. However it is only applied to the exterior syndrome due to invasion of cold in winter". It is not suitable for those with yin-yang, qi and blood deficiency or for syndrome of yang deficiency manifested as aversion to cold, pain and heavy sensation of the body, as well as deep pulse. Prepared Daughter Root of Common Monkshood(附子, Fuzi) must be used simultaneously to invigorate yang and disperse the exterior syndrome. It should not be used for influenza due to wind-heat.

Ephedra(麻黄, Mahuang) has the function of relieving asthma. Its chemical composition includes ephedrine and pseudoephedrine, which can relax the smooth muscles of the bronchi.

Thus it is used for excessive asthma even if there is exterior syndrome due to wind-cold. It can be used for cold water retention without exterior syndrome manifested as dyspnea with cough, profuse and thin expectoration, a moist coating lack of thirst or manifested as dyspnea, cough, and rough breath. This includes flapping the wing of the nose, irritability, thirst, red tongue with thin or yellow coating, and superficial, full and rapid pulse, even if sweat is present.

Furthermore pseudoephedrine has the function of promoting diuresis. Ephedra(麻黄, Mahuang) is usually applied to severe edema in the upper body or edema in the face and limbs or acute edema with exterior syndrome due to wind-cold. The actions of Ephedra(麻黄, Mahuang) in the treatment of edema are as follows: ①to cause sweating; ②to increase the amount of urine; ③to cause slight sweating and significantly increase the amount of urine to reduce edema. When combined with Gypsum(生石膏, Shigao) large dosage of Ephedra (麻黄, Mahuang), is required in the treatment of edema, from 9g to 15g. The ratio of dosage of Gypsum (生石膏, Shigao) and Ephedra (麻黄, Mahuang) is used with a ration of approximtely 3 to 1. In this condition, the function of dysphoresis of Ephedra(麻黄, Mahuang) is reduced so that edema can be eliminated by promoting diuresis of Ephedra (麻黄, Mahuang).

Ephedra(麻黄, Mahuang) can be applied to phlegm due to yin and cold stagnation by warming and dispersing the pathogenic factors. However it is not suitable for carbuncle and furuncle manifested with redness, swelling, heat and pain.

Largehead Atractylodes Rhizome(白术, Baizhu) in combination with Ephedra(麻黄, Mahuang) can be applied to Bi syndrome due to wind-dampness. For Largehead Atractylodes Rhizome(白术, Baizhu) has the function of arresting perspiration which can inhibit the strong function of damaging healthy qi from dysphoresis of Ephedra(麻黄, Mahuang). Dampness can not be removed completely when healthy qi is deficient and combined with the drug for promoting eruption, Ephedra(麻黄, Mahuang) can also be applied to acute urticaria by warming and dispersing pathogenic factors.

Ephedra (麻黄, Mahuang) has side effects, such as excitement, insomnia, irritability, tremor, as it can stimulate the central nervous system. It can contract vessels to increase blood pressure and stimulate the heart. Thus it should not be used in those with hypertension or heart diseases. Ephedra(麻黄, Mahuang) also has the function of mydriasis. Thus it should not be used for those with glaucoma.

Ephedra(麻黄, Mahuang) is pungent in taste and has the strong function of dispersion. However, when fried with Honey (蜂蜜, Fengmi), the above-mentioned taste and it function of fresh are reduced, while the moistening of the lung appears. Therefore, it should be used for dyphoresis and relieving exterior syndrome. It will relieve asthma and cough.

2. 桂枝, Guizhi

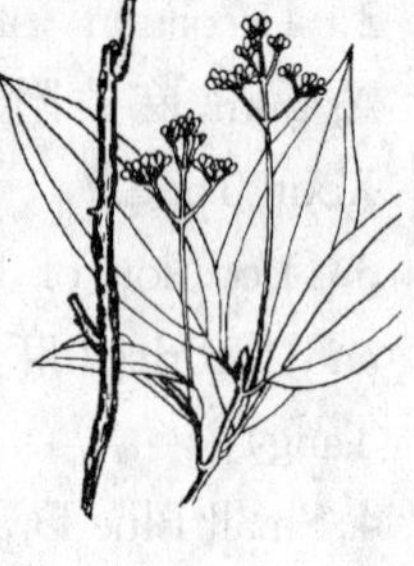
桂 枝

English name: Cassia Twig

Pharmaceutical name: Ramulus Cinnamomi

Botanical name: Cinnamomum cassia Presl

Properties and tastes: pungent, sweet, warm

Meridian tropism: the lung, heart and urinary bladder

Functions: 1. induce diaphoresis and disperse cold

2. warm the channels and move the yang

3. antipyretic, analgesia

4. bacteriostatic, inhibit influenza virus

5. tranquilizer, anticonvulsion

6. invigorate the stomach

7. diuresis and strengthen the heart

Indications: 1. wind cold for slight fever, aversion to cold, headache, stiff neck

2. rheumatic arthritis for excessive cold-dampness, pain and heavy sensation of the

joints, especially the shoulders

3. cold in the stomach and abdominal pain for cold pain in the epigastric regions relieved by pressure and warmth, pale or sallow complexion.

4. stagnation of cold evil and blood stasis syndrome in women for cold limbs and aversion to cold, cold pain in the lower abdomen with tenderness, irregular menstruation, dysmenorrhea, amenorrhea, hysteromyoma oophritic cyst

5. congested fluids syndrome for fullness, stuffiness and discomfort in the chest and hypochondriac regions, vertigo, palpitation, cough due to shortness of breath, etc, due to deficiency of the heart and the spleen yang, poor circulation of yang qi and water retention

6. water retention syndrome from urine retention, edema, headache, fever, irritability and thirst, vomiting right after drinking, a white and greasy coating of the tongue or a white and thick coating

7. obstruction in the chest due to hyperactivity of the heart yang, accompanied by chest congestion, shortness of breath, and radiating precardialgia

Dosage: 3～9g.

Contraindication: this drug is pungent and warm, easy to produce heat, damage yin and promote the circulation of the blood. It is forbidden for febrile disease, hyper-activity of yang due to yin deficiency and bleeding due to blood heat. Use cautiously in pregnant women and those women with excessive menses.

Combinations: 1. add Ephedra (麻黄, Mahuang)——wind-cold, headache, pain all over the body, pain in the joints, aversion to cold and absence of sweating

2. add Twotooth Achyranthes Root(牛膝, Niuxi)——pain of the back, lumbar and legs due to cold, amenorrhea and dysmenorrhea due to cold and stagnation of qi and blood

3. add Licorice Root(甘草, Gancao)——deficiency of the heart yang, palpitation of the heart and preference for pressure

4. add Fresh Ginger(生姜, Shengjiang)——pain in the epigastrium, vomiting of watery fluid, nausea, vomiting, and hiccups caused by cold in the stomach or water retention in the stomach

5. add White Peony Root (白芍药, Baishaoyao)——aversion to cold, fever, spontaneous perspiration, aversion to wind, superficial and slow pulse (The Taiyang meridian is affected by the wind) when externally contracted with wind-cold and disharmony of the Nutritive and Protective Qi

6. add Tuckahoe(茯苓, Fuling)——water retention, palpitation and shortness of breath due to heart yang deficiency

7. add Medicinal Evodia Root(吴茱萸, Wuzhuyu)——irregular menstruation and cold pain in the lower abdomen due to deficiency cold of Chong and Ren Meridians

8. add Peach Seed(桃仁, Taoren), Tree Peony Bark (牡丹皮, Mudanpi)——hysteromyoma

9. add Chinese Angelica Root(当归, Danggui), Manchurian Wildginger Herb(细辛, Xixin)——cold stagnation in the meridian, extremely cold hands and feet, pain of the lumbar region and knees

10. add Tuckahoe(茯苓, Fuling), Largehead Atractylodes Rhizome(白术, Baizhu)——urine retention

11. add Apricot Seed(杏仁, Xingren), Officinal Magnolia Bark(厚朴, Houpo)——

cough and asthma due to a reversed upward flow of qi

12. add Snakegourd Fruit(瓜蒌,Gualou), Longstament Oion Bulb(薤白,Xiebai)——radiating precardialgia, palpitation, knotty and regularly-intermittent pulse caused by hyparactivity of the heart yang

13. add White Peony Root (白芍药, Baishaoyao), Malt Sugar (饴糖, Yitang)——pain in the epigastrium due to insufficiency and coldness in the spleen and stomach

Prescriptions: 1. Decoction of Ramulus Cinnamomi(桂枝汤,Guizhi Tang)

2. Ephedra Decoction(麻黄汤, Mahuang Tang)

3. Pill of Cinnamom Twig and Poria(桂枝茯苓丸,Guizhi Fuling Wan)

4. Powder of Five Drugs with Poria(五苓散,Wuling San)

5. Decoction of Prepared Licorice(炙甘草汤,Zhigancao Tang)

Notes: Cassia Twig(桂枝,Guizhi)can not only be used for influenza due to wind-cold, but also widely applied to various diseases in the departments of internal medicine and gynecology. Cassia Twig(桂枝,Guizhi) is used for influenza due to wind-cold by warming WeiYang to disperse cold. Combination with White Peony Root (白芍药, Baishaoyao)and Cassia Twig(桂枝,Guizhi) can be used for influenza with sweating, while combination with Ephedra (麻黄, Mahuang) can be used to treat influenza without sweating.

Cassia Twig(桂枝,Guizhi) is used for Bi Syndrome in the chest manifested as pain in the chest by warming qi and blood, warming and activating yang in the chest. It can warm and activate the heart and vessels to restore a normal pulse beat. It is applied to phlegm retention syndrome by having the effect of warming and activating spleen-yang to remove dampness. It is applied to edema with difficult urination by warming qi of the urinary bladder; to pain of Bi syndrome, gastralgia and abdominal dysmenorrhea, mass and so on due to cold and blood stagnation. This is done by warming and activating blood vessels.

Both Cassia Twig (桂枝, Guizhi) and Ephedra(麻黄,Mahuang) can be used for exterior syndrome caused by wind-cold by way of dysphoresis. However Ephedra(麻黄,Mahuang) is pungent for dispersion and bitter for descent so that it can open the pores in the skin to cause profuse sweating, promote the dispersion of lung qi to relieve asthma and promote diuresis to eliminate edema. Being pungent and sweet in taste and warm in nature, Cassia Twig (桂枝, Guizhi) is good at warming and dredging Meridian to activate yang and relieve exterior syndrome, while the action of dysphoresis is weak. *Materia Medica of Decoction* (《汤液本草》, Tangyebencao) says: "Ephedra(麻黄, Mahuang) is the drug for excess syndrome in Wei stage, while Cassia Twig(桂枝, Guizhi) is the drug for deficiency. Although both of them are used for Tai Yang syndrome, they are actually the drugs for diseases in the ying or Wei stage. The lung controls the Wei stage and qi, while the heart controls the ying stage and blood. Therefore Ephedra(麻黄, Mahuang) is the drug for Hand Taiyin meridian (Lung meridian) and Cassia Twig(桂枝, Guizhi) is the drug for Hand Shaoyin Meridian(Heart meridian)."

3. 紫苏, Zisu

English name: Perilla Leaf

Pharmaceutical name: Folium Periliae Frutescentis

Botanical name: Perilla frutescens (L.) Britt. Var. Crispa (Thunb.) Hand.-Mazz. Or P. Frutescens (L.) Britt. Var. Acuta (Thunb.) Kudo

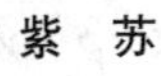

紫 苏

Properties and tastes: pungent, warm

Meridian tropism: lung and spleen

Functions: 1. relieve the exterior and disperse cold

2. promote qi circulation and provide harmony for the Middle-jiao

3. alleviate abdominal pain and vomiting due to fish and crab poisoning

Indications: 1. wind-cold, fever, aversion to cold, headache, nasal obstruction, accompanied by cough or congestion and discomfort in the chest

2. vomiting due to chest congestion, vomiting due to spleen and stomach qi stagnation. It can also be used in vomiting caused by pregnancy

3. abdominal pain, vomiting and diarrhea due to eating fish and crab

Dosage: 3～9g. It is not advisable to decoct it with water for a long time.

Contraindication: Used cautiously in exterior deficiency syndrome with excessive sweating.

Combinations: 1. add Fresh Ginger (生姜, Shengjiang)——externally contracted wind cold fever, aversion to cold, absence of sweating

2. add Apricot Seed (杏仁, Xingren), Whiteflower Hogfennel Root (前胡, Qianhu)——invasion of the pathogenic wind-cold factor, cough with profuse sputum

3. add Nutgrass Galingale Rhizome (香附, Xiangfu), Tangerine Peel (陈皮, Chenpi)——invasion of the pathogenic wind-cold factor, fever, aversion to cold, feeling of fullness in the chest

4. add Wrinkled Gianthyssop Herb (藿香, Huoxiang)——vomiting due to stomach cold and common cold in summer

5. add Coptis Rhizome (黄连, Huanglian)——vomiting due to stomach heat

6. add Ginseng (人参, Renshen)——deficiency of stomach qi, accompanied by exopathic disease

7. add Dahurian Angelica Root (白芷, Baizhi)——abdominal pain, vomiting and diarrhea due to eating fish and crab

8. add Tangerine Peel (陈皮, Chenpi), Villous Amomum Fruit (砂仁, Sharen)——threatened abortion due to qi stagnation

9. add Common Floweringquince Fruit (木瓜, Mugua), Officinal Magnolia Bark (厚朴, Houpo)——cholera, flaccidity of lower limbs

Prescriptions: 1. Powder of Cyperus Tuber and Perilla (香苏散, Xiangsu San)

2. Powder of Semen Armeniacae Amarum and Folium Perillae (杏苏散, Xingsu San)

Notes: Being pungent and warm, Perilla Leaf (紫苏, Zisu) is a mild drug for relieving exterior syndrome and regulating the flow of qi and gastrointestinal function. In the clinic it is suitable for influenza belonging to the gastrointestinal type or complicated by gastric diseases. Furthermore, Perilla Leaf (紫苏, Zisu), Perilla Seed (苏子, Suzi) and Perilla Stem (苏梗, Sugeng) belong to the same plant. Perilla Leaf(苏叶,Suye)is good at relieving exterior syndrome, Perilla Stem(苏梗,Sugeng)at regulating the flow of qi and Perilla Seed (苏子, Suzi) at removing phlegm.

Perilla Leaf(紫苏,Zisu)is the key drug for regulating the flow of qi. It is pungent in taste and acts on qi stage. It is said in *Collected Decoction of Herbals* (《本草汇言》,Bencaohuiyan) that it can"disperse cold qi, clear lung qi, regulate middle qi, benefit fetus qi, descend accumulated qi and remove phlegm qi. Thus it is a mysterious drug for qi imbalance".

The decoction of Perilla Leaf(紫苏,Zisu) can promote the secretion of digestive juice and can activate gastrointestinal peristalsis and inhibit colibacillus, bacillus dysenteriae and staphylococcus.

4. 生姜, Shengjiang

English name: Fresh Ginger

Pharmaceutical name: Rhizoma Officinalis Rencens

Botanical name: Zingiber officinal Rose

Properties and tastes: pungent, slightly warm

Meridian tropism: lung, spleen

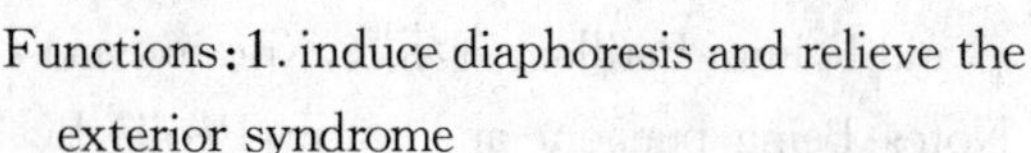

生 姜

Functions: 1. induce diaphoresis and relieve the exterior syndrome

2. warm the Middle-jiao and alleviate vomiting

3. warm the lung to arrest cough

4. reduce the poisonous effect of other herbs

Indications: 1. exterior wind-cold syndrome-Taiyang meridian affected by the wind, mild cases of cold. It is also used to prevent common cold.

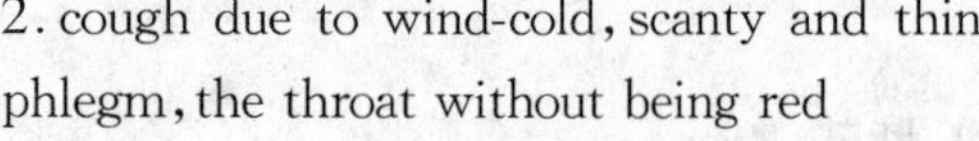

2. cough due to wind-cold, scanty and thin phlegm, the throat without being red

3. vomiting due to stomach-cold, It can be used for all kinds of vomiting when combined with different herbs

4. poisoning due to eating fish and crab, nausea, vomiting, abdominal pain. It can also reduce the poisonous and side effects of Pinellia Rhizome (半夏, Banxia), Jackinthepulpit Tuber(南星, Nanxing)

Dosage: 3~9g.

Contraindication: This herb is pungent and warm. Contraindicated in excessive heat syndrome and for cases of deficient yin with heat signs.

Combinations: 1. add Fineleaf Schizomepeta Herb (荆芥, Jingjie)——externally contracted wind cold, chills, fever, headache, nasal obstruction, and the absence of sweating

2. add Cassia Twig(桂枝, Guizhi)——the Taiyang channel affected by the wind, fever, aversion to wind, sweating, headache, and a floating-moderate pulse

3. add Pinellia Rhizome(半夏, Banxia)——retention of phlegm and fluid in the stomach, vomiting, and dizziness

4. add Perilla Leaf (苏叶, Suye), Apricot Seed (杏仁, Xingren)——cough due to wind-cold

5. add Lesser Galangal Rhizome(高良姜, Gaoliangjiang)——cold pain in the epigastric region due to stomach-cold

6. add Bamboo Shavings (竹茹, Zhuru), Coptis Rhizome (黄连, Huanglian)——vomiting due to heat phlegm

7. add Chinese Date (大枣, Dazao), Fresh Ginger(生姜, Shengjiang)——to adjust the nutritive ying qi and defensive wei qi. Combination with tonifying drugs can be used

for invigorating deficiency, and combination with purgative drugs can be used for purgation.

Prescription: Minor Decoction of Pinellia(小半夏汤, Xiaobanxia Tang)

Notes: Sun Simiao(孙思邈)said: "Fresh Ginger(生姜, Shengjiang) is a key drug for vomiting." It is pungent in taste and has the function of dispersing exterior pathogenic factor. Thus it can be used with drugs for relieving exterior syndrome in order to enhance the action of dysphoresis. Modern research shows that Fresh Ginger(生姜, Shengjiang) has a dual action for regulating the secretion of gastric acid and juice. It is an effective antiemetic, anti-inflammatory agent and analgesic. It can stimulate the vascular motor center and respiratory center. It is said in *Annotation on Shennong's Herbal Classic* (《本草经疏》, Bencaojingshu): "taking this drug for a long time may cause yin deficiency and eye injury." Therefore those with heat due to yin deficiency can not take a large dose or take it for a long time.

5. 荆芥, Jingjie

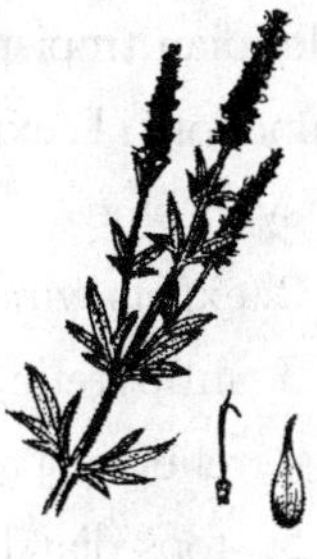

English name: Fineleaf Schizomepeta Herb

Pharmaceutical name: Herba Schizonepetae

Botanical name: Schizonepeta tenuifolia Briq.

荆 芥

Properties and tastes: pungent, slightly warm

Meridian tropism: lung, liver

Functions: 1. expel wind, release the exterior syndrome

2. promote the formation of eruption (encourage rash to surface)

3. stop bleeding and ablate boils

4. bacteriostatic

5. tranquilizer, analgesic

6. antiinflammation, antiallergy

Indications: 1. externally contracted wind cold——headache, fever, aversion to cold, lack of sweating

2. rubella, measles——skin eruptions with itching or measles without complete erupting

3. initial stages of carbuncles or boils——carbuncles and boils, especially when they are accompanied by chills, fever, lack of sweating, etc.

4. epistaxis, hematochezia, metrorrhagia and metrostaxis

Dosage: 3～9g. It is not advisable to decoct it in water for a long time. When used to stop bleeding, the herb is toasted ash.

Contraindication: Use cautiously in patient with spontaneous sweating due to exterior deficiency.

Combinations: 1. add Divaricate Saposhnikovia Root(防风, Fangfeng)——cold, diarrhea, dysentery, early stages of carbuncles and boils, hematochezia, metrorrhagia and metrostaxis, menorrhagia due to wind, cold and dampness evils

2. add Wild Mint(薄荷, Bohe)——diseases of the face and head, incomplete eruption of measles, itching skin due to wind evils

3. add Perilla Leaf(苏叶, Suye)——externally contracted wind cold, aversion to cold, fever, absence of sweating

4. add Gypsum(石膏, Shigao)——headache due to wind-heat

5. add Japanese Pagodatree Flower(槐花, Huaihua), Chinese Arborvitae Leafy Twig (侧柏叶, Cebaiye)-hematochezia

6. add Wild Mint (薄荷, Bohe), Chinese

Thorowax Root(柴胡,Chaihu)——invasion of the body surface by wind heat, headache, fever, nasal obstruction, sore throat,etc.

7. add Shunk Bugbane Rhizome(升麻, Shengma),Great Burdock Achene(牛蒡子, Niubangzi)——incomplete eruption of mealses

8. add Cicada Slough(蝉蜕,Chantui), Lobed Kudzuvine Root(葛根,Gegen)——skin eruptions with itching,etc.

9. add Great Burdock Achene(牛蒡子,Niubangzi), Honeysuckle Flower(金银花, Jinyinhua)——the initial stages of carbuncles and boils accompanied by exterior syndrome

10. add Red Peony Root(赤芍药, Chishaoyao), Swordlike Atractylodes Rhizome(苍术,Cangzhu), Chinese Corktree Bark(黄柏,Huangbai)——rubella,eczema, scabies

Prescriptions: 1. Powder of Lonicerae and Forsythiae(银翘散,Yinqiao San)

2. Powder of Schizonepeta and Ledebouriella (荆防败毒散,Jingfangbaidu San)

Notes: Fineleaf Schizomepeta Herb(荆芥, Jingjie)is a mild drug. Li Shizhen called it as a principal drug for diseases due to pathogenic wind, blood imbalance, skin and external diseases. It is said in *Collected Decoction of Herbals* (《本草汇言》,Bencaohuiyan): it "disperses wind and regulates blood. Thus it is a drug for dispersing wind in the blood." Using different combinations it can be used for exterior syndrome due to wind-cold or wind-heat. The spike of it is good at alleviating headache. Fineleaf Schizomepeta Herb(荆芥,Jingjie)and it is good at stopping bleeding in the upper body after being carbonized.

Both Fineleaf Schizomepeta Herb(荆芥, Jingjie)and Perilla Leaf(紫苏,Zisu)can relieve the exterior syndrome by dysphoresis. Perilla Leaf(紫苏,Zisu)has a strong action for dispersing cold. It mainly acts on qi stage and regulates qi in the Middle-jiao while Fineleaf Schizomepeta Herb(荆芥, Jingjie)has a strong function for dispersing wind. It mainly acts on the blood stage. Therefore Perilla Leaf(紫苏,Zisu)is usually used for regulating qi and Fineleaf Schizomepeta Herb(荆芥,Jingjie)for regulating blood.

6. 防风, Fangfeng

English name: Divaricate Saposhnikovia Root

Pharmaceutical name: Radix Ledebouriellae Sesloidis

Botanical name: Ledebouriella sesloides (Hoffm) Wolff; this plant is also known as Saposhinikovia divaricata(turcz)Schishk

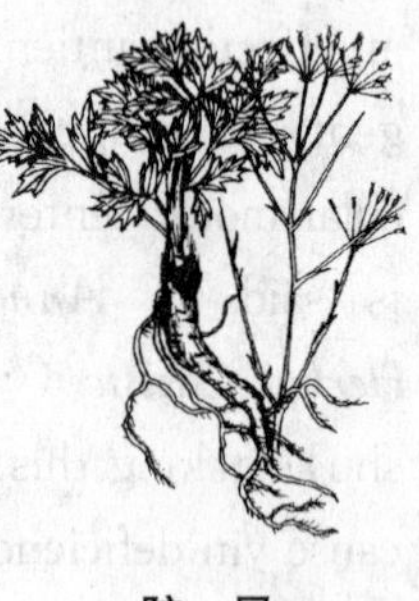

防 风

Properties and tastes: pungent, sweet, slightly warm

Meridian tropism: urinary bladder, liver, spleen

Functions: 1. expels wind and relieves exterior syndrome

2. expels wind dampness and alleviatess pain

3. antipyretic, anti-inflammatory, analgesic

4. relieves spasm

5. stops diarrhea

Indications: 1. externally contracted wind-cold——headache, generalized body ache, aversion to cold, nasal obstruction

2. arthralgia due to wind cold and dampness——pain in the joints, contracture of four limbs

3. tetanus for lockjaw, convulsion associated with rabies

4. abdominal pain, diarrhea, hematochezia, metrorrhagia and metrostaxis

Dosage: 3～9g.

Contraindication: Contraindicated in blood deficiency syndrome with spasm, and for case of yin deficiency with heat signs.

Combinations: 1. add Fineleaf Schizomepeta Herb(荆芥, Jingjie)——exterior syndrome from externally contracted wind cold. It can also be used for wind cold and damp painful obstruction with early stages of carbuncles and boils

2. add Largeleaf Gentian Root(秦艽, Qinjiao)——wind cold and damp painful obstruction

3. add Swordlike Atractylodes Rhizome(苍术, Cangzhu)——diarrhea due to spleen deficiency with excessive dampness evils and water diarrhea due to spleen deficiency attacked by wind evils

4. add Scorpion(全蝎, Quanxie)——tetanus

5. add Membranous Milkvetch Root(黄芪, Huangqi)——spontaneous perspiration due to exterior deficiency syndrome

6. add charred Fineleaf Schizomepeta Herb (荆芥炭, Jingjietan)——bleeding due to hemorrhoid, hematochezia, metrorrhagia and metrostaxis

7. add Largehead Atractylodes Rhizome(白术, Baizhu)——intermittent abdominal pain, borborygmus and diarrhea

8. add Chrysanthemum Flower(菊花, Juhua)——slight aversion to wind, fever, headache, eye itching caused by external attack of wind heat

9. add Fineleaf Schizomepeta Herb(荆芥, Jingjie), Perilla Leaf(苏叶, Suye) Wild Mint (薄荷, Bohe)——skin itching, eruptions, etc.

10. add Rhizome or Root of Forbes Notopterygium(羌活, Qianghuo)——headache in the Taiyang meridians, posterior part of the brain

Prescription: Powder of Schizonepeta and Ledebouriella(荆防败毒散, Jingfangbaidu San)

Notes: Divaricate Saposhnikovia Root(防风, Fangfeng) functions to disperse the wind and alleviate pain. It can relieve exterior syndrome as well as eliminate wind-dampness to alleviate pain. It is a mild drug and can be used for exterior syndrome due to either wind-cold or wind-heat Zhang Yuan Su called it "an immortal drug for dispersing wind-dampness." Divaricate Saposhnikovia Root(防风, Fangfeng) is usually combined with Fineleaf Schizomepeta Herb(荆芥, Jingjie) to enhance the function of dysphoresis and alleviate pain.

Our ancestors believed that "drugs for dispersing wind can remove dampness". Thus fried Divaricate Saposhnikovia Root(防风, Fangfeng) is usually used for diarrhea due to spleen deficiency. After being carbonized, Divaricate Saposhnikovia Root(防风, Fangfeng) can be used for metrorrhagia and metrostaxis to stop bleeding.

Divaricate Saposhnikovia Root(防风, Fangfeng) is a common drug for dispersing wind. However, it is said in *Collected Decoction of Herbals* (《本草汇言》, Bencaohuiyan): "Divaricate Saposhnikovia Root(防风, Fangfeng) may not succeed in treating diseases caused by pathogenic wind. Some drugs do not conduct it to the affected area. Thus with the conduction of Dahurian Angelica Root(白芷, Baizhi), Szechwan Lovage Rhizome (川芎, Chuanxiong) and Dahurian Angelica Root(白芷, Baizhi), it goes upward to disperse wind in the face and eyes; with the conduction of Whiteflower Hogfennel Root(前胡, Qianhu) and Doubleteeth Pulbescent Angelica Root(独活, Duhuo), it goes downward to disperse wind in the lumbus and knee; with Chinese Angelica Root(当归, Danggui), it can disperse wind in the blood; Largehead Atractylodes Rhizome(白术, Baizhu), it can disperse wind of the spleen; with Perilla Leaf(苏叶, Suye) and Ephedra(麻黄, Mahuang), it can disperse cold-wind; with Baikal Skullcap Root(黄芩, Huangqin) and Coptis Rhizome (黄连, Huanglian), it can disperse heat-wind; with Fineleaf Schizomepeta Herb(荆芥, Jingjie) and Chinese Corktree Bark(黄柏, Huangbai), it is used for hematochezia; with Olibanum, Frankincense(乳香, Ruxiang) and Cassia Bark(肉桂, Rougui), it can cure gout, adult apoplexy and infantile convulsion. For leprosy it should be comibined with the drugs for killing intestinal parasites and treating blood diseases."

Both Divaricate Saposhnikovia Root(防风, Fangfeng) and Fineleaf Schizomepeta Herb(荆芥, Jingjie) can eliminate wind to relieve exterior syndrome and disperse exterior pathogenic factors. Fineleaf Schizomepeta Herb(荆芥, Jingjie) is light in mass and has the function of dispersion. Thus it can disperse wind in the superficial area of the body and disperse wind-heat in the blood. While Divaricate Saposhnikovia Root(防风, Fangfeng) has strong action for dispersing wind and can be used for all kinds of diseases due to the mind. Furthermore, Divaricate Saposhnikovia Root(防风, Fangfeng) has the functions of eliminating dampness and alleviating pain.

7. 羌活, Qianghuo

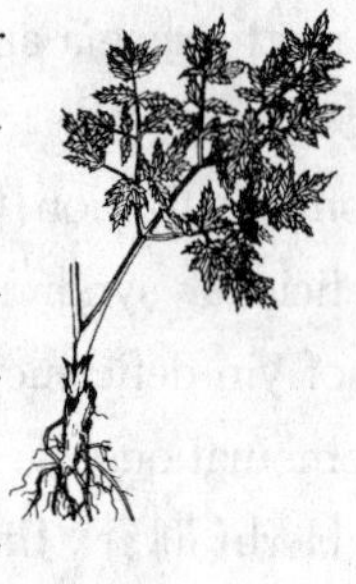

English name: Rhizome or Root of Forbes Notopterygium

Pharmaceutical name: Rhizoma et Radix Notopterygii

Botanical name: Notopterygium incisium Ting Mss., (N. Forbesii) Boiss. or (N. Franchetii) Boiss

羌活

Properties and tastes: pungent, bitter, warm

Meridian tropism: kidney, urinary bladder

Functions: 1. relieve the exterior and disperse cold

2. expels the wind and remove dampness

3. relieve pain

4. antipyretic, anti-inflammation

5. inhibit brucella and dermatomyces

Indications: 1. externally contracted wind cold——aversion to wind while with a slight fever, headache, generalized body ache

2. wind cold damp painful obstruction——pain in the limbs and joints, soreness and pain of the shoulder and back, expecially in the upper limbs and back

Dosage: 3～9g.

Contraindication: Do not use for patients with painful obstruction due to blood deficiency or headache due to yang deficiency. In addition, if used in too large dose, the herb can cause vomitting. Pay attention to the food and drink of the patients when using it.

Combinations: 1. add Doubleteeth Pulbescent Angelica Root(独活, Duhuo)——wind-cold dampness, painful obstruction, wandering pain of the whole body, pain of neck and back

2. add Divaricate Saposhnikovia Root(防风,

Fangfeng)——migraine, heaviness of the body and pain in the joints

3. add Swordlike Atractylodes Rhizome(苍术, Cangzhu)——headache as if the head was tightly bandaged

4. add Tumeric Rhizome (姜黄, Jianghuang), Cassia Twig (桂枝, Guizhi)——arthralgia due to wind damp in the shoulder, arms, palms and fingers

5. add Fineleaf Schizomepeta Herb(荆芥, Jingjie), Divaricate Saposhnikovia Root(防风, Fangfeng)——wind-cold type of common cold and painful obstruction due to wind cold damp

6. add Chrysanthemum Flower (菊花, Juhua), Puncturevine Caltrap Fruit(白蒺藜, Baijili) and Shrub Chastetree Fruit(蔓荆子, Manjingzi)——conjunctivitis due to wind-heat

7. add Szechwan Lovage Rhizome(川芎, Chuanxiong)——Taiyang headache and Jueyin headache

Prescription: Decoction of Notopterygium for Rheumatism (羌活胜湿汤, Qianghuoshengshi Tang)

Notes: Rhizome or Root of Forbes Notopterygium(羌活, Qianghuo) has the functions of dysphoresis to relieve exterior syndrome and eliminating wind-dampness to alleviate pain. Thus it may be used for exterior syndrome due to wind-cold, complicated with severe headache and joint pain. For the syndrome manifested as joint pain. Whiteflower Hogfennel Root (前胡, Qianhu) should be used with or without exterior syndrome. It is said in *Revelation of Medicine* (《医学启源》, Yixueqiyuan), "It has five functions as follows: conducting other drugs to work on the Hand and Foot Taiyang meridians, blending pathogenic wind and dampness, alleviating pain in the limbs and joints, removing stale blood in the focus of carbuncle and phlegm and curing headache due to wind-dampness."

8. 白芷, Baizhi

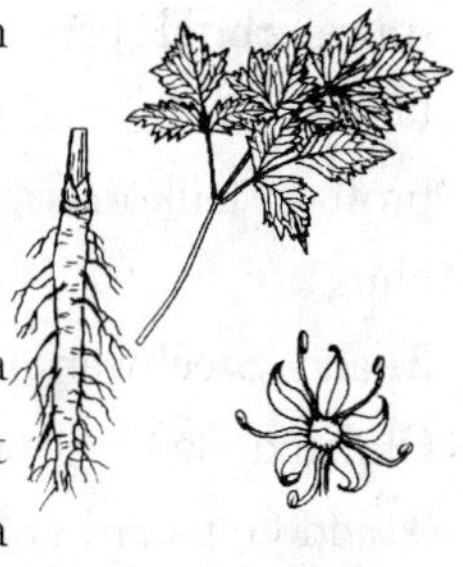

English name: Dahurian Angelica Root

Pharmaceutical name: Radix Angelicae

Botanical name: Angelica dahurica Benth. Et Hook. A. Anomala Lallem. or A. Taiwaniana Boiss.

白芷

Properties and tastes: pungent, warm

Meridian tropism: lung, stomach

Functions: 1. expel the wind and release exterior syndromes

2. alleviate pain

3. reduce swelling and expel pus discharge

4. expel dampness and alleviate discharge, stop leukorrhea

5. open up the nasal passages

Indications: 1. common cold due to wind cold——headache, absence of sweating, nasal obstruction

2. headache in Yangming Meridian, pain in the Supra-orbital Bone, headache caused by wind, toothache

3. nasosinusitis——rhinorrhea with turbid discharge, headache, sinusitis with turbid nasal discharge

4. pyogenic infection of the skin——used in the early stages of surface sores and carbuncles to reduce swelling and stop pain if the sore, ulcer, or carbuncles has already formed pus

5. cold damp leukorrhea in women, for thin and large quantity of leukorrhea, cold pain

in the lower abdomen

Dosage: 3～9g

Contraindication: Use cautionsly for patients with deficiency of qi.

Combinations: 1. add Silkworm with Batrytis Larva(白僵蚕,Baijiangcan)——pain in the supra-orbital bone due to invasion of the Upper-jiao by the wind heat evils, women's profuse leukorrhea with continuous dribbling

2. add Szechwan Lovage Rhizome(川芎, Chuanxiong)——wind-cold headache

3. add Gypsum(石膏,Shigao)——stomach-heat toothache

4. add Licorice Root(甘草, Gancao)——mastadenitis and suppurative ulcer with swelling and pain, pain of gastroduodencal ulcer

5. add Manchurian Wildginger Herb(细辛, Xixin)——headache associated with nasosinusitis

6. add Mantis Egg-Case(海螵蛸,Haipiaoxiao), Largehead Atractylodes Rhizome(白术,Baizhu)——cold damp leukorrhea

7. add Chinese Corktree Bark(黄柏,Huangbai)——damp heat leukorrhea

8. add Dandelion(蒲公英, Pugongying), Zhejiang Tendrilleaf Fritillary Bulb(浙贝母, Zhebeimu) Snakegourd Fruit(瓜蒌, Gualou)——swelling mastadenitis pain

Notes: Dahurian Angelica Root(白芷,Baizhi) is pungent in taste, warm in nature and fragrant in smell. It has the functions of diminishing cold, drying dampness and removing obstruction in the orifices. It acts on the superficial area of the body and disperses wind in Wei stage. It is a drug for relieving exterior syndrome of Yangming Meridian as well as a key drug for headache due to rhinorrhea. It is said in *Herbals for Easy Approaching* (《本草便读》, Bencaobiandu), "it not only clears pathogenic factors of the head and eyes, but also cures metrorrhagia, leucorrhea and hematochezia, for it can act on the lung in the upper body as well as in the large intestine in the lower body." Although it is pungent in taste and warm in nature, it can be used for heat syndrome in combination with other drugs, such as headache due to wind-heat, pyogenic infection of the skin, leucorrhea due to damp heat and so on. It is said in *Hunderd Herbs Selected from the Shennong's Herbal Classic* (《本草经百种录》, Bencaojingbaizhonglu), "All drugs for dispersing wind will consume essence and body fluid. Dahurian Angelica Root(白芷,Baizhi) is extremely fragrant so that it can eliminate wind and dry dampness. It is strongly lubricant in nature so it can regulate blood vessels without consuming essence. That is why Dahurian Angelica Root(白芷,Baizhi) performs its actions without side effects."

The decoction of Dahurian Angelica Root (白芷,Baizhi) can inhibit colibacillus, Bacillus dysenteriae, typhoid bacillus, pseudomonas aeruginosa and proteus.

9. 藁本, Gaoben

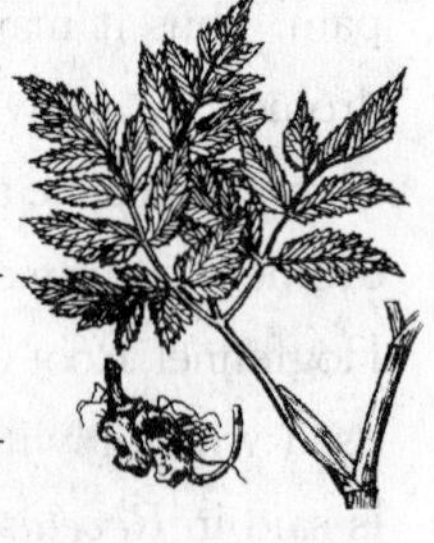
藁本

English name: Chinese Ligusticum Rhizome

Pharmaceutical name: Rhizoma Radix Ligustici Sinensis

Botanical name: Ligusticam sinense Oliv.

Properties and tastes: pungent, warm

Meridian tropism: urinary bladder

Functions: 1. relieve the exterior and expel

cold

2. expel wind and remove dampness

3. alleviate pain

Indications: 1. headache, pain at the vertex or pain that travels from the vertex down to the cheeks, teeth and migrane due to invasion of the pathogenic wind-cold

2. obstructive pain of limbs and joints from invasion of wind cold damp

Dosage: 3～9g.

Contraindication: This herb is pungent in taste and warm in nature, and has the function of expelling and dispersing. Do not use it for headache due to blood deficiency and heat syndrome.

Combinations: 1. add Dahurian Angelica Root (白芷, Baizhi)——herpes on the head and face due to wind damp, rosacea, acne and scalp desquamation etc.

2. add Manchurian Wildginger Herb(细辛, Xixin)——headache, stiffness of the neck and toothache

3. add Swordlike Atractylodes Rhizome(苍术, Cangzhu)——back pain and joint pain resulting from the initial stage of obstructive pain

4. add Medicinal Evodia Root (吴茱萸, Wuzhuyu)——abdominal pain and pain in the testicle due to stagnation of cold-dampness

5. add Shrub Chastetree Fruit (蔓荆子, Manjingzi)——headache and wind syndrome of head

Notes: Chinese Ligusticum Rhizome (藁本, Gaoben) is an analgesic antipyretic drug. Zhang Yuansu(张元素) said: "it is a necessary drug for headache. Pain in the top of head can not be relieved without it." It can also relieve the pain caused by arthritis.

All of Chinese Ligusticum Rhizome (藁本, Gaoben), Rhizome or Root of Forbes Notopterygium (羌活, Qianghuo) and Dahurian Angelica Root (白芷, Baizhi) are pungent and warm and have the functions of dispersing pathogenic factors, removing dampness and relieving pain. However the action of Rhizome or Root of Forbes Notopterygium(羌活, Qianghuo) is strong and tends to ascend. The main functions of it are dispersing wind in the superficial area of the body and eliminating wind-cold and wind-dampness in Taiyang Meridian. It has a better effect on pain of the shoulder and back. It is usually used for the Bi syndrome, for it can act on joint and remove wind-cold-dampness between tendon and bone. Dahurian Angelica Root (白芷, Baizhi) is pungent, fragrant and warm. It can disperse pathogenic factors remove obstruction in meridian and dry dampness. It also tends to ascend. Thus it can be used for diseases of the face and head, such as pain in the forehead and superficial area, pain and swelling of the gum, rhinorrhea due to wind-cold invading Taiyin and Yangming meridians. It also has the function of promoting subsidence of swelling and pus discharge, and drying dampness to cure leucorrhea. Chinese Ligusticum Rhizome (藁本, Gaoben) has a strong action of ascending and dispersing. It can go to the top of the head and relieve headache which radiates to the cheek and teeth. It is also applied to abdominal pain, diarrhea, and mass in the abdomen of women due to cold dampness.

10. 香薷, Xiangru

English name: Haichow Elsholtzia Herb

Pharmaceutical name: Herba Elsholtziae Splendentis

Botanical name: Elsholtzia splendens Nakai ex Maekwa. This plant is also known as E. Haichowensis Sun.

Properties and tastes: pungent, slightly warm

香 薷

Meridian tropism: lung, stomach

Functions: 1. induce diaphoresis and release exterior

2. transform dampness and expel summer-heat

3. promote urination and reduce swelling

Indications:

1. external wind cold in summer——aversion to cold, fever, headache, lack of sweating

2. edema and difficult urination

3. heliosis in summer for thirst, irritability, vomiting and diarrhea

Dosage: 3～9g.

Contraindication: This herb has strong effect of causing sweating. Not to be used for those who have spontaneous sweating accompanied by exterior syndrome of deficiency type.

Combinations: 1. add Wrinkled Gianthyssop Herb(藿香, Huoxiang)——common cold with dampness in summer, manifested as fever and aversion to cold, oppressive feeling in the chest, vomiting, abdominal pain, etc.

2. add Hyacinth Bean(扁豆, Biandou)——cold, vomiting and diarrhea caused by externally contracted cold disorders in summer time

3. add Largehead Atractylodes Rhizome(白术, Baizhu)——edema and urine retention resulting from accumulated damp cold

4. add Lalang Grass Rhizome(白茅根, Baimaogen), Motherwort Herb(益母草, Yimucao)——fever, lack of sweating, difficult urination, edema

5. add Coptis Rhizome(黄连, Huanglian), Talc(滑石, Huashi)——irritability and urine retention

6. add Hindu Lotus Leaf(荷叶, Heye), Hyacinth Bean(扁豆, Biandou), Foutune Eupatorium Herb(佩兰, Peilan)——acute nephritis edema

Prescription: Herbal Elsholtziae seu Moslae Decoction with Additions(新加香薷饮, Xinjiaxiangru Yin)

Notes: Haichow Elsholtzia Herb(香薷, Xiangru) has the function of dysphoresis and relieving exterior syndrome, clearing away summer heat and removing dampness. Thus it is a necessary drug for fever, aversion to cold, lack of sweating, vomiting and diarrhea due to over enjoying, cool temperatures in the summer. Because Haichow Elsholtzia Herb(香薷, Xiangru) is good at causing sweating to clear away summer-heat and promoting diuresis, and is similar to the function of Ephedra(麻黄, Mahuang), it is called "Ephedra(麻黄, Mahuang) in summer". The difference between Ephedra(麻黄, Mahuang) and Haichow Elsholtzia Herb(香薷, Xiangru) is as follows: Haichow Elsholtzia Herb(香薷, Xiangru) disperses stagnated yang qi, causing sweat to clear away summer-heat and regulates the spleen to remove dampness. While Ephedra(麻黄, Mahuang) promotes the dispersion of lung qi, opens the pore, causes sweating to relieve exterior syndrome, relieves asthma and promotes diuresis. The function of causing sweating and eliminating cold is strong. However it can not regulate the Middle-jiao to remove dampness.

11. 辛夷, Xinyi

English name: Biond Magnolia Flower-bud

Pharmaceutical name: Flos Magnoliae Liliflorae

Botanical name: Magnolia liliflora Desr.

辛 夷

Properties and tastes: pungent, warm

Meridian tropism: lung, stomach

Functions:

1. expel wind-cold and open the nasal passages
2. bacteriostatic, tranquilizer, analgesic
3. reduce blood pressure
4. stimulate the uterine smooth muscle

Indications: 1. wind cold, nasal obstruction or congestion, headache, thin nasal discharge

2. rhinitis, paranasal sinusitis, nasal polyp
3. vertigo, and nausea caused by hypertension

Dosage: 3～9g.

Contraindication: Not to be taken by patients with deficiency of yin leading to hyperactivity of fire and those women during pregnancy.

Combinations: 1. add Siberian Cocklebur Fruit (苍耳子, Cangerzi)——headache, nasal obstruction, toothache

2. add Dahurian Angelica Root (白芷, Baizhi)——spasm of face, swollen boils on face
3. add Manchurian Wildginger Herb (细辛, Xixin)——headache caused by rhinitis, paranusal sinusitis and nasal polyp, or headache, feeling of distension in the head, nasal obstruction, turbid nasal discharge and a poor sense of smell due to invasion of the pathogenic wind-cold factor
4. add Chrysanthemum Flower (菊花, Juhua), India Madder Root (茜草, Qiancao)——maxillary sinusitis
5. add Coptis Rhizome (黄连, Huanglian), Weeping Forsythia Capsule (连翘, Lianqiao)——distention in the nose and presence of sores in the nose
6. add Common Aucklandia Root (木香, Muxiang), Common Anemarrhea Rhizome (知母, Zhimu), Chinese Corktree Bark (黄柏, Huangbai)——acute rhinitis, paranusal sinusitis
7. add Fineleaf Schizomepeta Herb (荆芥, Jingjie), Baikal Skullcap Root (黄芩, Huangqin)——paranasal sinusitis or chronic rhinitis
8. add Mulberry Twig (桑枝, Sangzhi), Cassia Twig (桂枝, Guizhi)——inability of the joints to move
9. add Pinellia Rhizome (半夏, Banxia), Tall Gastrodia Rhizome (天麻, Tianma)——hypertension and vertigo

Notes: Biond Magnolia Flower-bud (辛夷, Xinyi) is pungent, warm, fragrant and light. It tends to ascend and disperse pathogenic factors including wind-cold in the Wei stage and stagnated fire of the lung. It is a special drug for diseases of the nose. Combined with other drugs, it may be used for all kinds of rhinitis and rhinorrhea manifested as headache, stuffed nose, turbid nasal discharge and loss of sense of smell. Li Shizhen (李时珍) said: "Biond Magnolia Flower-bud (辛夷, Xinyi) is pungent and warm and acts on qi stage and the lung. It can help clear yang of the stomach to ascend. As it warms the Middle-jiao and is used for diseases of head, face, eyes and nose." Biond Magnolia Flower-bud (辛夷, Xinyi) is also called Biond

Magnolia Immature Flower(木笔花,Mubihua).

12.葱白,Congbai

English name: Fistular Onion Stalk

Pharmaceutical name: Herba Allii Fistulosi

Botanical name: Allium fistulosum L.

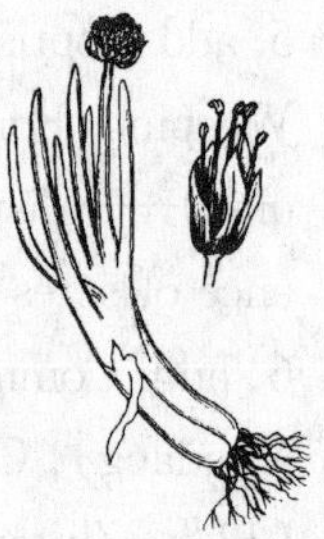

Properties and tastes: pungent, warm

葱 白

Meridian tropism: lung, stomach

Functions: 1. induce diaphoresis and release the exterior

2. disperse cold and penetrate yang

3. remove toxic substances and scatter blockage

Indications: 1. exterior wind-cold syndrome

2. diarrhea and abdominal pain due to overabundance of yin, deficiency of yang, and blockage of yang qi

3. wrap it in cloth and apply it to the skin below the navel after it is fried. It can treat qi stagnation by cold, cold-pain of the abdomen, or difficult urine resulting form hypofunction of the urinary bladder

Dosage: 3～9g.

Contraindication: Do not take it with Honey (蜂蜜, Fengmi).

Combinations: 1. add Prepared Soybean(淡豆豉, Dandouchi)——fever and chills, absence sweating during the initial stage of the exterior syndrome

2. add Fresh Ginger(生姜, Shengjiang)——intolerable headache caused by invasion by cold

3. add Chinese Date (大枣, Dazao)——cholera, irritability, inability to sleep soundly

4. add human milk——urine retention in newborn

5. add Olibanum, Frankincense(乳香, Ruxiang)——swelling and pain of the penis, pound all drugs into paste and apply topically to the penis.

6. add Tumeric Root-tuber (郁金, Yujin)——hematuria

7. add Prepared Daughter Root of Common Monkshood(附子, Fuzi), Dried Ginger(干姜, Ganjiang)——abdominal pain, diarrhea and dysentery, indistinct pulse

8. add Chinese Angelica Root(当归, Danggui)——externally used for sores, carbuncles and boils, which need to drain.

Prescription: Decoction of Fistular Onion Stalk and Prepared Soybean (葱豉汤, Congchi Tang)

Notes: Fistular Onion Stalk(葱白, Congbai) is pungent and warm. It can disperse pathogenic factors in the upper body and remove obstructions in the lower body. It can also dispel cold to relieve exterior syndrome and activate interior yang to stop pain. Thus it acts on both the interior and exterior of the body. It can be taken orally or applied externally. It can expel the poison of fish, crabs and earthworm.

The volatile oil of Fistular Onion Stalk (葱白, Congbai) can inhibit corynebacterium diphtheriae, bacillus tuberculosis, Bacillus dysenteria, staphylococcus, streptococcus and skin fungus. It also has the functions of dysphoresis and relieving exterior syndrome, promoting diuresis, invigorating the stomach and eliminating phlegm.

Both Fistular Onion Stalk (葱白, Congbai) and Cassia Twig(桂枝, Guizhi) are pungent and warm, they can disperse pathogenic factors and remove obstructions. The differences between them are as follows: Cassia Twig (桂枝, Guizhi) promotes the flowing of qi and blood and warms yang qi. It is usually applied to cases due to deficiency of yang qi, water and phlegm retention, and stagnated cold in meridian and obstruction in meridian and collaterals. Fistular Onion Stalk (葱白, Congbai) can only activate yang and is usually applied to Daiyang (戴阳) or Geyang (格阳) syndrome manifested as a red face, abdominal pain, diarrhea and weak pulse due to failure of yang qi to circulate in the body smoothly.

Section 2
Drugs of Pungent Taste and Cool Nature for Relieving the Exterior Syndromes

1. 薄荷, Bohe

English name: Wild Mint

Pharmaceutical name: Herba Menthae

Botanical name: Mentha haplocalyx Briq. Or M. Arvensis L.

Properties and tastes: pungent, cool

薄 荷

Meridian tropism: lung, liver

Functions: 1. disperse wind-heat

2. clear the head and eyes
3. benefit the throat
4. encourage rashes to come to the surface
5. smooth liver qi to alleviate mental depression (allow constrained liver qi to flow freely)
6. bacteriostatic, anti-virus
7. relieve spasm of gastrointestinal smooth muscle
8. externally used for alleviating pain and itching

Indications: 1. wind-heat syndrome and early stage of warm-febrile disease, manifested as headache, fever, slight aversion to wind

2. headache, conjunctival congestion, swelling and pain of the throat due to upward disturbance of wind heat
3. early stage of measles, measles without adequate eruption
4. constrained liver qi with such symptoms as pressure in the chest and distending pain in hypochondrium

Dosage: 3 ~ 6g. Proper amount for external use.

Contraindication: It is not advisable for patients with spontaneous perspiration due to exterior deficiency and those breast feeding women, for this drug has the side effect of arresting milk.

Combinations: 1. add Fineleaf Schizomepeta Herb (荆芥, Jingjie), Weeping Forsythia Capsule (连翘, Lianqiao)——common cold of wind heat type

2. add Chrysanthemum Flower (菊花, Juhua), Mulberry Leaf (桑叶, Sangye)——upward disturbance of wind heat leading to a headache, redness in the eyes
3. add Balloonflower Root (桔梗, Jiegeng), Silkworm with Batrytis Larva (白僵蚕, Baijiangcan)——swelling and pain of the throat due to upward disturbance of wind heat
4. add Cicada Slough (蝉蜕, Chantui), Great Burdock Achene (牛蒡子, Niubangzi)——

measles without adequate eruption

5. add White Peony Root(白芍药, Baishaoyao), Chinese Thorowax Root(柴胡,Chaihu)——stagnation of liver qi(constrained Liver qi)

6. add Common Selfheal Fruit-spike(夏枯草,Xiakucao)——conjunctivitis due to heat in the liver and lymphoid tuberculosis

7. add Silkworm with Batrytis Larva(白僵蚕, Baijiangcan), Scorpion(全蝎, Quanxie)——infantile convulsion and rebella itching

8. add White Mulberry Root-bark(桑白皮, Sangbaipi)——cough due to lung heat

9. add Gambirplant Hooked Stem and Branch(钩藤,Gouteng)——wind-heat type of common cold or early stages of febrile disease, fever and chills, absence of sweating, headache, vertigo, and morbid night crying

Prescriptions: 1. Powder of Lonicerae and Forsythiae(银翘散,Yinqiao San)

2. Decoction of Folium Mori and Flos Chrysanthemi(桑菊饮,Sangju Ying)

Notes: Wild Mint(薄荷,Bohe) a taste spicy, smells fragrant, and has the properties of slightly cold and penetrating. It may pierce through the layers of the bones, tendons, flesh, and skin and may remove blockage in the viscera and meridian system. It is commonly selected for use in febrile diseases without respiration thanks to its effect of promoting cool sweating. When used in a low dosage, it is also suitable for noninfectious diseases, such as pains from the stagnancy of liver-gallbladder or qi or fire and convulsion from liver-wind. This herb is also effective in the treatment of the disorders from wind, fire, or heat-stagnancy. The symptoms usually include headache, opthalmalgia(pain in the eyes), rhinorrhea(free release of mucus from the nose) with turbid discharge, nasal obstruction, throat inflammation, etc. Li Shizhen said(李时珍): "Wild Mint(薄荷, Bohe) is an advisable choice for the disorders of headache(even the long-standing intermittent type), various pains involving the eyes, throat and teeth, infantile convulsion with fever, scrofula, and skin diseases."

This herb has similar functions and often goes with burdock fruit. In comparison, Wild Mint(薄荷,Bohe) is better in promoting respiration and resolving superficial syndrome, while burdock fruit is more effective in clearing away toxic heat.

2. 牛蒡子, Niubangzi

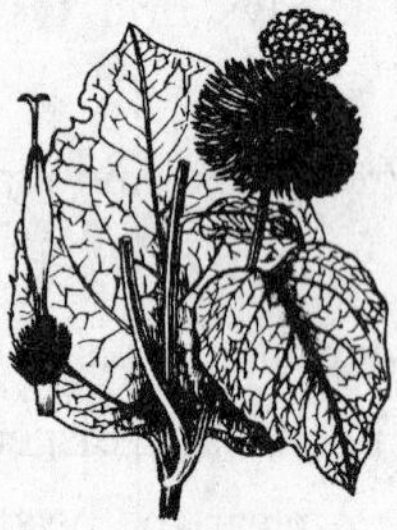

English name: Great Burdock Achene

Pharmaceutical name: Fructus Arctii Lappae

Botanical name: Fructus Arctii

Properties and tastes: pungent, bitter, cold

牛蒡子

Meridian tropism: lung, stomach

Functions: 1. disperse wind-heat

2. detoxify fire poison and relieve swelling

3. benefit the throat

4. encourage rashes to surface

Indications: 1. common cold of wind-heat type——fever in sever condition, slight aversion to cold, slight thirst, a floating and rapid pulse

2. acute pharyngitis, tonsillitis

3. cough due to wind-heat——externally contracted wind heat patterns with such symptoms as cough, sticky yellowish sputum with difficulty in expectorating

4. rebella itching, urticaria, measles

5. mumps

6. swelling of sore due to toxic heat

Dosage: 6~12g.

Contraindication: Contraindicated in patients with diarrhea due to qi deficiency, as this herb has the function of moistening the intestines.

Combinations: 1. add Fineleaf Schizomepeta Herb (荆芥穗, Jingjieshui)——common cold of wind-heat type

2. add Weeping Forsythia Capsule (连翘, Lianqiao)——swelling and pain of the throat, presence of ulcer in the mouth and tongue

3. add Common Ducksmeat Herb (浮萍, Fuping)——rebella itching

4. add Balloonflower Root (桔梗, Jiegeng)——cough due to wind-heat evil

5. add Shunk Bugbane Rhizome (升麻, Shengma)——mumps

6. add Indian Chrysanthemum Flower (野菊花, Yejuhua)——toxic heat, sore and swelling

7. add Rhizome or Root of Forbes Notopterygium (羌活, Qianghuo), Membranous Milkvetch Root (黄芪, Huangqi)——fever and migratory arthralgia of wind-heat type, redness, swelling and numbness in the fingers

8. add Common Yam Rhizome (山药, Shanyao)——cough lasting for a long time

Prescription: Universal Relief Decoction for Disinfection (普济消毒饮, Pujixiaodu Yin)

Notes: Great Burdock Achene (牛蒡子, Niubangzi) is quite effective in treatment of throat inflammation. When used in acute cases, it combines with Honeysuckle Flower (金银花, Jinyinhua) and Weeping Forsythia Capsule (连翘, Lianqiao), and with Figwort Root (玄参, Xuanshen) and Sichuan Tendrilleaf Fritillary Bulb (川贝母, Chuanbeimu) in chronic cases. It is described in *Herbals for Easy Approaching* (《本草便读》, Bencaobiandu) that Great Burdock Achene (牛蒡子, Niubangzi) is suitable for the lung diseases, and also effective for liver disorders. It has various functions of dispersing, humidifying, and descending. In treatment of the diseases related to lungs, ranging from sore throat to smallpox, this herb is an excellent choice. Furthermore, Great Burdock Achene (牛蒡子, Niubangzi) is capable of clearing away toxic heat and promoting the eruption of measles. Therefore, for the early febrile diseases due to wind-heat, this herb is always selected. Recent research has shown that, this herb has a powerful antibacterial effect and a function in reducing blood sugar.

3. 蝉蜕, Chantu

English name: Cicada Slough

Pharmaceutical name: Periostracum Cicadae

Botanical name: Cryptotympana pustulata Fabricius

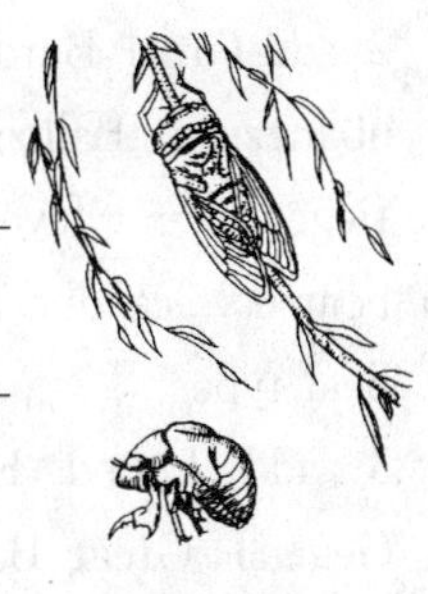
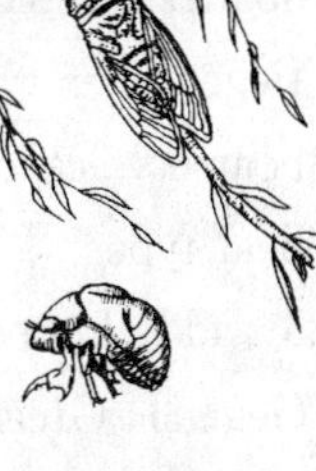

蝉 蜕

Properties and tastes: sweet, cold

Meridian tropism: lung, liver

Functions: 1. disperse wind and clear heat

2. detoxify poison and encourage rashes to surface

3. clear away the heat to benefit the throat

4. dissipate blockage to promote subsidence of swelling

5. disperse wind evil to alleviate itching

6. anticonvulsion

7. tranquilization

Indications: 1. common cold of wind-heat type or early stage of warm febrile disease——fever, headache, pain of the throat, hoarse voice

2. early stages of measles——fever, measles without adequate eruption

3. rubella——skin itching

4. wind heat evils in liver channel——conjunctival congestion, nebula, profuse gum of the eyes, vertigo and blurred vision

5. morbid night crying

6. tetanus

7. infantile convulsion

Dosage: 3～9g.

Contraindication: Use with caution for women during pregnancy.

Combinations: 1. add Chrysanthemum Flower (菊花, Juhua)——externally contracted wind heat patterns and early stage of warm febrile disease, manifested as fever and headache

2. add Great Burdock Achene (牛蒡子, Niubangzi), Balloonflower Root (桔梗, Jiegeng)——fever, pain of the throat, hoarse voice due to common cold of wind-heat type

3. add Lobed Kudzuvine Root (葛根, Gegen), Great Burdock Achene (牛蒡子, Niubangzi)——early stage of measles, incomplete manifestation of measles

4. add Puncturevine Caltrap Fruit (白蒺藜, Baijili), Fineleaf Schizomepeta Herb (荆芥, Jingjie)——rubella itching

5. add Chrysanthemum Flower (菊花, Juhua), Common Scouring Rush Herb (木贼, Muzei)——conjunctival congestion, nebula profuse gum of the eyes

6. add Scorpion (全蝎, Quanxie), Silkworm with Batrytis Larva (白僵蚕, Baijiangcan), Gambirplant Hooked Stem and Branch (钩藤, Gouteng)——tetanus, infantile convulsion and morbid night crying

7. add Gypsum (生石膏, Shengshigao)——facial paralysis (Cicada Slough (蝉蜕, Chantui) 3 pieces, Gypsum (生石膏, Shengshigao) of 3g, grind them into powder, and take it with Shaoxing wine before sleep

8. add Wild Mint (薄荷, Bohe)——cutaneous pruritus, urticaria

Notes: Cicada Slough (蝉蜕, Chantui) is light and cold in property with the main functions of dispersing lung-heat and calming liver-wind by cooling. It is thus suitable for the treatment of superficial heat syndrome and liver heat syndrome complicated by evil wind. It is said in *Herbals for Easy Approaching* (《本草便读》, Bencaobiandu), Cicada Slough (蝉蜕, Chantui) is especially effective in the treatment of the superficial wind-heat syndromes and the diseases of the upper part, including those of the head, eyes, teeth and gum, and in promoting eruption of measles. This drug has several records of treating difficult labor in *Transaction of Famous Physicians* (《名医别录》, Mingyibielu). It should be used cautiously for pregnant women.

According to recent research, Cicada Slough (蝉蜕, Chantui) has the functions of tranquilizing, abating tension of striated muscle, reducing reflex activities, and blocking ganglions.

4. 淡豆豉, Dandouchi

English name: Prepared Soybean

Pharmaceutical name: Semen Sojae Praeparatum

Botanical name: Glycine max (L.) Merr.

Properties and tastes: pungent, sweet, slightly

bitter and cold

Meridian tropism: lung, stomach

Functions: 1. disperse the external evil from the body surface

2. clear away heat and alleviate irritability

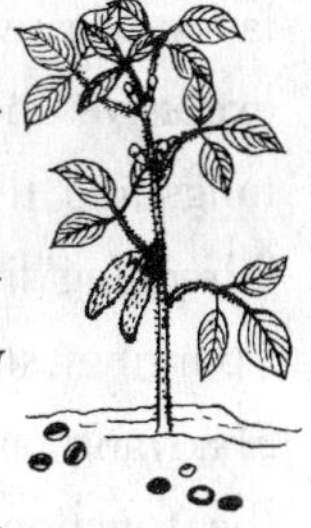

淡豆豉

Indications: 1. used for both heat and cold exterior syndrome patterns-fever, aversion to wind and cold, headache, etc.

2. chest congestion and restlessness, insomnia as sequelae of febrile disease

Dosage: 9～15g (the earliest stage of externally contracted wind cold)

Combinations: 1. add Fistular Onion Stalk (葱白, Congbai)——a mild case of affection by wind-cold exopathogen

2. add Wild Mint (薄荷, Bohe), Great Burdock Achene (牛蒡子, Niubangzi)——common cold of wind-heat type

3. add Cape Jasmine Fruit (栀子, Zhizi)——chest congestion, restlessness, insomnia in the early stage or late stage of febrile disease

Prescriptions: 1. Decoction of Fistular Onion Stalk and Prepared Soybean (葱豉汤, Congchi Tang)

2. Decoction of Capejasmine and Fermented Soybean (栀子豉汤, Zhizichi Tang)

Notes: Prepared Soybean (淡豆豉, Dandouchi) has properties of dispersing and lifting and also distributing in the lungs and the stomach. The effects include dispersing evil-stagnancy in both superficial and deep layers, removing moldy stagnancy from the chest. In treatment of the early febrile diseases from wind-cold or wind-heat, this drug is commonly used accompanied by other superficial syndrome-resolving herbs. It is also given for sorts of epidemic with internal evil stagnancy, which leads to the complication of internal-external syndromes. This drug is made of mature zymotic soybeans with the auxiliary materials of mulberry leaves and fresh sweet wormwood or with those of Perilla Leaf (苏叶, Suye) and Ephedra (麻黄, Mahuang). Its property turns slightly cold when combined with the first pair of herbs, and warm when used with the second pair. Attention should be paid to this difference.

5. 桑叶, Sangye

English name: Mulberry Leaf

Pharmaceutical name: Folium MoriAlbae

Botanical name: Morus alba L.

Properties and tastes: bitter, sweet and cold

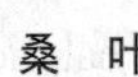

桑 叶

Meridian tropism: lung, liver

Functions: 1. expel wind and clear heat from the lungs

2. clear the liver and the eyes

3. remove heat from blood to arrest bleeding

4. bacteriostatic

5. lower blood pressure, reduce blood lipids

Indications: 1. externally contracted wind heat——fever, dizziness and headache, cough, pain and swelling of the throat

2. conjunctivitis with redness, swelling and pain of the eyes, profuse tears due to excessive heat or wind-heat in the liver meridian

3. mild cases of bleeding due to heat in the blood

Dosage: 6 ～ 12g. When decocted in water it can be used for washing eyes to treat diseases of the eye.

Combinations: 1. add Chrysanthemum Flower

(菊花, Juhua)——common cold of wind-heat type and early stage of wind-warm syndrome. It can also treat dizziness, headache, conjunctivitis congestion due to ascending of liver yang

2. add Chinese Wolfberry Root-bark(地骨皮,Digupi), Licorice Root(甘草, Shengancao)——cough due to lung heat

3. add Chrysanthemum Flower(菊花, Juhua), Cassia Seed(决明子, Juemingzi)——conjunctivitis

4. add Apricot Seed(杏仁, Xingren), Coastal Glehnia Root, and Fourleaf Ladybell Root(沙参, Shashen)——impairment of lung yin due to dry-heat, cough and dry throat

5. add Black Sesame(黑芝麻, Heizhima)——failing of eyesight and blurred vision due to deficiency of liver yin. They can also be used to treat premature greying of hair, baldness, etc.

6. add Barbary Wolfberry Fruit(枸杞子, Gouqizi), Cassia Seed(决明子, Juemingzi)——vertigo, dizziness, blurred vision

7. add Areca Pee(大腹皮, Dafupi), Tangerine Peel(陈皮, Chenpi)——edema and scanty urination

8. add Mulberry Twig(桑枝, Sangzhi)——wind-damp-heat arthritis, contracture of four limbs and rebulla itching due to wind heat

Prescriptions: 1. Decoction of Folium Mori and Flos Chrysanthemi(桑菊饮, Sangju Ying)

2. Decoction for Relieving Dryness of the Lungs(清燥救肺汤, Qingzaojiufei Tang)

Notes: Mulberry Leaf(桑叶, Sangye) is commonly used for superficial syndrome due to wind-heat, owing to its properties of lifting, cooling, clearing and dispersing as well as the function of clearing and scattering wind-heat evil in both the lungs and superficial layer. Meanwhile, its usage in treatment of excessive heat syndromes involving the lungs and the liver is due to the effects of "dredging liver-collateral of wind evil" and 'purging stagnant qi and fire from the Shaoyang area'. Furthermore, because of the functions of clearing heat from blood and arresting bleeding, it is also used in slight cases of hematemesis from blood heat. Described by Zhang Bingcheng(张秉成), "wind-heat diseases, ranging from the eye diseases to protracted headache, are all indications of Mulberry Leaf(桑叶, Sangye)." In addition, Li Shizhen(李时珍) wrote that, Mulberry Leaf(桑叶, Sangye) have an effect of relieving unquenchable thirst, if boiled and taken as beverage. Having same distribution of the lungs and liver and same functions of dispersing wind-heat and clearing-purging the lungs and liver, Mulberry Leaf(桑叶, Sangye) and Chrysanthemum Flower(菊花, Juhua) are generally used together for febrile diseases from wind-heat, fever, headache, conjunctival congestion and ophthalmalgia. In comparison, Mulberry Leaf(桑叶, Sangye) is used for lung injury from dryness-heat with cough but not phlegm because of the superior functions of clearing away lung-heat. As it is more effective in calming and clearing heat from liver and nourishing liver-yin, rather than Mulberry Leaf(桑叶, Sangye). Chrysanthemum Flower(菊花, Juhua) is used for abnormally up-flowing of liver-yang or liver-fire, and liver-yin deficiency manifested as vertigo, conjunctival congestion, nebula and hypopsia.

6. 菊花, Juhua

English name: Chrysanthemum Flower

Pharmaceutical name: Flos Chrysanthemi Morifolii

Botanical name: Chrysanthemum morifolium Ramat.

Properties and tastes: pungent, sweet, bitter and slightly cold

菊 花

Meridian tropism: lung, liver

Functions: 1. disperse wind and clear heat

2. clear away the heat and disperse wind

3. clear away liver heat and brighten the eyes

4. calm the liver to stop the wind

5. bacteriostatic, anti-inflammation

6. increase volume of blood flow of coronary artery

7. increase oxygen consumption of heart

8. reduce blood pressure

Indications: 1. externally contracted wind heat and early stage of warm-febrile disease-headache, fever, and dizziness (usually found in flu)

2. wind-heat in the liver channel or upward disturbance of liver fire——conjunctivitis

3. hypertention——dizziness, blurred vision, headache, and distention in the head due to hyperactivity of liver yang

4. furuncles

Dosage: 9～15g.

Contraindication: Use cautiously for patients with stomachache due to deficiency of qi or poor appetites, and diarrhea with loose stools.

Combinations: 1. add Szechwan Lovage Rhizome (川芎, Chuanxiong)——headache due to wind-heat stagnation of blood

2. add Barbary Wolfberry Fruit (枸杞子, Gouqizi)——vertigo and blurred vision due to deficiency of liver and kidney

3. add Tall Gastrodia Rhizome (天麻, Tianma)——headache and vertigo due to upward disturbance of liver yang and infantile colon convulsion due to liver wind moving internally

4. add Honeysuckle Flower (金银花, Jinyinhua)——furuncles

5. add Silkworm with Batrytis Larva (白僵蚕, Baijiangcan)——rubella itching

6. add Cicada Slough (蝉蜕, Chantui)——nebula after disease

7. add Common Selfheal Fruit-spike (夏枯草, Xiakucao)——conjunctivitis

8. add Honeysuckle Flower (金银花, Jinyinhua), Mulberry Leaf (桑叶, Sangye)——hypertention manifisted as evident vertigo

9. add Honeysuckle Flower (金银花, Jinyinhua), Hawthorn Fruit (山楂, Shanzha)——patients with arteriosclerosis, hyperlipidemia

10. add Baikal Skullcap Root (黄芩, Huangqin), Cape Jasmine Fruit (栀子, Zhizi)——irritability caused by excessive heat evils

Prescriptions: 1. Decoction of Folium Mori and Flos Chrysanthemi (桑菊饮, Sangju Yin)

2. Bolus of Fruit Lycii, Flos Chrysanthemi and Radix Rehmanniae (杞菊地黄丸, Qijudihuang Wan)

Notes: *Hundred Herbs Selected from the Shennong's Herbal Classic* (《神农本草经百种录》, Shennongbencaojingbaizhonglu) says: "Most fragrant herbs are capable of treating diseases involving the head, eyes and superficial layer but are all spicy and drying. Chrysanthemum Flower (菊花, Juhua) is neither dry nor strong, hence especially suitable for the cases from evil wind or fire."

Several different sorts of this herb include yellow, white and wild Chrysanthemum Flowers(菊花,Juhua), which share the functions of dispersing wind-heat, calming the liver to improve eyesight, and eliminating toxic heat. Bitter in taste, the yellow ones have a special function of purging heat; therefore, it is generally used to disperse wind-heat. Having a sweet taste, the white ones are less effective in eliminating heat but more in calming the liver to improve eyesight. The taste of the wild ones is extremely bitter. They are usually used for furuncle and pyogenic infections because of its capability of removing toxic heat.

7. 蔓荆子, Manjingzi

English name: Shrub Chastetree Fruit

Pharmaceutical name: Fructus Viticis

Botanical name: Vitex rolundifolia L. Or. V. Trifolia L.

蔓荆子

Properties and tastes: pungent, bitter and cool

Meridian tropism: liver, stomach, urinary bladder

Functions: 1. disperse wind and clear heat

2. clear and benefit the head and eyes

3. expel wind to relieve pain

Indications: 1. headache, dizziness, migraine for caused by wind heat

2. blurred vision, conjunctivitis, excessive tearing due to upward disturbance of wind heat

3. pain and stiffness of limbs due to wind damp painful obstruction

Dosage: 6～12g.

Contraindication: Do not use for patients with yin deficiency and excessive fire.

Combinations: 1. add Weeping Forsythia Capsule(连翘, Lianqiao)——headache due to wind-fire, epidemic hemorrhagic conjunctivitis

2. add Chrysanthemum Flower(菊花, Juhua)——headache and dizziness due to upward disturbance of wind heat

3. add Szechwan Lovage Rhizome(川芎, Chuanxiong)——headache and pain of the general body

4. add Divaricate Saposhnikovia Root(防风, Fangfeng)——externally contracted headache and pain of the general body, back and shoulder resulting from wind dampness

5. add Dang-shen Root(党参, Dangshen), Membranous Milkvetch Root(黄芪, Huangqi)——deafness and dizziness due to insufficiency of qi in the middl-jiao and failure of lucid yang to ascend

6. add Common Selfheal Fruit-spike(夏枯草, Xiakucao), Gambirplant Hooked Stem and Branch(钩藤, Gouteng)——headache and dizziness due to liver wind moving internally

7. add Fineleaf Schizomepeta Herb(荆芥, Jingjie), Puncturevine Caltrap Fruit(白蒺藜, Baijili)——chronic headache

8. add Membranous Milkvetch Root(黄芪, Huangqi), Chinese Corktree Bark(黄柏, Huangbai), White Peony Root(白芍药, Baishaoyao)——cataract

Notes: Shrub Chastetree Fruit(蔓荆子, Manjingzi) is frequently used for acute and chronic headaches in different forms. Crude drug is more effective in dispersing wind-heat, resolving superficial syndrome and alleviating pain. Therefore, it is suitable for headaches due to exterior evils. Parched herb is more effective in clearing away heat from the head and eye, used in headaches and migraine, blurred vision and epiphora. Described by Li Shizhen(李时珍),"Shrub Chastetree Fruit(蔓荆子, Manjingzi) is spicy in taste, clear in smell and light, floating, ascending, and dispersing in property. As a consequence, its indications revolve around wind-relaxation syndromes of the head."

8. 葛根, Gegen

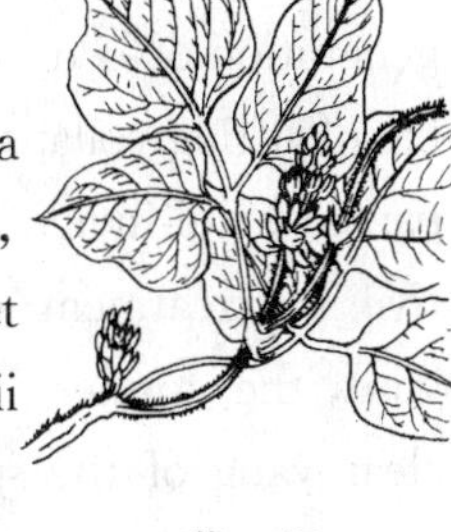

葛 根

English name: Lobed Kudzuvine Root

Botanical name: Pueraria lobota (Willd) ohwi., P. Omeiensis Wang et Tang, or P. Thomsanii Benth.

Properties and tastes: sweet, pungent and cool

Meridian tropism: spleen, stomach

Functions: 1. reduce fever
2. encourage the rash of measles to surface
3. control diarrhea
4. relieve spasm
5. invigorate vital function and promote the production of body fluid
6. reduce blood pressure
7. relieve CHD and AP(coronary heart disease and angina pectoris)
8. improve cerebral circulation

Indications: 1. exopathic heat syndrome——fever, headache, stiffness and pain of the neck and back due to evil heat invading the exterior
2. early stage of measles——fever, aversion to cold, measles without adequate eruption, which belong to wind heat stagnation in the exterior
3. damp heat diarrhea or dysentery with exterior syndrome——fever, aversion to cold, stool with foul smell, yellowish greasy tongue coating, which belong to unrelieved exterior and interior syndrome
4. early abrupt onset deafness
5. hypertensive encephalopathy——stiffness and pain of neck, headache, dizziness, tinnitus, numbness of limbs
6. intoxicated person who cannot awaken
7. CHD and AP
8. diabetes mellitus thirst and wasting syndrome, and thirst of febrile disease

Dosage: 9~15g.

Contraindication: Use cautiously for patients with yin deficiency and excessive fire, or upper excessive and lower deficiency.

Combinations: 1. add Chinese Thorowax Root (柴胡, Chaihu)——exterior syndrome of wind-heat, fever, stiffness and pain of the neck, headache
2. add Shunk Bugbane Rhizome (升麻, Shengma), Wild Mint (薄荷, Bohe)——headache due to wind-heat, measles without adequate eruption, conjunctivitis
3. add Coptis Rhizome(黄连, Huanglian), Baikal Skullcap Root(黄芩, Huangqin)——fever and aversion to cold, sweating and asthma, diarrhea with foul smelling stools
4. add Largehead Atractylodes Rhizome(白术, Baizhu)——poor appetite, loose stools, lack of fluid and dry throat due to deficiency of spleen qi and qi in Middle-jiao collapse
5. add Dwarf Lilyturf Root (麦门冬, Maimendong), Rehmannia Dried Root (生地黄, Shengdihuang)——wasting and thirsting syndrome, thirst and excessive drinking(diabetes)
6. add Medicated Leaven (神曲, Shenqu)——drunk, headache, vertigo, irritability and thirst, vomiting

Prescriptions: 1. Bupleurum and Pueraria Decoction for Dispelling Pathogenic Factors from Superficial Muscle (柴葛解肌汤, Chaigejieji Tang)

2. Decoction of Puerariae, Scutellariae and Coptidis (葛根黄芩黄连汤, Gegen Huangqin Huanglian Tang)

Notes: Lobed Kudzuvine Root (葛根, Gegen) usually acts on the spleen and the stomach. Its functions are to promote generation of body fluid and to activate and lift stomach qi. When used to quench thirst, it is the best type where fluids fail to ascend. Its other functions, such as dispelling evils from the superficial layers, reducing fever, lifting yang to promote eruption for measles are utilized in treatment of measles without adequate eruption, fever, headache with protracted superficial syndrome. Being able to lift qi of the spleen and stomach, the herb is also used for chronic diarrhea or dysentery. In treatment of cases with heat in both superficial and deep layers, crude herb is generally used, while baked ones used for the type of qi-collapse from spleen deficiency. After it is baked, the herb can no longer disperse in property and usually functions in the intestines instead of the stomach, which means it acts on the interior layer instead of the exterior layer of Yangming area. Li Gao (李杲) entitled the herb as "a great herb to treat diarrhea due to spleen-stomach deficiency".

As it is proved in some modern research, Lobed Kudzuvine Root (葛根, Gegen) has the functions as follows: to reduce fever, lower blood pressure, improve blood circulation of brain and coronary artery, relieve spasm of smooth muscle of the gastrointestinal tract, and to reduce blood sugar. The function of improving blood circulation is generally used to treat spasm (of muscles over the head and back of the neck) accompanying fever, hypertension, early sudden deafness, and coronary heart disease.

Lobed Kudzuvine Roots (葛根, Gegen) are similar to each other in properties of being light, ascending, clear, and dispersing and are usually used together to resolve superficial syndrome and reduce fever. However, the latter is effective in resolving liver-qi stagnancy, but has no effect on improving generation of body fluid. Besides, it is capable of lifting collapsed yang qi while accompanied by qi-invigorating drugs, and is effective in treatment of visceroptosis. Otherwise, the former has functions of lifting clear yang of the spleen and the stomach, improving generation of body fluid and quenching thirst and can be used for diarrhea.

9. 柴胡, Chaihu

English name: Chinese Thorowax Root

Pharmaceutical name: Radix Bupleuri

Botanical name: Bupleurum scorzoneraefolium Wild. Or B. Chinense D.C.

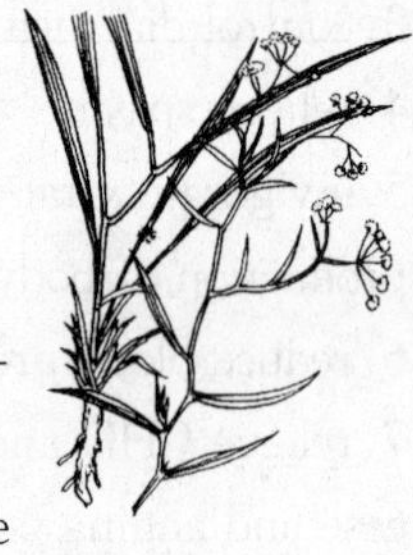
柴胡

Properties and tastes: pungent, bitter and slightly cold

Meridian tropism: liver, pericardium, san-jiao, gall bladder

Functions: 1. reduce fever, dispersing

2. relax constrained liver qi and alleviate mental depression

3. raise the yang qi

4. regulate the flow of qi to relieve pain

5. tranquilize the mind, stop coughing
6. anti-inflammation, anti-influenza, anti-mycobacterium, tuberculosis
7. reduce plasma cholesterol
8. prevent fatty liver, regulate function of the gallbladder, reduce transaminase
9. strengthen body immunity

Indications: 1. Shaoyang heat syndrome——alternating chills and fever, a sensation of constriction in the chest, vertigo, dizziness due to pathogenic changes located in the part between exterior and interior
2. wind cold exterior syndrome——fever and slight aversion to cold, general pain of the body, sore throat, a floating and rapid pulse
3. stagnation of liver qi——distention and fullness in the chest and hypochondrium, irregular menstruation due to qi stagnation and failure in flowing
4. sinking of qi due to qi deficiency——shortness of breath, fatigue, organs prolapse belonging to qi deficiency and inability to lift

Dosage: 3～9g.

Contraindication: Contraindicated in cases of tidal fever due to yin deficiency and liver-fire ascending to the upper portions of the body.

Combinations: 1. add Baikal Skullcap Root(黄芩, Huangqin)——alternating chills and fever, pathogenic changes located in the part between exterior and interior
2. add Nutgrass Galingale Rhizome(香附, Xiangfu), Green Tangerine Peel(青皮, Qingpi)——dysmenorrhea, hypochondriac pain due to contrained of liver qi
3. add Membranous Milkvetch Root(黄芪, Huangqi), Bitter Orange(枳壳, Zhiqiao)——gastroptosis and hysteroptosis
4. add Antifebrile Dichroa Root(常山, Changshan)——malaria
5. add Lobed Kudzuvine Root(葛根, Gegen)——fever due to pathogenic factors in the exterior
6. add Weeping Forsythia Capsule(连翘, Lianqiao), Capillary Wormwood Herb(茵陈蒿, Yinchenhao)——acute hepatitis
7. add Rhubarb(大黄, Dahuang)——cholecysitis, acute pancreatitis
8. add White Peony Root(白芍药, Baishaoyao)——stomachache due to attack on the stomach by liver qi

Prescriptions: 1. Minor Decoction of Bupleurum(小柴胡汤, Xiaochaihu Tang)
2. Xiaoyao Powder(逍遥散, Xiaoyao San)
3. Decoction for Strengthening Middle-jiao and Benefiting Vital Energy(补中益气汤, Buzhongyiqi Tang)
4. Powder for Treating Cold Limbs(四逆散, Sini San)

Notes: Chinese Thorowax Root(柴胡, Chaihu) is an effective herb to harmonize functions of the Shaoyang system and can reduce fever of febrile diseases even if it is used solely. It acts on the liver, therefore, it is the first choice for relieving depressed liver in clinic. It leads to the effects of relieving depression, regulating menstruation, and smoothing qi-circulation in different combinations. Li Shizhen(李时珍) said: "Chinese Thorowax Root(柴胡, Chaihu) is chosen when one wants to lead clear qi or to reduce fever." When the herb is taken for a long term, its shortcoming of having a drying property will result in an injury of yin.

Chinese Thorowax Root(柴胡, Chaihu) is simply the most frequently used herb and used widely. In Japanese medical circles, pharmaceutics are used very frequently, too.

Some modern research showed that, the herb has an antiviral effect. Therefore, pharmaceutics of bupleurum root is commonly selected to suppress the hepatitis virus, influenza virus, and mumps virus. Furthermore, the herb has antipyretic, anti-inflammatory, and antibiotic functions, which are utilized to cure or relieve various types of high fever or pains. Its liver-yin damaging shortcoming was described in ancient time, it is prohibited in the syndrome of flaring-up of yang from yin-deficiency. However, if the dose is not large, and used in combination with large amount of yin-nourishing herbs, such as White Peony Root(白芍药, Baishaoyao), the herb may be used in this kind of cases. It is advisable to give Chinese Thorowax Root(柴胡, Chaihu) with qi-reinforcing drugs in treatment of qi-collapse syndrome of deficient type. Meanwhile, it is forbidden in conditions of qi-exhaustion(e.g. Shock) due to its property of being dispersing and consumptive. A large dose of this drug will result in vomiting, which may be relieved by Pinellia Rhizome (半夏, Banxia) and Fresh Ginge (生姜, Shengjiang).

Chinese Thorowax Root(柴胡, Chaihu) and Lobed Kudzuvine Root(葛根, Gegen) share the effects of dispersing superficial evils, lifting yang-qi and resolving qi-depression. They, hence, also share the indications such as superficial heat syndrome, qi-collapse syndrome, and liver spleen qi-stagnancy. However, the former is effective in resolving evil of the Shaoyang system(boundary between the exterior and the interior layers) and in treating the syndrome manifested as cycling of fever and chill. The latter is slightly cold in property and effective in reducing superficial wind-heat or toxic heat of the Yangming system. In its yang-lifting function, the former is characterized by elevating the liver-yang, while the latter by elevating spleen-yang. In the aspect of dissolving qi depression or stagnancy, they have the same interrelationship. As a sequence, in treatment of the qi stagnancy syndrome involving the liver and spleen, the two may be used together.

10. 升麻, Shengma

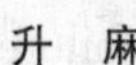

升 麻

English name: Shunk Bugbane Rhizome

Pharmaceutical name: Rhizomn Cimicifugae

Botanical name: Cimicifuga foetida L. Or C. Dahurica (Turcz.) or C. Heracleifoliz Kom.

Properties and tastes: pungent, sweet and slightly cold

Meridian tropism: lung, spleen, large intestine, and stomach

Functions: 1. disperse wind and encourage the rash of measles to surface

2. clear away heat and detoxify fire poison

3. elevate yang to ascend sinking of Middle-jiao qi

Indications: 1. headache in the places related to yangming meridian, marked by headache in the forehead

2. flaming up of stomach-fire, swelling and pain of tooth and gum, aphthosis, ozostomia

3. upward disturbance of wind-heat conjunctivitis

4. early stage of measles, measles without adequate eruption

5. sinking of qi in the Middle-jiao for shortness of breath, lassitude, chronic diarrhea,

anorexia, prolapse of rectum, metrorrhagia and metrostaxis due to deficiency of spleen qi and failure in restricting blood

6. warm febrile disease, skin eruptions caused by virulent heat evil

Dosage: 3~9g.

Contraindication: Contraindicated in heat conditions due to yin deficiency or other syndrones when the upper is excessive and the lower is deficient.

Combinations: 1. add Dahurian Angelica Root (白芷, Baizhi)——Yangming meridian headache

2. add Coptis Rhizome (黄连, Huanglian)——swelling and pain of tooth and gum

3. add Figwort Root(玄参, Xuanshen)——conjunctivitis

4. add Lobed Kudzuvine Root (葛根, Gegen), Great Burdock Achene(牛蒡子, Niubangzi)——measles without adequate eruption

5. add Chinese Thorowax Root(柴胡, Chaihu)——sinking of qi in the Middle-jiao syndrome

Prescriptions: 1. Decoction for Strengthening Middle-jiao and Benefiting Vital Energy (补中益气汤, Buzhongyiqi Tang)

2. Powder for Clearing Away Spleen Heat (泻黄散, Xiehuang San)

Notes: Shunk Bugbane Rhizome(升麻, Shengma)'s effects generally acts on the yangming system. Its functions include regulating stomach movement, dispersing evil wind, lifting limpid spleen-stomach qi, and preventing its collapse. Another important function is to reduce toxic heat, and is commonly used to treat yang macula or toothache. Three herbs sharing the lifting effect are Shunk Bugbane Rhizome(升麻, Shengma), Chinese Thorowax Root(柴胡, Chaihu) and Lobed Kudzuvine Root(葛根, Gegen). However, the first reduces toxicant, the second relieves liver depression while the third improves generation of body fluid. Some researches have shown that Shunk Bugbane Rhizome(升麻, Shengma) has the antipyretic, anti-inflammation, antibiotic, analgesic, and anticonvulsive functions. Consequently, it is usually used for infectious diseases. Its regulating effect on smoothing muscles is applied to cure proctoptosis and hysteroptosis from deficiency of spleen qi.

Crude herb is capable of improving eruption in measles, clearing away heat and reducing toxicant, while parched drug is more effective in elevating yang-qi.

11. 浮萍, Fuping

English name: Common Ducksmeat Herb

Pharmaceutical name: Herba Lemnae seu Spirodelae

Botanical name: Spirodela polyrrhiza Schield. Or Lemna minor L.

浮 萍

Properties and tastes: pungent and cold

Meridian tropism: lung, urinary bladder

Functions: 1. induce diaphoresis to relieve exterior syndrome

2. expel the wind evil to alleviate itching

3. detoxicate to encourage rashes to surface

4. remove water to reduce swelling

Indications: 1. common cold of wind-heat type——fever and slight aversion to cold, absence of sweating

2. urticaria of wind-heat type——itching, urticaria

3. measles without adequate eruption

4. superficial edema accompanied by exterior syndrome(wind-edema syndrome)

Dosage:3～9g.

Combinations: 1. add Fineleaf Schizomepeta Herb(荆芥,Jingjie),Wild Mint(薄荷,Bohe), Weeping Forsythia Capsule (连翘, Lianqiao)——common cold of wind-heat type

2. add Wild Mint(薄荷,Bohe),Great Burdock Achene(牛蒡子,Niubangzi), Cicada Slough(蝉蜕,Chantui)——measles without adequate eruption and urticaria of wind-heat type

3. add Belvedera Fruit(地肤子,Difuzi), Densefruit Pittany Root-bark(白鲜皮, Baixianpi), Puncturevine Caltrap Fruit(白蒺藜, Baijili)——urticaria of wind-heat type

4. add Lalang Grass Rhizome(白茅根, Baimaogen),Honeysuckle Flower(金银花, Jinyinhua), Rice Bean (赤小豆, Chixiaodou)——edema,urine retention accompanied by exterior syndrome

5. add Ephedra(麻黄,Mahuang)——acute nephritis,wind-edema syndrome and rebulla itching syndrome

Notes:Common Ducksmeat Herb(浮萍,Fuping) and Ephedra(麻黄, Mahuang) both have the functions of regulating lung qi, opening sweat pores and dredging the water passages to induce sweat and eliminate dampness. This combination can be used for fever without sweat, difficulty of micturation and edema. However, Ephedra(麻黄, Mahuang)is pungent in taste and warm in property,suitable for affection of exogenous wind-cold, exterior excess syndrome with the function of arresting asthma and stopping cough. Common Ducksmeat Herb(浮萍,Fuping)is cold in property,and used for affection of exogenous wind-heat without sweat accompanied with dysuria and edema or damp-heat syndrome. It has the function of eliminating wind to arrest itching.

12. 木贼, Muzei

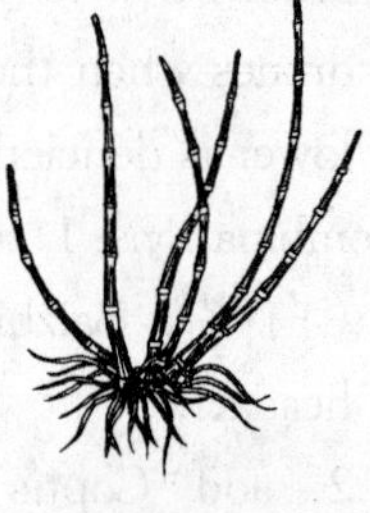

English name: Common Scouring Rush Herb

Pharmaceutical name: Herba Equiseti Hiemails

Botanical name: Equisetum hiemale L.

木 贼

Properties and tastes: sweet,bitter and medium

Meridian tropism:lung,liver

Functions:1. dispel wind-heat

2. clear eyes and remove superficial visual obstruction

3. arrest bleeding

Indications:1. redness of eyes,excessive tears, nebula due to wind-heat or liver fire and gallbladder stagnation

2. hematochezia and hemorrhoid bleeding

Dosage:3～9g.

Combinations: 1. add Cicada Slough(蝉蜕, Chantui), Baikal Skullcap Root(黄芩, Huangqin)——red eyes, profuse discharge from the eyes nebula

2. add Baikal Skullcap Root(黄芩, Huangqin), Garden Burnet Root(地榆, Diyu)——hematochezia and hemorrhoid bleeding

3. add Buerger Pipewort Flower(谷精草, Gujingcao), Pig liver(猪肝, Zhugan)——redness of eyes,superficial visual obstruction due to liver deficiency

4. add Swordlike Atractylodes Rhizome(苍术,Cangzhu),Common Selfheal Fruit-spike (夏枯草,Xiakucao)——blurred vision and

excessive tears

Notes: Common Scouring Rush Herb(木贼, Muzei), although it has the function of expelling wind-heat, it is seldom used for exterior wind-heat syndrome. It is mainly used for redness of eyes and lacrimation due to wind-heat. Common Scouring Rush Herb (木贼, Muzei) can soothe the liver and regulate the lung. It acts on the blood stage to stop bleeding. Parching Common Scouring Rush Herb (木贼, Muzei) can treat blood diseases due to pathogenic wind invading blood, or stagnation of liver blood, they may be manifested as metrohrragia and metrostaxis, hemorrhoid and dysentery due to pathogenic wind.

13. 西河柳, Xiheliu

English name: Chinese Tamarish Twig

Pharmaceutical name: Cacumen Tamaricis

Botanical name: Tamarix chinensis Lour.

Properties and tastes: pungent and medium

西河柳

Meridian tropism: lung, heart stomach

Functions: 1. induce diaphoresis and encourage rashes to surface

2. expel the wind to alleviate itching

Indications: 1. early stage of measles, incomplete appearance of measles and aggravated lay interior syndrome or due to wind cold stagnating in the exterior

2. itching rubella

3. wind-damp arthritis syndrome

Dosage: 3～9g.

Contraindication: Not to be taken by patients with fully erupted measles, In addition, too large dose can cause irritability.

Combinations: 1. add Bamboo leaf (竹叶, Zhuye), Great Burdock Achene (牛蒡子, Niubangzi)——the early stage of measles, measles without adequate eruption, or measles toxin entering into the interior or itching rubella

2. add Largeleaf Gentian Root (秦艽, Qinjiao), Divaricate Saposhnikovia Root (防风, Fangfeng)——wind-damp arthritis syndrome

Notes: Effects of Chinese Tamarish Twig (西河柳, Xiheliu) largely focus on lifting, expelling and penetrating, which enables it to promote eruption of rashes and release toxic heat. As proved in some modern research, this drug promotes perspiration and reduces fever by influencing the heat regulating center of the brain and dilating superficial vessels.

Chapter 2 Purgatives

Definition: Purgatives are herbs that can cause diarrhea, lubricate the large intestine and induce bowel movement.

Functions: Purgatives can induce bowel movement, remove food and water retention and poisonous materials. They may expel pathogenic heat, promote blood circulation, expel toxic substance, etc.

Indications: They are used for interior excessive syndromes, such as constipation, food retention in the intestines, excessive heat accumulated in the interior, edema and phlegm retention and so on.

Some of these herbs have the functions of clearing heat and expelling fire. Thus they may be used for febrile diseases due to invasion of exterior pathogenic factors, manifested as high fever, unconsciousness, delirium and mania. They can also be used in cases of headache, red eyes, sore throat, swelling and pain of the gum, hemoptysis, apostaxis and so on caused by ascending of pathogenic heat and fire. These herbs are bitter and cold and have a purgative function. Thus whether there is constipation or not, they can be used in order to purge pathogenic heat and expel heat, similar to taking away the firewood from under the cauldron. In the light of the theories, which include"the functions of six fu organs based on no obstruction" and"no obstruction no pain", the purgatives together with the herbs for clearing heat and expelling toxic substance, can be used for promoting blood circulation to remove blood stasis and acute abdomen diseases.

Classification: Purgatives are usually classified into three categories including potent purgatives, lubricant purgatives and drastic purgatives. The functions of potent and drastic purgatives are stronger than that of lubricant ones, especially drastic purgatives. Lubricant purgatives can moisten the intestines and they have a mild action.

Notes: 1. For interior excessive syndromes with invasion of exterior pathogenic factors, firstly the treatment principle of relieving exterior syndrome should be followed, then eliminating interior pathogenic factors. The herbs for relieving exterior and interior syndromes can be applied simultaneously to avoid exterior pathogenic factors invading interior body.

2. For interior excessive syndromes with deficiency of healthy qi, purgatives and tonifying should be used together to avoid impairment of healthy qi caused by purgation.

3. Those having strong purgative function may damage healthy qi. Thus they should be used carefully for chronic diseases, weak constitutions, pregnant women, and women after childbirth or during menstruation. Sometimes they can not be used in above cases.

4. Purgatives are prone to damage stomach qi. Therefore over dosage of the drug should be avoided.

Section 1
Drugs of Potent Purgatives

1. 大黄, Dahuang

English name: Rhubarb
Pharmaceutical name: Rhizoma Rhei
Botanical name: Rheum tanguticum Maxim. et Reg, R. Palmatum L., or R. Officinale Baill.
Properties and tastes: bitter, cold
Meridian tropism: spleen, stomach, large, intestine, liver and heart
Functions: 1. induce bowel movement
2. clear away heat, purge fire and remove toxins
3. promote blood circulation to remove blood stasis
4. dispel heat from the blood to stop bleeding
5. diminish inflammation

6. improve functions of the gallbladder

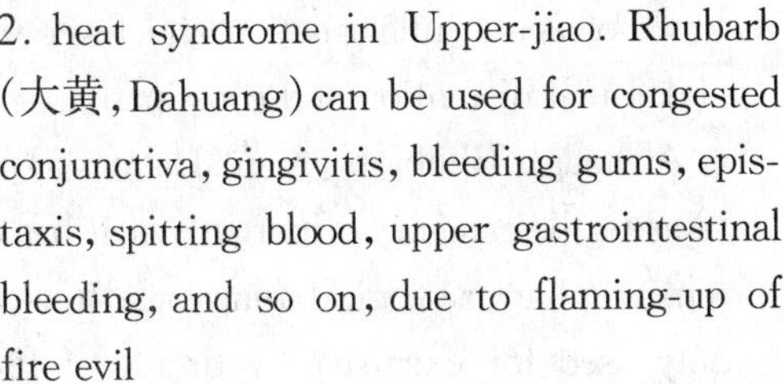

大 黄

Indications: 1. constipation accompanied by other herbs. Rhubarb (大黄, Dahuang) can be used for all types of constipation, especially for cases of excessive heat

2. heat syndrome in Upper-jiao. Rhubarb (大黄, Dahuang) can be used for congested conjunctiva, gingivitis, bleeding gums, epistaxis, spitting blood, upper gastrointestinal bleeding, and so on, due to flaming-up of fire evil

3. pyogenic infection and ulceration of skin caused by virulent heat, burn and scald, and injury from falls, fractures, contusions and strains. Take Rhubarb(大黄, Dahuang) orally or use it externally

4. acute appendicitis and acute ileus

5. acute cholecystitis and acute icterohepatitis with constipation

6. blood stasis in Lower-jiao of women: manifested as amenorrhea, lochiostasis, blood stasis after childbirth, abdominal pain due to blood stasis, pelvic tumor and bleeding after artificial abortion

7. thrombopenia

8. stranguria of heat type: manifested as frequent, difficult and painful discharge of urine due to accumulation of damp-heat in Lower-jiao

Dosage: Take 3 to 12 grams orally. Proper amount for external use.

Contraindication: Do not use for women during pregnancy, menstruation or the breast-feeding period. Use carefully. Combine it with other herbs for cases with weak constitutions and cold.

Combinations: 1. add Mirabilite(芒硝, Mangxiao)——constipation and high fever caused by excessive heat of fu yangming. A large dosage can be used for acute ileus

2. add Prepared Daughter Root of Common Monkshood(附子, Fuzi)——constipation of cold type manifested as constipation, abdominal angina and chilliness

3. add Hemp Seed(火麻仁, Huomaren) and Chinese Angelica Root(当归, Danggui)——constipation caused by blood deficiency

4. add Coptis Rhizome (黄连, Huanglian) and Baikal Skullcap Root (黄芩, Huangqin)——heat syndrome in Upper-jiao and epigastric fullness and oppression

5. add Oriental Wormwood (茵陈蒿, Yinchen)——jaundice due to damp-heat accumulation

6. add Moutan Bark(牡丹皮, Danpi)——acute appendicitis

7. add Ground Beetle(䗪虫, Zhechong) and Peach Seed(桃仁, Taoren)——blood stasis in Lower-jiao, amenorrthea and hysteromyoma

8. add Garden Burnet Root (地榆, Diyu)——burns and scalding by extenmal use

9. add Dahurian Angelica Root (白芷, Baizhi)——pyogenic infection and ulceration of skin caused by heat

10. add Red Peel of Peanut (花生红衣, Huashenghongyi)——thrombopenia

11. add Akebia Stem (木通, Mutong) and Plantain Seed (车前子, Cheqianzi)——stranguria of damp-heat type

12. add Medicinal Magnolia Bark (Houpo) and Immature Bitter Orange (枳实, Zhishi)——fullness and distention in chest and abdomen

13. add Ginseng (人参, Renshen)——con-

stipation caused by qi deficiency

14. add Common Aucklandia Root(木香, Muxiang)——dysentery

Prescriptions: 1. Timely-purging and yin-preserving Decoction(大承气汤, Dachengqi Tang)

2. Rhubarb and Peony Decoction(大黄牡丹皮汤, Dahuangmudanpi Tang)

3. Rhubarb and Ground Deetle Decoction (大黄䗪虫汤, Dahuangzhechong Tang)

Notes: Rhubarb(大黄, Dahuang) is a major herb for clearing heat and purgation. "Its property and flavour are strong. Its functions are purging and descending and exerted all over the body." So in ancient times it was known as "General" because of the analogy of its functions such as opening anus and purging evils.

Rhubarb(大黄, Dahuang) also has the function of cooling blood and promoting blood circulation. So it pertains to the categories of both qi fen and xue fen herbs. Along with other herbs, Rhubarb(大黄, Dahuang) is used widely. But it can't be used for asthenia and cold syndrome without combination of other herbs, because of its cold property and liable to damage yang qi.

The functions of Rhubarb(大黄, Dahuang) are different according to different preparation and boiling method. The purgation of crude Rhubarb(大黄, Dahuang) is stronger, so it is suitable for purging evils. Put Rhubarb(大黄, Dahuang) in the decoction when it is nearly done. Or make Rhubarb(大黄, Dahuang) into powder and take it after pouring liquid on it. The purgation of Rhubarb(大黄, Dahuang) will be reduced after long time boiling. After being prepared with wine, the purgation power of Rhubarb(大黄, Dahuang) is weak. But its function of promoting blood circulation becomes stronger, so it is suitable for cases with blood stasis. Stir-baked Rhubarb(大黄, Dahuang) is usually used for hemorrhage.

Modern research shows that Rhubarb(大黄, Dahuang) has good antibiotic, antiviral, anti-inflammatory and hemostatic functions. It can be extensively used for various kinds of acute inflammation and fever with abdominal distention and constipation.

Although Rhubarb(大黄, Dahuang) pertains to the category of purgatives, it has extensive pharmacological functions. It is not only used for excessive syndrome of fu of yangming, but also according to different combinations and dose, it can be used for various syndromes in clinic. Just as what is said by Zhang Jingyue(张景岳), "use Rhubarb(大黄, Dahuang) with Ginseng(人参, Renshen) in Yellow Dragon Decoction (黄龙汤, Huanglong Tang) for qi deficiency; with Chinese Angelica Root(当归, Danggui) in Jade Candle Powder(玉烛散, Yuzhu San) for blood deficiency. Accompanies with Licorice Root(甘草, Gancao) and Platycodon Root(桔梗, Jiegeng), its function will exert slowly; with Mirabilite(芒硝, Mangxiao) and Officinal Magnolia Bark (厚朴, Houpo), its function will become stronger. The dosage of it is different according to different conditions of patients. Do not use for asthenia syndrome in appearance but asthenia syndrome in nature. For asthenia syndrome, Rhubarb(大黄, Dahuang) is like a poison."

2. 芒硝, Mangxiao

English name: Mirabilite
Pharmaceutical name: Mirabilitum

Properties and tastes: salty, bitter, and cold

Meridian tropism: stomach, large intestine

Functions: 1. drain heat and move stool

2. soften and resolve hard mass

3. clear heat and reduce edema

芒 硝

Indications: 1. constipation for excess heat in the stomach and intestines, retention of feces, accompanied with restlessness, delirium, dry mouth, a dry and yellow tongue coating, a prickly tongue, a forceful and deep pulse

2. sore throat, aphthosis, redness of eyes, skin and external disease (usually for external use)

Dosage: 9 ~ 15g. It is taken after being dissolved into the strained decoction of boiled water. Proper amount for external use.

Contraindication: Contraindicated for pregnant women.

Combinations: 1. add Rhubarb (大黄, Dahuang)——excessive heat in the stomach and intestine, retention of feces

2. add Borneol (冰片, Bingpian)——treat swelling and pain of the throat and aphthosis. Used in powders and apply to the affected area

3. add Pinellia Rhizome (半夏, Banxia), Bitter Orange (枳壳, Zhiqiao)——pain in arms and numbness of the limbs due to stagnation of phlegm and qi

4. add Indigwoad Root (板蓝根, Banlangen), Honeysuckle Flower (金银花, Jinyinhua), Rhubarb (大黄, Dahuang)——cholecysitis

5. add Chinese Angelica Root (当归, Danggui), Safflower (红花, Honghua)——amenorrhea due to blood stasis

Prescriptions: 1. Timely-purging and yin-preserving Decoction (大承气汤, Dachengqi Tang)

2. Decoction for Regulating stomach and Purging down Digestive qi (调胃承气汤, Tiaoweichengqi Tang)

Notes: Mirabilite (芒硝, Mangxiao) which is salty and cold, has the functions of softening hard mass and moistening and purgation. It is commonly used for constipation due to excessive heat. Being cold and able to moisten the dryness, Mirabilite (芒硝, Mangxiao) is also, mostly used externally, for cases of red eyes, sore throat, mouth ulcers and so on. Furthermore, Mirabilite (芒硝, Mangxiao) can be externally used for mammary abscess in order to remove the mass. It also has the function of stopping lactation while being externally used around the nipples. After dissolving in water, Mirabilite (芒硝, Mangxiao) can be applied to sores, which are either swelling or red and hot, or painful and itching.

The main chemical ingredients of Mirabilite (芒硝, Mangxiao) are $Na_3SO_4 \cdot 10H_2O$. In ancient times there were several kinds of Mirabilite (芒硝, Mangxiao), such as sodium sulphate, exsiccated sodium sulphate… Their indications are slightly different; however, all of them are salty in taste, cold in nature and have the functions of moistening and purgation. They are only used for excessive heat accumulated in the stomach and intestines. Exsiccated sodium sulphate is used externally.

3. 番泻叶, Fanxieye

English name: Senna Leaf

Pharmaceutical name: Folium Sennae

Botanical name: Cassia angustifolia Vahl

Properties and tastes: sweet, bitter, cold

Meridian tropism: large intestine

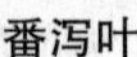

番泻叶

Functions: 1. drain downward and move stool

2. bacteriostasis

Indication: constipation

Dosage: Mild function of purgation with 1.5～3g, intense function of purgation with 6～9g. This herb is taken as a tea, decoct it after the other drugs boiled in the prescription.

Contraindication: Contraindicated in women during pregnancy, in the postpartum period, and during menstruation. Excessive use can cause side effect manifested as vomiting, nausea and abdominal pain.

Combination: add Immature Bitter Orange(枳实, Zhishi), Officinal Magnolia Bark(厚朴, Houpo)——to improve the effect of purging heat and moving stool

Notes: Senna Leaf(番泻叶, Fanxieye) has the functions of purgation and eliminating excessive heat. Thus it is especially suitable for constipation due to excessive heat. Senna Leaf(番泻叶, Fanxieye) is usually taken after soaking in water for some time. Small amount of Senna Leaf(番泻叶, Fanxieye) has the function of slow purgation while large amount may induce drastic purgation. Senna Leaf(番泻叶, Fanxieye) is used not only for constipation but also for acute pancreatitis, cholecystitis and digestive tract hemorrhage. It can clear the intestines by inducing defecation prior to roentgenograph and operation.

4. 芦荟, Luhui

English name: Aloes

Pharmaceutical name: Herba Aloes

Botanical name: Aloe vera L. Or A. Ferox Mill.

Properties and tastes: bitter, cold

芦 荟

Meridian tropism: liver, large intestine

Functions: 1. drain downward and move stool

2. clear away liver-fire

3. destory parasites and treat tinea

4. inhibit dermatomyces and mycobacterium tuberculosis

Indications: 1. constipation——habitual constipation and constipation due to heat accumulation in the large intestine accompanied by restlessness, insomnia, headache, vertigo, and susceptibility to anger

2. infantile ascariasis——abdominal pain due to parasitic infestation, sallow complexion, emaciation

3. tinea, comedo, acne, freckle. It can benefit the skin by external application

Dosage: 1～2g usually used in pills, not in decoction, proper amount for external use.

Contraindication: Not to be used in patients with deficiency cold of the spleen and stomach, poor appetite and loose stools. Not to be used by pregnant women.

Combinations: 1. add Cinnabar (朱砂, Zhusha)——constipation due to accumulation of heat in the large intestines, manifested as restlessness, insomnia

2. add Chinese Gentian Root (龙胆草, Longdancao), Cape Jasmine Fruit (栀子,

Zhizi)——retention of feces and excessive heat in liver meridian, manifested as headache, dizziness, restlessness, susceptibility of anger

3. add Rangooncreeper Fruit(使君子, Shijunzi)——make into powder and take after mixing with rice soup. It is used to treat ascariasis

4. add Licorice Root(生甘草, Shenggancao)——make it into powder and use as a topical application for treating tinea

5. add Borneol(冰片, Bingpian)——external use for treating swelling and pain of hemorrhoid complicated by anal fistual

6. add Licorice Root(生甘草, Shenggancao)——external use for tinea

Notes: Aloes(芦荟, Luhui) is extreme bitter and cold, and has the functions of cooling the liver and purgation. Thus it can be used for cases due to excessive liver-fire. However bitter taste and cold nature are harmful to the Stomach. Its smell is terrible and may cause vomiting and diarrhea for patients with stomach deficiency. Therefore Aloes (芦荟, Luhui) should not be used for cases of stomach and spleen deficiency. on, Aloes (芦荟, Luhui) is one of the most important herbs for eliminating heat and killing intestinal parasites.

Section 2
Drugs of Lubricant Purgatives

1. 火麻仁, Huomaren

English name: Hemp Seed

Pharmaceutical name: Semen Cannabis Sativae

Botanical name: Cannabis sativa L.

Properties and tastes: sweet, medium

Meridian tropism: spleen, large intestine

火麻仁

Functions: relieve constipation with laxation due to dryness of the intestine

Indication: Constipation for the aged and the women after delivery and persons in weak condition. Constipation and dryness are due to deficiency of fluid and blood.

Dosage: 9～30g.

Combinations: 1. add Chinese Angelica Root (当归, Danggui)——constipation due to

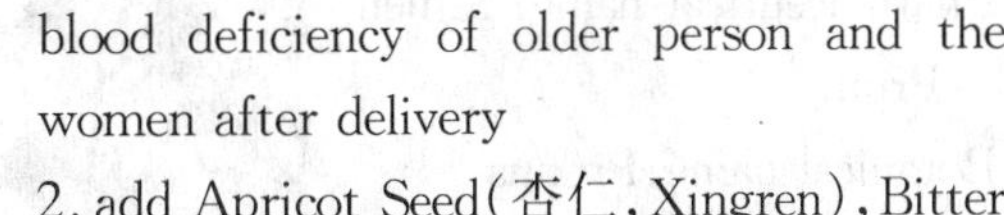

blood deficiency of older person and the women after delivery

2. add Apricot Seed(杏仁, Xingren), Bitter Orange(枳壳, Zhiaiao)——constipation dryness and habitual constipation

3. add Rehmannia Dried Root(生地黄, Shengdihuang), Tuber Fleeceflower Root (何首乌, Heshouwu)——dry intestines due to deficiency of blood, palpitation and insomnia. Difficulty in discharging with force

4. add Greed Gram Seed(绿豆, Lüdou)——dysentery with blood in stool

Prescription: Fructus Cannabis Bolus(麻子仁丸, Maziran Wan)

Notes: Hemp Seed(火麻仁, Huomaren), being rich in oil, can moisten the intestines and is particularly used for constipation due to qi stagnation of large intestine. It can be used for constipation due to blood deficiency of the old, qi and blood deficiency after childbirth, primary qi deficiency after illness and congenital deficiency. While used with Tatarian Aster Root (紫苑, Ziyuan) and Apricot Seed (杏仁, Xingren), Hemp Seed (火麻仁, Huomaren) can promote the dispersing function of the lung and moisten the large intestine, which is usually described as "lifting the teapot and opening the lid" in TCM.

It is reported that large amount of Hemp Seed (火麻仁, Huomaren, 60 ~ 120g) are poisonous and may give rise to nausea, vomiting, diarrhea, numbness of the limbs and so on. Therefore over dosage of it should not be used in clinic.

2. 郁李仁, Yuliren

English name: Bushcherry Seed

Pharmaceutical name: Semen Pruni

Botanical name: Prunus gatonica Thunb.

Properties and tastes: pungent, bitter, mild

郁李仁

Meridian tropism: large intestine, small intestine

Functions: 1. relieve constipation with laxation
2. induce diuresis to remove edema

Indications: 1. constipation due to dryness of the intestine
2. edema and fullness of the abdomen
3. flaccidity of lower limbs and edema

Dosage: 6 ~ 12g.

Combinations: 1. add Hemp Seed (火麻仁, Huomaren)——constipation due to dryness of the intestine. Difficulty in discharging stool, and habitual constipation
2. add White Mulberry Root-bark (桑白皮, Sangbaipi), Rice Bean (赤小豆, Chixiaodou), Lalang Grass Rhizome (白茅根, Baimaogen)——edema and fullness of the abdomen
3. add Common Floweringquince Fruit (木瓜, Mugua)——flaccidity of lower limbs and edema
4. add Coix Seed (薏苡仁, Yiyiren)——fullness of the stomach and abdomen, constipation and diuresis, rapid respiration and dyspnea.

Prescription: Five-Seed Pills (五仁丸, Wuren Wan)

Notes: Bushcherry Seed (郁李仁, Yuliren) is acrid and bitter for dispersion and purgation. Being rich in oil and lubricant, it not only can disperse the lung to promote diuresis but also has the function of purgation through descending qi and moistening the large intestine. Therefore it is commonly used for constipation due to qi stagnation and large intestine dryness. It is also used for cases of edema in limbs, ascites and abdominal distention, tinea pedis and difficulty in urination. It is said in the book *Herbals for Easy Approaching* (《本草便读》, Bencaobiandu): Bushcherry Seed (郁李仁, Yuliren) "especially used for moistening and descending, and has the functions of purgation and moistening dryness so that it can cure cases of water retention, wind obstruction and qi stagnation."

Both Bushcherry Seed (郁李仁, Yuliren) and Hemp Seed (火麻仁, Huomaren) have the functions of moistening and lubricating the large intestine. There is mutual reinforcement between them for the treatment of constipation due to dryness of the large intestine. However Bushcherry Seed (郁李仁, Yuliren) is usually used for excessive constipation through descending qi, purgation and promoting diuresis without tonification. For constipation due to deficiency of essence and blood, the herbs of tonification should be used together. Hemp Seed(火麻仁,Huomaren)has the function of tonifying and moistening and is commonly used for constipation due to deficiency of body fluid and blood, which will be seen either in the old patients or those in weak constitutions or women after childbirth.

Section 3
Drugs of Drastic Purgation and Dispelling Retained Water

1.甘遂,Gansui

English name:Kansui Root
Pharmaceutical name: Radix Euphorbiae Kansui
Botanical name:Euphorbia kansui Liou
Properties and tastes: bitter, sweet, cold, and toxic
Meridian tropism: lung, kidney, large intestine

甘 遂

Functions: 1. remove water retention by purgation
2. diminish the swelling and scatter blockage
Indications: 1. edema in the body and head
2. edema in the whole abdomen
3. hydrops of thoracic cavity
4. intestinal obstruction
5. hydrops in the intestinal cavity
6. epilepsy due to wind-phlegm syndrome
7. carbuncle and sore
Dosage: This drug can not be disolved in water. It is advisable to use pills. Take 0.5～1g each time. Kansui Root(甘遂,Gansui) with vinegar can relieve toxicity and the function of purgation. Proper amount for external use with fresh herbs.
Contraindication: Contraindicated in weak patients and pregnant women, incompatiable with Licorice Root(甘草,Gancao).
Combinations: 1. add Pharbitis Seed(牵牛子,Qianniuzi)——edema and abdominal distention
2. add Peking Euphorbia Root(大戟,Daji), Lilac Daphne Flower-bud(芫花,Yuanhua), Chinese Date(大枣,Dazao)——edema in the chest and abdomen
3. add Rhubarb(大黄,Dahuang), Mirabilite(芒硝,Mangxiao)——accumulation of water-evil and heat-evil in the chest
4. add Rhubarb(大黄,Dahuang), Officinal Magnolia Bark(厚朴,Houpo), Peach Seed(桃仁,Taoren)——intestinal obstruction in severe condition, hydrops in the intestinal cavity
5. add Cinnabar(朱砂,Zhusha)——put the powder of Kansui Root(甘遂,Gansui) in the heart of pig and cook it over a slow fire, then make it into pills with the powder of Cinnabar(朱砂,Zhusha). Taking the pills can treat manic-depressive psychosis and convulsive syndrome
Prescription: Ten Jujube Decoction(十枣汤,Shizao Tang)
Notes: Kansui Root(甘遂,Gansui) can drastically remove water retention by continuous purgation. It can be taken with or without other herbs for removing water retention. The powder of Kansui Root(甘遂,Gansui)

dissolved in water is externally applied to sores to relieve swelling and dispersing mass. Kansui Root(甘遂, Gansui) is poisonous. Li Shizhen(李时珍) said: "Do not take it excessively. Take proper amount in all cases."

2. 大戟, Daji

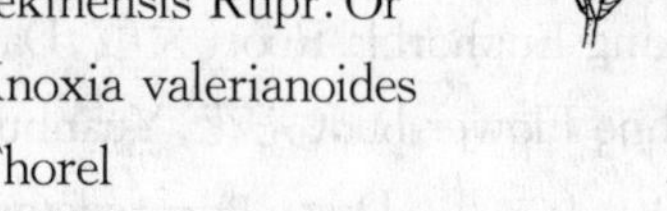

English name: Peking Euphorbia Root

Pharmaceutical name: Radix Euphorbiae seu Knoxiae

Botanical name: Euphorbia pekinensis Rupr. Or Knoxia valerianoides Thorel

Properties and tastes: bitter, pungent, cold and toxic

Meridian tropism: lung, kidney, large intestine

Functions: 1. expel extra fluids and eliminate water retention by purgation

2. diminish swelling and dissipate blockage

Indications: 1. edema in the body and head

2. edema in the whole abdomen

3. hydrops in the thoracic cavity

4. noxious heat, carbuncle and sore

5. scrofula and subcutaneous, nodule due to stagnation of phlegm-fire.

Dosage: 1.5～3g. Make it into powder, take 1g each time. Stir-baked Peking Euphorbia Root(大戟, Daji) with vinegar can relieve toxicity.

Contraindication: Contraindicated for pregnant women and weak patients. It is incompatible with Licorice Root(甘草, Gancao).

Combinations: 1. add Chinese Date (大枣, Dazao)——boil the date together with other drugs and eat the dates can treat edema

2. add Kansui Root(甘遂, Gansui), Lilac Daphne Flower-bud(芫花, Yuanhua)——edema in the whole abdomen, hydrops in the thoracic cavity

3. add Cinnabar(朱砂, Zhusha)——external application for carbuncle, sore, pyogenic infections, scrofula and subcutaneous nodule

Prescription: Ten Jujube Decoction(十枣汤, Shizao Tang)

Notes: Peking Euphorbia Root(大戟, Daji) is good at removing water retention and has the same functions as Kansui Root(甘遂, Gansui) does. However its effect is not so strong as that of Kansui Root(甘遂, Gansui). Modern research shows that the action of removing water retention of Peking Euphorbia Root(大戟, Daji) is mainly by drastic purgation whereas promoting diuresis is not obvious. It can be used for severe cases of edema and water retention in chest and abdomen, which will be seen in pleural effusion, cirrhosis ascites, schistosomial ascites and so on. However, Peking Euphorbia Root (大戟, Daji) is poisonous and its functions are extremely drastic. It should be used carefully to those with weak body and deficient Primary qi.

3. 芫花, Yuanhua

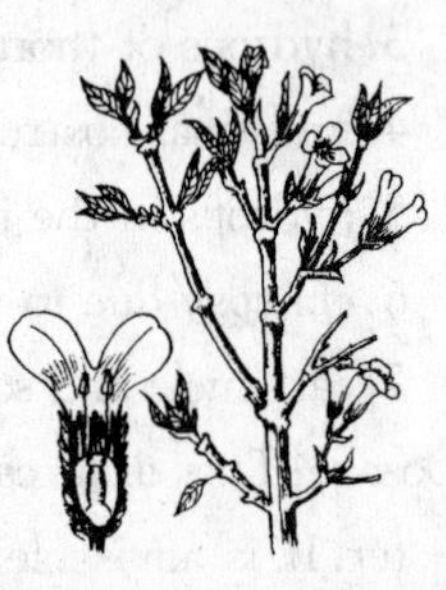

English name: Lilac Daphne Flower-bud

Pharmaceutical name: Flos Daphnes Genkwa

Botanical name: Daphne genkwa Sieb. Et Zuce.

Properties and tastes: pungent, bitter, warm and toxic

Meridian tropism: lung, kidney, large intestine

Functions: 1. expel extra fluids and eliminate water retention by purgation

2. expel phlegm for arresting cough

3. external application for destorying parasites and treating sores
4. antibacterial
5. promote urination
6. tranquilize, stop cough, expel phlegm

Indications: 1. edema in the body and head
2. edema in the whole abdomen
3. hydrops in the thoracic cavity
4. chronic tracheitis of cold type, fluid-retention
5. sore presenting in the head and obstinate tinea

Dosage: 1.5～3g. Taken of 0.6g each time, when put powder properly for external application. Stir-baked Lilac Daphne Flower-bud(芫花, Yuanhua) with vinegar can relieve toxicity.

Contraindication: Not to be taken for pregnant women and weak patients. Incompatible with Licorice Root(甘草, Gancao).

Combinations: 1. add Chinese Date (大枣, Dazao)——boil the dates together with other drugs and eat the dates for treating chronic tracheitis belonging to cold type fluid-retention
2. add Sulfur(雄黄, Xionghuang)——grind them into powder and mix them with fat of pigs. Apply the mixture to the diseased area for treating sores on the head and obstinate tinea

Prescription: Ten Jujube Decoction (十枣汤, Shizao Tang)

Notes: Lilac Daphne Flower-bud(芫花, Yuanhua) can remove water retention drastically. Modern research shows that Lilac Daphne Flower-bud(芫花, Yuanhua) may cause severe watery diarrhea and abdominal pain and promote diuresis. However large dosage of Lilac Daphne Flower-bud(芫花, Yuanhua) reduces urination.

Peking Euphorbia Root (大戟, Daji), Kansui Root (甘遂, Gansui) and Lilac Daphne Flower-bud (芫花, Yuanhua) have the functions of drastic purgation and removing water retention. Thus they are usually used together in order to enhance the effect of removing water retention in clinic. There is a saying in ancient time that "Kansui Root (甘遂, Gansui) removes water retention in the meridian, Peking Euphorbia Root(大戟, Daji) removes water retention in zang and fu organs and Lilac Daphne Flower-bud (芫花, Yuanhua) removes water retention in depressed areas." Modern research and clinical practice shows that all of them have the functions of drastic purgation and removing water retention. Lilac Daphne Flower-bud (芫花, Yuanhua) also promotes diuresis. All of them are rather poisonous, especially Lilac Daphne Flower-bud(芫花, Yuanhua). Therefore they can not be taken unless the constitution of patient is very strong and pathogenic factors are excessive. If water retention is so severe that distended abdomen is almost split and urine and stool can not discharge. Furthermore, the treatment of mild diuresis and purgation has no effect, these three herbs may be applied temporarily in spite of the weakness of patient. However the primary imbalance should be dealt with, based on an overall analysis of symptoms and signs, as soon as water retention is removed.

4. 牵牛子, Qianniuzi

English name: Pharbitis Seed

Pharmaceutical name: Semen Pharbitidis

Botanical name: Phabitis nil(L.) Choisy or P.

Purpurea(L.)Vogt

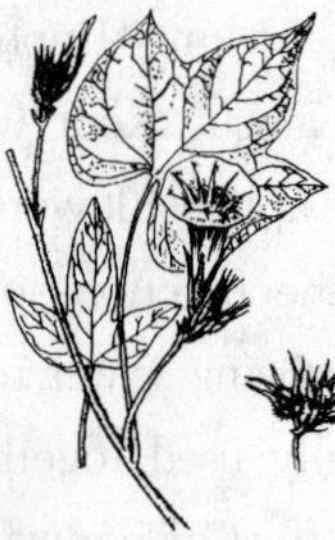

Properties and tastes: bitter, cold, toxic

Meridian tropism: lung, kidney, large intestine

Functions: 1. expel extra fluids and promote urination

2. relax the bowels, remove accumulation

3. destory ascarid and tenia

牵牛子

Indications: 1. edema and abdominal distention, urine retention due to stagnation of fluid-evil

2. retention of feces due to stagnation of damp-heat in the stomach and intestine

3. cough and asthma due to fluid-retention

4. ascariasis and taeniasis

Dosage: Decoct 3～9g with water after breaking it into pieces. Take powder of 1.5～3g. Crude drug or fried can be used. Fried drug is in mild property.

Contraindication: Contraindicated for patients with edema due to hypofunction of spleen and pregnant women. It is not advisable to use it with Croton Seed(巴豆, Badou).

Combinations: 1. add Rhubarb (大黄, Dahuang), Green Tangerine Peel (青皮, Qingpi)——edema, abdominal distention, thirst, short breath, difficult micturation constipation and stools due to excess of body structure and vital qi

2. add Immature Bitter Orange (枳实, Zhishi), Common Aucklandia Root (木香, Muxiang)——constipation and abdominal distention due to stagnation of qi in San-jiao and blockage of damp-heat

3. add Rhubarb (大黄, Dahuang), Areca Seed(槟榔, Binlang), Rangooncreeper Fruit (使君子, Shijunzi)——abdominal pain due to worm stagnation, abdominal distention, constipation

4. add Rhubarb(大黄, Dahuang), Mirabilite (芒硝, Mangxiao), Immature Bitter Orange (枳实, Zhishi)——ascites due to liver cirrhosis.

5. add Cushaw Seed (南瓜子, Nanguazi), Areca Seed(槟榔, Binlang)——taeniasis

6. add Hawthorn Fruit (山楂, Shanzha), Malt(麦芽, Maiya)——stagnation of food

Notes: Pharbitis Seed (牵牛子, Qianniuzi) tends to affect qi fen and dredge Sanjiao. It has the functions of purgation and promoting diuresis. Thus water retention in the body will disappear during urination and defecation. The function of Pharbitis Seed (牵牛子, Qianniuzi) is not so strong as that of either Kansui Root (甘遂, Gansui) or Peking Euphorbia Root(大戟, Daji) or Lilac Daphne Flower-bud(芫花, Yuanhua), however it is only applied to cases of edema and abdominal distention, without healthy qi deficiency, due to water retention. A small dosage of Pharbitis Seed(牵牛子, Qianniuzi) can promote defecation and be used for constipation. Together with Areca Seed(槟榔, Binlang) it has good effect on expelling intestinal parasites, such as ascaris and tenia.

5. 商陆, Shanglu

English name: Pokeberry Root

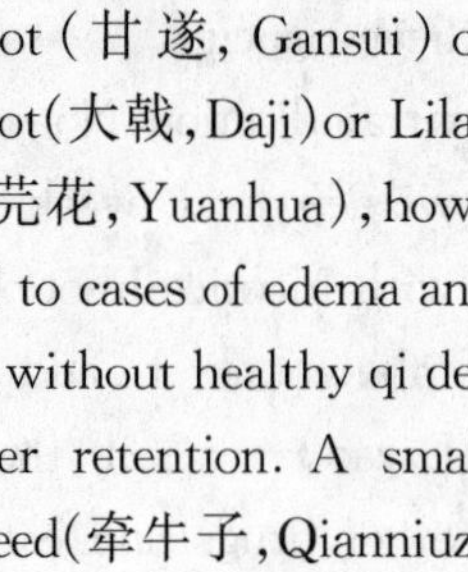

Pharmaceutical name: Radix Phytolaccae

Botanical name: Phytolacca acinosa Roxb. Or P. Esculenta Van Hout.

商 陆

Properties and tastes: bitter, cold, and toxic

Meridian tropism: lung, kidney, and large intestine

Functions: 1. remove retention by purgation

2. diminish swelling and scatter blockage

3. expel phlegm for arresting cough

Indications: 1. edema and abdominal distention-mostly accompanied by retention of feces and urine.

2. carbuncle, sore, pyogenic infections, scrofula

3. chronic tracheitis

Dosage: 6～9g. Proper amount for external application.

Contraindication: Contraindicated for patients with edema due to deficiency of spleen and pregnant women.

Combinations: 1. add Oriental Waterplantain Rhizome(泽泻, Zexie), Rice Bean(赤小豆, Chixiaodou), Tuckahoe(茯苓, Fuling)—— edema and abdominal distention

2. add salt——pound them into pieces for external use. It can treat all kinds of toxic swelling of the skin

Notes: Pokeberry Root(商陆, Shanglu) removes water retention by inducing bowel movement and promoting diuresis. Therefore it can be used for cases of edema, especially those with anuria and constipation. Furthermore it can induce swelling and disperse mass while externally applied to carbuncle. Thus fresh Pokeberry Root(商陆, Shanglu) and salt are pounded together into pieces and applied externally to carbuncle. They should be changed as soon as they become dry. Pharmacological research shows that Pokeberry Root(商陆, Shanglu) not only can cause severe diarrhea and promote diuresis but also has significant effect on alleviating cough and dispersing phlegm. Therefore it has been used successfully for chronic trachitis in recent years. However Pokeberry Root(商陆, Shanglu) is extremely poisonous. Its toxin gives rise to central nervous system paralysis, respiratory and motor disturbance, dysphasia, irritability, convulsion, even myocardial paralysis and death. Thus dosage should be limited.

Both Pokeberry Root(商陆, Shanglu) and Pharbitis Seed(牵牛子, Qianniuzi) can induce bowel movement and promote diuresis to remove water retention drastically. Thus they are applied to cases of edema with distention, asthma and cough due to phlegm retention, and anuria and constipation. Pokeberry Root(商陆, Shanglu) has the functions of expelling toxic subtance and inducing swelling by external application, however it is extremely poisonous while being taken orally. Pharbitis Seed(牵牛子, Qianniuzi) has the functions of promoting digestion and killing intestinal parasites. It is not so poisonous as Pokeberry Root(商陆, Shanglu). Therefore it can be used for children suffering from abdominal pain due to intestinal parasites, undigested food retention, poor appetite and so on.

6. 巴豆, Badou

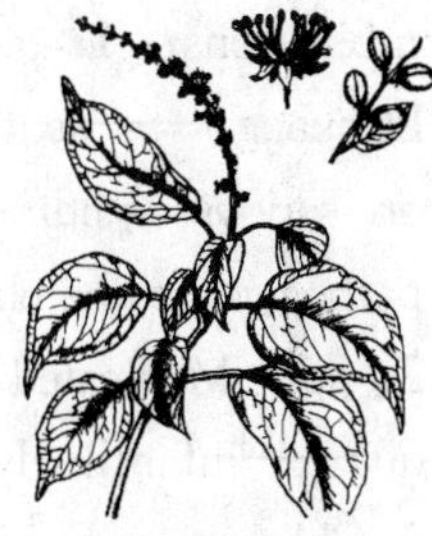
巴 豆

English name: Croton Seed

Pharmaceutical name: Fructus Crotonis

Botanical name: Croton tiglium L.

Properties and tastes: pungent, heat, extremely poisonous

Meridian tropism: lung, stomach, large intestine

Functions: 1. purge the accumulation of cold by purgation

2. dispel water retention and dissipate edema

3. expel phlegm for relieving sore throat

Indications: 1. fullness, distention and acute pain in the abdomen, constipation, even sudden syncope due to accumulation of cold stagnation in the intestine

2. edema in the abdomen, pharyngitis, stagnation of phlegm, even as phyxia when seems going to die

3. infantile dyspepsia, profuse phlegm even palpitation

4. throat obstruction due to diphtheria and inflammation of the throat

5. ulcerated sorves an tinea

Dosage: Pound it into powder and make it into pills, take 0.1～0.3g each time for internal use. Proper amount for external use.

Contraindication: Not to be taken with hot food in order to avoid intense purgation. Take the decoction of Chinese Goldthread Rhizome(黄连, Huanglian) and Amur Corktree Bark(黄柏, Huangbai) or cold porridge to relieve lingering purgation. Contraindicated for pregnant women and weak patients. Antagonistic to Pharbitis Seed(牵牛子, Qianniuzi)

Combinations: 1. add Rhubarb (大黄, Dahuang)——acute intestinal obstruction or serious syndrome of accumulation of pathogens in the chest

2. add Medicated Leaven (神曲, Shenqu)——infantile dyspepsia

3. add Apricot Seed(杏仁, Xingren)——ascites, fullness and distention of abdomen

4. add Ferrosisulfas Crudus (绛矾, Jiangfan)——late stage of schistosomiasis and ascites due to liver cirrhosis

5. add Balloonflower Root(桔梗, Jiegeng), Tendrilleaf Fritillary Bulb (贝母, Beimu)——pulmonary abscess, cough with discharging profuse thick phlegm

6. add Alum (白矾, Baifan)——emetic phlegm syndrome, and acute pharyngitis

7. add Bee Wax (蜂蜡, Fengla)——fry it with charcoal and make them into pills with wax can treat chronic diarrhea due to cold accumulation

8. add Sulfur (雄黄, Xionghuang)——externally used for treating malignant boil, itch, carbuncle.

Prescription: Pill of Three Drugs for Emergency(三物备急丸, Sanwubeiji Wan)

Notes: Croton Seed(巴豆, Badou) is pungent in taste, hot in nature and extremely poisonous. It is strong purgative and may stimulate mucosa of skin to form blister. There was a saying in ancient times that "it was like a brave soldier who always marched forward to capture an enemy stronghold." It should be used carefully in clinic. Proper amount of Croton Seed(巴豆, Badou) will be very effective. On the contrary it may bring disaster immediately. The preparation and the dosage must be stressed here. Unprepared Croton Seed(巴豆, Badou) is very effective. After being fried or frosted, its effect will appear slowly, and when being fried into brown material it can stop diarrhea. The regular dosage of Croton Seed(巴豆, Badou) causes diarrhea whereas small dosage(0.01～0.05g) will promote digestion, regulate Middle-jiao and eliminate phlegm.

Croton Seed(巴豆, Badou) may give rise to drastic purgation, however proper small dosage will be slow acting and not be harmful to healthy qi.

It is said in *Mystery of Herbology* (《本草通玄》, Bencaotongxuan) that: "both Croton

Seed (巴豆, Badou) and Rhubarb (大黄, Dahuang) are both purgatives. Rhubarb (大黄, Dahuang) is cold in nature and usually applied to cases of fu imbalance due to excessive heat, while Croton Seed (巴豆, Badou) is hot in nature and usually applied to cases of zang organs imbalance due to excessive cold."

Chapter 3
Drugs for Invigorating Deficiency

Definition: Herbs which are known to benefit the body or tonics, supplement necessary materials of the human body, strengthen functions, build up resistance to diseases and eliminate asthenia syndrome are drugs for invigorating deficiendy.

Indication: Tonics are suitable for all types of deficiency syndrome. They are used to support healthy qi and eliminate evils or protect healthy qi for cases characterized by both deficiency and excess syndrome.

Classification: There are four types of deficiency syndrome: qi deficiency, yang deficiency, blood deficiency and yin deficiency. According to different functions and indications of tonics, they are divided into four categories including drugs for replenishing qi, herbs for invigorating yang, drugs for enriching blood and drugs for nourishing yin.

Notes: It is not proper to use tonics for excess syndrome, since they will "close the door and keep the evils inside." For the cases of evils not being eliminated and healthy qi deficiency, some tonics with herbs for eliminating evils can be chosen in order to support healthy qi and eliminate evils.

Tonics, especially herbs for nourishing yin and blood are able to damage the stomach. So herbs for invigorating the stomach and regulating qi should be used properly with tonics to avoid damaging digestion and absorption of the stomach and spleen.

In the clinic, suitable tonics are chosen according to different types of deficiency syndrome. For instance, herbs for replenishing qi are used for tonifying yang deficiency syndrome, herbs for enriching blood are used for blood deficiency syndrome, herbs for nourishing yin are used for yin deficiency syndrome, etc. If herbs for tonifying yang are used for yin deficiency accompanied with heat syndrome, or herbs for nourishing yin are used for yang deficiency accompanied with cold syndrome, harmful results will be produced. During the process of the activities of human life, qi blood, yin and yang depend on each other. They also affect each other in deficiency situations. qi and yang refer to the decline of body activities. yang deficiency is usually combined with qi deficiency, while qi deficiency is liable to cause yang deficiency. Yin and blood deficiency refer to the damage and consumption of essence. Yin deficiency may accompany blood deficiency, while blood deficiency is liable to cause yin deficiency. Therefore, herbs for replenishing qi and for tonifying yang and herbs for nourshing blood and yin should be used simultaneously to increase the effect on each other. For the cases of qi and blood deficiency, or both yin and yang deficiency, the methods of replenishing qi and nourishing blood or tonifying yang and nourishing yin should be used in accordance with different situations.

Modern research shows that tonics influence immunity, the endocrine system, material and energy metabolism, cardiovascular system, etc; and can improve the adaptability of the body, resist fatigue, promote the ability to work, etc.

Section 1
Drugs for Replenishing Qi

1. 人参, Renshen

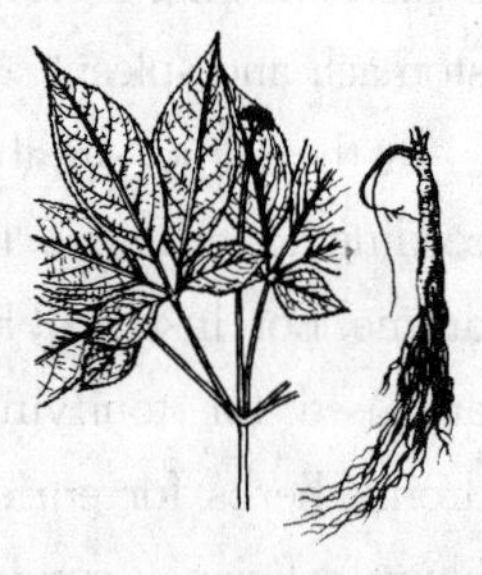
人 参

English name: Ginseng

Pharmaceutical name: inseng

Botanical name: Panax ginseng C. A. Mey

Properties and tastes: sweet, slightly bitter, and slightly warm

Meridian tropism: spleen, lung

Functions:

1. replenish the primary qi
2. tonify the spleen and lung
3. promote the secretion of body fluid
4. replenish qi and increase the production of blood
5. tranquilize and develop intelligence
6. support healthy qi to eliminate evils
7. replenish qi and tonify yang
8. lower blood sugar

Indications: 1. collapse syndrome due to qi deficiency: manifested as weak body with a tendency to faint, pale complexion, cold limbs, spontaneous perspiration, listlessness and fading pulse (coma state) caused by severe loss of blood, vomiting, diarrhea and other diseases with primary qi exhausted. Ginseng (人参, Renshen) can replenish qi and rescue collape. Modern medicine has proven that Ginseng (人参, Renshen) can give doctors an opportunity to rescue patients on the brink of death through stabilizing blood pressure and increasing the ability to resist diseases

2. deficiency of the spleen and stomach: Ginseng (人参, Renshen) can be used for the feeling of fullness and oppression in epigastrium, lassitude and weakness, anorexia, vomiting, diarrhea and so on caused by a lack of food essence. It is also suitable for diseases of the digestive system in modern medicine, such as chronic hepatitis, chronic gastritis, and gastric and duodenal ulcer caused by deficiency of the spleen and stomach qi

3. deficiency of the lung qi: manifested as shortness of breath, tiredness, frequent onset of asthma, weak pulse and spontaneous perspiration

4. thirst and diabetes due to deficiency of qi and impairment of body fluid

5. mental disturbance: manifested as insomnia, dream—disturbed sleep, amnesia, fright, palpitation, and so on, caused by deficiency of qi and blood and impaired nourishment of the heart spirit

6. anemia and hemorrhage

7. impotence and premature ejaculation due to deficiency of primary qi

8. supporting healthy qi to eliminate evils: taking the right amount of Ginseng (人参,

Renshen) orally and regularly can resist and prevent diseases. Use herbs for eliminating evils in combination, while healthy qi is deficient and evils are excess, Ginseng (人参, Renshen) can help the body to eliminate evils

Dosage: Small dosage is 1 to 9 grams, while the largest dosage is 30 grams (for coma)

Contraindication: Ginseng (人参, Renshen) can't be used for cases of hyperactivity of the liver yang, excess of internal heat and accumulation of damp-heat. Newborn babies and pregnant women can not take a large dose of Ginseng (人参, Renshen). Do not take it with Radish Seed (莱菔子, Laifuzi), radish and tea. It is incompatible with Black False Bellebore (藜芦, Lilu) and antagonistic to Trogopterus Dung (五灵脂, Wulingzhi).

Combinations: 1. add Prepared Daughter Root of Common Monkshood (附子, Fuzi)——collapse syndrome manifested as perspiration and cold limbs due to qi deficiency and yang exhaustion

2. add Lilyturf Root (麦冬, Maidong) and Chinese Magnoliavine (五味子, Wuweizi)——collapse syndrome manifested as thirst, hyperhidrosis and shortness of breath due to qi and yin deficiency

3. add Giant Gecko (蛤蚧, Gejie)——asthma due to deficiency of the lung and kidney qi

4. add Perilla leaf (苏叶, Suye)——diseases caused by exogenous evils and qi deficiency

5. add Rhubarb (大黄, Dahuang)——constipation resulting from qi deficiency

6. add Largehead Atractylodes Rhizome (白术, Baizhu)——deficiency of the stomach and spleen

7. add Snakegourd Root (天花粉, Tianhuafen)——diabetes

8. add Gypsum (石膏, Shigao)——febrile diseases with impairment of qi and body fluid manifested as fever, thirsty, hyperhidrosis and large and weak pulse

9. add Chinese Angelica Root (当归, Danggui)——anemia

10. add Longan Aril (龙眼肉, Longyanrou)——amnesia due to deficiency of the heart and spleen

11. add Spine Date Seed (酸枣仁, Suanzaoren)——mental disturbance due to deficiency of the heart and spleen

12. add Hairy Antler (鹿茸, Lurong)——impotence and premature ejaculation

13. add Membranous Milkvetch Root (黄芪, Huangqi) and Liquorice Root (甘草, Gancao)——which are sweet in taste and warm in nature, and can replenish primary qi, promote pus drainage and cure abscess

Prescriptions: 1. Decoction of Ginseng (独参汤, Dushen Tang)

2. Decoction of Four Mild Drugs (四君子汤, Sijunzi Tang)

3. Decoction for Strengthening Middle-Jiao and Benefiting Vital Energy (补中益气汤, Buzhongyiqi Tang)

4. Decoction for Invigorating the Spleen and Nourishing the Heart (归脾汤, Guipi Tang)

Notes: Since ancient times, Ginseng (人参, Renshen) has been known as precious herbal medicine which can prevent diseases, build up health and prolong life. In recent years, great attention has been paid to the pharmacological study of Ginseng (人参, Renshen) in many countries. Research shows that Ginseng (人参, Renshen) can regulate the central nervous system, increase adaptability of the body, Strengthen immunity of the body, relieve tiredness, improve blood circulation, regulate blood pressure, influence the pituitaryadrenocortical system, improve functions of gonad, alleviate damaging of hemopoietic system caused by radiation, inhibit growth of cancerous cells, etc.

Although Ginseng (人参, Renshen) pertains to herbs for replenishing qi, combined with other herbs, it can be used for various types of asthenia syndrome caused by yin, yang, qi and blood deficiency. Please note the following three points: ① Compatibility with Ginseng (人参, Renshen). Cases of yin deficiency, blood deficiency and those with evils, appropriate herbs should be used with Ginseng (人参, Renshen). Do not misuse Ginseng (人参, Renshen). ② Dosage of Ginseng (人参, Renshen). Use a small dosage, 6 to 9 grams per week for health care. Use about 9 grams per day for common diseases. Use 30 to 60 grams per day (2 to 3times) for coma. ③ Variety of Ginseng (人参, Renshen). Ginseng (人参, Renshen) includes Korean Ginseng (高丽参, Gaolishen), Jilin Ginseng (吉林参, Renshen), Tassel Ginseng (人参, Renshen), and Red Ginseng (红参, Renshen) and so on according to their different origins and processing in clinic.

Korean Ginseng, which is dry and strong, has the best functions of replenishing qi and restoring yang. However, it is liable to damage yin and invigorate fire. The function of replenishing qi of JiLin Ginseng (人参, Renshen) is not as good as that of Korean Ginseng, but JiLin Ginseng (人参, Renshen) can promote the production of body deficiency of qi and body fluid and upsurge of asthenia fire.

It was reported that a newborn baby and a pregnant woman suffered from arrhythmia after taking overdoses of Ginseng (人参, Renshen). Patients with internal fire will suffer bleeding from the gum and nose if it is misused. In the book of *A New Book of Materia Medica* (《本草新编》, Bencaoxinbian), there is a saying that "Ginseng (人参, Renshen) should be used with other herbal medicine in order to achieve a good effect. If the combination and dosage are proper, it can be used to eliminate evils or restore healthy qi in different situations. As mentioned above, it is clear that the method of combining Ginseng (人参, Renshen) with other herbs is very important in the clinic."

2. 西洋参, Xiyangshen

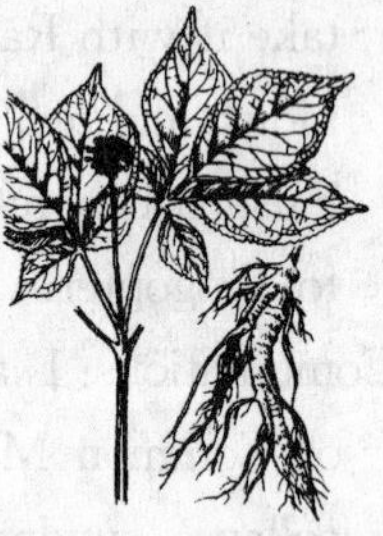

西洋参

English name: American Ginseng Root

Pharmaceutical name: Radix Panacis Quinquefolii

Botanical name: Panax quinquefolium L.

Properties and tastes: bitter, slightly sweet and cold

Meridian tropism: lung, kidney, heart

Functions: 1. benefit qi and nourish yin

2. reduce deficiency fire to promote the production of the body fluid

Indications: 1. cough, asthma, sputum with blood, hyperactivity of fire due to yin deficiency

2. impairment of fluids and qi during febrile disease, lassitude and restlessness and thirst

3. dry mouth and tongue due to deficiency of body fluid

4. hematochezia due to intestinal heat

Dosage: 3～6g.

Contraindication: This drug is cold in nature, it can impair yang and generate pathogenic dampness. Use cautiously for patients with yang deficiency of Middle-jao and cold damp in the stomach. The drug should not be fired in ironware. Incompatible with Black False Bellebore(藜芦, Lilu), antagonistic to Trogopterus Dung(五灵脂, Wulingzhi).

Combinations: 1. add Dwarf Lilyturf Root(麦门冬, Maimendong), Ass - hide Glue(阿胶, Ejiao), Common Anemarrhea Rhizome (知母, Zhimu), Tendrilleaf Fritillary Bulb (贝母, Beimu)——cough, asthma, sputum with blood, hyperactivity of fire due to yin deficiency

2. add Rehmannia Dried Root(生地黄, Shengdihuang), Dwarf Lilyturf Root(麦门冬, Maimendong), Figwort Root(玄参, Xuanshen)——impairment of yin and qi due to febrile disease, lassitude and restlessness, thirst and hematochezia due to intestinal heat

3. add Longan Aril(龙眼肉, Longyanrou)——take it for hematochezia due to intestinal heat

Notes: American Ginseng Root(西洋参, Xiyangshen) can reinforce not only qi but also yin. Hence, it is largely used in the syndrome of qi-yin deficiency. For the cases of qi deficiency with sensitivity to the warm-dry property of Ginseng(人参, Renshen), American Ginseng Root(西洋参, Xiyangshen) is a good substitution. Said in *Herbals for Easy Approaching* (《本草便读》, Bencaobiandu), "Being sweet, bitter in taste and cold in nature, American Ginseng Root (西洋参, Xiyangshen) can be used to clear away heat in the lungs and to strengthen the body. Being sweet, warm, and strong in nature, Japanese Ginseng(人参, Renshen) is good at invigorating qi to reinforce the body the spleen."

3. 黄芪, Huangqi

English name: Membranous Milkvetch Root

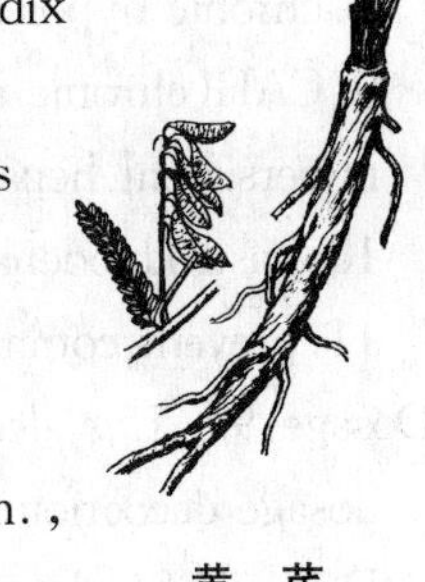

黄 芪

Pharmaceutical name: Radix Astragali

Botanical name: Astragalus membranaceus(Fisch.) Bge, A. mongholicus Bge., A. chrysopterus Bge., A. floridus Benth., or A. tongolensis Ulbr.

Properties and tastes: sweet and slightly warm

Meridian tropism: the lung and spleen meridian

Functions: 1. benefit the qi and raise the yang qi of the spleen and stomach

2. stabilizes the exterior and stop sweating

3. dissolve putrid tissues and promote the growth of new tissues (promote the discharge of pus and healing)

4. promote urination and remove edema

5. strengthen body immunity

6. remove urinary protein

7. protect the liver

8. increase white cells

Indications: 1. deficiency of both the spleen and lung syndrome-poor appetite and diarrhea with loose stools, shortness of breath and fatigue, etc.

2. sinking of the spleen and stomach qi syndrome-prolapsed of the rectum due to long term hysteroptosis and gastroptosis

3. hemorrhage due to failure of qi in controlling blood-hematochezia, metrorrhagia and metrostaxis

4. deficiency conditions with spontaneous perspiration syndrome

5. carbuncle failing to suppurate, or non-healing of boils

6. edema, scanty urine, for example, chronic diffuse glomerulone phritis

7. numbness of the limbs, pain of the joints, paralysis, qi deficiency and blood stagnation

8. chronic hypoleukocytosis

9. CAH(chronic active hepatitis) and chronic persistent hepatitis.

10. gastroduodenal ulcer

11. prevent common cold

Dosage: 9～15g, decocted 30～60g as a large dosage decoction. Toast it in Honey(蜂蜜, Fengmi) for benefiting qi and raising the yang of spleen and stomach. Use fresh herbs for other actions.

Contraindication: This herb has the actions of invigorating qi and ascending yang. It is easy to generate interior pathogenic fire for arresting sweating. It is not suggested for patients with exterior excess syndrome, retention of dampness due to stagnation of qi, retention of food, hyperactivity of yang due to deficiency of yin, the early stage of a carbuncle or external heat-toxin after ruptured abscess, etc.

Combinations: 1. add Ginseng(人参, Renshen) or Dang-shen Root(党参, Dangshen)——deficiency of qi in Middle-jiao, deficiency of spleen and stomach syndrome, weakness due to chronic disease

2. add Largehead Atractylodes Rhizome(白术, Baizhu)——poor appetite and loose stools, or diarrhea due to deficiency of spleen.

3. add Chinese Angelica Root(当归, Danggui)——deficiency of qi and blood

4. add Prepared Daughter Root of Common Monkshood(附子, Fuzi)——aversion to cold, polyhidrosis, deficiency of qi and declination of yang

5. add Ginseng(人参, Renshen), Shunk Bugbane Rhizome(升麻, Shengma)——sinking of the spleen and stomach qi syndrome

6. add Ginseng(人参, Renshen), Longan Aril(龙眼肉, Longyanrou), Spine Date Seed(酸枣仁, Suanzaoren)——hematochezia, metrorrhagia and metrostaxis, purpura due to failure of qi in controlling blood

7. add Oyster Shell(牡蛎, Muli), Blighted Wheat(浮小麦, Fuxiaomai)——spontaneous perspiration due to deficiency of qi

8. add Rehmannia Dried Root(生地黄, Shengdihuang), Chinese Corktree Bark(黄柏, Huangbai)——night sweating due to yin deficiency

9. add Chinese Angelica Root(当归, Danggui), Rice Bean(赤小豆, Chixiaodou)——carbuncle difficult to hasten suppuration

10. add Chinese Angelica Root(当归, Danggui), Ginseng(人参, Renshen), Cassia Bark(肉桂, Rougui)——carbuncle with nonhealing of boils

11. add Fourstamen Stephania Root(防己, Fangji), Largehead Atractylodes Rhizome(白术, Baizhu)——edema, scanty urine caused by diffuse glomerulonephritis, or heaviness and numbness of the limbs caused by arthralgia due to dampness

12. add Cassia Twig(桂枝, Guizhi), White Peony Root(白芍药, Baishaoyao)——numbness of the limbs

13. add Rhizome or Root of Forbes Notopterygium(羌活, Qianghuo), Divaricate Saposhnikovia Root(防风, Fangfeng)——pain of the shoulder and arm due to wind-cold-damp arthralgia, for example, periomethrisis

14. add Chinese Angelica Root(当归, Danggui), Szechwan Lovage Rhizome(川芎, Chuanxiong), Peach Seed(桃仁, Taoren)——apoplexy sequela and hemiplegia

15. add Chinese Angelica Root(当归, Danggui), Ginseng(人参, Renshen), Rehmannia

Dried Root (生地黄, Shengdihuang)——hypoleukocytosis and anemia

16. add Cassia Twig(桂枝, Guizhi), White Peony Root (白芍药, Baishaoyao), Malt Sugar (饴糖, Yitang)——gastroduodenal ulcer

17. add Prepared Rhizome of Adhesive Rehmannia(熟地黄, Shoudihuang), Ginseng(人参, Renshen)——uriedema due to glomerulonephritis has gone, but urinary protein remains positive after disappearance of edema due to nephritis

18. add Divaricate Saposhnikovia Root (防风, Fangfeng)——reinforcing without stagnation, activating without purgation, used for patients with spontaneous perspiration, or person who is easier to catch cold

19. add Earth Worm(地龙, Dilong)——reduce blood pressure

Prescriptions: 1. Decoction for Strengthening Middle-Jiao and Benefiting Vital Energy(补中益气汤, Buzhongyiqi Tang)

2. Decoction of Ten Powderful Tonics(十全大补汤, Shiquandabu Tang)

3. Jade Screen Powder (玉屏风散, Yupingfeng San)

Notes: Membranous Milkvetch Root (黄芪, Huangqi) is one of the most commonly used herbs to invigorate qi because it has the capacity to reinforce qi of the spleen and the lungs, to lift collapsed qi, to strengthen defensive qi and the superficial layer, as well as arrest sweating and promote pus discharge. It was entitled "the best reinforcing herb" by Li Shizhen (李时珍), the great ancient pharmacologist for its applicability to various qi deficient syndromes and the cases of chronic diseases complicated with qi deficiency. Recent research shows that Membranous Milkvetch Root(黄芪, Huangqi) has the functions to improve immunity, improve metabolism, promote urination, reduce blood pressure and improve cardiac function. Membranous Milkvetch Root (黄芪, Huangqi) is similar to Ginseng(人参, Renshen) in reinforcing qi but weaker. These two may go with each other in the treatment of the qi deficient syndromes involving the lungs and the spleen. Meanwhile, for cases with shock caused by severe loss of blood, vomiting, or diarrhea, Ginseng(人参, Renshen) is the first choice because of its functions of invigorating primordial qi and nourishing blood and fluid. According to *Origin of Shennong's Herbal Classic* (《本经逢源》, Benjingfengyuan), the feature of Membranous Milkvetch Root (黄芪, Huangqi) is "being able to drive through meridian and never causing stagnancy in spite of its property of warm and strengthening.' Furthermore, this herb is able to promote pus discharge and tissue regeneration and therefore has been called a great drug for skin and external diseases."

4. 白术, Baizhu

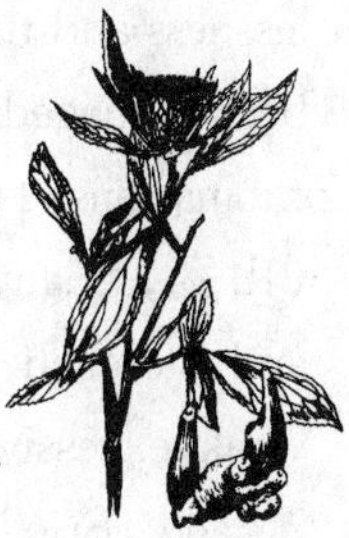

English name: Largehead Atractylodes Rhizome

Pharmaceutical name: Rhizoma Atractylodis macrocephalae

Botanical name: Atractylodes macrocephala Koidz.

白 术

Properties and tastes: bitter, sweet and warm

Meridian tropism: the spleen and stomach meridian

Functions: 1. invigorate the spleen and qi

2. eliminate dampness and promote diuresis

3. strengthen the superficial to promote uri-

nation

4. prevent miscarriage

Indications: 1. deficiency of spleen and stomach syndrome——poor appetite, loose stools, fullness and distention syndrome discussed above

2. phlegm and fluid syndrome——profuse phlegm, edema, dizziness, vomiting, accompanied with the spleen deficiency syndrome talked above

3. spontaneous sweating due to qi deficiency——profuse sweating upon exercises, accompanied with poor appetite and loose stools

4. threatened abortion

Dosage: 6～15g. Largehead Atractylodes Rhizome(生白术, Shengbaizhu) is used for eliminating dampness and inducing diuresis. While Stir-baked Largehead Atractylodes Rhizome(白术, Baizhu) is used for tonifying qi and spleen.

Contraindication: This herb can eliminate dampness to impair yin. It is used only for those with dampness retention in the Middle-jiao. Do not use for patients with interior-heat caused by deficiency of yin or restlessness and thirst due to body fluid that has been damaged.

Combinations: 1. add Common Yam Rhizome (山药, Shanyao)——deficiency of spleen and stomach, poor appetite, loose stools, weak, excessive leucorrhea, etc.

2. add Fried Malt (炒麦芽, Chaomaiaiy a)——vomiting and diarrhea due to spleen deficiency complicated by food stagnation

3. add Coix Seed(薏苡仁, Yiyiren)——diarrhea due to spleen deficiency

4. add Ginseng (人参, Renshen)——all kinds of syndromes due to deficiency of the spleen and stomach

5. add Prepared Licorice Root(炙甘草, Zhigancao)——vomiting due to disharmony of spleen and stomach

6. add Immature Bitter Orange (枳实, Zhishi)——dyspepsia, epigastria distention and fullness due to deficiency of the spleen and qi stagnation, it can also be used to treat hepatosplenomegaly, gastroptosis, hysteroptosis and prolapsed of rectum

7. add Baikal Skullcap Root (黄芩, Huangqin)——heat syndrome in newborn, threatened abortion, habitual abortion

8. add Prepared Daughter Root of Common Monkshood (附子, Fuzi)——pain of the body due to cold-dampness

9. add White Peony Root (白芍药, Baishaoyao)——borborygmus, abdominal pain, diarrhea

10. add Areca Peel (大腹皮, Dafupi)——epigastria distention and fullness, poor appetite, lassitude, edema and abdominal fullness

11. add Oyster Shell(牡蛎, Muli), Divaricate Saposhnikovia Root (防风, Fangfeng)——spontaneous sweating and night sweating

12. add Chinese Angelica Root(当归, Danggui), White Peony Root (白芍药, Baishaoyao)——threatened abortion due to blood deficiency

13. add Chinese Clematis Root (威灵仙, Weilingxian), Mulberry Twig (桑枝, Sangzhi)——pain of the limbs due to wind-dampness

14. add Rehmannia Dried Root (生地黄, Shengdihuang), Shunk Bugbane Rhizome (升麻, Shengma)——moisten the intestine to relax bowels(It is advisable to use a large amount of crude Largehead Atractylodes

Rhizome(白术,Baizhu))

15. add Swordlike Atractylodes Rhizome(苍术,Cangzhu)——the fluid and food can not be transported and transformed due to deficiency of the spleen, abdominal distention caused by chronic hepatitis

16. add Tuckahoe (茯苓, Fuling)——phlegm and fluid syndrome, Meniere's syndrome

Prescriptions: 1. Powder of Radix Gingeng, Poria and Rhizoma Atractylodis Macrocephalae(参苓白术散,Shenlingbaizhu San)

2. Decoction for Regulating Function of Middle-energizer(理中汤,Lizhong Tang)

3. Fructus Anrranttii Immaturus and Rhizoma Atractylodis Macrocep Halae Pill(枳术丸,Zhizhu Wan)

4. Decoction of Pineliae, Atractylodis Macrocephalae and Gastrodiae(半夏白术天麻汤,Banxia Baizhu Tianma Tang)

Notes: Largehead Atractylodes Rhizome (白术,Baizhu)and Swordlike Atractylodes Rhizome(苍术, Cangzhu) have similarities in their functions of drying up dampness and reinforcing the spleen. However, the former is stronger in reinforcing qi, while the latter in eliminating dampness and promoting sweating. Hence, the former is often used in the treatment of spleen deficient syndromes with the symptoms of diarrhea, spontaneous perspiration, and threatened abortion. The latter is often used to treat the cases of superficial dampness syndrome with the symptoms of migraine, a sensation of heaviness in the head with dull headache and arthralgia complicated with arthrocele. The two may be used in combination if the above syndromes accompany with each other. As it was described in *Tracing the Origin of Materic Medica* (《本草崇原》, Bencaochongyuan), "Largehead Atractylodes Rhizome(白术,Baizhu)and Swordlike Atractylodes Rhizome(苍术,Cangzhu)are different from each other in reinforcing and activating. The two proposes may go with each other by means of combination of the two herbs, while the proportion of the propose depends upon the proportion of the dosage. "This tells the essential utilization of them.

Largehead Atractylodes Rhizome(白术, Baizhu)is a herb for strengthening, especially effective for the spleen. However, if used improperly, it may make the fullness sensation even worse due to dampness-stagnancy. To avoid this, it is often used in combination with Immature Bitter Orange(枳实, Zhishi), Tangerine Peel (陈皮, Chenpi), Villous Amomum Fruit(砂仁,Sharen), etc in order to associate reinforcement and reduction together. In addition, if it is parched with soil, its stagnant property will be reduced. Furthermore, it has the functions of activating the spleen qi, moistening the intestine and relaxing the bowels if a large dosage of approximately 60 grams is used.

5. 山药, Shanyao

English name: Common Yam Rhizome

Pharmaceutical name: Radix Dioscoreae Oppositae

Botanical name: Dioscorea opposita Thunb.

山 药

Properties and tastes: sweet and mild

Meridian tropism: lung, kidney and spleen

Functions: 1. tonify qi and nourish yin

2. tonify the lung, spleen and kidney

3. arrest qi and astringe yin

4. reduce blood sugar

Indications: 1. poor appetite, loose stools or diarrhea due to deficiency of the spleen

2. cough and asthma due to deficiency of the lung

3. frequent seminal emission, premature ejaculation, frequency of urine, women have a large quantity of leukorrhea due to kidney deficiency

4. diabetes

Dosage: 9 ~ 30g, a large dosage about 60 ~ 250g can be used. Grind it into fine powder and take the powder 6 ~ 9g each time. Crude Common Yam Rhizome (生山药, Shengshanyao) is used for nourishing yin, and it is suitably used for invigorating the spleen to arrest diarrhea after being parched.

Contraindication: This herb has the action of nourishing yin, and may cause interior pathogenic dampness. It is not suggested for patients with dampness blockage in the Middle-jiao or stagnation in the interior.

Combinations: 1. add Dwarf Lilyturf Root (麦门冬, Maimendong) Chinese Magnoliavine (五味子, Wuweizi)——cough, asthma, general lassitude due to lung deficiency

2. add Largehead Atractylodes Rhizome (白术, Baizhu) Plantain Seed (车前子, Cheqianzi)——large quantity of leukorrhea due to deficiency

3. add Prepared Rhizome of Adhesive Rehmannia (熟地黄, Shoudihuang) Asiatic Cornelian Cherry Fruit (山茱萸, Shanzhuyu)——dizziness, vertigo, tinnitus and deafness, lumbar soreness, frequent seminal emission, premature ejaculation, frequency of urine due to excessive fire and deficiency of the kidney yin

4. add Membranous Milkvetch Root (黄芪, Huangqi) Snakegourd Root (天花粉, Tianhuafen)——diabetes

5. add Sharpleaf Galangal Fruit (益智仁, Yizhiren) Combined Spicebush Root (乌药, Wuyao)——frequency of urination due to kidney deficiency

6. add Largehead Atractylodes Rhizome (白术, Baizhu), Hindu Lotus Seed (莲子, Lianzi) and Tuckahoe (茯苓, Fuling)——poor appetite, loose stools due to deficiency of the spleen

7. add Swordlike Atractylodes Rhizome (苍术, Cangzhu)——deficient diarrhea due to damp heat in the large intestine

8. add Coix Seed (薏苡仁, Yiyiren) White Crystal On Dried Persimmon (柿霜, Shingshuang)——deficiency of spleen and lung yin, poor appetite, consumptive cough due to deficiency heat

Prescriptions: 1. Bolus of Six Drugs Containing Rhizome Rehmanniae Peaeparatae (六味地黄丸, Liuweidihuang Wan)

2. Rhizoma Dioscoreae (薯蓣丸, Shuyu Wan)

Notes: Common Yam Rhizome (山药, Shanyao), which was once used under the name of 薯蓣 (Shuyu), has the function of nourishing yin and qi and improving the functions of the spleen and the stomach. In addition, it is able to nourish lung-yin and arrest the exhaustion of the kidneys. Consequently, the deficient syndromes involving the spleen, the lungs, and the kidneys, the symptoms of diarrhea, cough, asthma, nocturnal emission, frequency of micturition and leukorrhagia are indications. It is commonly selected for the feature of treating the root (the kidneys) and secondary organs (the spleen and the stomach) together. It is acknowledged as a dietetic medication because of its good taste and mild property.

6. 扁豆, Biandou

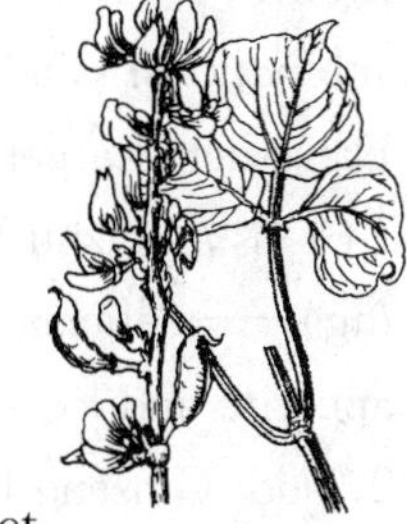
扁 豆

English name: Hyacinth Bean

Pharmaceutical name: Semen Dolichoris Lablab

Botanical name: Dolichos lablab L.

Properties and tastes: sweet and slight warm

Meridian tropism: liver, stomach

Functions: 1. promote the functions of the spleen and reduce dampness

2. expel toxin

Indications: 1. diarrhea due to deficiency of the spleen——poor appetite, loose stools, lassitude and fatigue (diarrhea of chronic enteritis or chronic hepatitis)

2. morbid leukorrhea due to spleen deficiency——a large quantity of leukorrhea, lassitude and fatigue

3. vomiting and diarrhea due to summer-dampness

4. detoxicate wines, arsenic poisoning, tetrodontoxism, poisoning of calomel

Dosage: 9～30g.

Contraindication: Hyacinth Bean (扁豆, Biandou) contains poisonous protein. Uncooked Hyacinth Bean (扁豆, Biandou) is poisonous. The toxicity of Hyacinth Bean (扁豆, Biandou) is greatly reduced when it is heated. Be cautious when taking powder of uncooked Hyacinth Bean (生扁豆, Shengbiandou).

Combinations: 1. add Common Yam Rhizome (山药, Shanyao)——diarrhea due to spleen deficiency, morbid leukorrhea

2. add Haichow Elsholtzia Herb (香薷, Xiangru) Officinal Magnolia Bark (厚朴, Houpo)——catching cold after enjoying the cool in hot summer months (yin-summer-heat syndrome)

3. add Lobed Kudzuvine Leaf (葛花, Gehua)——detoxicate wine

4. add Reed Rhizome (芦根, Lugen)——detoxicate tetrodontoxism

Prescription: Powder of Radix Gingeng, Poria and Rhizoma Atractylodis Macrocephalae (参苓白术散, Shenlingbaizhu San)

Notes: Hyacinth Bean (扁豆, Biandou) is said in *Developed Inferpretation of the Herbs* (《药品化义》, Yaopinhuayi), "to be effective in treatment of cholera, drastic vomiting, borborygmus, diarrhea, stomach injuries due to summer heat or alcohol. Therefore, it is a good choice for regulating the stomach and invigorating qi." It is best parched when used to invigorate the spleen and arrest diarrhea, and it is used fresh to remove summer heat and toxic substances.

7. 甘草, Gancao

甘 草

English name: Licorice Root

Pharmaceutical name: Radix Glycyrrhizae Uralensis

Botanical name: Glycyrrhiza uralensis Fisch.

Properties and tastes: sweet and medium

Meridian tropism: lung, heart, spleen and stomach

Functions: 1. invigorate the spleen and replenish qi

2. moisten the lung to relieve cough

3. relieve spasm and pain

4. coordinate the actions of various ingredients in a prescription

5. mitigate the properties of herbs
6. function as glucocorticoid hormone
7. function as mineralocorticoid hormone
8. prevent ulcer
9. relieve gastrointestinal spasm
10. inhibit gastric acid secretion
11. detoxicate
12. reduce blood fat
13. prevent cancer
14. protect the liver
15. antidiuresis

Indications: 1. spleen and stomach qi deficiency——shortness of breath, lassitude, poor appetite, loose stools, etc.
2. cough and asthma
3. carbuncle, sores, pyogenic infection
4. alimentary intoxication or medicine intoxication
5. pain of epigastrium and abdomen, spasm and pain of the limbs
6. addisonism
7. diabetes insipidus
8. Sheehan's syndrome
9. gastroduodenal ulcer
10. IH(infectious hepatitis)
11. purpura
12. suppurativetonsillitis

Dosage: 3~9g. Crude Licorice Root(生甘草, Shenggancao) is mostly used for detoxication, while stir-fried Licorice Root(炙甘草, Zhigancao) is used for tonifying qi and alleviating pain.

Contraindication: This herb is sweet in taste, and can cause interior pathogenic dampness and block qi, makes the person feel full in the epigastrium and abdomen. Use cautiously for patients with vomiting, fullness and distention in the chest and abdomen due to excessive dampness. Incompatible with Peking Euphorbia Root(大戟, Daji), Lilac Daphne Flower-bud(芫花, Yuanhua), Seaweed(海藻, Haizao). Taking a large dosage of this herb for a long time may cause edema. So pay attention to this point when using it.

Combinations: 1. add Dang-shen Root(党参, Dangshen) Largehead Atractylodes Rhizome (白术, Baizhu) Tuckahoe (茯苓, Fuling)——deficiency of the spleen qi, poor appetite and loose stools
2. add Ginseng (人参, Renshen), Cassia Twig (桂枝, Guizhi), Rehmannia Dried Root (生地黄, Shengdihuang)——qi and blood deficiency, a knotty or regularly-intermittent pulse, palpitation, shortness of breath
3. add Honeysuckle Flower(金银花, Jinyinhua), Dandelion(蒲公英, Pugongying)——carbuncle, scabies, pyogenic infection
4. add Balloonflower Root(桔梗, Jiegeng), Figwort Root (元参, Xuanshen)——swelling and pain of the throat
5. add Apricot Seed(杏仁, Xingren), Tendrilleaf Fritillary Bulb (贝母, Beimu) and Mulberry Leaf (桑叶, Sangye)——dry cough due to lung-heat, cough with little phlegm, difficult to expectorate or dry cough without phlegm caused by upper respiratory tract infrection, bronchitis
6. add Chinese Date(大枣, Dazao)——purpura
7. add Snakegourd Fruit (瓜蒌, Gualou) Baikal Skullcap Root(黄芩, Huangqin)——cough with expectoration of thick yellowish sputum
8. add Dried Ginger (干姜, Ganjiang) Manchurian Wildginger Herb (细辛, Xixin)——cough, profuse thin white sputum
9. add Cuttle-bone(乌贼骨, Wuzeigu) Tangerine Peel(陈皮, Chenpi)——gastroduode-

nal ulcer

10. add Ephedra(麻黄,Mahuang),Perilla Leaf(紫苏,Zisu)——invasion of the body surface by wind cold

11. add Talc(滑石,Huashi)——heliosis in summer,heat in both interior and exterior, irritability and thirst, difficult micturition, vomiting, diarrhea, infection of urinary system

12. add Greed Gram Seed (绿豆, Lüdou)——heat stroke, carbuncle, sores, pyogenic infection

13. add White Peony Root (白芍药, Baishaoyao)——stomachache and abdominal pain, spasm and pain of the limbs

14. add Capillary Wormwood Herb(茵陈蒿,Yinchenhao)——IH(infectious hepatitis)

15. add Oriental Waterplantain Rhizome(泽泻,Zexie)——arrhythmia

Prescriptions: 1. Decoction of Ramulus Cinnamomi and Radix Glycyrrhizae Constitution(桂枝甘草汤,Guizhigancao Tang)

2. Decoction of Prepared Licorice(炙甘草汤,Zhigancao Tang)

Notes: Licorice Root(甘草, Gancao) takes a supplementary role when taken to reinforce spleen-qi, to humidify the lungs to arrest cough, or to relieve convulsion and pain. Its distinguishing function is to harmonize. Actually, the harmonizing effect can be divided into two aspects. First, it has the function of detoxicating, and is effective in treatment of poisoning from food, drugs, or pesticides. It may be taken decocted solely or together with green beans. Second, the feature of Licorice Root(甘草, Gancao) is to alleviate or to dampen the actions of other herbs. For example, if given with Prepared Daughter Root of Common Monkshood(附子, Fuzi) and dried Fresh Ginge(生姜,Shengjiang), it may reduce their shortcoming of being hot, drying-up, and yin-damaging; if with Common Anemarrhea Rhizome (知母, Zhimu) and Gypsum(石膏; Shigao), it may reduce their cold property and protect stomach qi. If it is given with Rhubarb(大黄, Dahuang) and Mirabilite(芒硝, Mangxiao), the purgation will be milder. If with the reinforcing herbs such as Dang-shen Root(党参, Dangshen), Largehead Atractylodes Rhizome(白术, Baizhu), Chinese Angelica Root(当归, Danggui), and Prepared Rhizome of Adhesive Rehmannia (熟地黄, Shoudihuang), it can cause gradual effectiveness. Furthermore, if used in the group of cold-natured and hot-natured herbs, it will alleviate their actions.

In addition, this herb has similar action to cortical hormone according to recent pharmacological research. it is reported it is used for treatment of endocrinopathy. For example, its extract may be given at the dose of 15 ml per day for addison's disease; its powder may be given at the dose of 5 grams four times per day for diabetes insipidus; and 10 grams tid. For Sheehan's syndrome. If combined with western drugs, it may have a better effect.

8. 大枣, Dazao

English name: Chinese Date

Pharmaceutical name: Fructus Ziziphi Jujibae

Botanical name: Ziziphus jujuba Mill. var. inermis(Bge.)Rehd.

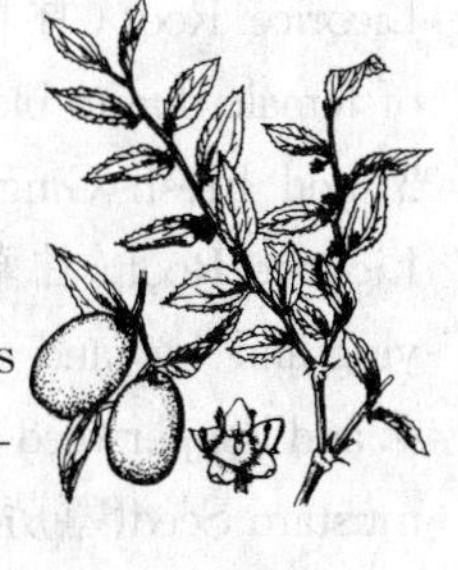
大 枣

Properties and tastes: sweet and warm

Meridian tropism: spleen, stomach

Functions: 1. strengthen the Middle-jiao and qi

2. nourish the blood to tranquilize

3. reinforce qi to arrest bleeding

4. harmonize the functions of different drugs

Indications: 1. deficiency of both the spleen and stomach syndrome——poor appetite, loose stools, lassitude with sallow complexion, thin body or muscles

2. hysteria due to blood deficiency in female——anxiety, sadness without reason. It can usually be seen in climacteric syndrome

3. failure of the spleen in controlling blood leads to the deficiency of spleen-qi——hematochezia, epistaxis, etc. For example TP(thrombocytolytic purpura)

4. relieve severe stimulation in the stomach and intestines after administration

5. can be used for improving constitution, strengthening myodynamia and protecting the liver

Dosage: 3～12 pieces.

Contraindication: It is not suggested for patients with damp-heat in Middle-jiao, cough due to phlegm-heat. A large dosage will moisten the intestines and relax the bowels.

Combinations: 1. add Dang-shen Root (党参, Dangshen) Largehead Atractylodes Rhizome(白术, Baizhu)——deficiency of both the spleen and stomach syndrome

2. add Blight Wheat(浮小麦, Fuxiaomai), Licorice Root (甘草, Gancao)——hysteria of female due to blood deficiency

3. add Fresh Ginger (生姜, Shengjiang), Licorice Root (甘草, Gancao)——regulate ying and wei, and to improve appetite

4. add Pepperweed Seed or Flixweed Tansymustard Seed(葶苈子, Tinglizi)——inability to lie on the back due to asthma, edema of the limbs, which belong to excessive syndrome

5. add Ass-hide Glue (阿胶, Ejiao)——all kinds of bleeding manifested as deficiency of ying-blood, and can also treat TP(thrombocy-tolytic purpura)

6. add Ephedra(麻黄, Mahuang), Prepared Daughter Root of Common Monkshood(附子, Fuzi)——Bi syndrome due to wind-cold-damp For example, rheumatic arthritis, sciatica

Prescriptions: 1. Decoction of Lepidium and Jujube for Removing Phlegm(葶苈大枣泻肺汤, Tinglidazaoxiefei Tang)

2. Decoction of Licorice, Wheat and Chinese-dates(甘麦大枣汤, Ganmaidazao Tang)

Notes: Chinese Date (大枣, Dazao) is mild in property. Hence, it is used as a supplementary herb to regulate and reinforce the spleen and the stomach. It is also used in diet to improve diseases with blood deficiency because it is tasty. In the clinic, it has been recently used for allergic purpura. It takes effect after a long period of administration.

9. 饴糖, Yitang

English name: Malt Sugar

Pharmaceutical name: Saccharum Granorum

Properties and tastess: sweet and warm

Meridian tropism: spleen, stomach and lung

Functions: 1. strengthen the spleen and replenish its qi

2. relieve spasm and pain

3. humidify lung to arrest cough

Indications: 1. deficiency cold of spleen and stomach——over working or over resting damages the spleen, shortness of breath, lassitude, poor appetite

2. abdominal pain due to deficiency cold, pain in the abdomen which is relieved after meals, and prefer heat and pressure

3. cough and asthma due to lung deficiency,

dry cough without phlegm, shortness of breath and asthma

Dosage: 30～60g, dissolved in decoction, 2～3 times for oral use

Contraindication: It can generate interior pathogenic dampness and heat, which makes the person feel full in the epigastrium and abdomen. It is unsuitable for patients with accumulation of damp-heat in the interior, vomiting due to stagnation of pathogens in the Middle-jiao, cough and asthma due to phlegm-heat, and malnutrition in children.

Combinations: 1. add Cassia Twig (桂枝, Guizhi), White Peony Root (白芍药, Baishaoyao), stir-fried Licorice Root (炙甘草, Zhigancao)——abdominal pain due to deficiency cold of spleen and stomach

2. add Pepertree (川椒, Chuanjiao), Dried Ginger (干姜, Ganjiang), Ginseng (人参, Renshen)——pain in the chest and abdomen due to excessive cold

3. add Apricot Seed (杏仁, Xingren), Sessile Stemon Root (百部, Baibu)——cough due to lung deficiency

Prescription: Minor Decoction for Strenthening Middle-energizer (小建中汤, Xiaojianzhong Tang)

Notes: Malt (麦芽, Maiya) extract is made from powder of polished glutinous rice, which is boiled. After well boiled, it is mixed with Malt (麦芽, Maiya) and the mixture is then boiled further with gentle fire. Despite its functions of reinforcing the stomach and relieving convulsion to ease pain, it has shortcomings such as promoting generation of damp-heat and dental caries if too much is eaten.

10. 蜂蜜, Fengmi

English name: Honey

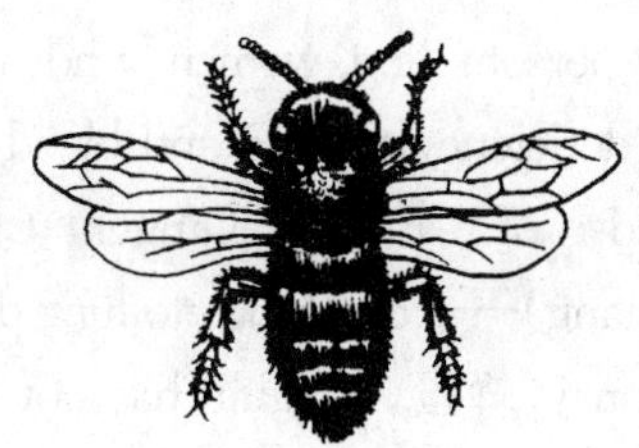

蜂 蜜

Pharmaceutical name: Mel

Properties and tastes: sweet and mild

Meridian tropism: lung, spleen and large intestine

Functions: 1. nourish the spleen and lung

2. arrest cough, relieve pain, detoxicate

3. lubricate the intestines to loosen bowels

Indications: 1. deficiency of the stomach and spleen syndrome, lassitude and poor appetite

2. deficiency cold in the Middle-jiao, pain in the epigastrium and abdomen

3. protracted cough due to lung deficiency, dry cough due to lung drying and dry throat

4. constipation due to intestinal drying

5. burn empyroaia for external use

Dosage: 15～30g, taken with water or used in bolus, or in orintment.

Contraindication: It can generate interior pathogenic dampness, which makes the person feel fullness in the epigastrium and abdomen, and having a loos stool. So use cautiously for patients with stagnation of dampness, heat and phlegm, oppressive feeling in the chest, diarrhea with loose stools.

Combinations: 1. add Rehmannia Dried Root (生地黄, Shengdihuang) Tuckahoe (茯苓, Fuling) Ginseng (人参, Renshen)——deficiency of the spleen and stomach syndrome, consumptive disease and dry cough or hemoptysis.

2. add Chinese Angelica Root (当归, Danggui) Black Sesame (黑芝麻, Heizhima)——

elderly persons and women who are weak due to deficiency of fluid and blood

3. add of Fresh Ginger (生姜, Shengjiang)——cough due to lung deficiency

Notes: Honey (蜂蜜, Fengmi) has not only the function of reinforcing the stomach and the spleen, but also the function of harmonizing the actions of other herbs. Therefore, it is used as a vehicle in pill or ointment medications of reinforcement. In addition, it will enhance the function of some of the nourishing herbs, such as astragalus root and Licorice Root (甘草, Gancao), if fried together. This herb also has the function of humidifying the lungs to arrest cough. As a result, herbs with similar functions, such as Common Coltsfoot Flower (款冬花, Kuandonghua) and Loquat Leaf (枇杷叶, Pipaye) are often processed with Honey (蜂蜜, Fengmi) to enhance their functions. Having the function of humidifying the intestine to free the movement of bowel, it is usually given for the constipation due to deficiency, especially as a dietetic medication.

It is said in *Compendium of Materia Medica* (《本草纲目》, Bencaogangmu), Honey (蜂蜜, Fengmi) has five basic functions: to clear away heat, strengthen the stomach and the spleen, reduce toxic effects, moisten dryness, and stop pain. The harmonizing may result in balance, so it has the similar effect with Licorice Root (甘草, Gancao) in balancing the actions of other herbs.

Section 2
Drugs for Invigorating Yang

1. 鹿茸, Lurong

English name: Hairy Antler

Pharmaceutical name: Cornu Cervi Pantotrichum

Botanical name: Cervus elaphus Linnaeus

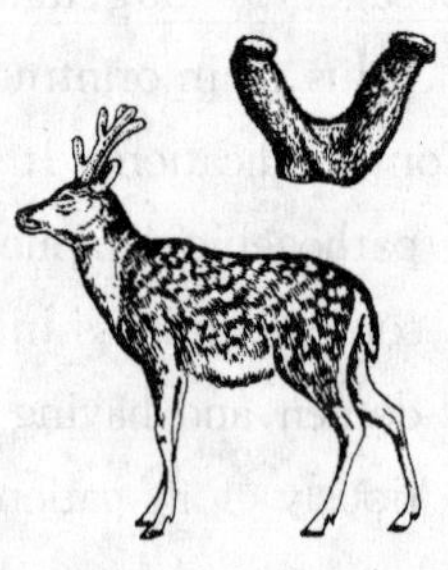
鹿 茸

Properties and tastes: sweet, salty and warm

Meridian tropism: liver, kidney

Functions: 1. reinforce kidney yang

3. strengthen the muscles and bones

4. regulate Chong and Ren meridions, stop metrorrhagia and leukorrhagia

5. treat chronic carbuncle of yin type

6. strengthen the body and fight fatigue

7. promote the production of red cells and hemoglobin, increase white cells and blood platelet

8. enhance the contracture of cardiac muscle, raise blood pressure

9. excite intestinal tract and uterine, smooth muscle

10. strengthen regeneration and shorten the healing time of wound and bone fracture

11. promote growth and development

Indications: 1. deficiency of kidney yang syndrome——aversion to cold and cold limbs, impotence and premature ejaculation, sterility due to retention of cold pathogen in the uterus, frequent micturition, soreness and pain of the lumbar region and knee joints, listlessness, etc

2. congenital defect, insufficiency of essence

and blood syndrome-deficiency of development in children, weak bones and walking retardation in children, delayed dentition, infantile metopism or aging before his(her) time

3. leukorrhagia due to deficiency of the kidney for metrorrhagia and metrostaxis, Leukorrhagia due to cold and deficiency of Chong and Ren meridians, which is accompanied with deficiency of the kidney yang syndrome as discussed above

4. a sore which has festered for a long period, sinking of chronic carbuncle of yin type, etc

5. severe anemia due to insufficiency of essence and blood, such as aplastic anemia

6. heat failure, especially used for patient with rheumatic heat disease manifested as palpitation, shortness of breath, dyspnea, difficulty in urination

7. neurosis or weakness after illness manifested as deficiency of kidney yang

8. thrombocytopenia, leukopenia, blood disease due to chronic benzene poisoning

Dosage: 1～3g, grind it into fine powder. Take three times a day.

Contraindication: Take small doses in the begining and increase the dosage grandually. Do not take a large dose suddenly in case of dizziness, red eyes, yang hyperactivity and convulsions, or impairment of yin and bleeding. Use causiously for patients with hyperactivity of yang due to deficiency of yin, heat in the blood system, excessive stomach-fire, phlegm-fire stagnating in the lung and febrile disease caused by exogenous pathogens.

Combinations: 1. add Ginseng (人参, Renshen)——tonify vital qi, nourish essence and blood-impotence, emission, male infertility, anemia etc

2. add Prepared Rhizome of Adhesive Rehmannia (熟地黄, Shoudihuang)——to replenish kidney essence and nourish liver blood. Use in children with delayed and deficient growth

3. add Chinese Angelica Root (当归, Danggui)——recuperate Chong and Ren meridians to stop metrorrhagia and metrostaxis, used for women whose metrorrhagia and metrostaxis is treated for a long time

4. add East Asian Tree Fern Rhizome (狗脊, Gouji)——long term female leukorrhagia and general debility due to consumption of Du meridian, debility of Dai meridian

5. add Membranous Milkvetch Root (黄芪, Huangqi)——chronic carbuncle of yin type being festered and unhealed, discharging clear and thin pus

6. add Chinese Caterpillar Fungus (冬虫夏草, Dongchongxiacao)——rheumatic heart disease

7. add Dried Human Placenta (紫河车, Ziheche)——thrombocytopenia, leukopenia and aplastic anemia.

Prescription: Pill of Cornu Cervi Pantotrichum for Expelling Cold Evil and Restoring Yang (鹿茸再造丸, Lurongzaizao Wan)

Notes: Hairy Antler (鹿茸, Lurong) is an animal-originated medication that replenishes essence and blood for the kidneys. Its effects can be divided into two aspects. Firstly, it includes invigorating kidney-yang and yang in the Du Meridian and stimulating growth of the body. Secondly, it involves nourishing marrow and blood, strengthening the bones and stimulating the generation of sperm. It is quite effective in the treatment of male and female infertility or male sexual dysfunction. Note that it is only for the cases with the kidney yang deficient syndrome, whose symptoms and signs are aversion to cold, coldness in the limbs, cold pain in the waist and knees, deep weak pulse, and pale tongue with white tongue coating. If used for a long term, it ought to be given with yin-nourishing herbs, such as Prepared Rhizome of Adhesive Rehmannia (熟地黄, Shoudihuang), Common Yam Rhizome (山药, Shanyao), Ass-hide Glue (阿胶, Ejiao), etc. There are other drugs from the same source, which are antler, antler glue, and deglued antler powder. See the following table for their features.

Name	Properties and taste	Meridian tropism	Functions	Indications	Dosage
Antler (鹿角, Lujiao)	salty and warm	Liver and kidney	① Invigorate kidney-yang (weaker than Hairy Antler (鹿茸, Lurong) ② Eliminate blood stasis, promote blood circulation and subsiding swelling	Skin and external diseases, acute mastitis, pain due to blood stasis, and aching in waist, spine and limbs; severe cases of yang-deficient syndrome involving the kidneys	6～9 g
Antler Glue (鹿角胶, Lujiaojiao)	sweet, salty and slightly warm	Liver and kidney	① Strengthen liver and kidney and nourish essence and blood ②Arrest bleeding	Abnormal leanness, consumptive diseases, hematemesis, epistaxis, metrorrhagia, metrostaxis, hematuria (cold-deficient type), and chronic phlegm; cases with deficiency of essence and blood that are unsuitable for "stagnant replenishing"	6～9 g
Deglued Antler Powder (鹿角霜, Lujiaoshuang)	salty and slightly warm	Kidney	① Invigorate kidney-yang (relatively weaker) ② Astringency	yang-deficient syndromes involving the kidneys and the spleen with the symptoms of diarrhea before dawn, metrorrhagia and metrostaxis and leukorrhagia due to coldness, exudative skin diseases, and unhealed ulcer, especially suitable for the patients who are sensitive to "stagnant replenishing."	9～15 g

Hairy Antler (鹿茸, Lurong), Prepared Daughter Root of Common Monkshood (附子, Fuzi) and Cassia Twig (桂枝, Guizhi) invigorate kidney-yang. Being hot spicy, dry, prompt-acting and strong in warming and eliminating coldness, aconite root and Cassia Twig (桂枝, Guizhi) bark are appropriate for the cases of severe yang-deficiency and coldness-excess rather than those with insufficiency of essence and blood. Hairy Antler (鹿茸, Lurong) is sweet and salty in taste and warm in property. Gradually acting and replenishing essence and blood, Hairy Antler (鹿茸, Lurong) is more effective in the cases of yang-deficiency involving the kidneys complicated with insufficiency of essence and blood rather than those of coldness excess.

2. 紫河车, Ziheche

English name: Dried Human Placenta

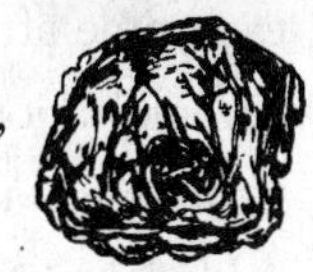

Pharmaceutical name: Placenta Hominis

Botanical name: Homo sapiens Linnaeus

Properties and tastes: sweet, salty, warm

Meridian tropism: lung, liver, kidney

Functions: 1. reinforce qi, replenish essence and nourish blood
2. promote the development of female mammary gland, genitals and ovary
3. strengthen body immunity and resistance
4. resist allergy

Indications: 1. insufficiency of kidney essence syndrome for sterility, impotence, emission, soreness of the back, dizziness, tinnitus, etc
2. deficiency of both qi and blood disease, consumptive disease due to overwork, weakness and emaciation due to deficiency of qi, sallow complexion or darkish and lusterless complexion
3. deficiency of both lung and kidney syndrome——dyspnea due to deficiency and prolonged cough, it can also be used in for pulmonary emphysema and tuberculosis
4. deficiency of qi and blood, unconsciousness caused by long-term epilepsy
5. lack of lactation after delivery

Dosage: 1.5～3g Grind it into powder and put the powder into a capsule and take it two or three times each day, take double dosage when it is used in serious syndrome, or used as an ingredient of bolus or powder. Eating fresh placenta after boiling the whole piece or half of it.

Contraindication: Not suitable for patients with hyperactivity caused by yin deficiency, if this material is used without adding other herbs.

Combinations: 1. add Dang-shen Root (党参, Dangshen)——anemia
2. add Indian Bread Hostwood (茯神, Fushen)——consumptive disease and overwork
3. add Dang-shen Root (党参, Dangshen), Membranous Milkvetch Root (黄芪, Huangqi)——deficiency of qi syndrome, manifested as spontaneous sweating, absence of strength, shortness of breath
4. add Prepared Rhizome of Adhesive Rehmannia (熟地黄, Shoudihuang), Chinese Angelica Root (当归, Danggui)——deficiency of blood syndrome, manifested as pale complexion, mental fatigue, palpitation, and dizziness
5. add Prepared Rhizome of Adhesive Rehmannia (熟地黄, Shoudihuang), Eucommia Bark (杜仲, Duzhong)——senile weakness, anemia
6. add Dang-shen Root (党参, Dangshen), Chinese Magnoliavine (五味子, Wuweizi)——cough and dyspnea due to lung deficiency
7. add Common Yam Rhizome (山药, Shanyao), Villous Amomum Fruit (砂仁, Sharen)——poor appetite due to spleen deficiency
8. add Siberian Solomonseal Rhizome (黄精, Huangjing), Giant Knotweed Rhizome (虎杖, Huzhang)——leukopenia
9. add Tortoise Shell and Plastron (龟版, Guiban), Chinese Corktree Bark (黄柏, Huangbai)——dizziness, tinnitus, soreness and weakness of the lumbar regions and knees, hectic fever due to deficiency of liver and kidney, flaming up of deficiency fire
10. add Asiatic Cornelian Cherry Fruit (山茱萸, Shanzhuyu), Barbary Wolfberry Fruit (枸杞子, Gouqizi), Common Yam Rhizome

(山药,Shanyao)——insufficiency of kidney essence syndrome

Prescription: Wonder Pill of Placenta Hominis (河车大造丸,Hechedazao Wan)

Notes: Dried Human Placenta (紫河车, Ziheche) is human-originated, rich in both property and taste, and therefore is powerful and effective in nourishing qi and blood. It is mainly given to the patients who are physically weak(some are from chronic diseases)and low in immunity. It is also given to the patients with chronic diseases, such as asthma and epilepsy in resting stages in order to prevent or reduce attacks. This drug takes effect only after a long-term administration and it is advisable to suspend use when the patient gets cold, has diarrhea, or bitter taste in the mouth due to internal heat-evil.

3. 蛤蚧, Gejie

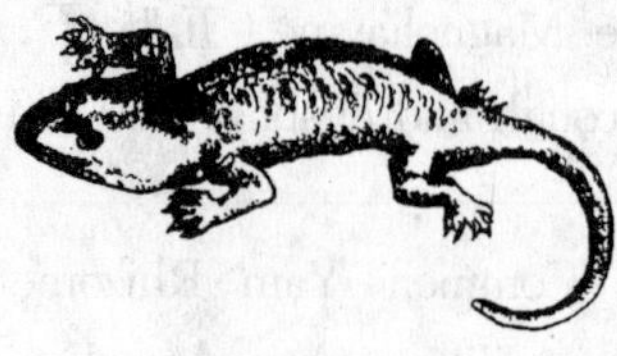

蛤 蚧

English name: Giant Gecko

Pharmaceutical name: Gecko

Properties and tastes: salty and medium

Meridian tropism: lung and kidney

Functions: 1. reinforce the lung, stop asthma

2. invigorate kidney yang, nourish blood and essence

Indications: 1. cough due to lung deficiency, dyspnea due to deficiency of the kidney, asthma and cough due to asthenia of viscera

2. impotence due to deficiency of kidney yang

Dosage: 3 ~ 6g, decocted with water. Make it into power and take 1 ~ 2g each time, three times a day. For oral use, take 1 ~ 2 pairs each time after it is soaked in the wine.

Contraindication: It is not advisable for patients with asthma and cough due to wind-cold or excess-heat.

Combinations: 1. add Ginseng (人参, Renshen), Apricot Seed (杏仁, Xingren), Tendrilleaf Fritillary Bulb (川贝母, Chuanbeimu)——cough and asthma due to deficiency of both lung and kidney

2. add Ginseng (人参, Renshen), Hairy Antler (鹿茸, Lurong), Shorthorned Epimediun Herb (淫羊藿, Yinyanghuo)——impotence

Prescription: Powder of Ginseng and Gecko (人参蛤蚧散, Renshengejie San)

Notes: Giant Gecko (蛤蚧, Gejie) is capable of reinforcing the lungs and the kidneys, arresting asthma and cough, and is most effective in treatment of asthma due to failure of the kidney to attract qi deep. The whole Giant Gecko (蛤蚧, Gejie) is applicable except the head, legs and scales. Its tail, however, is the most powerful part, used under the name of Giant Gecko (蛤蚧, Gejie) tail. Li Shizhen (李时珍) said, Giant Gecko (蛤蚧, Gejie) reinforces lung-qi, arrests asthma, relieves unquenchable thirst, which resembles Ginseng (人参, Renshen), and those functions resembling mutton that are nourishing blood and essence, and relieve general weakness. Told by Zhang Bingcheng (张秉成), another great ancient physician, Giant Gecko (蛤蚧, Gejie) helps to cure consumptive diseases, improves sexual abilities, and attracts primary qi back to the kidneys.

Current recent research has shown that Giant Gecko (蛤蚧, Gejie) has anti-inflammatory and adrenocorticotropic functions, greatly improves immunity, reduces blood sugar, increases activity of radical enzyme and content of GSH, and significantly LPO. Furthermore, it also assists in the prevention of aging.

4. 胡桃仁, Hutaoren

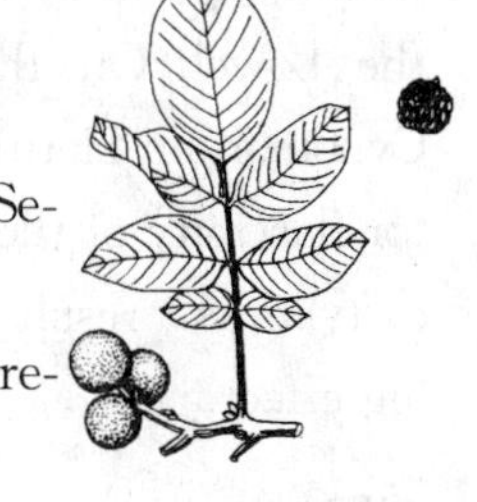

胡桃仁

English name: Walnut

Pharmaceutical name: Semen Juglandis Regiae

Botanical name: Juglans regia L.

Properties and tastes: sweet and warm

Meridian tropism: the kidney, lung and large intestine

Functions: 1. nourish the kidney and invigorate yang

2. strengthen the waist and knees

3. warm the lung to relieve asthma

4. invigorate the intestines and empty bowels

Indications: 1. lack of essence due to deficiency of kidney, lower-back pain and weakness of the foot, impotence and seminal emission, frequent and scanty urination

2. cough and asthma due to insufficiency cold, protracted cough due to lung deficiency

3. constipation due to dry intestine

Dosage: 9～30g.

Contraindication: It is not suggested for patients with hyperactivity of fire caused by deficiency of yin, cough due to phlegm for heat, and diarrhea.

Combinations: 1. add Eucommia Bark (杜仲, Duzhong)——lumbago pain and foot weakness due to deficiency of kidney

2. add Ginseng (人参, Renshen) Fresh Ginger (生姜, Shengjiang)——protracted cough and asthma due to lung deficiency

3. add Desertliving Gistanche (肉苁蓉, Roucongrong), Chinese Angelica Root (当归, Danggui)——constipation of elderly person due to deficiency of body fluid

Notes: Disorders mentioned above can be treated with Walnut (胡桃仁, Hutaoren). It is given as a dietetic herb with the following method: Put 1 kilogram of it and 1 kilogram of Honey (蜂蜜, Fengmi) in a pot in boiling water untill the Honey (蜂蜜, Fengmi) is well cooked. Take it without strict timing regularity, the honey and Walnut (胡桃仁, Hutaoren) is also mixed in boiling water.

It is said in *Dietary Materia Medica* (《食疗本草》, Shiliaobencao), Walnut (胡桃仁, Hutaoren) has the effects of promoting blood circulation and humidifying the meridian. After long-term administration, the results can be seen as black hair and fair skin conditions.

5. 肉苁蓉, Roucongrong

肉苁蓉

English name: Desertliving Cistanche

Pharmaceutical name: Herba Cistanches

Botanical name: Cistanche salsa (C. A. Mey.) G. Beck, C. deserticola Y. C. Ma, or C. ambigua (Bge.) G. Beck

Properties and tastes: sweet, salty and warm

Meridian tropism: kidney and large intestine

Functions: 1. reinforce kidney and strengthen yang

2. nourish the essence and blood

3. moisten the intestine and regulate defecation

4. lower blood pressure

Indications: 1. deficiency of kidney yang——

impotence infertility due to retention of cold in the uterus and cold pain in the waist and knees.

2. deficiency of blood and essence for soreness and weakness of the waist and knees, flaccidity of tendons and bones

3. constipation due to dry intestine, especially for individuals who are older and weak with constipation due to fluid exhaustion with yang deficiency

Dosage: 9～30g.

Contraindication: It is not suggested for patients with diarrhea due to spleen deficiency or constipation due to excess-heat.

Combinations: 1. add Dodder Seed (菟丝子, Tusizi)——impotence, aphoria

2. add Hairy Antler (鹿茸, Lurong), Common Yam Rhizome (山药, Shanyao)——seminal emission due to kidney deficiency enuresis (incontinence of urine)

3. add Antler Glue (鹿角胶, Lujiaojiao) Dried Human Placenta (紫河车, Ziheche)——infertility due to retention of cold in the uterus

4. add Eucommia Bark (杜仲, Duzhong), Himalayan Teasel Root (续断, Xuduan)——weakness of the bones and tendons

5. add Hemp Seed (火麻仁, Huomaren), Bitter Orange (枳壳, Zhiqiao)——constipation of people with weak consititution

Notes: In a mild manner, Desertliving Gistanche (肉苁蓉, Roucongrong) nourishes yin of the kidneys, stimulates its yang and frees movement of the bowel. Invigorate yang without causing dryness and nourishing yin without causing stagnancy. Therefore, pharmacological books suggest that the herb is be used for preserving health, prolonging lives, improving skin conditions and sexual ability. It is suggested that it be taken continuously in larger dosage, for it is mild in its function. Compared to Songaria Cynomorium Herb (锁阳, Suoyang), which has the similar functions and strong in warming and drying, it is better in exciting yang, as well as sexual activities, and freeing movement of the bowel. On the other hand, Songaria Cynomorium Herb (锁阳, Suoyang) is good for flaccidity of the limb of kidney deficiency type, as a result of its tendon-strengthening effect.

6. 锁阳, Suoyang

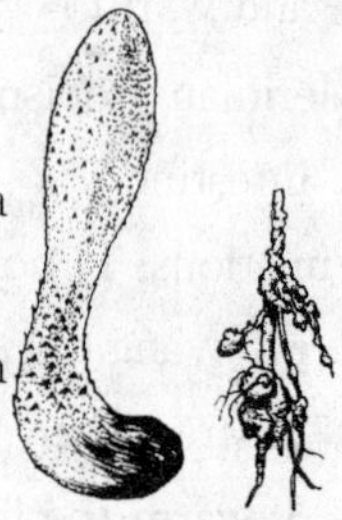

English name: Songaria Cynomorium Herb

Pharmaceutical name: Herba Cynomorii Songarici

Botanical name: Cynomorium songaricum Rupr.

Properties and tastes: sweet and warm

锁阳

Meridian tropism: liver, kidney and large intestine

Functions: 1. reinforce the kidney and invigorate yang

2. moisten the intestines and promote bowel movement

Indications: 1. deficiency of kidney yang, deficiency of both blood and essence——male impotence, female infertility, weakness and flaccidity of the waist and knees

2. constipation due to dry intestines and depleted fluid

Dosage: 9～15g.

Contraindication: Do not use for patients with hyperactivity of yang caused by yin deficiency, diarrhea due to spleen deficiency, and costipation due to excess-heat.

Combinations:

1. add Prepared Rhizome of Adhesive

Rehmannia(熟地黄, Shoudihuang), East Asian Tree Fern Rhizome(狗脊, Gouji)——male impotence

2. add Dodder Seed(菟丝子, Tusizi), Tuber Fleeceflower Root (何首乌, Heshouwu)——female infertility

3. add Prepared Rhizome of Adhesive Rehmannia(熟地黄, Shoudihuang), Tortoise Shell and Plastron(龟版, Guiban)——weakness and flaccidity of the waist and knees, weakness of the bones and tendons

4. add Hemp Seed(火麻仁, Huomaren), Chinese Angelica Root(当归, Danggui)——constipation

Notes: Songaria Cynomorium Herb(锁阳, Suoyang) is sweet, warm and humidifying in property and is capable of nourishing yin of the kidney and liver and exciting yang(including sexual ability) as well. Other functions involve strengthening tendons and relieving flaccidities. It is used in the treatment of flaccidities of the lower limbs of the deficient syndrome involving the kidney and liver. Similar to Desertliving Gistanche(肉苁蓉, Roucongrong), it is humidifying in effect and appropriate for constipation of senile patients, whose yang deficiency has already affected yin.

7. 巴戟天, Bajitian

English name: Medicinal Indian-mulberry Root

Pharmaceutical name: Radix Morindae Officinalis

Botanical name: Morinda officinalis How

巴戟天

Properties and tastes: pungent, sweet and slightly warm

Meridian tropism: kidney

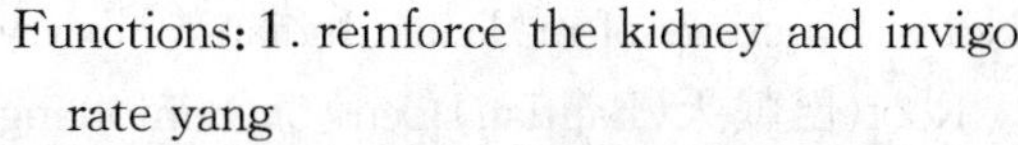

Functions: 1. reinforce the kidney and invigorate yang

2. strengthen bones and tendons

3. expel wind and eliminate dampness

Indications: 1. deficiency of the kidney yang syndrome——impotence frequent urination, infertility due to retention of cold in the uterus, irregular menstruation, and cold pain in the lower abdomen

2. soreness in the lumber region due to consumption of kidney essence and osteomalacia aching and limp bones

3. wind-cold-dampness Bi syndrome——contracture and spasm of muscles(pain in the joints, limited movement of limbs), severe stabbing and fixed pain in the joints, limited movement of the joints

Dosage: 9~15g.

Contraindication: It is not suggested for using by itself for patients with hyperactivity of fire caused by deficiency of yin or damp heat in the interior.

Combinations: 1. add Ginseng(人参, Renshe n), Common Yam Rhizome(山药, Shanyao), Palmleaf Raspberry Fruit(覆盆子, Fupenzi)——impotence, infertility

2. add Sharpleaf Galangal Fruit(益智仁, Yizhiren), Dodder Seed(菟丝子, Tusizi)——dilute urination(enuresis)

3. add Cassia Bark(肉桂, Rougui), Medicinal Evodia Root(吴茱萸, Wuzhuyu)——irregular menstruation; cold pain in the lower abdomen

4. add Twotooth Achyranthes Root(牛膝, Niuxi)——when decocted with wine it can treat impotence

5. add Hypoglaucous Collett Yam Rhizome(萆薢, Bixie), Eucommia Bark(杜仲, Duzhong)——pain or lassitute of the lumbar region and knees.

Notes: Functions of medicinal Indian-mulberry Root(巴戟天, Bajitian) focus on reinforcing kidney-yang and dispelling wind-dampness evils. It is humidifying and mild, nourishing both yin and yang, but not stagnant, expelling but not drying. It shows good results in the treatment of impotence, high frequency of micturition, sterility and irregularity of menstruation of kidney-qi deficiency complicated with wind-dampness evils, which has the typical symptoms of pain or weakness in the waist and knee joints. As a substitution of Cassia Bark(肉桂, Rougui), Prepared Daughter Root of Common Monkshood(附子, Fuzi), it is applicable to edema due to kidney deficiency so as to avoid their side-effects of drying-up and yin impairment.

8. 杜仲, Duzhong

English name: Eucommia Bark

Pharmaceutical name: Cortex Eucommiae Ulmoidis

Botanical name: Eucommia ulmoides Oliv.

Properties and tastes: sweet and warm

杜 仲

Meridian tropism: liver and kidney

Functions: 1. reinforce both the liver and kidney

2. strengthen bones and tendons

3. stop metrorrhagia and prevent miscarriage

4. reduce blood pressure

5. dilate blood vessels and reduce serum cholesterol

6. resist inflammation

7. tranquilize and stop pain

8. strengthen body immunity

Indications: 1. soreness and pain of the lumbar and knees or flaccidity and weakness of the lumbar and knees

2. impotence, frequent urination due to cold deficiency of the liver and kidney

3. threatened abortion, habitual abortion

Dosage: 9 ~ 15g, stir-barked Eucommia Bark (杜仲, Duzhong) has better effect than fresh Eucommia Bark(生杜仲, Shengduzhong).

Contraindication: Use cautiously with patients with hyperactivity of fire caused by deficiency of yin.

Combinations: 1. add Prepared Rhizome of Adhesive Rehmannia (熟地黄, Shoudihuang), Twotooth Achyranthes Root (牛膝, Niuxi)——deficiency of liver and kidney, soreness and pain of the lumbar region and knees, flaccidity and weakness of the lumbar and knees

2. add Asiatic Cornelian Cherry Fruit(山茱肉, Shanyurou), Dodder Seed(菟丝子, Tusizi)——cold deficiency of liver and kidney, impotence, frequent urination

3. add Himalayan Teasel Root(续断, Xuduan), Common Yam Rhizome (山药, Shanyao)——threatened abortion, habitual abortion.

4. add White Peony Root (白芍药, Baishaoyao), Common Selfheal Fruit-spike (夏枯草, Xiakucao)——dizziness due to hyperactivity of liver yang and hypertension

Notes: As a consequence of its liver-kidney-fortifying and tendon-bone-strengthening functions, Eucommia Bark(杜仲, Duzhong) is one of the commonly selected herbs for the liver-kidney deficiency syndrome that has the symptoms of aching, flaccidities of waist, knee joints, enuresis, threatened abortion, vertigo, and so on. *Essentials of Materia Medica* (《本草备要》, Bencaobeiyao) says that it takes effect in the qi aspect of the liver, humidifies it to correct its dryness syndrome, and nourishes to cure its insufficiency. By means of the mother-child relationship from Five-element theory, a "child" is able to help the "mother" to regain its strength, it helps the kidney. Accordingly, the herb's functions focus on the liver. Another book, *Herbals for Easy Approaching* (《本草便读》, Bencaobiandu) says, however, Eucommia Bark (杜仲, Duzhong) is more for evil-eliminating than for reinforcing, which should be taken into account in clinical practice.

9. 续断, Xuduan

English name: Himalayan Teasel Root

Pharmaceutical name: Radix Dipsaci

Botanical name: Dipsacus japonica Miq. Or D. Asper Wall.

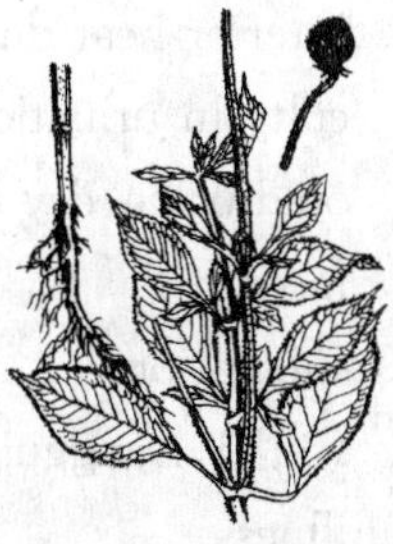

续 断

Properties and tastes: bitter, sweet, pungent and slightly warm

Meridian tropism: liver and kidney

Functions: 1. reinforce both the liver and kidney

2. miscarriage prevention

3. promote the circulation of blood, promote reunion of fractured bones

Indications: 1. lumbar pain, soreness of the foot due to deficiency of both the liver and kidney

2. seminal emission, metrorrhagia and metrostaxis, vaginal bleeding during pregnancy of habitual abortion due to deficiency of liver and kidney

3. traumatic injury, injury of muscles and fractured bones

4. carbuncle, deep rooted carbuncle, pyogenic infection and ulceration of skin

Dosage: 9 ~ 15g, stir-baked Himalayan Teasel Root (续断, Xuduan) is used for metorrhagia metrosaxis, and hematochezia. For external use, grind it into powder and apply it to the affected area.

Combinations: 1. add Eucommia Bark (杜仲, Duzhong)——soreness and pain of the lumbar and knees, which have weakness and lassitute, wind-cold-dampness Bi syndrome, metrorrhagia and metrastaxis, threatened aborition

2. add Membranous Milkvetch Root (黄芪, Huangqi), Prepared Rhizome of Adhesive Rehmannia (熟地黄, Shoudihuang)——metrorrhagia and metrostaxis, and excessive menses

3. add Chinese Taxillus Twig (桑寄生, Sangjisheng), Dodder Seed (菟丝子, Tusizi), Ass-hide Glue (阿胶, Ejiao)——vaginal bleeding during pregnancy, habitual abortion

4. add Olibanum, Frankincense (乳香, Ruxiang), Myrrh (没药, Moyao)——traumatic injury from fracure bone

5. add Dandelion (蒲公英, Pugongying)——acute mastitis

6. add Siberian Solomonseal Rhizome (黄精, Huangjing)——treat consumptive disease and relieve lumbar pain

Prescription: Pills for Preventing Habitual Abortion (寿胎丸, Shoutai Wan)

Notes: Himalayan Teasel Root (续断, Xuduan)'s feature is reinforcing without being stagnant, for it has two functions. One is as reinforcing the liver-kidney system and warming the uterus; the other is promoting blood circulation and strengthening the functions of joints. Therefore, it is commonly given for threatened abortions, ligament injuries, fractures, and skin diseases as well. Similar to Himalayan Teasel Root(续断, Xuduan) and Chinese Taxillus Twig(桑寄生, Sangjisheng), have the functions to reinforce the liver and kidney, strengthen tendons and bones, and nourish blood to cure threatened abortions. The two herbs are used interchangeably or together to cure knee-waist aching and weakness from liver-kidney deficiency, threatened abortions and vaginal bleeding during pregnancy from insufficiency of essence and blood. The difference lies in the fact that Himalayan Teasel Root(续断, Xuduan) is a dredger of vessels without rendering hemorrhage, and helps to cure fractures and ligament injuries, hence, is given for fracture and metrorrhagia and metrostaxis, while Chinese Taxillus Twig (桑寄生, Sangjisheng) is an eliminator of wind-dampness evils and is given for aching (especially of waist) from wind-dampness evils and liver-kidney deficiency.

This herb resembles Twotooth Achyranthes Root(牛膝, Niuxi) in properties and functions and indications. However, Twotooth Achyranthes Root(牛膝, Niuxi) acts more on descending blood while Himalayan Teasel Root(续断, Xuduan) is more effective in warming and reinforcing.

10. 狗脊, Gouji

English name: East Asian Tree Fern Rhizome

Pharmaceutical name: Rhizoma Cibotii Barometz

Botanical name: Cibotium barometz (L.) J. Sm.

Properties and tastes: bitter, sweet and warm

Meridian tropism: liver and kidney

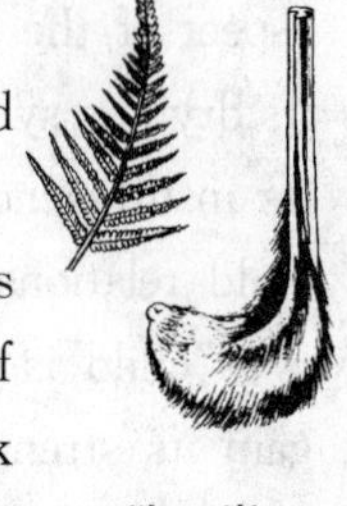

狗脊

Functions: 1. reinforce liver and kidney

2. strengthen the waist and knees

3. eliminate wind-dampness

Indications: 1. deficiency of liver and kidney and attack of wind-cold-dampness pathogens for lumbar pain and stiffness of back, inability to bend or lift readily, weakness of the knees and feet

2. failure of kidney qi deficiency to store for incontinence of urine, excessive leukorrhea of women

Dosage: 9～15g

Contraindication: Do not use for patients with interior-heat due to kidney deficiency, difficulty in urination, or oligura with deep colored urine, dry mouth and bitter taste in the mouth.

Combinations: 1. add Chinese Angelica Root (当归, Danggui)——edema of the feet after illness

2. add Dodder Seed(菟丝子, Tusizi)——waist pain of kidney disease

3. add Chinese Taxillus Twig(桑寄生, Sangjisheng), Eucommia Bark(杜仲, Duzhong), Twotooth Achyranthes Root(牛膝, Niuxi)——deficiency of the kidney and liver, lumbar pain and stiffness of the back, inability to bend or lift freely, weakness of the knees and foot

4. add Dodder Seed(菟丝子, Tusizi), Chinese Magnoliavine(五味子, Wuweizi), Mantis Egg-case(桑螵蛸, Sangpiaoxiao)——frequent urination due to kidney deficiency

5. add Largehead Atractylodes Rhizome(白术, Baizhu), Japanese Ampelopsis Root(白敛, Bailian) Swordlike Atractylodes Rhizome

(苍术, Cangzhu)——a large quantity of leukorrhea

6. add Leatherleaf Mahonia Leaf(十大功劳, Shidagonglao)——deficiency of liver and kidney, dizzness, tinnitus, soreness and pain of the lumbar, weakness of the feet and knees

It can also be used for treating Bi syndrome due to wind-cold-damp.

Notes: Ancient people considered East Asian Tree Fern Rhizome(狗脊, Gouji) was capable of strengthening spine and the Du Meridian originally because of the similarity between it and a dog's spine in shape. In fact, it works. Its functions include nourishing liver, kidney and removing wind-dampness evils. Consequently, arthritis, especially spinal diseases, is its main indication. It is told in *Shennong's Herbal Classic* (《神农本草经》, Shennongbencaojing), the herb is used for stiffness of the spine, spasm of various joints, general obstruction syndrome, knee pain from cold-dampness and varied senile diseases. The functions of reinforcing liver, kidney and bone-tendon are found in East Asian Tree Fern Rhizome(狗脊, Gouji), Eucommia Bark(杜仲, Duzhong) and Medicinal Indianmulberry Root(巴戟天, Bajitian). Eucommia Bark (杜仲, Duzhong), however, is more effective on liver kidney deficiency, while Medicinal Indianmulberry Root(巴戟天, Bajitian) on yang-strengthening rather than drying or wind-dampness-removing. In addition, the herb can be used for hemorrhage due to skin diseases, lingering blockage of circulation, while the black species for parasitosis, according to *Supplement to the Compendium of Materia Medica* (《本草纲目拾遗》, Bencaogangmushiyi).

11. 益智仁, Yizhiren

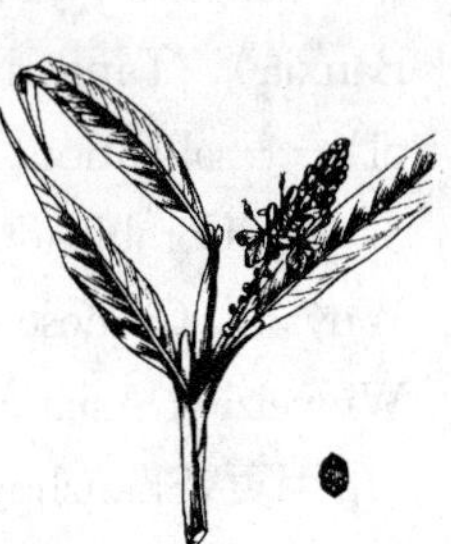
益智仁

English name: Sharpleaf Galangal Fruit

Pharmaceutical name: Furctus Alpiniae Oxyphyllae

Botanical name: Alpinia oxyphlly Miq.

Properties and tastes: pungent and warm

Meridian tropism: spleen and kidney

Functions: 1. warm the kidney to invigorate yang

2. control essence and decrease urination(arrest enuresis)

3. warm the spleen to arrest diarrhea

4. warm the stomach to control saliva

Indications: 1. cold deficiency of kidney qi, seminal essence, enuresis, profuse urination during the night, dribbling of urine

2. invasion of pathogenic cold to the spleen and stomach, abdominal pain, vomiting and diarrhea

3. deficiency in the cold spleen and stomach, poor appetite and profuse saliva

Dosage: 3～6g

Contraindication: This herb is pungent in taste and warm in property. It can invigorate fire to impair yin. It is not used for patients with hyperactivity of fire caused by deficiency of yin, impotence, frequent urination, metrorrhagia and metrostaxis due to heat.

Combinations: 1. add Largehead Atractylodes Rhizome (白术, Baizhu), Membranous Milkvetch Root(黄芪, Huangqi), Common Aucklandia Root(木香, Muxiang)——deficiency cold of spleen and stomach, cold pain in the abdomen, vomiting and diarrhea, profuse saliva and acid regurgitation

2. add Swordlike Atractylodes Rhizome(苍术, Cangzhu), Pinellia Rhizome(半夏, Banxia), Tangerine Peel(陈皮, Chenpi)——salivation

3. add Combined Spicebush Root(乌药, Wuyao), Chinese Magnoliavine(五味子, Wuweizi), Asiatic Cornelian Cherry Fruit (山茱萸,Shanzhuyu)——enuresis, frequent urine, profuse urination at night, etc.

4. add Hypoglaucous Collett Yam Rhizome (萆薢,Bixie)——mildy turbid urine, woman with morbid leukorrhea.

It can also treat high uric acid

5. add Largehead Atractylodes Rhizome(白术,Baizhu), Officinal Magnolia Bark(厚朴, Houpo)——spleen deficiency, poor appetite, diarrhea with loose stools

Prescription: Pill for Arresting Enuresis(缩泉丸,Suoquan Wan)

Notes: Sharpleaf Galangal Fruit(益智仁, Yizhiren) acts in reinforcement of the yang of spleen and kidney, and in the arresting of yin generation, urination and saliva. Very spicy, Sharpleaf Galangal Fruit(益智仁, Yizhiren) is an activator of yang and a reducer of yin evils according to Li Shizhen (李时珍). Poor appetite, hypersalivation, enuresis, high frequency of micturition, lethargy, and so on, which are symptoms of spleen-kidney deficiency of cold type are its main indications. A considerably helpful ancient description says, Sharpleaf Galangal Fruit(益智仁, Yizhiren) is hot and fragrant in property, and able to improve appetite, and scatters stagnation and cold evil.

12. 沙苑子, Shayuanzi

English name: Flatstem Milkvetch Seed

Pharmaceutical name: Semen Astragali

Botanical name: Astragalus complanatus R. Br., A. chinensis L., or A. adsurgens Pall.

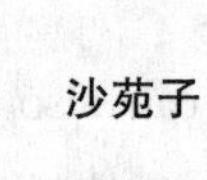

沙苑子

Properties and tasates: sweet and warm

Meridian tropism: liver and kidney

Functions: 1. warm and invigorate the kidney yang

2. control essence and decrease urination

3. nourish liver to promote eye-slight

Indications: 1. lumbar pain due to kidney deficiency

2. impotence and seminal emission

3. enuresis and frequent urine

4. a large quantity of leukorrhea

5. poor vision

Dosage: 9～18g

Contraindication: It is a herb for warming, tonifying, and astringing. Use cautiously with patients with hyperactivity of fire caused by deficiency of yin and difficulty in urination.

Combinations: 1. add Prepared Rhizome of Adhesive Rehmannia(熟地黄, Shoudihuang), Eucommia Bark(杜仲, Duzhong), Himalayan Teasel Root(续断, Xuduan)——lumbar pain due to kidney deficiency

2. add East Asian Tree Fern Rhizome(狗脊, Gouji), Hairy Antler(鹿茸, Lurong)——impotence

3. add Calcining Dragen's Bone(煅龙骨, Duanlonggu), Hindu Lotus Seed(莲子, Lianzi), Gordon Euryale Seed(芡实, Qianshi)——seminal emission, spermatorrhea

4. add Sharpleaf Galangal Fruit(益智仁, Yizhiren), Common Yam Rhizome(山药, Shanyao)——enuresis, frequent urine

5. add Ginkgo Seed(白果, Baiguo), Plantain

Seed(车前子,Cheqianzi)——a large quantity of leukorrhea

6. add Cassia Seed(决明子,Juemingzi), Abalone Shell(石决明,Shijueming)——poor vision

7. add Barbary Wolfberry Fruit(枸杞子, Gouqizi), Chrysanthemum Flower(菊花, Juhua)——dizziness and poor vision

8. add Puncturevine Caltrop Fruit(刺蒺藜, Cijili)——mildly benefits the spleen and kidney, to be used in treating deficiency of the liver and kidney, blurred vision and hysteria seen in women

Prescription: Golden Lock Pill for Keeping Kidney Essence(金锁固精丸,Jinsuogujing Wan)

Notes: Flatstem Milkvetch Seed(沙苑子, Shayuanzi) reinforces kidney, controls seminal emission, nourishes liver, improves eyesight and especially conditions of the pupils, frequent seminal emission, premature ejaculation, and urinary bleeding from instability of the Lower-jiao and deficiency of kidney, and diminution of vision, vertigo and dimness of eyesight from deficiency syndrome involving both liver and kidney are its applications.

Flatstem Milkvetch Seed(沙苑子, Shayuanzi) is the seed part of the same species of Membranous Milkvetch Root(黄芪, Huangqi), which is the root. The two herbs have the same functions of reducing blood pressure, heart rate, cardiac muscular tension and time exponent, increasing cerebral blood flow, and reducing cerebrovascular resistance, improving immunity, diminishing blood lipid and transaninase.

Eye diseases are indications of both Flatstem Milkvetch Seed(沙苑子, Shayuanzi) and Puncturevine Caltrop Fruit(刺蒺藜, Cijili), however, the former reinforces the liver and kidney with a mildness and finds its way in treatment of those from yin deficiency of the two organs. The latter, meanwhile, is able to smooth liver-qi, remove stagnancy and wind evil and improve eyesight rather than to reinforce.

13. 菟丝子, Tusizi

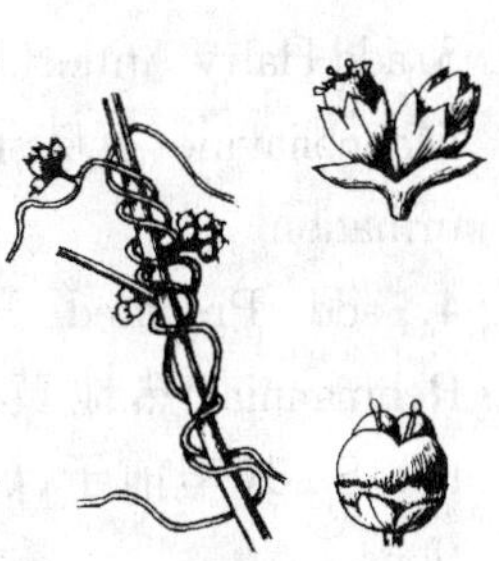

English name: Dodder Seed

Pharmaceutical name: Semen Cuscutae

Botanical name: Cuscuta chinensis Lam. Or C. japonica Choisy

菟丝子

Properties and tastes: pungent, sweet and medium

Meridian tropism: liver and kidney

Functions: 1. invigorate yang and nourish yin

2. control essence and decrease urination

3. nourish the liver to promote eyesight

4. stop diarrhea

5. miscarriage abortion

Indications: 1. kidney deficiency syndrome——soreness and pain of the lumbar and knees, impotence, spermatorrhea, frequent urination, a large quantity of leukorrhea

2. deficiency of kidney and liver essence——blurred vision, dusky eye, poor vision

3. diarrhea or loose stools due to spleen deficiency

4. threatened abortion due to deficiency of kidney and liver

Dosage: 9～15g

Contraindication: Use cautiously with patients with hyperactivity of fire caused by deficiency of yin, constipation, oliguria with deep colored urine.

Combinations: 1. add Eucommia Bark(杜仲, Duzhong), Common Yam Rhizome(山药, Shanyao)——soreness and pain of the lumbar region and knees

2. add Barbary Wolfberry Fruit(枸杞子, Gouqizi), Chinese Magnoliavine(五味子, Wuweizi)——impotence and seminal emission

3. add Hairy Antler(鹿茸, Lurong), Chinese Magnoliavine(五味子, Wuweizi)——dilute urination

4. add Prepared Rhizome of Adhesive Rehmannia(熟地黄, Shoudihuang), Plantain Seed(车前子, Cheqianzi)——poor vision

5. add Membranous Milkvetch Root(黄芪, Huangqi), Dang-shen Root(党参, Dangshen), Largehead Atractylodes Rhizome(白术, Baizhu)——diarrhea or loose stools due to spleen deficiency

6. add Himalayan Teasel Root(续断, Xuduan), Chinese Taxillus Twig(桑寄生, Sangjisheng), Ass-hide Glue(阿胶, Ejiao)——vaginal bleeding during pregnancy, threatened abortion

Notes: Both yin and yang of the kidney can be reinforced by this herb, which is also good in arresting and is a necessary drug in treatment of importance, frequent seminal emission, high frequency of micturition, profuse leukorrhea, threatened abortion, etc from the kidney's failure to arrest due to deficiency. It had been clinically proved to be effective for diabetes mellitus, which was originally described in *Formulas for Guidance in Saving Life* (《全生指迷方》, Quanshengzhimifang).

The same functions, as reinforcing liver and kidney, arresting seminal emission and frequent micturition, and improving eyesight, are found in both Dodder See(菟丝子, Tusizi) and Flatstem Milkvetch Seed(沙苑子, Shayuanzi). The former, however, can also reinforce the spleen to cure diarrhea and threatened abortion, while the latter is better in astringing.

14. 胡芦巴, Huluba

English name: Common Fenugreek Seed

Pharmaceutical name: Semen Trigonellae Foeni-graeci

Botanical name: Trigonella foenum-graecum L.

胡芦巴

Properties and tastes: bitter, warm

Meridian tropism: liver, kidney

Functions: 1. warm kidney yang

2. expel cold-dampness

Indications: 1. testagia due to cold evil, abdomial pain for cold pain in the lower abdomen which radiates to the scrotum, stagnation of qi, sensation of fullness and distention

2. cold pain of the knees and feet, unable to walk

Dosage: 3～9g

Contraindication: Use cautiously with patients with hyperactivity of fire caused by deficiency of yin, damp for heat in the interior.

Combinations: 1. add Prepared Daughter Root of Common Monkshood(附子, Fuzi), Sulfur(硫黄, Liuhuang)——fullness and distention in the abdomen and hypochondriac region due to kidney deficiency

2. add Common Floweringquince Fruit(木瓜, Mugua), Malaytea Scurfpea Fruit(补骨脂, Buguzhi)——flaccidity of the lower legs due to pathogenic cold and dampness, pain

of knees and feet

3. add Medicinal Evodia Root (吴茱萸, Wuzhuyu), Fennel Fruit(小茴香, Xiaohuixiang)——testagia due to cold evil, pain in the lower abdomen which radiates to the scrotum

Notes: Similar to Prepared Daughter Root of Common Monkshood(附子, Fuzi) and Common Cruculigo Rhizome(仙茅, Xianmao), though less strong in effect, activates kidney yang and expels cold evil from the lower part of the body, and is commonly given in combination with these two herbs to accomplish the functions. Its usual distribution is the liver system. Cold stagnancy, mass, and cold-dampness syndrome are consequently its indications.

It is reported that after a course of 21 days, 25 grams per day for some patients of diabetes mellitus. Prepared Daughter Root of Common Monkshood(附子, Fuzi) can reduce the content of blood sugar and urine sugar.

15. 阳起石, Yangqishi

English name: Actinolite

Pharmaceutical name: Actinolitum

Properties and tastes: salty, slightly warm

Meridian tropism: kidney

Function: warm the kidney and invigorate yang

阳起石

Indications: 1. declination of the kidney-yang, impotence of male and infertility of female due to retention of cold in the uterus

2. cold pain of the lumbar regions and knees

Dosage: 3～6g. used as an ingredient of bolus or powder.

Contraindication: Use cautiously with patients with hyperactivity of fire caused by deficiency of yin. It is not recommended to be taken for a long time.

Combinations: 1. add Prepared Rhizome of Adhesive Rehmannia (熟地黄, Shoudihuang), Chinese Angelica Root (当归, Danggui)——impotence

2. add Hairy Antler(鹿茸, Lurong)——infertility due to retention of cold in the uterus

3. add Medicinal Indian-mulberry Root(巴戟天, Bajitian)——cold pain of lumbar regions and knees

4. add Prepared Daughter Root of Common Monkshood(附子, Fuzi), Stalactite(钟乳石, Zhongrushi)——spermatorrhea, diarrhea with loose stools

Notes: Able to activate kidney qi and to warm the lower part of the body. It is salty in taste and warm in property, it is useful in impotence, frequent seminal emission, premature ejaculation, sterility of yang deficiency, metrorrhagia and metrostaxis, cold pain of waist and knees, resulted from insufficiency of kidney qi. Its primary ingredient is asbestos(calcium, magnesium and iron silicate), which is carcinogenic, based upon recent research. Therefore, its use is not recommended.

16. 淫羊藿, Yinyanghuo

English name: Shorthorned Epimedium Herb

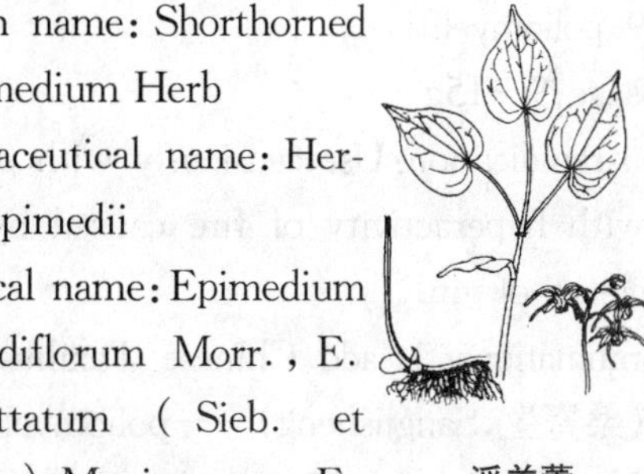

Pharmaceutical name: Herba Epimedii

Botanical name: Epimedium grandiflorum Morr., E. Sagittatum (Sieb. et Zucc.) Maxim., or E. Brevicornum Maxim.

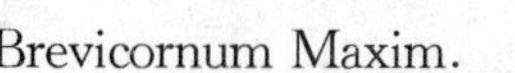

淫羊藿

Properties and tastes: pungent, sweet and warm

Meridian tropism: liver and kidney

Functions: 1. reinforce kidney and invigorate yang

2. strengthen bones and tendons

3. expel wind and eliminate dampness

4. lower blood pressure

5. increase the flow of coronary artery and improve hypoxia tolerance

6. remove blood fat and reduce blood sugar

7. stop cough, expel phlegm, and arrest asthma

8. tranquilize the mind

9. inhibit bateria and resist inflammation

10. improve immunity

11. function as rogenic hormones

Indications: 1. declination of the kidney-yang for impotence, infertility, enuresis, weakness of the lumbar region and knees, climacteric syndrome

2. wind-cold-damp Bi syndrome for cold pain of the limbs, numbness of hands and feet, spasm of muscles

3. windstroke, paralysis

4. climacteric hypertension due to deficiency of both yin and yang

5. CHD(coronary heart disease)

6. chronic bronchitis

7. neurasthenia

8. hypoleukocytosis

9. poliomyelitis

Dosage: 9～15g

Contraindication: Use causiously with patients with hyperactivity of fire caused by deficiency of yin.

Combinations: 1. add Chinese Taxillus Twig (桑寄生, Sangjisheng)——poliomyelitis

2. add Medicine Terminalia Fruit (诃子, Hezi)——hypoleukocytosis

3. add Common Cruculigo Rhizome (仙茅, Xianmao)——climacteric hypertension

4. add Medicinal Indian-mulberry Root (巴戟天, Bajitian), Songaria Cynomorium Herb (锁阳, Suoyang)——impotence, infertility

5. add Songaria Cynomorium Herb (锁阳, Suoyang), Prepared Rhizome of Adhesive Rehmannia (熟地黄, Shoudihuang)——infertility due to retention of cold in the uterus

6. add Asiatic Cornelian Cherry Fruit (山茱萸, Shanzhuyu), Flatstem Milkvetch Seed (沙苑子, Shayuanzi)——depressive state of neurasthenia

7. add Chinese Taxillus Twig (桑寄生, Sangjisheng), Perilla Leaf (紫苏 Zisu)——wind-cold-dampness Bi syndrome

8. add Chinese Magnoliavine (五味子, Wuweizi), Walnot (胡桃肉, Hutaorou)——chronic bronchitis

9. add Slenderstyle Acanthopanax Root-bark (五加皮, Wujiapi), Divaricate Saposhnikovia Root (防风, Fangfeng)——windstroke in women and hemiplegia

Prescription: Decoction of Two Immortals (二仙汤, Erxian Tang)

Notes: It is said in *Materia Medica of Ri Hua-zi* (《日华子本草》, Rihuazibencao) that Shorthorned Epimedium Herb (淫羊藿, Yinyanghuo) cures all sorts of wind, cold or exhaustive syndromes, strengthens waist and knee joints, activates heart functions. It can be used for impotence, sterility, spasm of tendons and bones, limb flaccidities, senile dementia, middle-aged-amnesia. As it has the effect of exciting the heart, it is how used for coronary heart disease, and cardiomyopathy. Similar functions, like exciting kidney yang, eliminating wind-dampness evils, and same indications, like impotence, sterility, arthritis, Shorthorned Epimedium Herb(淫羊藿,Yinyanghuo)Medicinal Indian-mulberry Root(巴戟天, Bajitian) and Common Cruculigo Rhizome(仙茅, Xianmao). Medicinal Indian-mulberry Root(巴戟天,Bajitian)is less effective but nourishes essence and blood. Common Cruculigo Rhizome(仙茅,Xianmao)is effective, especially on dispelling cold-dampness evil. Shorthorned Epimedium Herb (淫羊藿, Yinyanghuo) is more reliable in fortifying kidney yang and is useful in hemiparalysis.

17. 补骨脂, Buguzhi

English name: Malaytea Scurfpea Fruit

Pharmaceutical name: Fructus Psoraleae Corylifoliae

Botanical name: Psoralea corylifolia L.

补骨脂

Propertiese and tastes: bitter, pungent and extremly warm

Meridian tropism: kidney, spleen

Functions: 1. reinforce kidney and invigorate yang

2. control essence and arrest urination

3. warm the spleen to arrest diarrhea

4. nourish the kidney to hold qi and stop asthma

5. expand coronary artery

6. increase the white cells

7. inhibit bacteria

8. resist aging and lengthen the life span

9. resist cancer

10. increase pigment of skin

11. contract the uterus and shorten the bleeding time

12. function as estrogenic hormones

Indications: 1. deficiency of kidney yang-cold pain of the waist and knees, impotence, diarrhea enuresis

2. deficiency of both the spleen and kidney-morning diarrhea, poor appetite, abdominal distention.

3. deficiency of both the lung and the kidney-asthma, shortness of breath, breathe out more and breathe in less

4. vitiligo, pelada

5. psoriasis

6. endometrorrhagia

7. nocturnal enuresis in children

8. hypoleukocytosis

Contraindication: It is not suggested for patients with hyperactivity of fire caused by deficiency of yin, and constipation.

Combinations: 1. add Eucommia Bark(杜仲, Duzhong), Walnot(胡桃肉, Hutaorou)-lumbago due to deficiency of the kidney

2. add Medicinal Indian-mulberry Root(巴戟天, Bajitian)——impotence and seminal emission

3. add Sharpleaf Galangal Fruit(益智仁, Yizhiren)——enuresis, frequent urination

4. add Nutmeg Seed(肉豆蔻, Roudoukou)——morning diarrhea and chronic diarrhea

5. add Giant Gecko(蛤蚧, Gejie), Chinese Eaglewood Wood(沉香, Chenxiang)——asthma of deficiency type which is due to the kidney's failure to hold qi

6. add Red Halloysite (赤石脂, Chishizhi)——endometrorrhagia

Prescription: Pill of Four Miraculous Drugs(四神丸, Sishen Wan)

Notes: In comparison to Malaytea Scurfpea Fruit (补骨脂, Buguzhi) and Sharpleaf Galangal Fruit(益智仁, Yizhiren), has the effects of warming and reinforcing spleen and kidney and arresting seminal emission and micturition. They are principal drugs for spleen-kidney-yang insufficiency and failure to control sperm and urination. Malaytea Scurfpea Fruit(补骨脂,Buguzhi) is stronger in fortifying yang and focuses more on the kidney rather than, on warming the spleen to cure diarrhea. The main purpose of it includes impotence, frequent seminal emission, cold pain in the waist and knee joints, enuresis, asthma, cough and lingering diarrhea from spleen-kidney-yang insufficiency, when dissolved in alcohol, and applied externally. Sharpleaf Galangal Fruit (益智仁, Yizhiren), meanwhile, is less effecting on exciting yang and focuses more on warming the spleen, expelling cold, arresting excessive saliva, which are more reliable than warming the kidney, arresting sperm and urination, usually used for abdominal pain of cold type, vomiting, diarrhea, anorexia, hypersalivation, frequent seminal emission, enuresis, etc.

18. 冬虫夏草, Dongchongxiacao

English name: Chinese Caterpillar Fungus

Pharmaceutical name: Cordyceps Sinensis

Botanical name: Cordyceps sinensis(Berk.)Sacc.

Properties and Tastes: sweet and warm

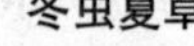

冬虫夏草

Meridian tropism: kidney and lung

Functions: 1. tonify the brain and invigorate yang

2. nourish the lung to relieve asthma

3. stop bleeding and remove phlegm

4. function of androgenic hormones

5. slow down heart rate, and lower blood pressure

6. resist arrhythmia and myocardial oxygen consumption

7. reduce cholesterol and triglyceride

8. improve kidney function

9. strengthen and adjust the function of immunity

10. tranquilize the mind and benefit sleep

11. resist cancer, inhibit bacteria virus and inflammation

Indications: 1. declination of the kidney-yang for soreness and weakness of the lumbar region and knees, impotence and spermatorrhea, tinnitus and amnesia

2. deficiency of both the lung and the kidney for asthma of deficiency type, protracted cough or cough due to asthenia of viscera, with discharge phlegm and weak blood constitution after illness

3. aversion to cold, spontaneous sweating, poor appetite, lassitute

4. chronic renal failure

5. arrhythmia

6. chronic bronchitis

7. tumors

8. allergic rhinitis

9. thrombocytopathic thrombocytopenia

Dosage: 6~9g, decocted in water or made into bolus or powder.

Contraindication: Do not use with patients with exterior syndrome, hemoptysis due to lung-heat.

Combinations: 1. add Shorthorned Epimedium Herb(淫羊藿, Yinyanghuo)——impotence due to kidney deficiency

2. add Ass-hide Glue(阿胶, Ejiao), Tendrilleaf Fritillary Bulb (川贝母, Chuanbeimu)——cough due to asthenia of viscera, cough with discharge of blood

3. add Chinese Magnoliavine (五味子, Wuweizi), Walnot(胡桃肉, Hutaorou)——asthma of deficiency type, protracted cough

4. add Ginseng(人参, Renshen)——weak constitution after illness

Notes: Because Chinese Caterpillar Fungus(冬虫夏草, Dongchongxiacao) excites the kidney yang as well as nourish the lung yin, arrest hemorrhage and eliminate phlegm. It is particularly suitable for pulmonary tuberculosis with hemoptysis, and impotence due to kidney deficiency. According to Li Shizhen (李时珍), Chinese Caterpillar Fungus(冬虫夏草, Dongchongxiacao) controls seminal emission, fortifies qi and especially reinforces the life gate. It is mild and may be cooked with chicken, duck, beef and mutton. Since it is rare and expensive, it is usually taken solely in capsules. Cultivated Chinese Caterpillar Fungus(冬虫夏草, Dongchongxiacao) is generally used in mass procession, which is a product of recent research on cultivation.

Appendix: Other Drugs For Tonifying Yang

Name	Properties and tastes	Meridian tropism	Functions	Indications	Dosage	Contraindication
Common Cruculigo Rhizome (仙茅, Xianmao)	pungent, hot, poisonous	kidney	Warm kidney, tonify yang, expel cold, eliminate dampness	Impotence, enuresis, cold sperm, cold pain of back and knee joint, numbness of the limb	3~9g	Hyperactivity of fire due to yin deficiency
Baron's Drynaria Rhizome (骨碎补, Gusuibu)	bitter, warm	liver, kidney	Tonify kidney, strengthen bones and teeth, tendons, stop pain	Lumbago due to kidney deficiency, weakness in the legs, teeth shaking, bones fracture, traumatic injury	3~9g	Hyperactivity of fire due to yin deficiency and toothache due to excess fire
Testes and Penis of an Ursine Seal (海狗肾, Haigoushen)	salty, hot	kidney	Reinforce kidney, tonify yang, reinforce essence, tonify marrow	Impotence, infertility due to cold uterus, cold and little sperm	1~3g /time, grind into fine powder,	Hyperactivity of fire due to yin deficiency
Sea Horse (海马, Haima)	sweet, salty and warm	kidney, liver	Reinforce kidney, tonify yang, activate blood by eliminating stasis, eliminate swelling and stop pain	Impotence, little sperm, infertility abdominal mass, traumatic injury	1~1.5g /time grind into fine powder	Hyperactivity of fire due to yin deficiency
Tuber Onion Seed (韭子, Jiuzi)	pungent, sweet and warm	liver, kidney	Reinforce liver and kidney, warm lower back and knee joint, tonify yang and strengthen essence	Cold pain in lower back and knee joint due to insufficiency of liver and kidney, seminal emission, frequent urine, profuse leukorrhea	6~9g	Hyperactivity of fire due to yin deficiency

Section 3
Drugs for Enriching Blood

1. 当归, Danggui

Botanical name: Angelica sinensis(Oliv.)Diels

English name: Chinese Angelica Root

Pharmaceutical name: Radix Angelicae Sinensis

Properties and tastes: sweet, pungent and warm

当 归

Meridian tropism: heart, liver and spleen

Functions: 1. nourish blood

2. promote the circulation of blood

3. regulate menstruation

4. stop pain

5. moisten the intestine to loosen the bowels

6. dual regulatory function on uterus

7. lower blood pressure, expand blood vessels, increase blood flow and prevent arteriosclerosis

8. protect the liver

9. alleviate water retention

10. resist inflammation

Indications: 1. blood deficiency of the heart and liver syndrome for manifested as a pale complexion, pale tongue, lip, dizziness, blurring of vision palpitation, etc.

2. blood phase syndrome of women for irregular menstruation, amenorrhea, dysmenorrhea, etc.

3. pain syndrome for abdominal pain due to cold deficiency, pain due to blood stasis, traumatic injury, numbness due to arthralgia syndrome

4. carbuncle, skin and external disease, it can offer benefit by relieving swelling and pain

5. constipation due to blood deficiency and dry intestines

6. thromboangiitis obliterans

7. acute and chronic nephritis

8. cerebral arteriesclerosis

9. chronic hepatitis, cirrhosis

Dosage: 6~15g

Contraindication: Use cautiously with patients with retention of excessive dampness in the Middle-jiao, diarrhea with loose stools, deficiency of blood accompanied with dryness due to heat.

Combinations: 1. add Nutgrass Galingale Rhizome(香附, Xiangfu), Yanhusuo(延胡索, Yanhusuo)——dysmenorrhea

2. add Szechwan Lovage Rhizome(川芎, Chuanxiong), Prepared Rhizome of Adhesive Rehmannia(熟地黄, Shoudihuang), White Peony Root(白芍药, Baishaoyao)——irregular menstruation, a basic prescription for regulating menstruation in gynecology

3. add Peach Seed(桃仁, Taoren), Safflower(红花, Honghua)——amenorrhea

4. add Olibanum, Frankincense(乳香, Ruxiang), Myrrh(没药, Moyao)——pain of the limbs due to blood stasis, thromboangitis obliterans

5. add Rhubarb(大黄, Dahuang), Peach Seed(桃仁, Taoren)——traumatic injury

6. add Rhubarb(大黄, Dahuang)——arthralgia pain in the joints, or skin numb-

ness

7. add Fresh Ginger(生姜, Shengjiang), mutton (羊肉, Yangrou)——abdominal pain due to deficiency of cold

8. add Membranous Milkvetch Root(黄芪, Huangqi)——blood deficiency syndrome

9. add Pangolin Scales(穿山甲, Chuanshanjia), Honeysuckle Flower(金银花, Jinyinhua)——carbuncle and ucler

10. add Membranous Milkvetch Root(黄芪, Huangqi), Rice Bean(赤小豆, Chixiaodou)——unulcered carbuncle or non-healing of boils due to blood and qi deficiency

11. add Dan-shen Root (丹参, Danshen)——cerebral arteriosclersis

12. add Chinese Magnoliavine (五味子, Wuweizi), Chinese Thorowax Root(柴胡, Chaihu)——chronic hepatitis, cirrhosis

13. add Motherwort Herb(益母草, Yimucao)——chronic nephritis

14. add Desertliving Gistanche (肉苁蓉, Roucongrong)——constipation of elderly and weak persons and postpartum women who are in the condition of consumption of body fluid and dry blood

15. add Szechwan Lovage Rhizome(川芎, Chuanxiong)——pain due to blood staiss, for example dysmenorrhea, swelling and pain due to carbuncle, althralgic pain, headache, etc.

Prescriptions: 1. Decoction Containing Four Drugs(四物汤, Siwu Tang)

2. Powder of Radix Angelicae Sinensis and Radix Paeoniae (当归芍药散, Danggui Shaoyao San)

3. Decoction for Warming Channels(温经汤, Wenjing Tang)

Notes: Chinese Angelica Root(当归, Danggui) is able to regulate menstruation and to nourish blood and it is frequently used in various gynecopathies. Its emphasis varies from nourishing blood to promoting blood circulation with different combinations. Zhang Yuansu(张元素), a great ancient physician, said:" It is an essential drug for all blood disorders. Attaching motivating to replenishing, it is a qi-regulating herb that acts upon blood system". said Zhang Jingyue(张景岳), another famous ancient physician," It is reinforcing when put together with reinforcing herbs and applicable to all deficient syndromes, while it is also blockage-removing when with reducing drugs, and appropriate to manage pain and free movement of bowls." In spite of these, it is advisable to give this herb to the cases of blood deficiency of stasis with cold syndromes, for it is warming and drying in properties.

It was said in ancient times that the ending part of the root is better in promoting blood circulation, when the main part in replenishing blood. Yet, no significant difference has been observed.

Recent research shows that Chinese Angelica Root(当归, Danggui) increases the flow of coronary artery, reduces oxygen consumption of myocardium, lowers blood pressure, reduces platelet aggregation, prevents thrombosis, decreases level of blood-lipid, hinders arteriosclerosis, and is usually given for cardio-cerebral-vascular diseases.

Chinese Angelica Root(当归, Danggui) and White Peony Root (白芍药, Baishaoyao), have the effect of nourishing blood, and stoping pains. They are generally used in combination. Chinese Angelica Root (当归, Danggui) is sweet in taste for strengthening, but also bitter for purgation, leave alone spicy to expel and warm to remove blockage. Based upon this two-way effect, it can be used for irregular menstruation and pains due to blood stasis that was induced both by blood deficiency accompanied by cold evil, and injuries. White Peony Root(白芍药, Baishaoyao) is sour in taste, and effective in controlling yin substances, tenderizing liver, relieving spasm, managing pain and tranquilizing hyperactive liver-yang. It can be used for irregular menstruation, dysmenorrhea, fullness and distension in chest and hypochondrium, muscular contraction, which result from blood deficiency and stagnation of liver, as well as headache and vertigo due to hyperactivity of liver-yang.

2. 熟地黄, Shoudihuang

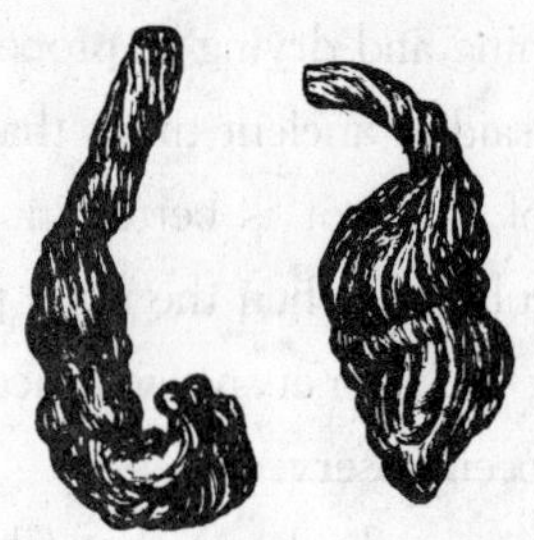

熟地黄

English name: Prepared Rhizome of Adhesive Rehmannia

Pharmaceutical name: Radix Rehmanniae Glutinosae Conquitae

Botanical name: Rehmannia glutinosa (Gaertn.) Libosch. Or R. Glutinosa Libosch. f. hueichingensis (Chao et Schih) Hisao

Properties and tastes: sweet and slightly warm

Meridian tropism: liver and kidney

Functions: 1. nourish blood and yin

2. replenish vital essence and benefit marrow

3. lower blood pressure

4. reduce blood sugar

Indications: 1. blood deficiency syndrome for a sallow complexion, dizziness, palpitation, insomnia, irregular menstruation

2. deficiency of the kidney yin syndrome-tidal fever, night sweating and seminal emission

3. deficiency of blood and essence syndrome-soreness and weakness of the lumbar region and feet, dizziness and blurred vision, tinnitus and deafness, early greying of the retarded development of children

4. asthma and cough due to kidney deficiency

5. hypertension

6. diabetes

Dosage: 9～30g, large dosage may be used of 30～60g.

Contraindication: This herb is sticky in property, which may affect normal digestion. Do not use with patients with profuse phlegm, stagnation of qi, distention and pain in the epigasrium and abdomen, poor appetite and those with loose stool.

Combinations: 1. add Asiatic Cornelian Cherry Fruit(山茱萸, Shanzhuyu), Common Yam Rhizome(山药, Shanyao)——deficiency of the liver and kidney yin syndrome, manifested as soreness and weakness of the waist and knees, dizziness and tinnitus and deafness, tidal fever and night sweating, seminal emission, etc

2. add Tortoise Shell and Plastron(龟版, Guiban), Common Anemarrhea Rhizome (知母, Zhimu), Chinese Corktree Bark(黄柏, Huangbai)——yin deficiency and hyperactivity of fire, tidal fever, night sweating, hemoptysis

3. add Chinese Angelica Root(当归, Danggui)——palpitation, insomnia and protract-

ed cough and asthma due to yin and blood deficiency in women

4. add Chinese Angelica Root(当归,Danggui), White Peony Root (白芍药, Baishaoyao), Szechwan Lovage Rhizome(川芎,Chuanxiong)——blood deficiency, a sallow complexion, dizziness, palpitation, insomnia and irregular menstruation, metrorrhagia and metrostaxis

5. add Tangerine Peel (陈皮, Chenpi), Pinellia Rhizome(半夏,Banxia), Tuckahoe (茯苓, Fuling)——deficiency of both the lung and kidney, cough and asthma with a profuse phlegm

6. add Common Yam Rhizome (山药, Shanyao), Chinese Magnoliavine(五味子, Wuweizi), Heterophylla Falsestarwort Root (太子参,Taizishen)——wasting and thirst syndrome, excessive drinking and eating

7. add Chinese Angelica Root(当归,Danggui), Membranous Milkvetch Root(黄芪, Huangqi), Ass-hide Glue(阿胶,Ejiao)——all kinds of anemia

8. add Coastal Glehnia Root, and Fourleaf Ladybell Root (沙参, Shashen), Barbary Wolfberry Fruit(枸杞子,Gouqizi), Szechwan Chinaberry Fruit(川楝子,Chuanlainzi)——chronic hepatitis

9. add Chinese Taxillus Twig (桑寄生, Sangjisheng), Baikal Skullcap Root(黄芩, Huangqin), Largehead Atractylodes Rhizome(白术, Baizhu)——threatened abortion

10. add White Peony Root (白芍药, Baishaoyao), Divaricate Saposhnikovia Root (防风, Fangfeng)——deficiency of liver blood, blurred vision of both eyes

11. add Ass-hide Glue(阿胶,Ejiao), Argy Wormwood Leaf(艾叶, Aiye)——metrorrhagia and metrostaxis

12. add Ephedra(麻黄, Mahuang)——yin deep-rooted ulcer subcutaneous nodule due to stagnation of cold-dampness, asthma and protracted cough without sputum during menstrual period

13. add Manchurian Wildginger Herb (细辛,Xixin)——all kinds of lumbar pain

Prescriptions: 1. Decoction Containing Four Drugs(四物汤,Siwu Tang)

2. Bolus of Six Drugs Containing Rhizome Rehmanniae Peaeparatae(六味地黄丸,Liuweidihuang Wan)

Notes: As a frequently used herb for insufficiency of blood, kidney yin and essence, Prepared Rhizome of Adhesive Rehmannia(熟地黄,Shoudihuang) is important for nourishing yin substances, blood, essence and marrow/brain, and said to be a essential drug for all categories of blood deficiency.

It is usually used in combination with Prepared Daughter Root of Common Monkshood(附子, Fuzi), Cassia Bark (肉桂,Rougui) which are drugs for invigorating, such as Jin Gui's Bolus for Tonifying the Kidney Yin(金匮肾气丸,Jinguishenqi Wan).

As it is not easy to digest, it is advisable to get it stir-baked with Fresh Ginger(生姜,Shengjiang) juice, or together with digestion-promoting drugs, like Tangerine Peel(陈皮,Chenpi), Villous Amomum Fruit (砂仁,Sharen) to compensate its digestion-blocking side-effect.

The difference, between Adhesive Rehmannia Dried Root(干地黄, Gandihuang) and Prepared Rhizome of Adhesive Rehmannia (熟地黄,Shoudihuang) leads to variances in functions. The former is, sweet, bitter, and cold, with the function of clearing away heat to cool the blood, nourishing yin substances to humidify, and used for the syndromes related to heat evil invaded blood and heat-dryness syndrome. The latter replenishes the yin aspect of liver and kidney, essence and blood, and is suitable for blood deficiency syndromes. If the condition appears to be the combination of the two, the two herbs can be used together.

3. 何首乌, Heshouwu

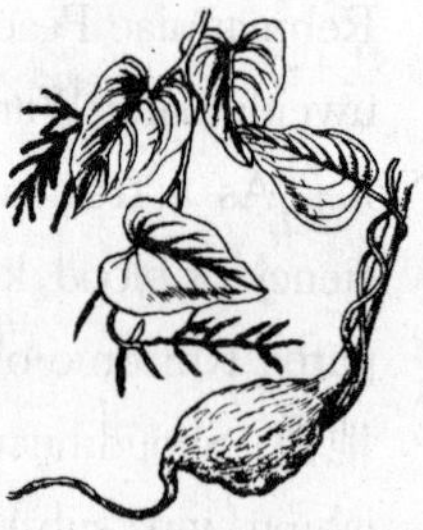

English name: Tuber Fleeceflower Root

Pharmaceutical name: Radix Polygoni Multiflori

Botanical name: Polygonum multiflorum Thunb.

何首乌

Properties and tastes: bitter, sweet, astringent and slightly warm

Meridian tropism: liver and kidney

Functions: 1. reinforce the liver and kidney, reinforce essence
2. treat malaria
3. detoxicating
4. moisten the intestine to loosen the bowels
5. reduce cholesterol
6. resist arteriosclerisis
7. excite the nervous system

Indications: 1. deficiency of blood and essence for dizziness, blurred eyes, early greying of the beard and hair, soreness and weakness of the waist and feet, seminal emission, metrorrhagia and metrostaxis, and morbid leukorrhea
2. prolonged malaria
3. carbuncle, furuncle and abscess, scrofula and pyogenic disease in the deep area
4. constipation due to dry intestines

Dosage: 9～30g. when prepared Tuber Fleeceflower Root(何首乌, Heshouwu) is used for tonifying the kidney and liver, while when fresh the herb is used for other functions.

Contraindication: It is not suggested for patients with diarrhea, loose stools, phlegm damp of severe case.

Combinations: 1. add Ginseng (人参, Renshen)——prolonged malaria, deficiency of both qi and blood
2. add Prepared Rhizome of Adhesive Rehmannia(熟地黄, Shoudihuang)——be used in treating beard and hair
3. add Black Sesame (黑芝麻, Heizhima)——constipation due to blood deficiency and dry intestines
4. add Barbary Wolfberry Fruit(枸杞子, Gouqizi)——deficiency of liver and kidney, soreness and pain of the waist and knees, grey and rusterless hair
5. add Achyranthis Root(怀牛膝, Huainiuxi)——dizziness vertigo and numbness of the limbs due to deficiency of liver blood
6. add Mulberry Solomonseal(桑椹, Sangshen)——dizziness due to deficient blood yin, palpatition and insomnia
7. add Puncturevine Caltrop Fruit(刺蒺藜, Cijili)——neurosism, dizziness, headache, vertigo, insomnia and hypertension
8. add Gambirplant Hooked Stem and Branch(钩藤, Gouteng)——arteriosclerosis, hypertension, coronary heart disease
9. add Lucid Ganoderma(灵芝, Lingzhi), Dan-shen Root(丹参, Danshen)——hypercholesterolemia
10. add Weeping Forsythia Capsule(连翘, Lianqiao), Common Selfheal Fruit-spike(夏枯草, Xiakucao)——lymphoid tuberculosis
11. add Lightyellow Sophora Root(苦参, Kushen), Densefruit Pittany Root-bark(白鲜皮, Baixianpi)——itching due to rubella
12. add Honeysuckle Flower(金银花, Jiny-

inhua), Fineleaf Schizomepeta Herb(荆芥, Jingjie)——ulcer due to damp-heat

13. add Coastal Glehnia Root, and Fourleaf Ladybell Root(沙参, Shashen), Dwarf Lilyturf Root(麦门冬, Maimendong)——myocardial infarction of yin deficiency type

14. add Magnetite(磁石, Cishi), Chinese Magnoliavine(五味子, Wuweizi)——inhibitory neurosism

15. add Chinese Angelica Root(当归, Danggui), Ass-hide Glue(阿胶, Ejiao)——all kinds of anemia

16. add Siberian Solomonseal Rhizome(黄精, Huangjing), Tumeric Root-tuber(郁金, Yujin) Yanhusuo(延胡索, Yanhusuo)——angina pectoris

Notes: Tuber Fleeceflower Root(何首乌, Heshouwu) is not cold, dry or sticky, and it is a good drug for reinforcement. Although less effective in reinforcement, the dry herb is able to remove toxic substances, purge, and cure malaria. When baked, it is stronger in reinforcement and able to control essence and qi from being lost, hence, it is beneficial for the syndromes of liver-kidney deficiency.

Tuber Fleeceflower Root(何首乌, Heshouwu) and Prepared Rhizome of Adhesive Rehmannia(熟地黄, Shoudihuang) are similar in function. The former is not sticky and does not affect digestion while the latter is sticky and easy to impair the stomach, but it has strong effect on reinforcing blood essence.

The variance between Tuber Fleeceflower Root(何首乌, Heshouwu) and Chinese Angelica Root(当归, Danggui) was best described in Chong Qing Tang Jottings(重庆堂随笔, Chongqingtangsuibi). Tuber Fleeceflower Root(何首乌, Heshouwu) regulates conditions of qi and blood, improves eruption of skin infections. This is quite similar to Chinese Angelica Root(当归, Danggui), which is spicy(smelly), and suitable for wind-cold-rendered disorders of the blood system. Tuber Fleeceflower Root(何首乌, Heshouwu) is not spicy and appropriate for windi-heat-rendered disorders of the same system. The two drugs, however, are both principal drugs for gynecopathies.

Add: 夜交藤, Yejiaoteng

English name: Tuber Fleeceflower Stem and Leaf

Pharmaceutical name: Caulis Polygoni Multiflori

Botanical name: Polygonum multiflorum Thunb.

Properties and tastes: sweet and medium

Meridian tropism: heart and liver

Functions: 1. nourish heart and tranquilize the wind

2. nourish blood and dredge the collaterals

3. relieve itching

Indications: 1. restlessness of deficiency type, insomnia

2. soreness and pain all over the body

3. skin itching due to rebuttal

Dosage: 15～30g

Combinations: 1. add Spine Date Seed(酸枣仁, Suanzaoren), Chinese Arborvitae Seed(柏子仁, Baiziren), Thinleaf Milkwort Root(远志, Yuanzhi)——restlessness of deficiency type, insomnia

2. add Chinese Angelica Root(当归, Danggui), Prepared Rhizome of Adhesive Rehmannia(熟地黄, Shoudihuang), Suberect Satholobus Stem(鸡血藤, Jixueteng)——soreness and pain all over the body

3. add Cicada Slough(蝉蜕, Chantui),

Belvedera Fruit(地肤子,Difuzi),Densefruit Pittany Root-bark(白鲜皮,Baixianpi)——itching due to rebuttal on the skin

Notes:Effective in nourishing blood and tranquilizing,Tuber Fleeceflower Stem and Leaf (夜交藤,Yejiaoteng)is mainly used for insomnia resulted from deficiency of blood and yin. Besides,it has the functions of improving blood circulation,and dredging the collaterals. So it can be used for general aching due to blood deficiency. It is said in *Compendium of Materia Medica* (《本草纲目》,Bencaogangmu),"It is quite effective if the decoction is used in bathing to relieve itching due to skin diseases."

4.白芍药,Baishaoyao

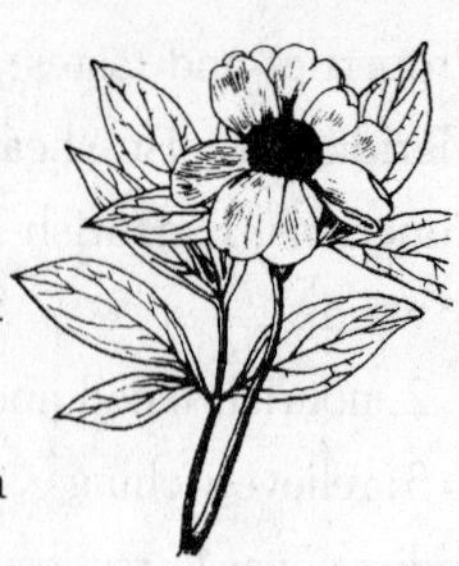

English name:White Peony Root

Pharmaceutical name: Radix Paeoniae Lactiflorae

Botanical name: Paeonia lactiflora Pall.

白芍药

Properties and tastes: bitter,soul and slightly cold

Meridian tropism:liver and spleen

Functions: 1. nourish the blood and astringe yin

2. smooth the liver to stop pain

3. subdue the hyperactive liver-yang

4. relieve muscular spasm, tranquilize the mind

5. lower blood pressure

6. promote urination

7. inhibit bacteria (Bacillus dysenteriae, etc.)

Indications: 1. pain in the abdomen and epigast, hypochondriac pain caused by disharmony between the liver and stomach or stagnation of liver qi. For example, used for peptic ulcer, gastritis, enteritis, pain due to gastrointestinal spasm.

2. dysentery for has a good effect in relieving abdominal pain and tenesmus

3. menstruation disease for irregular mentstruation,metrorrhagia

4. pain and spasm of the four limbs for due to blood deficiency which fail to nourish muscles and tenons

5. hypertension and arteriosclerosis for dizziness, tinnitus, numbness of the limbs, and muscular spasm

6. due to deficiency of liver yin.

Dosage: 6～9g, large dosage can be used as high as 15～30g. White Peony Root(白芍药,Baishaoyao) is used for smoothing liver and astringing yin, while stir for barked White Peony Root(白芍药, Baishaoyao) with wine is used for harmony in the middle for jiao, relieving spasm, nourishing the blood, parched White Peony Root(白芍药, Baishaoyao)is used for arresting bleeding.

Contraindication: It is not recommended that it be singularly for exhaustion of yang and deficiency for cold, incompatible with Black False Bellebore(藜芦,Lilu).

Combinations: 1. add Common Aucklandia Root(木香, Muxiang)——dysentery, abdominal pain, tenesmus

2. add Cassia Twig(桂枝,Guizhi)——spontaneous sweating and night sweating

3. add Licorice Root(甘草, Gancao)——pain in the abdomen and spasm of the four limbs, whooping cough, asthma, etc

4. add Silktree Albiziae Bark(合欢皮, Hehuanpi)——mental depression, ankiety, insomnia, nervousness

5. add Gambirplant Hooked Stem and Branch(钩藤,Gouteng)——hypertension

6. add Barbary Wolfberry Fruit (枸杞子, Gouqizi)——dizziness, dry mouth and eyes, palpitation, insomnia or a profused menstruation in women

7. add Fresh Ginger(生姜, Shengjiang)——blood deficiency with pathogenic cold, dysmenorrhea or postpartum abdominal pain

8. add Chinese Thorowax Root(柴胡, Chaihu)——relieve stagnation and stop pain, abdominal pain, distension and pain in the hypochondriac region

9. add Dwarf Lilyturf Root (麦门冬, Maimendong), Chinese Angelica Root (当归, Danggui), Prepared Rhizome of Adhesive Rehmannia (熟地黄, Shoudihuang)——chronic hepatitis, anemia, hypertension, arteriosclerosis

10. add Chinese Angelica Root(当归, Danggui), Prepared Rhizome of Adhesive Rehmannia(熟地黄, Shoudihuang), Szechwan Lovage Rhizome (川芎, Chuanxiong)——irregular menstruation, dysmenorrhea, metrorrhagia and metrostaxis

11. add Licorice Root(甘草, Gancao), Common Floweringquince Fruit (木瓜, Mugua)——spasm of gastrocnemius muscle due to consumption of body fluid

12. add Chinese Taxillus Twig (桑寄生, Sangjisheng), Largehead Atractylodes Rhizome (白术, Baizhu), stir-barked Baikal Skullcap Root(黄芩, Huangqin)——threatened abortion

Prescriptions: 1. Decoction Containing Four Drugs(四物汤, Siwu Tang)

2. Decoction for Collapse (四逆汤, Sini Tang)

3. Powder of Radix Angelicae Sinensis and Radix Paeoniae (当归芍药散, Dangguishaoyao San)

Notes: White Peony Root (白芍药, Baishaiyao) is a dominant herb for diseases of the liver meridian with the functions of soothing and tranquilizing the liver, and fortifying spleen, by nourishing liver-yin. "White Peony Root (白芍药, Baishaiyao) has six functions," said in *The Revelation of Medicine* (《医学启源》, Yixueqiyuan), "firstly, it protects the spleen; secondly, it relieves soreness; thirdly, it collects stomach qi; fourthly, to cure diarrhea; fifthly, to harmonize blood circulation, and finally, to tighten superficial layers."

In comparison to another blood-reinforcing herb, Chinese Angelica Root (当归, Danggui), White Peony Root (白芍药, Baishaiyao) is slightly cold in property and more suitable for blood insufficiency of the heat type, Chinese Angelica Root (当归, Danggui) is warm and appropriate for cold type. They both can be used to stop pain. Chinese Angelica Root(当归, Danggui) acts via improving qi and blood circulation, while White Peony Root(白芍药, Baishaiyao) does by relieving spasm.

The same application of "tendon" (ligament) illnesses, e. g. spasm, finds its way in both Common Flowering quince Fruit (木瓜, Mugua) and White Peony Root(白芍药, Baishaoyao). These two differ from one another as follows. White Peony Root (白芍药, Baishaiyao) acts through nourishing blood, astringing yin fluid and soothing the liver, with the indications of failure of the insufficient blood to moisten "tendons", manifested as spasm, contracture pain, etc. Common Floweringquince Fruit (木瓜, Mugua) performs its functions by removing dampness and is helpful for cramp in cholera morbus, ankylosis in arthritis (dampness type), which are caused by dampness accumulation. In addition, White Peony Root(白芍药, Baishaiyao) is effective in the treatment of abnormal yang-flushing due toyin deficiency and gynecopathies, while Common Floweringquince Fruit(木瓜, Mugua) is effective in treating vomiting complicated by diarrhea and edema in beriberi, because it has the functions of removing dampness and harmonizing the spleen.

5. 阿胶, Ejiao

English name: Ass-hide Glue

Pharmaceutical name: Gelatinum Asini

Botanical name: Equs asinus L.

阿 胶

Properties and tastes: sweet and medium

Meridian tropism: lung, liver and kidney

Functions: 1. nourish blood to stop bleeding

2. nourish yin and moisten the lung

Indications: 1. blood deficiency syndrome for a pale or sallow complexion, dizziness, palpitation

2. hemorrhagic syndrome for hematemesis, epistaxis, hematochezia, hematuria metrorrhagia and metrostaxis, a large quantity of menses, postpartum persistent lochia

3. yin deficiency syndrome for irritability, insomnia, amenorrhea

4. cough and asthma due to asthenia of viscera and dry cough due to yin deficiency

5. constipaton due to deficiency of blood and yin

6. TP, thrombocytolytic purpura

7. AA, aplastic anemia

8. hypoleukocytosis

9. incipient abortion

Dosage: 6 ~ 9g, dissoved in boiling water or yellow rice wine before eating, or melting in decoction. stir for baked Ass-hide Glue(阿胶, Ejiao) with Cattail Pollen(蒲黄, Puhuang) solution is good at arresting bleeding, while stir-baked Ass-hide Glue(阿胶, Ejiao) with powder of Giant Gecko(蛤蚧, Gejie) is good at moistening the lung.

Contraindication: This drug is sticky and greasy in property, which may affect digestion. It is unsuitable for patients with deficiency of the spleen and stomach, poor appetite, indigestion, vomitting and diarrhea.

Combinations: 1. add Membranous Milkvetch Root(黄芪, Huangqi), Dragon's Bone(龙骨, Longgu), Oyster Shell(牡蛎, Muli)——metrorrhagia and metrostaxis

2. add Chinese Angelica Root(当归, Danggui), Prepared Rhizome of Adhesive Rehmannia(熟地黄, Shoudihuang)——all kinds of anemia

3. add Rehmannia Dried Root(生地黄, Shengdihuang), Lalang Grass Rhizome(白茅根, Baimaogen)——hematemesis due to blood heat, epistaxis, hematuria

4. add Membranous Milkvetch Root(黄芪, Huangqi), Chinese Angelica Root(当归, Danggui)——a sallow complexion due to blood deficiency, dizziness, palpatation

5. add Apricot Seed(杏仁, Xingren), Loquat Leaf(枇杷叶, Pipaye)——dry cough without sputum, dry throat due to acute trachitis

6. add Coptis Rhizome(黄连, Huanglian), Rehmannia Dried Root(生地黄, Shengdihuang), White Peony Root(白芍药, Baishaoyao)——irritability of deficiency type, insomnia due to febrile disease damaging yin

7. add Garden Burnet Root(地榆, Diyu),

Janpanese Pagodatree Flower(槐花, Huaihua)——hematochezia

8. add Dwarf Lilyturf Root (麦门冬, Maimendong), Ginseng(人参, Renshen), Membranous Milkvetch Root (黄芪, Huangqi)——TP, thrombocytolytic purpura

9. add Dried Human Placenta(紫河车, Ziheche), Cassia Bark(肉桂, Rougui)——AA aplastic anemia

10. add Barbary Wolfberry Fruit(枸杞子, Gouqizi), Dan-shen Root (丹参, Danshen)——hypoleukocytosis

11. add Argy Wormwood Leaf (艾叶, Aiye), Chinese Angelica Root(当归, Danggui), Prepared Rhizome of Adhesive Rehmannia(熟地黄, Shoudihuang)——incipient abortion

12. add Immature Bitter Orange (枳实, Zhishi), Honey (蜂蜜, Fengmi)——postpartum thin body, constipation

Prescriptions: 1. Decoction of Colla Corii Asini and Artemisiae Argyi(胶艾汤, Jiaoai Tang)
2. Decoction of Rhizoma Coptidis and Colla Corii Asini (黄连阿胶汤, Huanglian Ejiao Tang)

Notes: Ass-hide Glue(阿胶, Ejiao) is most effective in replenishing blood, accompanied by styptic effect, thus, it is mostly used for diseases of the hematopoietic system. It can nourish yin and moisten the lungs and also can stop bleeding, enable it to cure, most suitable for, cough, and asthma from dryness involving the lungs, which are complicated by a dryness sensation of the throat with little or bloody sputum.

"Ass-hide Glue(阿胶, Ejiao) harmonizes blood, nourishes yin, eliminates wind evil and dryness," said in *Compendium of Materia Medica* (《本草纲目》, Bencaogangmu), "clears lungs, dissolves phlegm, and improves retarded urination and defecation." Said in *Herbals for Easy Approaching* (《本草便读》, Bencaobiandu). Ass-hide Glue(阿胶, Ejiao) is a commonly used herb for consumptive diseases, cough and all sorts of bleeding disorders.

6. 龙眼肉, Longyanrou

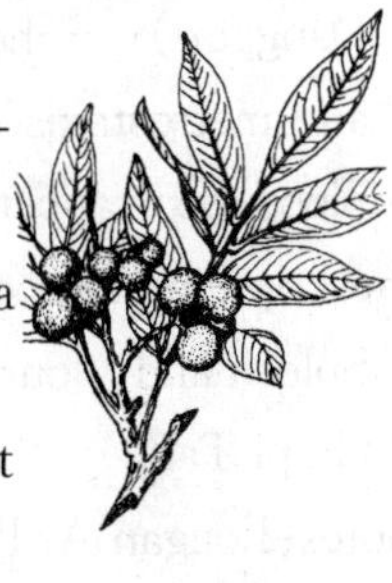

English name: Longan Aril

Pharmaceutical name: Arillus Euphoriae Longanae

Botanical name: Euphoria longan(Lour.)Steud.

Properties and tastes: sweet and slightly warm

Meridian tropism: heart and spleen

龙眼肉

Functions: 1. tonify the heart and spleen
2. nourish qi and blood

Indications: 1. deficiency of the heart and spleen syndrome for palpitation due to fright, insomnia, amnesia
2. deficiency of qi and blood syndrome for lassitude, shortness of breath, spontaneous sweating, a sallow complexion

Dosage: 9 ~ 15g, large dose may be used for 30g. It can be decocted in water and made into medical paste, saked in wine, and made into a bolus. Steaming or boiling it with sugar and dissolving it in boiling water before taking. It can also be soaked in wine for a hundred days before eating.

Contraindication: Not to be taken for patients with retention of dampness in Middle-jiao, fullness in the epigastrium and abdomen, or for retention of fluid, sputum and fire.

Combinations: 1. add Spine Date Seed(酸枣仁, Suanzaoren)——overanxiety, overstain damaging the spleen and heart, a sallow complexion, palpitation, amnesia, insomnia, bad dreams frightened easily

2. add Lily Bulb(百合,Baihe)——sleeplessness, over excitement

3. add Grassleaf Sweetflag Rhizome(石菖蒲,Shichangpu)——amnesia, dizziness, lassitude due to deficiency of qi and blood

4. add Membranous Milkvetch Root(黄芪,Huangqi), Chinese Angelica Root(当归,Danggui)——hematochezia, metrorrhagia and metrostaxis due to deficiency of qi and blood, poor appetite, lassitude

Prescription: Decoction for Invigorating the Spleen and Nourishing the Heart(归脾汤,Guipi Tang)

Notes: Longan Aril(龙眼肉,Longyanrou) is an advisable drug for reinforcement, and useful for palpitations due to heart-spleen impairment due to excessive mental activities, Since it has the functions of improving appetite, fortifying spleen, replenishing heart blood and ameliorating intelligence, and the feature of being neither digesting-disturbing nor qi-blocking, it is also used as a dietetic herb because of its mild property. Different from Spine Date Seed(酸枣仁,Suanzaoren), which also cures uneasiness of the mind. The type of irritability due to liver-blood insufficiency, while Longan Aril(龙眼肉,Longyanrou) treats poor appetite and lassitude from heart-spleen deficiency.

Section 4
Drugs for Nourishing Yin

1. 沙参, Shashen

English name: Coastal Glehnia Root, and Fourleaf Ladybell Root

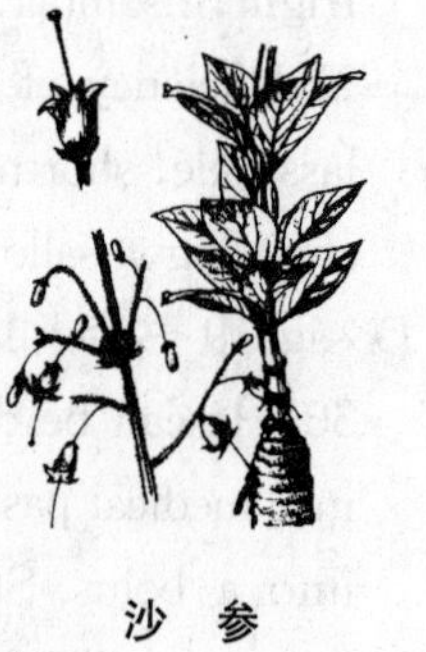

Pharmaceutical name: Radix Glehniae littoralis

Botanical name: Glehnia littoralis F. Schmidt ex Miq.

沙 参

Properties and tastes: sweet, slightly cold

Meridian tropism: lung and stomach

Functions: 1. clear away the pathogenic heat in the lung and nourish yin

2. tonify the stomach and promote the production of body fluid

Indications: 1. dry cough or cough due to asthenia of viscera, hempotysis due to accumulation of heat in the lung and yin deficiency

2. dry tongue and thirst due to febrile disease which damaging body fluid

Dosage: 9～15g, fresh herb may be used for 15～30g.

Contraindication: Not to be taken for patients with deficiency cold. Incompatible with Black False Bellebore(藜芦,Lilu).

Combinations: 1. add Mulberry Leaf(桑叶,Sangye), Dwarf Lilyturf Root(麦门冬,Maimendong)——impairment of yin due to dry-heat, dry cough with little sputum, dry throat and thirst

2. add Common Anemarrhea Rhizome(知母,Zhimu), Tendrilleaf Fritillary Bulb(贝母,Beimu)——fever in chronic consumptive disease due to yin deficiency, cough and hempotysis

3. add Dwarf Lilyturf Root(麦门冬,Maimendong), Rehmannia Dried Root(生

地黄, Shengdihuang)——febrile disease damaging the body fluid, dry tongue and thirst.

4. add Rehmannia Dried Root(生地黄, Shengdihuang), Figwort Root(玄参, Xuanshen)——dry cough due to deficiency of lung yin, protracted cough which a coarseness of voice

5. add Lobed Kudzuvine Root(葛根, Gegen), Cape Jasmine Fruit(栀子, Zhizi)——early stage of cold, aoute caugh(infection of upper respiratory tract)and cough caused by acute bronchitis

6. add Chinese Angelica Root(当归, Danggui), Barbary Wolfberry Fruit(枸杞子, Gouqizi), Szechwan Chinaberry Fruit(川楝子, Chuanlainzi)——pain in the chest and hypochondriac regions, vomiting with sore water, dry tongue and throat due to deficiency of liver and kidney yin

Prescription: Decoction of Glehnia and Ophipogon(沙参麦门冬汤, Shashen Maimendong Tang)

Notes: There are two kinds of Coastal Glehnia Root, and Fourleaf Ladybell Root(沙参, Shashen), which are found in northern and southern of China. They almost have the same functions. The former has a better effect on replenishing yin substances, while the latter has a phlegm-resolving effect. "Being sweet, bitter, warm, and solid, Ginseng(人参, Renshen) focuses its Functions: on reinforcing genuine qi of spleen and stomach, through which it reinforces lungs and kidneys, and is recommended for syndromes of primary qi deficiency." Discussing the difference between Coastal Glehnia Root, and Fourleaf Ladybell Root(沙参, Shashen) and Ginseng(人参, Renshen), Li Shizhen(李时珍) says, "Sweet(tasteless), cold, light and hollow as it is, its functions emphasizes on reinforcing lung-qi, through which it fortifies the spleen and kidneys, and is advisable for syndromes of heart-fire invading lungs." An important difference lies in the fact that Ginseng(人参, Renshen) replenishes yin substances by fortifying yang, while Coastal Glehnia Root, and Fourleaf Ladybell Root(沙参, Shashen) nourishes yin substances to balance yang activities.

2. 麦门冬, Maimendong

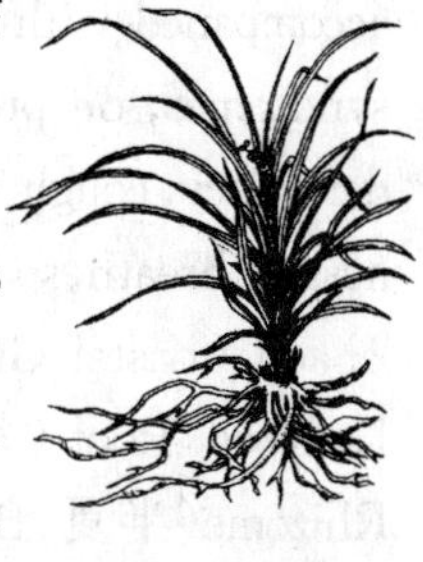

English name: Dwarf Lilyturf Root

Pharmaceutical name: Tuber Ophiopogonis Japonici

Botanical name: Ophiopogon japonicus ker-Gawl. In some parts of China Liriope spicata Lour., L. platyphylla Wang et Tang, or L. minor(Maxim) Mak are used instead.

麦门冬

Properties and tastes: sweet, slightly bitter and slightly cold

Meridian tropism: lung, heart and stomach

Functions: 1. moisten lung and nourish yin

2. tonify and stomach and promote the production of body fluid

3. clear away pathogenic evil heat in the heart

4. moisten intestines to loose the bowels

Indications: 1. lung yin deficiency syndrome——cough with a small amount of thick sputum, hemoptysis, cough due to asthenia of viscera

2. stomach yin deficiency syndrome——dry tongue and thirst, wasting and thirsting syndrome

3. deficiency syndrome——irritability, insomnia, palpitation, and shortness of breath.

4. constipation due to dry intestines

Dosage: 9～15g

Contraindication: Not to be taken for patients with cough due to cold by wind-cold or due to fluid retention or turbid phlegm, and diarrhea due to deficiency cold of the spleen and stomach.

Combinations: 1. add Ginseng (人参, Renshen), Chinese Magnoliavine (五味子, Wuweizi)——a profuse sweating of a patient, who has collapsed due to deficiency, accompaned with tachycardia, hypotension, syndromes, or protracted cough and lung deficiency, cough with little sputum, shortness of breath, spontaneous sweating, etc

2. add Coastal Glehnia Root, and Fourleaf Ladybell Root (沙参, Shashen), Pinellia Rhizome (半夏, Banxia), Licorice Root (甘草, Shenggancao)——deficiency of lung and stomach yin, inflammation of deficiency fire, dry throat and tongue, cough with little sputum.

3. add Honeysuckle Flower (金银花, Jinyinhua), Figwort Root (玄参, Xuanshen)——swelling with pain of the throat, dry mouth and tongue

4. add Coastal Glehnia Root, and Fourleaf Ladybell Root (沙参, Shashen), Ass-hide Glue (阿胶, Ejiao), Loquat Leaf (枇杷叶, Pipaye)——dry cough with a small amount of sputum, hemoptysis.

5. add Rehmannia Dried Root (生地黄, Shengdihuang), Rhubarb (大黄, Dahuang)——constipation due to dry intestines caused by febrile disease which damaging the body fluid

6. add Rehmannia Dried Root (生地黄, Shengdihuang), Figwort Root (玄参, Xuanshen)——yin deficiency and dry intestines, constipation

7. add Bamboo Leaf (竹叶, Zhuye), Coptis Rhizome (黄连, Huanglian)——pathogenic heat entering ying and blood system due to febrile disease, fever aggravated at night, irritability, restlessness

8. add Spine Date Seed (酸枣仁, Suanzaoren), Rehmannia Dried Root (生地黄, Shengdihuang)——yin deficiency and excessive heat, irritability, insomnia

9. add Cochinchinese Asparagus Root (天门冬, Tianmendong)——nourish fluid of the lung, stomach and kidney, and used in all kinds of deficiencies of body fluid and body fluid syndromes

10. add Smoked Plum (乌梅, Wumei)——wasting and thirsting syndrome, excessive drinking

Prescription: Decoction of Radix Ophiopogonis (麦门冬汤, Maimendong Tang)

Notes: Similar to Cochinchinese Asparagus Root (天门冬, Tianmendong), Dwarf Lilyturf Root (麦门冬, Maimendong) nourishes lung-yin, moistens dryness, stimulates generation of vital fluid, and is used for insufficiency of fluid, dryness of the throat, thirst, dry cough (phythisical) and constipation from dryness in intestines. Slightly cold in property, in contrast to Cochinchinese Asparagus Root (天门冬, Tianmendong), which replenishes kidney-yin and is stronger in yin-nourishment. It serves to humidify, cool and provide fluid. It clears away heat from the heart to relieve irritability and replenishes stomach yin as well.

Recent experiments have shown that it, increases the activities of the reticuloendothelial system, number of peripheral white blood cells, immunity, hypoxia tolerance and coronary flow, protects ischemic cardiac muscle, prevents arrhythmia, dilates peripheral vessels, improves functions of pituitary-adrenocortical system, and suppresses staphylococcusalbus, colibacillus, corynebacterium typhi, etc with a strong effect.

3. 天门冬, Tianmendong

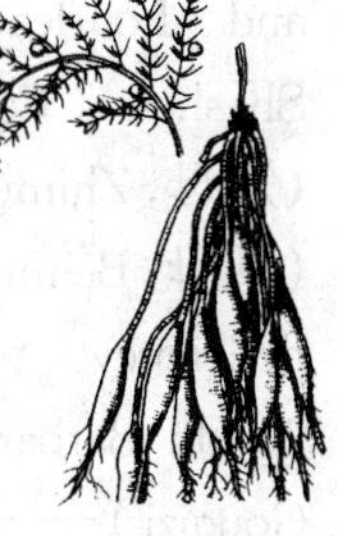
天门冬

English name: Cochinchinese Asparagus Root

Pharmaceutical name: Tuber Asparagi Cochinchinensis

Botanical name: Asparagus cochinchinensis (Lour.) Merr.

Properties and tastes: sweet, bitter and extremely cold

Meridian tropism: lung and kidney

Functions: 1. remove heat from the lung
 2. nourish yin to moisten dryness
 3. moisten the lung and loosen the bowels
 4. inhibit bacteria
 5. inhibit mouse sarcoma-180 and leukemia cells

Indications: 1. dry cough with thick sputum, hemoptysis, cough due to asthenia of viscera.
 2. febrile disease damaging the body fluid, dry tongue, thirst or wasting and thirsting syndrome due to consumption of body fluid
 3. constipation due to dry intestines

Dosage: 6～15g

Contraindication: Not to be taken for patients with deficiency cold of the spleen and stomach, poor appetite.

Combinations: 1. add Rehmannia Dried Root (生地黄, Shengdihuang), Ginseng (人参, Renshen)——yin deficiency and interior heat, dry cough and hemoptysis
 2. add Figwort Root (玄参, Xuanshen), Chinese Angelica Root (当归, Danggui)——constipation due to dry intestines
 3. add Ginseng (人参, Renshen), Prepared Rhizome of Adhesive Rehmannia (熟地黄, Shoudihuang) Cochinchinese Asparagus Root (天门冬, Tianmendong), Snakegourd Root (天花粉, Tianhuafen)——febrile disease damaging the body fluid, thirst, dry throat, constipation
 4. add Dwarf Lilyturf Root (麦门冬, Maimendong), Snakegourd Fruit (瓜蒌, Gualou), Tangerine Peel (陈皮, Chenpi)——whooping cough
 5. add Chinese Corktree Bark (黄柏, Huangbai), Prepared Rhizome of Adhesive Rehmannia (熟地黄, Shoudihuang)——yin deficiency and excessive fire, seminal emission during sleep

Notes: Cohinchinese Asparagus Root (天门冬, Tinmendong), Dwarf Lilyturf Root (麦门冬, Maimendong) and Coastal Glehnia Root, and Fourleaf Ladybell Root (沙参, Shashen), have the same functions of nourishing yin and moistening dyness. Substances and humidifies. Among them, Cohinchinese Asparagus Root (天门冬, Tinmendong) is very cold in property, juicy and humidifying, effective in suppressing lung fire, and thus, It is most helpful for hemoptysis in phthisical cough. Its kidney-yin-replenishing function enables it to cure the high frequency of seminal emission, hyperactivity of fire due to yin deficiency. Dwarf Lilyturf Roo (麦门冬, Maimendong) and Coastal Glehnia Root, and Fourleaf Ladybell Root (沙参, Shashen) are usually used in combination to moisten the lungs, reinforce yin substances, stimulate generation of vital fluid and to fortify stomach functions. Cohinchinese Asparagus Root(天门冬, Tinmendong)is specifie for it is slightly bitter, distributed in the heart system to meridian, clear away heart fire, so it is mostly used to relieve irritability and insomnia due to heat syndrome resulted from yin deficiency.

It is have been given recent in the treatment of hyperplasia of mammary glands and malignant lymphoma.

4. 黄精, Huangjing

English name: Siberian Solomonseal Rhizome

Pharmaceutical name: Thizoma Polygonati

Botanical name: Polygonatum sibiricum Redoute, P. Cyrtonema Hua, p. Macropodium Turcz., P. Kingianum Coll. Et Hemsl., P. Cirrhifolium(Wall.) Royle, or many other varieties of Polygonatum

黄精

Properties and tastes: sweet and medium

Meridian tropism: spleen, lung and kidney

Functions: 1. moisten the lung and nourish yin

2. tonify spleen and supplement qi

3. lower blood pressure

4. reduce blood fat

5. prevent arteriosclerosis

6. reduce blood sugar

Indications: 1. dry cough due to lung deficiency

2. kidney deficiency and insufficiency of essence——soreness in the lumbar region, dizziness, weakness of the feet, etc.

3. deficiency of the spleen and stomach syndrome——lasstitude or fatigue, poor appetite, a weak and soft pulse

4. coronary heart disease

5. hypertension

6. diabetes

7. pulmonary tuberculosis

Dosage: 9~18g

Contraindication: Not to be taken for patients with fluid retention due to spleen deficiency, cough with profuse phlegm, diarrhea with loose stools caused by deficiency cold of the Middle-jiao.

Combinations: 1. add Coastal Glehnia Root, and Fourleaf Ladybell Root (沙参, Shashen), Common Anemarrhea Rhizome (知母, Zhimu), Tendrilleaf Fritillary Bulb (贝母, Beimu)——dry cough due to lung deficiency

2. add Barbary Wolfberry Fruit(枸杞子, Gouqizi)——kidney deficiency and consumption of essence syndrome

3. add Dang-shen Root(党参, Dangshen), Tuckahoe(茯苓, Fuling), Largehead Atractylodes Rhizome(白术, Baizhu)——deficiency of the spleen and stomach qi syndrome

4. add Coastal Glehnia Root, and Fourleaf Ladybell Root(沙参, Shashen), Dwarf Lilyturf Root(麦门冬, Maimendong), Rice Germinating Fruit Sprout(谷芽, Guya)——spleen and stomach yin deficiency

5. add Membranous Milkvetch Root(黄芪, Huangqi), Snakegourd Root(天花粉, Tianhuafen), Dwarf Lilyturf Root(麦门冬, Maimendong), Rehmannia Dried Root(生地黄, Shengdihuang)——diabetes

6. add Red Peony Root(赤芍药, Chishaoyao), Dan-shen Root(丹参, Danshen)——coronary heart disease

7. add Oriental Waterplantain Rhizome(泽泻, Zexie), Tuber Fleeceflower Root(何首乌, Heshouwu)——atherosis

8. add Common Selfheal Fruit-spike(夏枯草, Xiakucao), Chrysanthemum Flower(菊花, Juhua)——hypertension

Notes: Sweet in taste, medium and humidifying in property, Siberian Solomonseal Rhizome(黄精, Huangjing) activates qi and nourishes yin substances such as essence and blood. It is generally used for the syndromes of qi-yin insufficiency involving spleen and lungs, and inadequacy of essence and blood, whose manifestations consist of reduction of appetite, lassitude, cough (from lung deficiency), diabetes mellitus, and general weakness after long-term illness. It is especially used for damage of qi resulted from febrile diseases, after pathogenic heat has been cleared away. It is said in *Herbals for Easy Approaching* (《本草便读》, Bencaobiandu) "Even healthy people may take it as a balanced herb to replenish spleen yin."

Similar to Siberian Solomonseal Rhizome (黄精, Huangjing), Chinese yam is a sweet, medium and qi-yin reinforcing herb and usually given for deficient syndromes of spleen, lungs, heart and kidneys. Chinese yam, however, is viscous in property and cures uncontrollable exhaustion of qi and yin, when Siberian Solomonseal Rhizome (黄精, Huangjing) is used more for humidifying and yin replenishing, and most suitable for damage of qi and yin after febrile diseases as mentioned above.

5. 百合, Baihe

English name: Lily Bulb

Pharmaceutical name: Bulbus Lilii

Botanical name: Lilium brownii F. E. Brown var. colchesteri Wils., L. pumilium DC., or L. longiflorum Thunb.

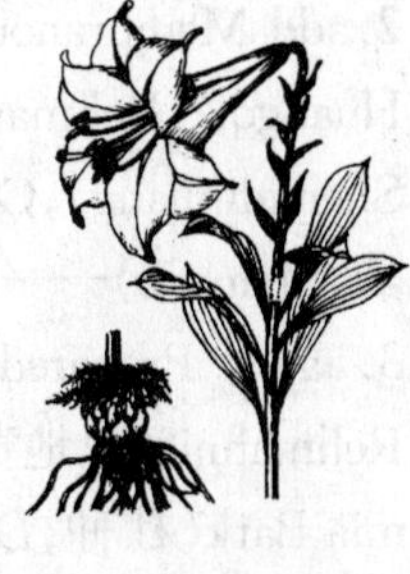

百合

Properties and tastes: sweet, slightly bitter and slightly cold

Meridian tropism: heart and lung

Functions: 1. moisten lung to arrest cough
2. tranquilize the mind

Indications: 1. cough, hemoptysis for due to lung heat, dry lung, yin deficiency and excessive fire, which can be accompanied with dry throat, coarseness of voice
2. palpitation, insomnia for the later stage of febrile disease, failure to clear away excessive heat or neurosis with symptoms of heart yin deficiency. May be accompanied with tidal fever and night sweating

Dosage: 9～30g

Contraindication: This herb is cold and moistening in property. It is not to be taken for patients with cough caused by affection of exogenous wind cold, diarrhea with loose stools due to spleen deficiency.

Combinations: 1. add Common Coltsfoot Flower (款冬花, Kuandonghua)——protracted cough due to lung heat, bloody sputum, or cough with yellow and thick sputum
2. add Figwort Root (玄参, Xuanshen)——yin deficiency and excessive fire, hemoptysis
3. add Common Anemarrhea Rhizome (知母, Zhimu)——the late stage of febrile disease, palpitation, insomnia due to excessive heat
4. add Prepared Rhizome of Adhesive Rehmannia (熟地黄, Shoudihuang)——neurosis, palpitation, insomnia, spontaneous sweating, irritability due to heart yin deficiency

Prescription: Bubus Lily Pill for Strengthening the Lung (百合固金汤, Baihegujin Tang)

Notes: Used to suppress evil fire in heart, protect lungs, relieve cough and tranquilize the mind, it is commonly used for palpitation, thirst and irritability resulted from insufficiency of yin or blood without any obvious side effect. Taking advantage of its reinforcing, heat-suppressing and tranquilizing functions, Zhang Zhongjing(张仲景), the greatest ancient physician, used it for treatment of Lily Bulb(百合, Baihe) complex, which was probably named after Lily Bulb(百合, Baihe). It is caused by stay of the heart and lungs after illness.

Generally used for weakness child birth, or diseases, and for mental disturbances in climacteric, Lily Bulb(百合, Baihe), boiled with Lotus Seed(莲子, Lianzi), it is used for dietetic therapy. Especially for weak persons after illness and the women after delivery and mented disturbance in dimacteric. Pathogenic heat in Lily Bulb(百合, Baihe) and sessile Stemon Root (百部, Baibu), both have the functions of lowering qi to arrest cough Sessile Stemona Root(百部, Baibu) is commonly used for cough, regardless of duration of illness, marked by cold evil, Lily Bulb(百合, Baihe) it emphasizes its functions on humidifying lungs and arresting cough, with an indication of chronic cough of deficient-heat-type due to lung deficiency.

6. 枸杞子, Gouqizi

English name: Barbary Wolfberry Fruit

Pharmaceutical name: Fructus Lycii Chinensis

Botanical name: Lycium chinense Mill. In some parts of China L. barbarum L. is used locally as this herb.

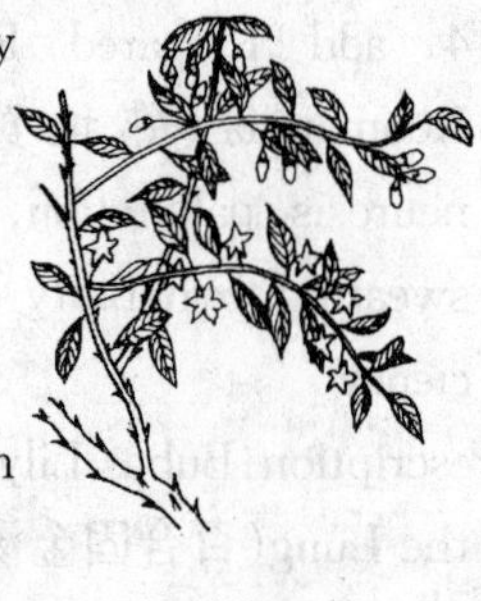

枸杞子

Properties and tastes: sweet and medium

Meridian tropism: liver, kidney and lung

Functions: 1. nourish liver and kidney

2. improve visual acuity

3. moisten the lung

4. strengthen nonspecific immunity

5. hematopoiesis

6. growth stimulating

7. reduce blood fat

8. protect the liver and prevent fatty liver

9. lower blood pressure

10. reduce blood sugar

Indications: 1. liver and kidney yin deficiency syndrome for dizziness, blurred vision soreness and weakness of the waist and knees, seminal emission.

2. cough due to asthenia of viscera and yin deficiency

3. anemia

4. hypertension

5. diabetes

6. chronic hepatic disease

Dosage: 6～9g

Contraindication: It is not advisable for patients with diarrhea due to spleen deficiency.

Combinations: 1. add Chrysanthemum Flower (菊花, Juhua), Asiatic Cornelian Cherry Fruit(山茱萸, Shanzhuyu), Prepared Rhizome of Adhesive Rehmannia (熟地黄, Shoudihuang)——dizziness, blurred eyes due to deficiency of the liver and kidney, hypertension

2. add Membranous Milkvetch Root(黄芪, Huangqi), Rehmannia Dried Root(生地黄, Shengdihuang), Common Yam Rhizome(山药, Shanyao)——diabetes

3. add Prepared Rhizome of Adhesive Rehmannia(熟地黄, Shoudihuang), Eucommia Bark(杜仲, Duzhong)——soreness and weakness of the waist and knees due to kidney deficiency and body weakness.

4. add Chrysanthemum Flower (菊花, Juhua)——eye dizziness and blurred vision, failing of eyesight and headache due to yin deficiency

5. add Dodder Seed(菟丝子, Tusizi)——deficiency of liver and kidney, soreness and pain of the waist and knees, impotence, dark eyes

6. add Longan Aril (龙眼肉, Longyanrou)——palpitation, amnesia, insomnia, irritability, dizziness, lasstitude, soreness and weakness of the waist and knees of the old weak constitution or nonnourishment after illness

7. add Chinese Angelica Root(当归, Danggui)——early greying of the beard and hair, anernia

8. add Chinese Magnoliavine (五味子, Wuweizi), Prepared Rhizome of Adhesive Rehmannia (熟地黄, Shoudihuang)——cough due to consumptive disease

9. add Coastal Glehnia Root, and Fourleaf Ladybell Root(沙参, Shashen), Dwarf Lilyturf Root(麦门冬, Maimendong), Szechwan Chinaberry Fruit (川楝子, Chuanlainzi)——chronic hepatic disease

Prescriptions: 1. Bolus of Fruit Lycii, Flos Chrysanthemi and Radix Rehmanniae(杞菊地黄丸, Qijudihuang Wan)

2. Kidney Ying Reinforcing Bolus(左归丸, Zuogui Wan)

Notes: Barbary Wolfberry Fruit (枸杞子, Gouqizi) is an effective drug for yin deficiency syndrome of liver and kidney for it has the functions of nourishing the liver and kidney and improving eyesight.

It is sweet and tasteful and a dietetic benefit results, in which it can be taken stemmed or made into tea. 9 grams each time, 2～3 times per day. It is used for liver-kidney deficiency. Barbary Wolfberry Fruit(枸杞子, Gouqizi) reinforces yin and yang without obvious imbalance and is commonly used for fortifying kidney. So does Dodder Seed (菟丝子, Tusizi). Barbary Wolfberry Fruit(枸杞子, Gouqizi) provides more yin-replenishing, blood-nourishing and lung-humidifying, and is helpful for consumptive cough from deficiency of lungs and kidneys. Dodder Seed (菟丝子, Tusizi) is more yang-activating, with essence solidifying, and applicable for aching of waist and knee joints, impotence, male sterility, frequent seminal emission, nebulous urination, urinary stuttering, etc. from deficiency of liver and kidneys.

7. 石斛, Shihu

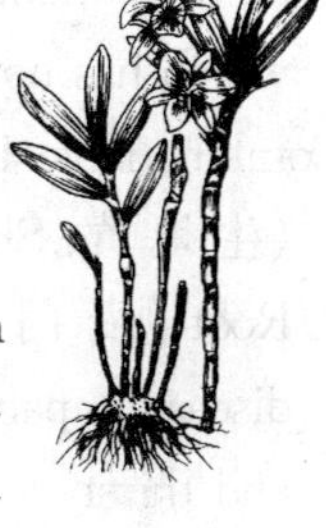
石斛

English name: Dendrobium Herb

Pharmaceutical name: Herba Dendrobii

Botanical name: Dendrobium nobile Lindl., D. Linawianum Reichb. f., D. Officinale K. Kimura et Migo, D. Moniliforme (L.) Sw., D. Hercoglossum Reichb. f., D. Aduncum Wall. Et Lindl., or D. Wilsonii Rolfe, D. Hancockii Rolfe

Properties and tastes: sweet, tasteless and slightly cold

Meridian tropism: the lung, stomach and kidney Meridian

Functions: 1. nourish yin and remove heat

2. tonify the stomach and promote the production of body fluid

3. improve acuity of vision

4. strengthen the waist and knees

5. promote secretion of gastric juice, benefit digestion

Indications: 1. febrile disease impairing the body fluid——dry mouth and tongue, irritability, thirst, sweating

2. deficiency of stomach yin——dry mouth and throat, poor appetite, dry bowels, a red tongue and scanty body fluid

3. yin deficiency and interior heart for prolonged low fever

4. consumption of liver and kidney yin for weakness of the waist and knees, failing of eyesight

Dosage: 6～15g, fresh herb of 15～30g may be used for decoction.

Contraindication: This herb has the action of astringing pathogens, it is not advisable to use in early stage of the epidemic febrile disease. It is sweet and cool, which can generate the pathogenic dampness. Not to be taken for patients with damp-warm pathogens which has not turned into dryness.

Combinations: 1. add Rehmannia Dried Root (生地黄, Shengdihuang), Dwarf Lilyturf Root (麦门冬, Maimendong)——febrile disease impairing the body fluid, irritability and thirst

2. add Ginseng (人参, Renshen), Dwarf Lilyturf Root (麦门冬, Maimendong)——consumption of both qi and yin, lassitude, unwilling to speak, dry mouth and lip

3. add Coastal Glehnia Root, and Fourleaf Ladybell Root (沙参, Shashen), Fragrant Solomonseal Rhizome (玉竹, Yuzhu)——deficiency of stomach yin

4. add Rehmannia Dried Root (生地黄, Shengdihuang), Sweet Wormwood (青蒿, Qinghao)——yin deficiency and interior heat

5. add Prepared Rhizome of Adhesive Rehmannia (熟地黄, Shoudihuang), Twotooth Achyranthes Root (牛膝, Niuxi)——deficiency of kidney yin, soreness and weakness of the waist and knees

6. add Cassia Seed (决明子, Juemingzi), Barbary Wolfberry Fruit (枸杞子, Gouqizi)——deficiency of liver and kidney, blurred vision

Prescription: Eyesight Improving Bolus of Nobles Dendrobium (石斛夜光丸, Shihuyeguang Wan)

Notes: Dendrobium Herb (石斛, Shihu) is characterized by suppressing dissociated heat in the Yangming system, and generally used to improve appetite, nourish stomach-yin and recover intestinal flora balance. Stronger in suppressing heat and stimulating fluid generation, the fresh herb is more suitable for fluid scarcity and lingering heat. This herb is sweet, salty and slightly cold. Ancient books say that it cools lungs and kidneys, replenishes yin substances, improves eyesight and strengthens waist and knees.

8. 桑椹, Sangshen

English name: Mulberry Solomonseal

Pharmaceutical name: Fructus Mori Albae

Botanical name: Mori Alba L.

Properties and tastes: sweet and cold

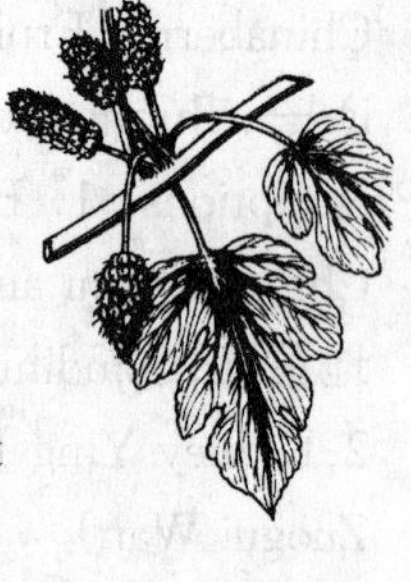
桑椹

Meridian tropism: the heat, liver and kidney Meridian

Functions: 1. nourish yin and moisten lung

2. promote the production of body fluid

3. moisten intestines

Indications: 1. consumption of yin and blood deficiency for dizziness, blurring (vision), tinnitus, insomnia, early greying of the beard and hair

2. thirst due to impairment of body fluid, wasting an thirsting syndrome

3. constipation due to dry intestines

4. diabetes

Dosage:9～15g, use paste of this herb for 15～30g, take it with boiled water.

Contraindication: Not to be taken for patients with diarrhea due to deficiency cold of the spleen and stomach.

Combinations: 1. add Prepared Fleece-flower Root (制首乌, Zhishouwu), Yerbadetajo Herb (墨旱莲, Mohanlian)——yin consumption and blood deficiency, early greying of the beard and hair

2. add Coastal Glehnia Root, and Fourleaf Ladybell Root (沙参, Shashen), Fragrant Solomonseal Rhizome (玉竹, Yuzhu)——dry mouth due to an impairment of body fluid, wasting and thirsting syndrome

3. add Desertliving Gistanche (肉苁蓉, Roucongrong), Hemp Seed (火麻仁, Huomaren)——constipation due to dry intestines

Notes: Being sweet and cold, Mulberry Solomonseal (桑椹, Sangshen) suppresses heat evils, cools heat invaded blood, nourishes blood and yin substances. Mild and tasty as it is, the herb, when taken for a long time, may treat and prevent early greying of hair, improve eyesight, nourish blood, reinforce liver and kidneys, remove dampness-wind evils, improve the movement of the legs, and clear wind or fire of deficiency type. It was proved recently that the 100% decoction of Mulberry Solomonseal (桑椹, Sangshen) stimulates transformation of lymphocyte in a medium level.

9. 玉竹, Yuzhu

English name: Fragrant Solomonseal Rhizome

Pharmaceutical name: Rhizoma Polygonati Odorati

Botanical name: Polygonatum odoratum (Mill.) Druce var. pluriflorum (Miq.) Ohwi (also known as p. Officinale All.). In some parts of China P. Involucratum Maxim., P. Inflatum Komar., or P. Macropodium Turcz. Are used instead.

玉竹

Properties and tastes: sweet and medium

Meridian tropism: the lung and stomach Meridian

Functions: 1. nourish yin and moisten lung

2. promote the production of the body fluid and tonify the stomach

3. reduce blood pids

4. reduce arteriosclerosis cicatrization

5. increase tolerance of oxygen deficit

Indications: 1. consumption of yin and lung dryness for dry cough without sputum or with scanty and sticky sputum, yin deficiency and cough due to consumptive disease.

2. deficiency of stomach yin for hunger with disinclination of a patient for food although suffering from hunger, dry tongue and thirst

3. weak constitution of yin deficiency type, attack of exogenous cold for fever, dry cough with little sputum, irritability, dry mouth

4. wasting and thirsting syndrome due to interior heat

Dosage: 9～15g, it is advisable to use fresh for heat due to deficiency of yin, use streamed Fragrant Solomonseal Rhizome (玉竹, Yuzhu) for patients with mild heat.

Contraindication: It is not advisable for patients with excessive sputum due to spleen deficiency.

Combinations: 1. add Coastal Glehnia Root,

and Fourleaf Ladybell Root(沙参, Shashen), Dwarf Lilyturf Root(麦门冬, Maimendong)——dry cough due to lung dryness or dry-heat in the stomach and lung, irritability and thirst due to an impairment of body fluid

2. add Wild Mint(薄荷, Bohe), Balloonflower Root(桔梗, Jiegeng)——cold due to yin deficiency, fever, cough, etc.

3. add Common Anemarrhea Rhizome(知母, Zhimu), Chinese Wolfberry Root-bark(地骨皮, Digupi), Sichuan Fritillary Bulb(川贝母, Chuanbeimu)——cough due to yin deficiency prolonged low fever

4. add Ginseng(人参, Renshen) for Fragrant Solomonseal Rhizome(玉竹, Yuzhu) in combination with Ginseng(人参, Renshen) benefit body strength, and fortify the courage of people. It is useful for reinforcing qi.

Prescription: Modified Decoction of Fragrant Solomonseal(加减葳蕤汤, Jiajianweirui Tang)

Notes: Being sweet, cold and juicy, Fragrant Solomonseal Rhizome(玉竹, Yuzhu), is mild in effect, does not obstruct the expelling of evils when nourishing yin substances and given for dry-heat syndrome resulting from yin deficiency involving lungs and stomach. It is so mild that it takes effects only after long-term administration.

10. 墨旱莲, Mohanlian

English name: Yerbadetajo Herb

Pharmaceutical name: Herba Ecliptae Prostratae

Botanical name: Eclipta prostrata L.

Properties and tastes: sweet, sour and cold

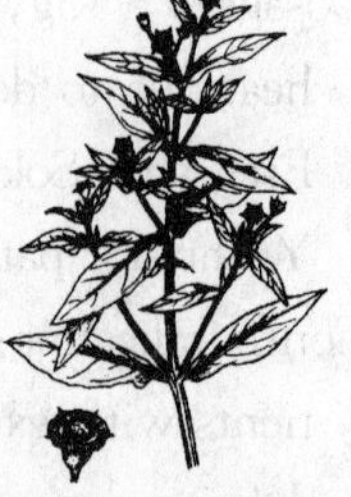
墨旱莲

Meridian tropism: the liver and kidney Meridian

Functions: 1. nourish yin and tonify the kidney

2. remove heat from blood and stop bleeding

3. expand coronary artery, increase the flow of coronary

4. increase tolerance of oxygen deficit

5. tranquilize the mind stop pain

6. inhibit bacteria

7. promote growth and blackening of hair

Indications: 1. deficiency of liver and kidney yin for dizziness, blurring vision, early greying of the beard and hair, soreness and weakness of the waist and knees

2. failure of blood circulation in the vessels due to blood heat for hematemesis, epistaxis, hematochezia, hematuria, metrorrhea and metrostaxis, and suboutaneous hemorrhage

Dosage: 9～15g, proper amount for external use.

Contraindication: It is not advisable for patients with diarrhea due to deficiency cold of spleen and stomach and those in the condition of deficiency cold of kidney qi.

Combinations: 1. add Glossy Privet Fruit(女贞子, Nuzhenzi), Mulberry Solomonseal(桑椹, Sangshen)——early greying of the beard and hair

2. add Rehmannia Dried Root(生地黄, Shengdihuang), Lalang Grass Rhizome(白茅根, Baimaogen)——hemorrhagic syndrome due to yin deficiency and heat in blood

Prescription: Two Solstices Pill(二至丸, Erzhi Wan)

Notes: It is said in *Annotation on Shennong's Herbal Classic* (《本草经疏》, Bencaojingshu), Yerbadetajo Herb(墨旱莲, Mohanlian) is good at cooling blood. Early greying of hair suggests heat evil in blood, loose teeth shows kidney deficiency with heat. This herb has the function: of nourishing yin, cooling blood, and arresting hemorrhage. Therefore, it is regarded as an essential herb for dealing with the disorder in blood system.

11.女贞子,Nuzhenzi

English name: Glossy Privet Fruit

Pharmaceutical name: Fructus Ligustri Lucidi

Botanical name: Ligustrum lucidum Ait

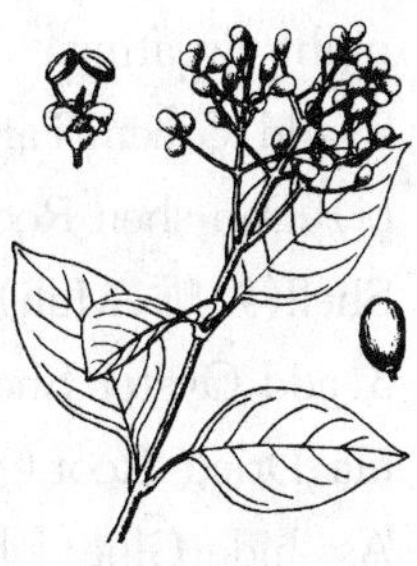

女贞子

Properties and tastes: sweet, bitter and cool

Meridian tropism: the liver and kidney Meridian

Functions: 1. tonify the liver and kidney

2. clear away the heat and improve visual acuity

3. increase the flow of coronary artery

4. protect the liver

5. reduce blood fat pids

6. inhibit bacteria

7. improve the immunity of body fluid

Indications: 1. deficiency of liver and kidney yin for dizziness, blurring vision, early greying of the beard and hair, failing of eyesight, soreness and weakness of the waist and knees

2. fever due to yin deficiency for tidal fever, night sweating, five-center heat

3. chronic hepatitis

4. hyperlipidemia

5. hypoleukocytosis——usually used for prevention and treatment of hypoleukocytosis of cancer patients caused by radiotherapy and chemotherapy

Dosage: 9～15g

Contraindication: It is not advisable for patients with diarrhea due to deficiency cold of spleen and stomach and those in condition of yin deficiency.

Combinations: 1. add Yerbadetajo Herb(墨旱莲, Mohaolian), Prepared Rhizome of Adhesive Rehmannia (熟地黄, Shoudihuang)——deficiency of liver and kidney yin

2. add Chinese Wolfberry Root bark(地骨皮, Digupi), Sweet Wormwood(青蒿, Qinghao)——fever due to yin deficiency

3. add Barbary Wolfberry Fruit(枸杞子, Gouqizi), Dodder Seed (菟丝子, Tusizi)——failing of eyesight

4. add Cassia Seed(决明子, Juemingzi), Feather Cockscomb Seed(青葙子, Qingxiangzi)——fasciculitis optica

5. add Fragrant Solomonseal Rhizome(玉竹, Yuzhu), Barbary Wolfberry Fruit(枸杞子, Gouqizi)——hyperlipidemia

6. add Chinese Thorowax Root(柴胡, Chaihu)——chronic hepatitis

7. add Himalayan Teasel Root(续断, Xuduan)——hyposexuality of women

Prescription: Two Solstices Pill(二至丸, Erzhi Wan)

Notes: Sweet, bitter in taste and slightly cold in property, Glossy Privet Fruit(女贞子, Nuzhenzi) replenishes yin aspect of liver and kidney, through which it cures early greying of hair and improves eyesight. It is similar to Barbary Wolfberry Fruit (枸杞子, Gouqizi) in unctions, both of them nourish yin of liver and kidney, cures the soreness and weakness of waist and knees, and blurred vision due to yin deficiency of liver and kidney. Barbary Wolfberry Fruit(枸杞子, Gouqizi) is more effective in replenishing yin while Glossy Privet Fruit (女贞子, Nuzhenzi), clears away heat with nourishment at the same time and can be used for hectic fever due to tuberculosis, and early greying of hair due to deficiency fire stirring up.

12. 鳖甲, Biejia

English name: Turtle Carapace

Pharmaceutical name: Carapax Amydae Sinensis

Properties and tastes: salty and cold

Meridian tropism: the liver meridian

鳖 甲

Functions: 1. nourish yin and suppress yang
2. soften and resolve hard mass

Indications: 1. consumption of yin and blood, stirring-up of deficiency in the late stage of febrile disease for dry tongue, black teeth wriggling of the limbs or even spasm and contracture of the four limbs
2. fever due to yin deficiency——night fever which is serious at night with recovery in the morning, emaciation, rapid pulse, a red tongue with less coating
It can also be used for hectic fever due to yin deficiency, fever in chronic consumptive disease or tidal fever and night sweating, prolonged lower fever
3. amonorrhea, fibroid, abdominal mass in women
4. hepatolienomegaly
5. prolonged malaria with splenomegaly

Dosage: 9～30g for decoction. Turtle Carapace (鳖甲, Biejia) is advisable for nourishing yin and suppressing hyperactive of yang, and stir-backed Turtle Carapace (鳖甲, Biejia) with vinegar for softening and resolving hard mass.

Contraindication: Not to be taken for patients with deficiency cold of the spleen and stomach, poor appetite, diarrhea and pregnant women.

Combinations: 1. add Sweet Wormwood (青蒿, Qinghao), Rehmannia Dried Root (生地黄, Shengdihuang)——fever due to yin deficiency, hectic fever due to yin deficiency, night sweating
2. add Green Tangerine Peel (青皮, Qingpi), Dan-shen Root (丹参, Danshen), Oyster Shell (牡蛎, Muli)——hepatosplenomegaly
3. add Oyster Shell (牡蛎, Muli), Rehmannia Dried Root (生地黄, Shengdihuang), Ass-hide Glue (阿胶, Ejiao)——stirring-up of edopathic wind due to yin deficiency
4. add Rhubarb (大黄, Dahuang), Amber (琥珀, Hupo)——amenorrhea, fibroid
5. add Membranous Milkvetch Root (黄芪, Huangqi), Oyster Shell (牡蛎, Muli)——pyogenic infection and ulceration of skin and a delay in wound healing
6. add Ass-hide Glue (阿胶, Ejiao), Argy Wormwood Leaf (艾叶, Aiye), White Peony Root (白芍药, Baishaoyao)——profuse menstruation, metrorrhagia and metrostaxis
7. add Ground Beetle (䗪虫, Zhechong), Peach Seed (桃仁, Taoren), Rhubarb (大黄, Dahuang)——malaria with splenomegaly

Prescriptions: 1. Decoction of Three Jia for Restoring Pulse (三甲复脉汤, Sanjiafumai Tang)
2. Bolus for Serious Endogenous Wind-syndrome (大定风珠, Dadingfengzhu)

Notes: Both Tortoise Shell and Plastron (龟版, Guiban), have the functions of nourishing yin to control the hyperactive yang. Turtle Carapace (鳖甲, Biejia) is less effective in nourishment, but more effective in clearing away heat. The two, therefore, are frequently used together to enhance the effect in treatment of fever and stirring up of generated wind, caused by yin deficiency.

Furthermore, Turtle Carapace (鳖甲, Biejia) increases blood circulation and, resolves blood stasis and hard mass. while, Tortoise Shell and Plastron(龟版, Guiban), arrests hemorrhage, reinforces blood, invigorates liver and kidney and strengthens bones and tendons.

13. 龟版, Guiban

English name: Tortoise Shell and Plastron

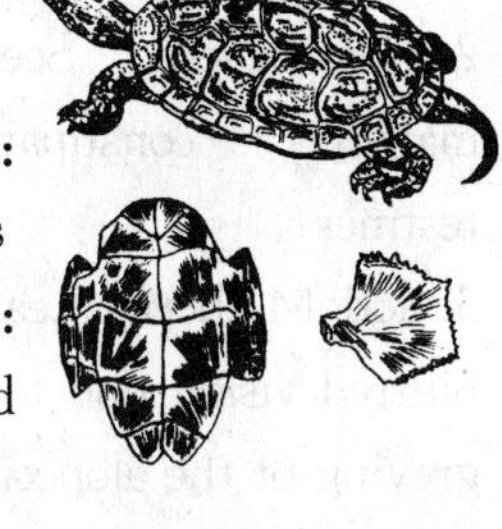

龟 版

Pharmaceutical name: Plastrum Testudinis

Properties and tastes: sweet, salty and cold

Meridian tropism: the liver, kidney and heart Meridian

Functions: 1. nourish yin and suppress yang

2. tonify the kidney and strengthen the bones

3. nourish blood and tonify the heart

4. stop bleeding

5. eliminate blood stasis and relieve pain

6. lower plasma viscosity

7. a dual-regulation of DNA synthetic ratio

8. reduce fever

9. tranquilize to get angry

Indications: 1. yin deficiency and hyperactivity of yang for dizziness, blurred vision, irritability inclined to get angered

2. internal stirring up of deficiency wind wriggling of the limbs, contracture and spasm of muscles and tendons

3. yin deficiency and hyperactivity of fire for hectic fever due to yin deficiency and tidal fever, night sweating, seminal emission

4. kidney yin deficiency for flaccidity of the waist and legs, five delays of children

5. yin deficiency and blood heat syndrome for profuse bleeding, metrorrhagia and metrostaxis

6. deficiency of heart blood syndrome for palpitation, insomnia, amnesia

7. carbuncle and sores (grind it into fine powder for external use)

Dosage: 9～30g, for decoction. Proper amount for external use.

Contraindication: Not to be taken for patients with deficiency cold of spleen and stomach, retention of cold-dampness in the body, exterior syndrome being not relieved.

Combinations: 1. add White Peony Root(白芍药, Baishaoyao), Twotooth Achyranthes Root(牛膝, Niuxi)——yin deficiency and hyperactivity of yang syndrome

2. add Chinese Corktree Bark(黄柏, Huangbai), Common Anemarrhea Rhizome(知母, Zhimu)——fever due to yin deficiency

3. add Rehmannia Dried Root (生地黄, Shengdihuang), Ass-hide Glue (阿胶, Ejiao)——bleeding due to yin deficiency and blood heat

4. add Dragon's Bone (龙骨, Longgu), Thinleaf Milkwort Root (远志, Yuanzhi)——palpitation due to fright, insomnia

5. add Prepared Rhizome of Adhesive Rehmannia (熟地黄, Shoudihuang), Deglued Antler Powder (鹿角霜, Lujiaoshuang)——lack of strength in the muscles and bones due to kidney deficiency

6. add Turtle Carapace(鳖甲, Biejia), Oyster Shell(牡蛎, Muli)——internal stirring up of deficiency wind syndrome

7. add Antler(鹿角,Lujiao),Ginseng(人参,Renshen)——excessive consumption and impairment of blood and essence, deficiency of both yin and yang syndrome

8. add Antler Glue(鹿角胶,Lujiaojiao), Ass-hide Glue(阿胶,Ejiao)——remove obstruction in Ren and Du Meridians, nourish the brain, relieve spasm epilepsy and all kinds of deficiency syndromes

Prescriptions: 1. Tranquilizing Liver-wind Decoction(镇肝息风汤,Zhenganxifeng Tang)

2. Bolus for Serious Endogenous Wind Syndrome(大定风珠,Dadingfengzhu)

Notes: Tortoise Shell and Plastron (龟版, Guiban) is effective in reinforcing the kidney and nourishing yin substances. Suppress deficient yang in the condition of sufficiency of kidney yin. If the two herbs are used in combination, the therapeutic effect will be amplified.

The glue of Tortoise Shell and Plastron (龟版,Guiban), made by its decoction and concentration, is stronger in effect, on nourishing blood and yin substances, and arresting hemorrhage. 3~9 grams of gluey drugs can be melted for internal use.

14. 黑脂麻, Heizhima

English name: Black Sesame

Pharmaceutical name: Semen Sesami Indici

Botanical name: Sesamum indicum Dc

Properties and tastes: sweet and medium

黑脂麻

Meridian tropism: the liver and kidney Meridian

Functions: 1. nourish essence and blood

2. moisten dryness and loosen the bowels

3. reduce cholesterol in blood

Indications: 1. consumption and deficiency of blood and essence syndrome, early greying of the beard and hair, dizziness, blurred vision, tinnitus

2. constipation due to dry intestines

3. arteriosclerosis

Dosage: 9~30g, stir-baked drugs for internal use.

Contraindication: It is not advisable for patients with diarrhea with loose stools.

Combinations: 1. add Yerbadetajo Herb(墨旱莲,Mohanlian), Glossy Privet Fruit(女贞子, Nuzhenzi)——early greying of the beard and hair

2. add Hemp Seed (火麻仁, Huomare n)——constipation due to dry intestines

3. add Mulberry Leaf(桑叶, Sangye)——blurred vision due to liver deficiency, early greying of the alopecia

4. add Chinese Angelica Root(当归,Danggui), Pangolin Scales(穿山甲,Chuanshanjia)——post partum hypogalactia due to blood deficiency

5. add Walnut(胡桃仁,Hutaoren), Chinese Date(大枣, Dazao)——chronic gastritis, and protein urinary due to kidney disorder

Notes: Being mild in property, tasty and harmless to digestive system, Black Sesame(黑脂麻,Heizhima) can be used as a dietetic remedy for a long administration. Take solely after stemmed or stir-baked and ground into powder, or put into pills or pasted with Honey(蜂蜜, Fengmi) or date, or boiled with rice or baked with wheat flour into flat cake.

[Appendix] Astringent Drugs

Definition: Those drugs whose function is astringent are called astringent drugs.

Functions: Most of these drugs are sour and astringent in taste. Their functions comprise arresting perspiration, controlling diarrhea, solidifying sperm, arresting urination, relieving cough and asthma, preventing hemorrhage, etc.

Indications: Spontaneous perspiration, night sweating, prolonged diarrhea and dysentery, frequent seminal emission, enuresis, chronic deficient cough and asthma, metrorrhagia, profuse leukorrhea used to weak constitution after long duration of illness and deficiency of vital qi.

Cautions: These drugs are not advisable for unrelieved exterior evils, early stage of measles, internal accumulation of dampness or stagnant heat evils. It is not used solely for extreme deficiency leading to collapse.

The application of astringent drugs is to prevent continuous discharge leading to exhaustion of vital qi. As deficiency of vital qi is thought to be the principal cause astringent drugs are often combined with drugs for reinforcement in application to achieve the purpose of treating its symptoms and cause at the same time. Some astringent drugs have the function of nourishment that is why they are appended to drugs for replenishing yin.

1. 五味子, Wuweizi

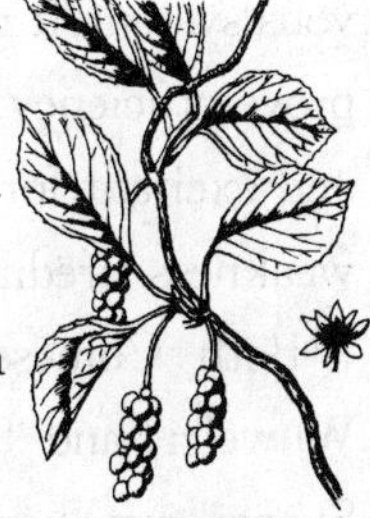
五味子

English name: Chinese Magnoliavine

Pharmaceutical name: Fructus Schisandrae Chinensis

Botanical name: Schisandra chinensis(Turcz.)Baill.

Properties and tastes: sour and warm

Meridian tropism: the lung, kidney and heart Meridian

Functions: 1. astringe the lung to stop coughing

2. promote the production of body fluid and astringe perspiration

3. tonify the kidney to consolidate the essence

4. relieve diarrhea

5. tranquilize the wind and calm the heart

6. reduce GPT protect the liver

7. excite the uterus

8. improve eyesight

Indications: 1. prolonged cough and asthma of deficiency type

2. thirst, spontaneous sweating, night sweating

3. seminal emission and premature ejaculation

4. prolonged diarrhea can not be arrested

5. palpitation, imsomnia, excessive dreams during sleep

6. chronic hepatitis

7. unbroken or broken before time of amniotic membrane of fetus and atonic labor

Dosage: 3～6g, grind it into fine powder, 1～3g each time. Cooked Chinese Magnoliavine (五味子, Wuweizi) is used for tonifying deficiency and fresh Chinese Magnoliavine(五味子, Wuweizi) for relieving cough.

Contraindication: This herb has the function of astringing pathogens, not to be used for patients with exterior syndrome not being relieved, excess heat in the interior, early stage of cough, or measels. Improper for pregnant women

Combinations: 1. add Asiatic Cornelian Cherry Fruit(山茱萸, Shanzhuyu), Common Yam Rhizome(山药, Shanyao)——asthma of deficiency type, prolonged cough

2. add Ephedra(麻黄, Mahuang), Gambirplant Hooked Stem and Branch (钩藤,

Gouteng)——senile(as thmatic)bronchitis

3. add Ginseng(人参, Renshen), Dwarf Lilyturf Root(麦门冬, Maimendong)——heat evil impairing qi and yin, palpitation, a weak pulse, thirst and sweating

4. add Membranous Milkvetch Root(黄芪, Huangqi), Rehmannia Dried Root(生地黄, Shengdihuang), Snakegourd Root(天花粉, Tianhuafen)——diabetes marked by thirst with excessive drinking

5. add Chinese Arborvitae Seed(柏子仁, Baiziren), Ginseng(人参, Renshen), Oyster Shell(牡蛎, Muli)——night sweating due to yin deficiency, spontaneous sweating due to yang deficiency

6. add Mantis Egg-case(桑螵蛸, Sangpiaoxiao), Dragon's Bone(龙骨, Longgu)——seminal emission, lingering diarrhea

7. add Medicinal Evodia Root(吴茱萸, Wuzhuyu), resh Ginger(生姜, Shengjiang)——prolonged diarrhea

8. add Dwarf Lilyturf Root(麦门冬, Maimendong), Dan-shen Root(丹参, Danshen), Spine Date Seed(酸枣仁, Suanzaore n)——palpitation, insomnia, amnesia, anxiety, lassitude, impotence

9. add Dried Ginger(干姜, Ganjiang), anchurian Wildginger Herb(细辛, Xixin)——cough with dyspnea due to cold phlegm attacking the lungs, watery and excessive sputum due to cough of lung cold type.

10. add Capillary Wormwood Herb(茵陈蒿, Yinchenhao), Chinese Date(大枣, Dazao)——chronic hepatitis

11. add Twotooth Achyranthes Root(牛膝, Niuxi), Ginseng(人参, Renshen)——unbroken or broken before time of amniotic membrane of fetus and atonic labor

12. add Ginseng(人参, Renshen), Giant Gecko(蛤蚧, Gejie)——asthma of deficiency type and prolonged cough due to deficiency of the lung and kidney

13. add Cherokee Rose Fruit(金樱子, Jinyingzi), Mantis Egg-case(桑螵蛸, Sangpiaoxiao)——seminal emission due to kidney deficiency

14. add Chinese Gall(五倍子, Wubeizi)——spontaneous sweating, night sweating prolonged cough, asthma, diarrhea, dysentary, seminal emission, morbid leukorrhea, mentrorrhagia and mentrostaxis, prolapse of rectum, and prolapse of uterus

Prescription: Powder for Restoring Pulse Beat (生脉散, Shengmai San)

Notes: Chinese Magnoliavine(五味子, Wuweizi) is very sour, in taste with functions of astringing and warm, nourishing yin, it astrings lung qi in the upper pant and nourishes kidney yin in the lower, arrests perspiration, stimulates fluid generation, controls diarrhea and seminal emission, tonifies the kidney to consolidate the essence. It is a warm drug with strong astringent functions.

Ancient people said that Chinese Magnoliavine(五味子, Wuweizi) is applicable for all sorts of exhaustion syndromes of qi and blood, without the exterior evils, in combination with tonifying drugs.

By a dual regulation of the central nervous system, it relieves tiredness so as to improve efficiency. It is used as a rehabilitation and excitant for those patients with general weakness tiredness.

Both Chinese Magnoliavine(五味子, Wuweizi) and Spine Date Seed(酸枣仁, Suanzaoren) have the functions of astringing, stimulating fluid generation, relieving over-thirst and arresting perspiration. Combination of the two drugs is suitable for profuse perspiration, night perspiration, and over-thirst due to fluid scarcity. In comparison, Chinese Magnoliavine (五味子, Wuweizi) tranquilizes through reinforcing the kidney, astringing qi and relieving restlessness, while, Spine Date Seed (酸枣仁, Suanzaoren) through reinforcing the liver and replenishing blood, is used together with Chinese Magnoliavine (五味子, Wuweizi), for irritability, palpitation and insomnia. Chinese Magnoliavine (五味子, Wuweizi) has a wider extent of application, especially for solidifying the kidney to control spermatorrhea, calming lungs to relieve cough, etc.

2. 乌梅, Wumei

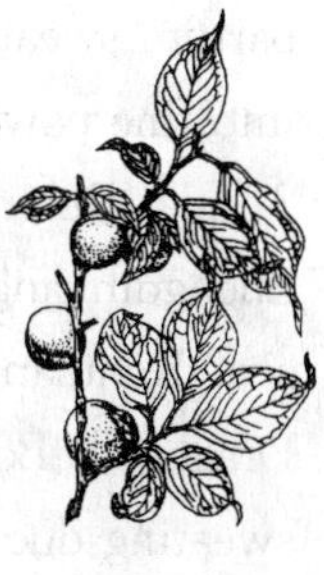

English name: Smoked Plum

Pharmaceutical name: Fructus Pruni Mume

Botanical name: Prunus mume (Sieb.) Sieb. et Zucc.

Properties and tastes: sour and medium

乌 梅

Meridian tropism: the liver, spleen, lung and large intestine Meridian

Functions: 1. astringe the lung to stop coughing
2. astringe the intesines to stop diarrhea
3. promote the production of body fluid to relieve thirst
4. harmonize the stomach to relieve colic caused by ascaris
5. stop bleeding
6. relax Oddi's sphincter
7. inhibit tumor

Indications: 1. prolonged cough due to lung deficiency
2. prolonged diarrhea and dysentery
3. irritabiltiy, thirst due to deficiency heat
4. colic caused by ascariasis, abdominal pain and vomiting for biliary ascariasis, ascaris intestinal obstruction
5. mentrorrhagia and mentrostaxis
6. polyps
7. carcinoma of the rectum, hysterocarcinoma

Dosage: 3 ~ 9g, large dosage may be used for 30g, properly amount for external use. Pound it into pieces or carbonize and grind it into fine powder before it is applied to the affected parts.

Contraindication: This herb is sour in taste and astringing in property. It is not advisable for patients with exterior pathogens, or stagnation of the excess-heat in the interior.

Combinations: 1. add Pinellia Rhizome (半夏, Banxia), Apricot Seed (杏仁, Xingren), Ass-hide Glue (阿胶, Ejiao)——prolonged cough due to lung deficiency
2. add Medicine Terminalia Fruit (诃子, Hezi), Nutmeg Seed (肉豆蔻, Roudoukou)——prolonged diarrhea
3. add Coptis Rhizome (黄连, Huanglian), Hawthorn Fruit (山楂, Shanzha)——prolonged dystentery
4. add Snakegourd Root (天花粉, Tianhuafen), Lobed Kudzuvine Root (葛根, Gegen)——diabetes marked by thirst
5. add Manchurian Wildginger Herb (细辛, Xixin), Dried Ginger (干姜, Ganjiang), Coptis Rhizome (黄连, Huanglian)——abdominal pain, vomiting caused by ascariasis
6. add Garden Burnet Root (地榆, Diyu), Ass-hide Glue (阿胶, Ejiao)——hematochezia, mentrorrhagia and mentrostaxis
7. add Areca Seed (槟榔, inlang), Common Aucklandia Root (木香, Muxiang), Bitter Orange (枳壳, Zhiqiao)——biliary ascariasis
8. add Turtle Carapace (鳖甲, Biejia)——hepatolienomegaly

9. add Rehmannia Dried Root(生地黄, Shengdihuang)——diabetes, diabetes insipidus and achlorhydria

10. add Spreading Hedyotis Herb(白花蛇舌草, Baihuasheshecao) - carcinoma of the rectum, hysterocarcinoma

11. add Silkworm with Batrytis Larva(白僵蚕, Baijiangcan)——esophagopolypus, proctopoly pus colpopoly pus, metropolypus

12. add Chinese Magnoliavine(五味子, Wuweizi)——spontaneous sweating, night sweating diabetes, high urinary sugar

Prescription: Dark Pulm Pill(乌梅丸, Wumei Wan)

Notes: "Smoked Plum(乌梅, Wumei) corrals lung qi, calms intestinal movement," described by Huang Gongxiu(黄宫绣), an ancient physician, "relieves spasm of the limbs, calms irritated intestinal ascarides, removes necrotic tissue, malignant nevi, and helps to remove splinters from tissue." It is reported that Smoked Plum(乌梅, Wumei) is used for removing vaginal and rectal polyps, etc with evident effect. To use this take Smoked Plum(乌梅, Wumei, carbonize the pure pulp) and Silkworm with Batrytis Larva(白僵蚕, Baijiangcan, baked slightly brown), 248 grams of each, grind them into fine powder and make into pills with 500 grams of Honey(蜂蜜, Fengmi). Take 6 grams each time, 3 times a day for internal use. It is reported that it is also effective for rectum polyp and vaginal polyps.

3. 麻黄根, Mahuanggen

English name: Ephedra Root

Pharmaceutical name: Radix Ephedrae

Botanical name: Ephedra sinica Staph or E. Equisetina Bge.

Properties and tastes: sweet and medium

Meridian tropism: the lung meridian

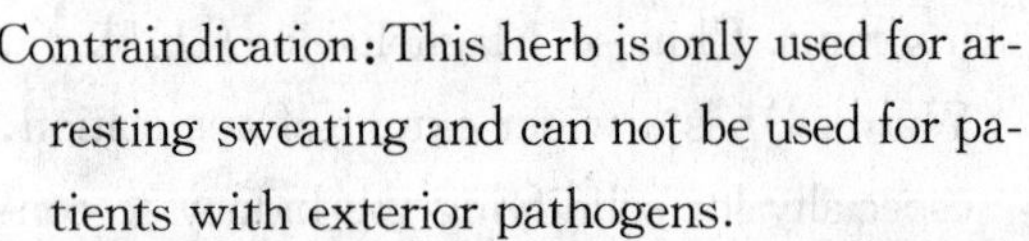
麻黄根

Function: astringe sweating

Indications: 1. spontaneous sweating

2. night sweating

Dosage: 3～9g, proper amounts for external use, grind it into fine powder and then make into face powder.

Contraindication: This herb is only used for arresting sweating and can not be used for patients with exterior pathogens.

Combinations: 1. add Membranous Milkvetch Root(黄芪, Huangqi)——spontaneous sweating

2. add Oyster Shell(牡蛎, Muli)——postpartum sweating due to deficiency, grind it into fine powder and apply it to the body.

3. add Rehmannia Dried Root(生地黄, Shengdihuang), Prepared Rhizome of Adhesive Rehmannia(熟地黄, Shoudihuang), Dragon's Bone(龙骨, Longgu)——night sweating due to yin deficiency

Notes: Acting on lung meridian, Ephedra Root (麻黄根, Mahuanggen) is sweet, and intacte and medium in property. Ephedra Root(麻黄根, Mahuanggen) performs its functions, for arresting perspiration, in the superficial layer to cure sweat syndromes of deficiency type, such as, spontaneous perspiration due to qi deficiency and night sweating due to yin deficiency.

Another drug, Oyster Shell(牡蛎, Muli), also astrings perspiration and frequently takes its effect together with Ephedra Root (麻黄根, Mahuanggen) in sweat syndromes of deficiency type. However, Ephedra Root (麻黄根, Mahuanggen) focus its functions on mere perspiration-arresting, white Oyster

Shell(牡蛎,Muli)acts through calming the hyperactive yang and astringing yin, and hence, is widely used. Furthermore, these functions of Oyster Shell(牡蛎,Muli)enable it to relieve restlessness of yin deficiency with hyperactivity of yang, insomnia or sleep with dreams, vertigo, stirring up of deficiency wind stirring up of deficiency, frequent seminal emission, profuse leukorrhea, etc.

4. 石榴皮, Shiliupi

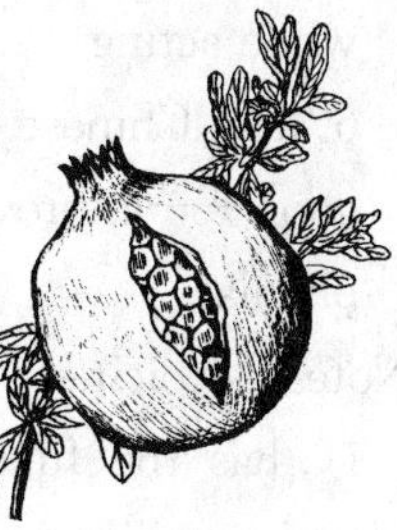

English name:
Pomegranate Rind Peel

Pharmaceutical name:
Pericarpium Punicae Granati

Botanical name: Punica granatum L.

石榴皮

Properties and tastes:
sour, astringent and warm

Meridian tropism: the stomach and large intestine meridian

Functions: 1. astringe the intestines to stop diarrhea
2. control the essence and keep the semen
3. cure leukorrhagia
4. kill ascaris
5. stop bleeding

Indications: 1. prolonged diarrhea, prolonged dysentery, prolapsed of the rectum
2. ascariasis
3. seminal emission, premature ejeculation (prospermia)
4. mentrorrhagia and mentrostaxis, morbid leukorrhea
5. amibic dysentery

Dosage: 3 ~ 9g, proper amount for external use. Use fresh drugs for decoction stir-baked Pomegranate Rind Peel(石榴皮, Shiliupi) is used as powder, carbonized Pomegranate Rind Peel(石榴皮, Shiliupi) is used for arresting bleeding.

Contraindication: Not to be taken for patients in early stage of diarrhea and dysentery.

Combinations: 1. add brown sugar——chronic dysentery
2. add Areca Seed(槟榔, Binlang)——ascariasis, taeniasis, enterobiasis
3. add Nutmeg Seed(肉豆蔻, Roudoukou u)—— prolonged diarrhea, prolonged dysentery prolapse of the rectum
4. add Membranous Milkvetch Root(黄芪, Huangqi), Shunk Bugbane Rhizome(升麻, Shengma), Largehead Atractylodes Rhizome(白术, Baizhu)——prolonged diarrhea, prolapse of rectum accompanied with shortness of breath, lassitude
5. add Ass-hide Glue(阿胶, Ejiao), Chinese Angelica Root(当归, Danggui)——mentrorrhagia and mentrostaxis
6. add Plantain Seed(车前子, Cheqianzi)——morbid leukorrhea
7. add Chinese Magnoliavine(五味子, Wuweizi)——seminal emission
8. add Coptis Rhizome(黄连, Huanglian), Chinese Corktree Bark(黄柏, Huangbai), Ass-hide Glue(阿胶, Ejiao)——prolonged dysentery due to damp-heat not being relieved

Notes: Pomegranate Rind Peel(石榴皮, Shiliupi) is sour and astringeant in tastes which suggests its astringent function, It is suitable for prolonged diarrhea or dysentery, profuse leukorrhea, and prolapse of rectum. To avoid evils being retained, Pomegranate Rind Peel(石榴皮, Shiliupi) can not be used in the early stages of diarrhea or dysentery, when remaining evils still exist.

Grind Carbonize Pomegranate Rind Peel (石榴皮, Shiliupi) into powder and mix it with oil, it can be externally applied for psoriasis.

5. 诃子, Kezi

English name: Medicine Terminalia Fruit

Pharmaceutical name: Fructus Terminaliae Chebulae

Botanical name: Terminalia chebula Retz. or T. Chebula Retz. var. gangetica Roxb.

诃 子

Properties and tastes: bitter, sour, astringent, medium

Meridian tropism: the lung and large intestine meridians

Functions: 1. astringe the interstine to stop diarrhea

2. astringe lung qi to arrest cough

3. clear away heat in the lung, easy on the throat and voice

Indications: 1. prolonged diarrhea, prolonged dysentery, prolapse of the rectum

2. cough and asthma due to lung deficiency

3. prolonged cough, aphonia

Dosage: 3 ~ 9g, fresh Medicine Terminalia Fruit(诃子, Hezi) is good at astringing lung-qi, roasted in ashes is good at relieving diarrhea with astringents.

Contraindication: Not to be taken for patients with exterior pathogens, interior stagnation of damp-heat, and early stage of cough.

Combinations: 1. add Coptis Rhizome(黄连, Huanglian), Common Aucklandia Root(木香, Muxiang)——prolonged dysentery, abdominal pain with heat.

2. add Dried Ginger(干姜, Ganjiang), Poppy Capsule(罂粟壳, Yingsuqiao)——prolonged diarrhea due to deficiency cold or prolapse of rectum

3. add Balloonflower Root(桔梗, Jiegeng), Licorice Root(甘草, Gancao)——aphonia, failure to speak

4. add Apricot Seed(杏仁, Xingren), Ricepaperplant Pith(通草, Tongcao), Dried Ginger (干姜, Ganjiang)——prolonged cough and a husky voice

5. add Ginseng(人参, Renshen), Chinese Magnoliavine(五味子, Wuweizi), Giant Gecko(蛤蚧, Gejie)——cough and asthma due to lung deficiency, shortness of breath while acting

6. add Chinese White Olive(青果, Qingguo)——improve clearness of voice, treat aphonia

Notes: Medicine Terminalia Fruit(诃子, Hezi), has the functions of arresting diarrhea and expelling intestinal gas to relieve distention, it is applicable to most cases in different combination according to varied cold or heat types of the syndromes.

Medicine Terminalia Fruit(诃子, Hezi) calms the lungs to relieve cough, purges the lungs and relieves sore throat to cure hoarseness. It is applicable to either deficiency or excess type.

Both Medicine Terminalia Fruit(诃子, Hezi) and Smoked Plum(乌梅, Wumei) are sour and astringent in taste with the functions of astringing arresting cough and diarrhea. The former reduces evil fire, relieves sore throat and hoarseness, while the latter balances movement of the stomach, stimulates fluid generation and relieves colic via calming ascarides.

6. 肉豆蔻, Roudoukou

English name: Nutmeg Seed

Pharmaceutical name: Semen Myristicae Fragranticis

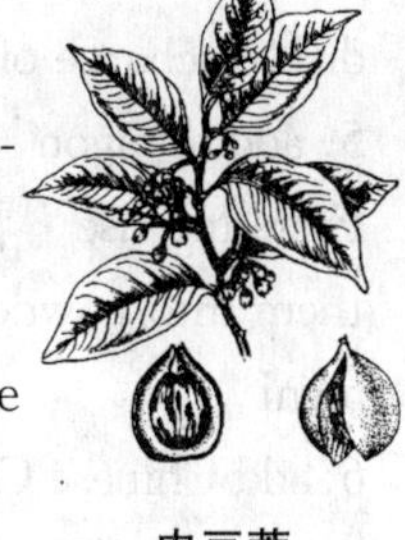
肉豆蔻

Botanical name: Myristica fragrans Houtt.

Properties and tastes: pungent and warm

Meridian tropism: the spleen stomach and large intestine Meridian

Functions: 1. warm the Middle-jiao and activate the vital energy

2. astringe the intestine to stop diarrhea

Indications: 1. prolonged diarrhea

2. poor appetite and vomiting due to stomach cold

3. pain in the chest and epigastrium due to qi stagnation

Dosage: 3 ~ 9g, 1.5 ~ 3g used in bolus and powder, it can strengthen the action of warming the Middle-jiao and arresting diarrhea after it is roasted in ashes.

Contraindication: This herb has the action of warming the Middle-jiao and astringing, It cannot be used for patients with diarrhea due to damp-heat. Fresh Nutmeg Seed(肉豆蔻, Roudoukou) can cause diarrhea, overtaking can cause poisoning, manifested as dizziness, delirium, lethargy, illusion.

Combinations: 1. add Nutgrass Galingale Rhizome(香附, Xiangfu), Medicated Leaven (神曲, Shenqu), Malt(麦芽, Maiya)——improper diet of children, vomiting milk and dyspepsia

2. add Ginseng(人参, Renshen), Largehead Atractylodes Rhizome(白术, Baizhu), Dried Ginger(干姜, Ganjiang)——prolonged diarrhea and dysentery due to deficiency cold of spleen and stomach

3. add Common Aucklandia Root(木香, Muxiang), Pinellia Rhizome(半夏, Banxia), Dried Ginger(干姜, Ganjiang)——distension and pain in the abdomen and epigastrium, vomiting due to deficiency cold of spleen and stomach.

4. add Medicinal Evodia Root(吴茱萸, uzhuyu), Chinese Magnoliavine(五味子, Wuweizi)——diarrhea just before dawn due to deficiency cold of spleen and kidney

5. add Malaytea Scurfpea Fruit(补骨脂, Buguzhi)——diarrhea just before dawn, chronic colitis, diarrhea of tuberculosis

6. add Sharpleaf Galangal Fruit(益智仁, Yizhiren)——profuse saliva due to spleen deficiency, and enuresis due to kidney deficiency

Prescription: Pill of Four Miraculous Drugs(四神丸, Sishen Wan)

Notes: Nutmeg Seed(肉豆蔻, Roudoukou) is particularly effective for prolonged diarrhea and dysentery of deficiency cold type, achieving the purpose of treating both symptoms and causes at the same time.

It is said in *Orthodox Interpretation of Materia Medica* (《本草正义》, Bencaozhengyi) "Nutmeg Seed (肉豆蔻, Roudoukou) eliminates cold evil, dries up dampness, removes stagnancy, promotes qi circulation, balances movement of digestive system, and arrests uncontrollable diarrhea."

7. 赤石脂, Chishizhi

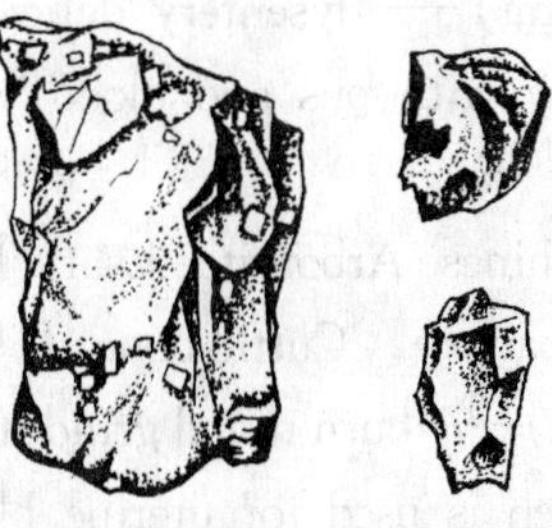
赤石脂

English name: Red Halloysite

Pharmaceutical name: Halloysitum Rubrum

Properties and tastes: sweet, sour, astringent and warm

Meridian tropsim: large intestine and stomach Meridian

Functions: 1. astringe the intestine to stop diarrhea

2. stop bleeding

3. remove dampness, promote tissue regeneration and ulcer healing (for external use)

Indications: 1. prolonged dysentery for dysentery, hematochezia, prolapse of the rectum due to failure of Lower-jiao

2. mentrorrhagia and mentrostaxis

3. morbid leukorrhea

4. unhealing ulcer

5. watery discharge of ulcer

6. bleeding due to injury

Dosage: 9 ~ 18g, proper amounts for external use, grind it into fine powder and apply it to the affected areas.

Contraindication: Not to be taken for patients with stagnation of damp-heat in the interior. Take cautions for pregnant women in application.

Combinations: 1. add Limonite (禹余粮, Yuyuliang) —— protracted dysentery, protracted diarrhea, excessive mense of women.

2. add Dried Ginger (干姜, Ganjiang), Polished Round-grained Nonglutinous Rice (粳米, Jingmi) —— dysentery deficiency cold, dysentery with pus and blood which does not stop

3. add Chinese Arborvitae Leafy Twig (侧柏叶, Cebaiye), Cuttle-bone (乌贼骨, Wuzeigu) —— burn it and grind it into powder, which is used for uterine bleeding for several years of women.

4. add White Peony Root (白芍药, Baishaoyao), Dried Ginger (干姜, Ganjiang) —— Leukorrhea with liagering reddish discharge of women

5. add Dragon's Bone (龙骨, Longgu), Frankincense (乳香, Ruxiang) —— grind them into powder for external use to treatment

6. add Chinese Corktree Bark (黄柏, Huangbai), Coptis Rhizome (黄连, Huanglian) —— external use to, treat damp scabies with watery discharge

7. add Rhubarb (大黄, Dahuang) —— put for external use into powder, treat bleeding due to injury

8. add Malaytea Scurfpea Fruit (补骨脂, Buguzhi) —— excessive menses.

Notes: Red Halloysite (赤石脂, Chishizhi) has the function of astringing (for it is a kind of heavy mineral). Red Halloysite (赤石脂, Chishizhi) cures "exhaustion" disorders, which includes diarrhea, a disorder of the digestive system, metrorrhagia and profuse leukorrhea, and disorders of the female reproductive system. In Addition, it promotes tissue regeneration and ulcer healing when it is applied externally.

8. 禹余粮, Yuyuliang

English name: Limonite

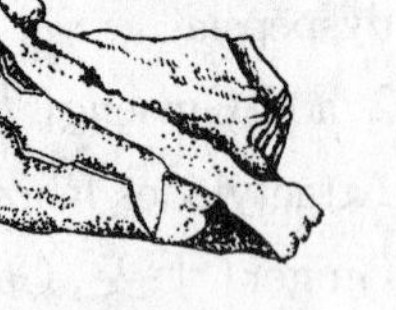
禹余粮

Pharmaceutical name: Limonitum

Properties and tastes: sweet, astrigent and medium

Meridian tropism: the stomach and large intestine Meridian

Functions: 1. astringe the intestine to stop diarrhea

2. astringe and arrest bleeding

Indications: 1. prolonged diarrhea and dysentery

2. mentrorrhagia and mentrostaxis

3. morbid leukorrhea

Dosage: 9～18g

Contraindication: This herb is only used for astringing, contraindicated in excess syndrome. Take cautions for pregnant women in application.

Combinations: 1. add Charred Human Hair(血余炭, Xueyutan)——protracted diarrhea and dysentary, chronic enteritis, impairment of intestinal mucosa

2. add Malaytea Scurfpea Fruit(补骨脂, Buguzhi), Largehead Atractylodes Rhizome (白术, Baizhu), Licorice Root(甘草, Gancao)——diarrhea due to spleen deficiency and deficiency diarrhea in older persons

3. add Cuttle-bone(乌贼骨, Wuzeigu), Oyster Shell(牡蛎, Muli), Cassia Bark(肉桂, Rougui)——grind equal share of the drug into fine powder and take it with wine for metrorrhagia and metrostaxis

4. add Dried Ginger(干姜, Ganjiang)——lingering leukorrhea of women

Notes: Heavy in property, Red Halloysite(赤石脂, Chishizhi) is characterized by astringing. It is an effective drug for astringing the Lower-jiao. When acting in the qi system, it arrests diarrhea; when in the blood system, it arrests hemorrhage. It can be used for prolonged or severe diarrhea, hematochezia, dysentery, metrorrhagia, profuse leukorrhea, etc.

Limonite(禹余粮, Yuyuliang) and Red Halloysite(赤石脂, Chishizhi) are similar in properties and functions, used for astringing diarrhea, metrorrhagia. They are usually used in combination in clinical treatment to enhance astringent functions.

9. 莲子, Lianzi

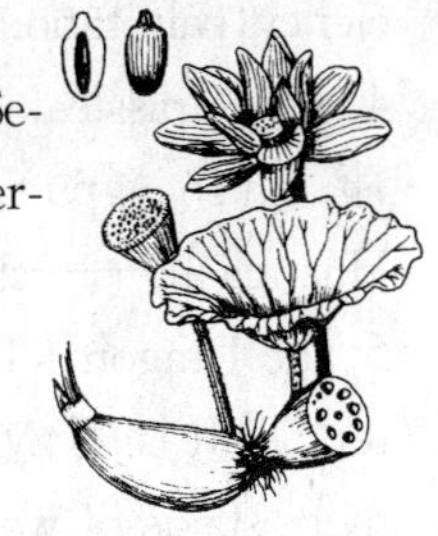
莲 子

English name: Lotus Seed

Pharmaceutical name: Semen Nelumbinis Nuciferae

Botanical name: Nelumbo nucifera Gaertn.

Properties and tastes: sweet, astringent and medium

Meridian tropism: the spleen, kidney and heart Meridian

Functions: 1. nourish the spleen to stop diarrhea

2. tonify the kidney to stop seminal emission

3. nourish heart and calm the wind

Indications: 1. protracted diarrhea due to spleen deficiency, poor appetite

2. seminal emission and lingering diarrhea due to kidney deficiency

3. irritability of deficiency type, palpitation, insomnia

4. metrorrhagia and metrostaxis, profuse leukorrhea of women

Dosage: 6～15g

Contraindication: It is not suitable for patients with costipation.

Combinations: 1. add Rehmannia Dried Root (生地黄, Shengdihuang), Asiatic Cornelian Cherry Fruit(山茱萸, Shanzhuyu), Chinese Magnoliavine(五味子, Wuweizi)——seminal emission, and lingering diarrhea due to kidney deficiency

2. add Common Yam Rhizome(山药, Shanyao), Tuckahoe(茯苓, Fuling)——diarrhea due to spleen deficiency, poor appetite

3. add Spine Date Seed(酸枣仁, uanzaoren),

Thinleaf Milkwort Root (远志, Yuanzhi)——insomnia due to heart deficiency, palpitation, amnesia

4. add Grassleaf Sweetflag Rhizome (石菖蒲, Shichangpu), Coptis Rhizome (黄连, Huanglian)——chronic dysentery

5. add Dragon's Bone (龙骨, Longgu), Oyster Shell (牡蛎, Muli)——metrorrhagia and metrostaxis of women, profuse leukorrhea

Prescription: Lotus Seed Decoction For Clearing Away The Heart-fire (清心莲子饮, Qingxin Lianzi Yin)

Notes: Being sweet and medium, Lotus Seed (莲子, Lianzi) takes its function of astringing and acts on the heart, spleen and kidney. It can treat both symptoms and cause at the same time, such as lingering diarrhea due to spleen deficiency, frequent seminal emission due to kidney deficiency and insomnia of deficiency type.

Comparision Among Lianxu, Lianzixin, Lianfang. Heye and Oujie

Name	Part used as herb	Properties and tastes	Functions	Indications and prescriptions	Dosage
Hindu Lotus Stamen (莲须, Lianxu)	Stamen of lotus	Sweet, stringing and medium	Clear heart heat, stregthen kidney, astringe essence and stop bleeding	Nocturnal emission, prospermia, enuresis, frequent urine, hematemesis and metrorrhagia. Often used with Dragon's Bone (龙骨, Longgu) and Oyster Shell (牡蛎, Muli)	1.5～6g
Hindu Lotus Plumule (莲子心, Lianzixin)	Plumule of lotus	Bitter and cold	Clear heart heat, reduce fever, stop bleeding and astringe essence	Restless heat and unconsciousness due to febrile disease, insomnia and seminal emission due to disharmony between heart and kidney, hematemesis due to blood heat. Together used with Scrophularia Root (玄参, Xuanshen), Ophiopogon Root (麦门冬, Maimendong) and Lophatherum (竹叶, Zhuye)	1.5～3g
Hindu Lotus Receptacle (莲房, Lianfang)	Mature receptacle of lotus	Bitter, stringing and warm	Remove blood stasis and stop bleeding	Uterine bleeding, haematuria, haemorrhoid, postpartum abstruction and lochiostasis	6～9g

Name	Part used as herb	Properties and tastes	Functions	Indications and prescriptions	Dosage
Hindu Lotus Leaf (荷叶, Heye)	Leaf of lot us	Bitter, stringing and medium	Clear away summer heat, remove dampness, raise yang and stop bleeding	Summer heat disease (used with Honey-suckle Flower (金银花, Jinyinhua), diarrhea due to spleen deficiency and various bleeding. For stopping bleeding often used with Oried Rehmannia Root (生地黄, Shendihuang) and Biota Tops (侧柏叶, Cebaiye)	3～9g
Lotus Rhizome Note (藕节, Oujie)	Node of rhizome of lotus	Sweet, stringing and medium	Fresh use for removing stasis and stopping bleeding. Praching into charcoal for astringing and stopping bleeding	Various bleeding, especially for hematemesis and haemoptysis. Often used with Hyacinth Bletilla (白及, Baije) and Biota Tops (侧柏叶, Ceibaiye)	9～15g

10. 山茱萸, Shanzhuyu

English name: Asiatic Cornelian Cherry Fruit

Pharmaceutical name: Fructus Corni Officinalis

Botanical name: Cornus officinalis Sieb. et Zucc.

Properties and tastes: sour and slightly warm

山茱萸

Meridian tropism: the liver and kidney Meridian

Functions: 1. nourish liver and kidney
2. astringency
3. reduce blood pressure and blood sugar
4. inhibit bacteria

Indications: 1. consumption of kidney and liver syndrome for dizziness, vertigo, soreness and weakness of the waist and knees, impotence, etc
2. seminal emission, lingering diarrhea
3. enuresis
4. sweating due to deficiency
5. metrorrhagia and metrostaxis, hypermentrorrhea

Dosage: 6～9g, large dosage may be used for 30g. Decoct it with water or make it into bolus powder.

Contraindication: This herb has the action of warming, reinforcing and astringing. It is not used for patients with hyperactivity of fire from the gate of life, damp-heat stagnation in the body and difficulty in urination.

Combinations: 1. add Ginseng (人参, Renshen), Dragon's Bone (龙骨, Longgu), Oyster Shell (牡蛎, Muli)——exhaustion of yang qi due to excessive perspiration, shock, coldness of the extremities
2. add Chinese Magnoliavine (五味子, Wuweizi), Membranous Milkvetch Root (黄芪, Huangqi)——night sweating
3. add Prepared Rhizome of Adhesive

Rehmannia(熟地黄, Shoudihuang), Asshide Glue(阿胶, Ejiao)——metrorrhagia and metrostaxis, hypermentrorrhea due to deficiency of qi and blood

4. add Prepared Rhizome of Adhesive Rehmannia(熟地黄, Shoudihuang), Common Yam Rhizome(山药, Shanyao), Tuckahoe(茯苓, Fuling)——lumbar pain due to kidney deficiency, vertigo and blurred vision

5. add Dodder Seed(菟丝子, Tusizi), Sharpleaf Galangal Fruit(益智仁, Yizhiren)——seminal emission, frequent urination

6. add Eucommia Bark(杜仲, Duzhong), Grassleaf Sweetflag Rhizome(石菖蒲, Shichangpu)——hypertension due to deficiency of the kidney and liver

7. add Hairy Antler(鹿茸, Lurong), Prepared Rhizome of Adhesive Rehmannia(熟地黄, Shoudihuang), Chinese Magnoliavine(五味子, Wuweizi)——serious spermatorrhea

Prescrition: Bolus of Six Drugs Containing Rhizome Rehmanniae Peaeparatae(六味地黄丸, Liuweidihuang Wan)

Notes: Slightly warm in property, Asiatic Comelian Cherry Fruit(山茱萸, Shanzhuyu) has the function of astringing. It not only replenishes blood and essence of liver and kidney, but also activates kidney yang and gains, its functions on both symptoms and cause in treatment of frequent seminal emission, enuresis, and spontaneous perspiration. Both Asiatic Comelian Cherry Fruit(山茱萸, Shanzhuyu) and Prepared Rhizome of Adhesive Rehmannia(熟地黄, Shoudihuang), replenish blood and essence of liver and kidney, and are used for insufficiency of liver kidney blood and essence. But Asiatic Comelian Cherry Fruit(山茱萸, Shanzhuyu) reinforces yang as well as yin, and is applicable to the cases of yin or yang deficiency, inability to astring, threatened yang exhaustion due to failure to attract yang by yin. White prepared Rhizome of Adhesive Rehmannia(熟地黄, Shoudihuan g), though stronger in nourishing essence and blood, does not reinforce or astring.

11. 金樱子, Jinyingzi

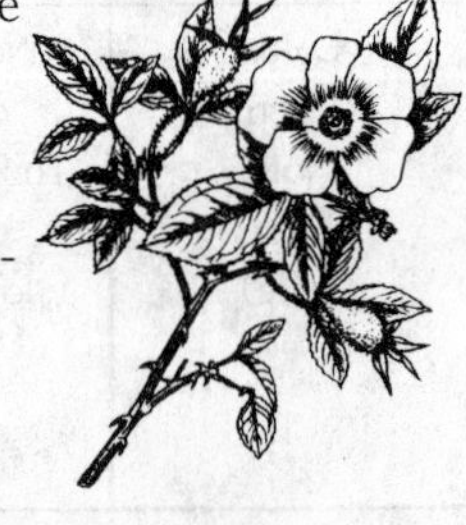

金樱子

English name: Cherokee Rose Fruit

Pharmaceutical name: Fructus Rosae laevigatae

Botanical name: Rosa laevigata Michx. In parts of northern China R. Bella Rehd. et Wils is used instead.

Properties and tastes: sour, astringent and medium

Meridian tropism: the kidney, urinary bladder, and large intestine Meridian

Functions: 1. stop noctural emission and astringe urinary function

2. astringe the intestine to stop diarrhea

Indications: 1. seminal emission and spermatrorrhea

2. enuresis and frequent urination

3. profuse leukorrhea

4. protraced diarrhea and dysentery

5. prolapse of the rectum

6. hysteroptosis

7. metrorrhagia and metrostaxis

Dosage: 6～18g

Contraindication: This herb is only used for astringing. It is not advisable for patients with excess-fire, excessive pathogens in the interior.

Combinations: 1. add Asiatic Cornelian Cherry Fruit(山茱萸, Shanzhuyu)——seminal emission, spermatrorrhea

2. add Dragon's Bone(龙骨, Longgu), Thinleaf Milkwort Root(远志, Yuanzhi)——enuresis, frequent urination

3. add Lotus Seed(莲子, Lianzi)——profuse leukorrhea

4. add Dang-shen Root(党参, Dangshen), Largehead Atractylodes Rhizome(白术, Baizhu), Common Yam Rhizome(山药, Shanyao)——protracted diarrhea and dysentery

5. add Membranous Milkvetch Root(黄芪, Huangqi), Chinese Thorowax Root(柴胡, Chaihu)——prolapse of rectum, hysteroptosis

6. add India Madder Root(茜草, Qiancao), Dragon's Bone(龙骨, Longgu)——metrorrhagia and metrostaxis

7. add Gordon Euryale Seed(芡实, Qianshi)——Lleukorrhea due to kidney deficiency, seminal emission, diarrhea

Notes: Cherokee Rose Fruit(金樱子, Jinyingzi) is sour and astringent in taste with the function of arresting collapse syndrome by astringents. Its can be used for diarrhea due to spleen deficiency, enuresis, frequent seminal emission, etc. It is only used for astringing without the function of reinforcement.

In the treatment of diarrhea, collapse etc, drugs for replenishing yin must be used in combination to treat the cause of disease according to the syndromes. An experiment proved that Cherokee Rose Fruit 金樱子, Jinyingzi) can be used for treating asterioslerosis, and its decoction can inhibit the virus of influenza.

Cherokee Rose Fruit(金樱子, Jinyingzi) and Asiatic Comelian Cherry Fruit(山茱萸, Shanzhuyu) are both sour and astringent in taste with astringing function. Cherokee Rose Fruit(金樱子, Jinyingzi) is only used for astringing whileAsiatic Comelian Cherry Fruit(山茱萸, Shanzhuyu) has the function of reinforcement at the time of actringing, so it has wider application than Cherokee Rose Fruit(金樱子, Jinyingzi).

Name	Properties and tastes	Meridian tropism	Functions	Indications	Dosage	Contraindication
Chinese Gall (五倍子, Wubeizi)	sour, stringing and cold	Lung, large intestine and kidney	Astringe lung, reduce fire, astringe intestine, keep essence, stop perspiration and bleeding. External use: detoxicate, reduce swelling, treat external diseases	Cough due to lung dificiency, prolonged diarrhea and dysentery, seminal emission, spermatorrhea, spontaneous sweating, night sweat and uterine bleeding. External use for carbuncle, ulcer, prolapse of anus and uterus.	1.5～6g for pill or powder. Proper amount for external use, like decoction for steaming and washing	Don't use for exogenous cough and diarrhea due to damp-heat.
Blighted Wheat (浮小麦, Fuxiaomai)	sweet and cool	Heart	Tonify qi, remove heat and stop perspiration.	Spontaneous sweating, night sweat and hectic fever	16～50g	

Name	Properties and tastes	Meridian tropism	Functions	Indications	Dosage	Contraindication
Gordon Euryale Seed(芡实, Qianshi)	sweet, stringing and medium	Spleen and kidney	Reinforce spleen to remove dampness and treat diarrhea, tonify kidney to keep essence and stop seminal emission	Diarrhea, seminal emission due to kidney deficiency, enuresis, morbid leckorhea.	9～15g	
Mantis Egg-case (桑螵蛸, Sangpiaoxiao)	sweet, salty and medium	Liver and kidney	Tonify kidney to support yang, keep essence, reduce urination	Impotence, seminal emission, spermatorrhea, enuresis, frequent urine and morbid leukorrhea caused by kidney yang deficiency	3～9g	Not use for yin deficiency with excessive fire and frequent urine due to gall bladder heat.
Cuttle-bone (乌贼骨, Wuzeigu)	salty, stringing and slightly warm	Liver and kidney	Astringe to stop bleeding, keep essence to stop leukorrhea, treat regurgitation, relieve pain, treat external diseases by removing dampness. Internal use: uterine bleeding, bleeding of lung and stomach, seminal emission, leukorrhea, stomach pain, regurgitation. External use: traumatic bleeding, carbuncle, eczema and ulcers with pus by external application.	6～12g. Proper amount for external use.	It's not proper for yin deficiency or with excessive fire case.	
Tree of Heaven Ailanthus Bark(椿皮, Chunpi)	bitter, stringing and cold	Large intestine, stomach and liver	Clear away heat, dry dampness, stop leukorrhea, control bleeding and anthelmintic function	Prolonged diarrhea and dysentery, bloody stool, uterine bleeding, leukorrhea, ascariasis and tinea.	3～6g. Proper amount for external use.	
Palmleaf Raspberry Fruit (覆盆子, Fupenzi)	sweet, sour and slightly warm	Liver and stomach	Tonify kidney, keep essence and reduce urination. seminal emission, impotence, frequent urine, enuresis and infertility.	3～9g	It's not proper for cases with kidney deficiency and excessive fire.	
Poppy Capsule (罂粟壳, Yingsuqiao)	sour, stringing, medium and poisonous	Lung, large intestine and kidney	Astringe lung and intestine, relieve pain	Prolonged cough, diarrhea and pain. Various pains which cannot be tolerated.	3～9g	Don't use in the early stage of disease. Don not take continuously for those with addiction

PART Ⅱ
Cold-natured Drugs and Hot-natured Drugs

The nature of diseases can be classified into heat and cold syndrome. Yang heat syndrome refers to fever or hyperactivity of Zang and fu organs. Yin cold syndrome refers to chills, aversion to cold or hypofunction of Zang and Fu organs. It is said that yin deficiency produces cold and yang excess produces heat. Heat syndrome is manifested as cold, aversion to heat, and cold syndrome manifested as warm, aversion to cold.

One of the principles of treatment in T. C. M. is to treat cold syndrome by warm drugs and to treat heat syndrome by cold drugs. But cold syndrome as well as heat syndrome can appear excess or deficiency. The differentiation of Wei, qi, Ying, Xue, Zang and Fu organs, meridians and collaterals must be clear when drugs are prescribed.

For the deficiency cold and deficiency heat syndromes, the treatment principle must include tonifying yin and yang. Cold syndrome and heat syndromes are very complicated in clinic. They can occur as complication of cold or heat, external heat and internal cold, external cold and internal heat, upper heat or lower cold, cold with false heat or heat with false cold. That is why we can say that it is not very easy to decide the correct method of treament. This is the key point.

Chapter 4
Drugs for Clearing Away Heat

Definition: The nature of these drugs is cold or slightly cold. Their main function is to clear away internal heat. It is called drugs for clearing away heat.

Functions: The main functions of these drugs are clearing away heat, purging internal heat, detoxicating and removing heat from the blood etc. Some drugs have the function of tranquilizing the mind, promoting urination, drying dampness and nourishing yin.

Indications: Heat syndromes includes febrile disease of external infection, fever from carbuncle, swelling and wound poison, the heat syndrome in viscera with imbalance of internal organs and overbearing yang heat. Some drugs are good at reducing deficiency heat syndrome in combination with drugs for tonifying yin.

Classification: According to the nature and indications of cold-natured drugs, they can be divided into following five types:

1. Heat-clearing and fire-purging drugs: They can clear away heat in the qi-stage, used

for syndrome of the yangming meridian in exogenous febrile disease, qi-stage syndrome in seasonal febrile disease and heat syndrome in viscera.

2. Heat-clearing and dampness-drying drugs: Bitter in taste and cold in nature, they have the functions of clearing away heat and drying dampness, used primarily for damp heat disease and syndrome.

3. Heat-clearing and heat-removing from the blood drugs: They can clear away heat in the blood-stage. When some drugs are used together, they have the function of nourishing yin and reducing fever.

4. Heat-clearing and toxin-expelling drugs: They have the functions of clearing away heat and expelling toxins, and are usually used to eliminate noxious heat disease of pestilence, toxin dysentery, carbuncle swelling, and wound poison, etc.

5. Fever-reducing drugs: These drugs can reduce fever and hectic fever, and are usually used for afternoon tidal fever, low fever failing to be reduced, children's fever due to malnutrition and so on.

Cautions:

1. Distinguishing the stages and position of Fever.

When you use a heat-clearing drug, you must make it clear in which part of the qi-stage and blood-stage the heat syndrome exists. The treatment principle should be decided according to the patient's condition. If it is a superficial syndrome, you should use diaphoresis to relieve super ficies. If heat of qi-stage is accompanied with that of blood-stage, you should clear away heat from both stages.

2. Distinguishing fever's nature of deficiency and excess.

Interior heat syndrome has two different types: deficient heat and excess heat. This type of drug was used mostly for the excess heat syndrome. Combinations of the tonic drugs with deficiency heat-clearing drugs are used for various deficient heat syndromes. Some drugs used together have coordinated kidney effect of nourishing Ying and reducing fever, reducing fever and strengthening renal yin. It can also be used for deficient heat syndrome like Rehmannia Dried Root(生地黄, Shengdihuang), Chinese Corktree Bark(黄柏, Huangbai) and so on.

3. Attending to stomach and protecting normal climate.

The nature of the heat-clearing drugs is cold and slightly cold. These drugs are easy to impair the spleen and stomach for the patient with stomach and spleen deficiency and long-term administration. Drugs for invigorating the stomach should be used in the prescription. Use it carefully for the patients with deficiency of speen and stomach yang, anorexia, slippery intestine and diarrhea. As febrile disease can easily impair the body fluid, the nature of heat-clearing and dampness-drying drugs are dry and easily relieves impairment of body fluid. Therefore, you should use drugs for nourishing Ying for patients with Ying asthenia. Using this kind drug properly, to avoid the vital qi being damaged.

Section 1
Heat-clearing Drugs in Qi Stage

1. 石膏, Shigao

English name: Gypsum

Pharmaceutical name: Gypsum

Properties and tastes: pungent, sweet, and extremely cold

Meridian tropism: lung, stomach

石 膏

Functions: 1. clear away heat-fire

2. relieve restlessness and thirst

3. clear away heat to heal sores

4. reduce fever by inhibiting thermogenic center

5. inhibit muscular excitability to relieve spasm

6. externally used for reducing vascular permeability to remove inflammation

Indications: 1. the sthenia pyrosyndrome in qi——seasonal febrile disease pathogen lives in qi-stage, exogenous febrile disease pathogen lives in yangming meridians, high fever, polydipsia, profuse sweating, bounding large pulse

2. the pyretic pulmonary syndrome——cough with sticky sputum, hoarse asthma, fever

3. the gastric heat syndrome——headache, toothache with gingival swelling

4. the eczema——when oozing fluid is more and sticky oily, powdered Gypsum (石膏, Shigao) may be used for external use

5. the diabetes——gastric heat, diabetes mellitus, excessive drinking, overeating

Dosage: 15～30g. Largest dosage may be used for 60～90g. Decoct it first.

Contraindication: Not to be used with patients with stomach cold, poor appetite, loose stool.

Combinations: 1. add Common Anemarrhea Rhizome (知母, Zhimu)——heat lives in qi-stage, polydipsia, taking fluids profusely, high fever, polyhidrosis

2. add Prepared Rhizome of Adhesive Rehmannia (熟地黄, Shoudihuang)——headache, toothache, thirst of asthenic yin causing excessive pyrexia

3. add Rehmannia Dried Root (生地黄, Shengdihuang)——febrile disease consuming body fluid due to excessive pyretic pathogenic factor

4. add Cape Jasmine Fruit (栀子, Zhizi)——aphtha, foul breath.

5. add Medicininal Cyathula Root (川牛膝, Chuanniuxi)——gastropyretic toothache

6. add Buffalo Horn (水牛角, Shuiniujiao)——thermy and heat with seasonal epidemic pathogen, high fever, coma, heamatemesis and rhinorrhagia

7. add Cassia Twig (桂枝, Guizhi), Chinese Corktree Bark (黄柏, Huangbai)——redness of the joint and swollen joints

8. add Ephedra (麻黄, Mahuang)——cough, asthma due to lung heat and general edema with wind-edema

9. add Shunk Bugbane Rhizome (升麻, Shengma)——parietal headache and toothache with gingival swelling due to hyperactivity of the stomach fire, which flaring

up along the meridian

10. add Ginseng(人参, Renshen)——qi asthenia, gastric heat, heat impairing qi and yin, diabetes

11. add Chinese Corktree Bark (黄柏, Huangbai)——the medical treatment for burns, scalding and eczema for external use

12. add Manchurian Wildginger Herb (细辛, Xixin)——the endopyretic toothache and anemopyretic headache

Prescriptions: 1. White Tiger Decoction(白虎汤, Baihu Tang).

2. Decoction of Ephedra, Apricot, Gypsum and Licorice (麻杏石甘汤, Maxingshigan Tang)

Notes: Gypsum(石膏, Shigao) is an important drug for clearing away heat in the qi-stage syndrome. Internally it may be clearing away heat of the lung and stomach. Externally it may be relieving heat in the muscles and superficies. It is used for pyreticosis the qi-stage sthenia pyrosyndrome of high fever, sweating, restlessness, thirst, bounding, large pulse etc. Cough and asthma with heat lives in the lung, toothache and gingival swelling with heat lives in the stomach, eruption with heat entering the blood-layer, therefore, these all may be used. As it is said in *Records of Traditional Chinese and Western Medicine in Combination* (《医学衷中参西录》, Yixuezhongzhongcanxilu): "The nature is cool and capable of dispersing. It has an ability of relieving superficies and relieving muscles. If it is exogenous excess pyrosyndrome, use it and get good results." This drug can clear away heat. The directions always indicate larger dosages. Dosages of 30g ~ 60g, or larger may be used. If there is high fever with abdominal distention and constipation (Yangming fu excess syndrome), Gypsum(石膏, Shigao) is not used. Use Rhubarb(大黄, Dahuang) act as leading or Rhubarb(大黄, Dahuang) and Gypsum(石膏, Shigao) are used together. After the Gypsum(石膏, Shigao) is forged, it can eliminate dampness and astringe wounds. It is used to treat skin disease with oozing of fluid which is better than Calcined Gypsum(煅石膏, Duanshigao). It can't be taken orally. It has been reported that Gypsum(石膏, Shigao) has the function of promoting the growth of callus. It is used to treat marrow inflammation, bone stone lead to bone defect and injury. It can promote healing.

2. 知母, Zhimu

English name: Common Anemarrhea Rhizome

Pharmaceutical name: Radix Anemarrhenae Asphodeloidis

Botanical name: Anemarrhena asphodeloides Bge

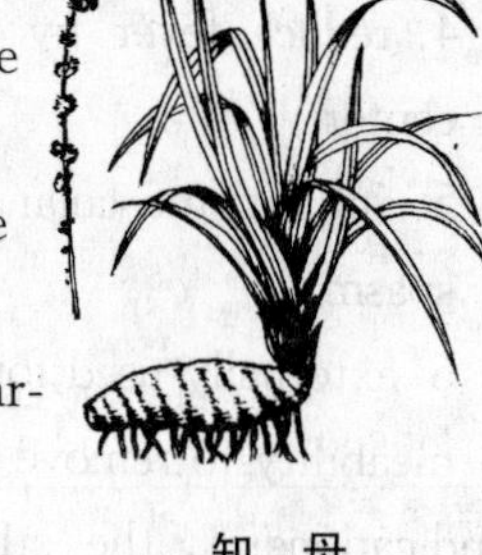

知 母

Properties and tastes: bitter, sweet, cold

Meridian tropism: lung, stomach, and kidney

Functions: 1. clear away heat and relieve restlessness

2. clear away lung-heat and moisten if dry

3. nourish yin to lower pathogenic fire

4. quench thirst

5. reduce fever and tranquilize the mind

6. function as broad-spectrum antibiotic

Indications: 1. yangming heat syndrome——high fever, sweating not relieve, restlessness, thirst, bounding large pulse of qi-layer with excessive heat

2. cough with lung heat——cough with yellow sticky sputum or bloody sputum, red

tongue with yellowish coating

3. yin asthenia dry cough——cough with sticky sputum, difficult expectoration or bloody sputum, manifested as hectic fever and night sweat at the same time

4. yin asthenia hectic fever——osteopyrexia, night sweat, dysphoria of asthenic yin causing excessive pyrexia

5. diabetes——this drug is suitable for thirst, diuresis belonging to gastric heat and yin asthenia

Dosage: 6～12g.

Contraindication: Do not use in condition of loose stool due to spleen deficiency.

Combinations: 1. add Gypsum (石膏, Shigao)——yangming heat syndrome

2. add Tendrilleaf Fritillary Bulb (川贝母, Chuanbeimu) and Coastal Glehnia Root, and Fourleaf Ladybell Root (沙参, Shashen)——dry cough due to yin deficiency

3. add Chinese Corktree Bark (黄柏, Huangbai)——hectic heat with yin asthenia

4. add Baikal Skullcap Root (黄芩, Huangqin)——cough with lung heat

5. add Snakegourd Root (天花粉, Tianhuafen)——diabetes

6. add Chinese Corktree Bark (黄柏, Huangbai) and Cassia Bark (肉桂, Rougui)——prostatic hyperplasia

7. add Prepared Rhizome of Adhesive Rehmannia (熟地黄, Shoudihuang)——yin deficiency, constipation due to intestinal dryness

Prescriptions: 1. Bolus for Replenishing Vital Essence (大补阴丸, Dabuyin Wan)

2. Bolus of Rhizoma Anemarrhenae, Cortex Phollodendri and Rhizoma Rehmanniae (知柏地黄丸, Zhibaidihuang Wan).

Notes: Common Anemarrhea Rhizome (知母, Zhimu) is bitter, cold and moist in nature. It can quench lung heat in the upper part clear away gastric heat in the middle part and renal fire in the lower part, moisturize dryness and nourish yin, treat fever with yin asthenia. One can say that Common Anemarrhea Rhizome (知母, Zhimu) has the function of clearing away both deficiency and excess. Common Anemarrhea Rhizome (知母, Zhimu), said Li Dongyuan (李东垣): "has four functions: purging deficiency fire of kidney, treating bone steaming with sweating, stopping deficient heat of consumptive disease and nourishing yin of vital genesis." Modern research has shown that Common Anemarrhea Rhizome (知母, Zhimu) has the function of reducing fever and resisting bacteria. It also affects the function of adrenal cortex hormones, and can reduce blood pressure.

Gypsum (石膏, Shigao) and Common Anemarrhea Rhizome (知母, Zhimu) can clear away heat and purge intense heat, relieve restlessness and relieve thirst. It produces an effect for the lungs and stomach; therefore it is usually used in combination. But Gypsum (石膏, Shigao) is good at clearing away sthenic heat of the lungs and stomach. Common Anemarrhea Rhizome (知母, Zhimu) is good at moisturizing dryness by nourishing yin, removing sthenic fire, and loosening the bowels to relieve constipation.

3. 芦根, Lugen

English name: Reed Rhizome

Pharmaceutical name: Rhizoma Phragmitis Communis

Botanical name: Phragmites communis

Properties and tastes: sweet, cold

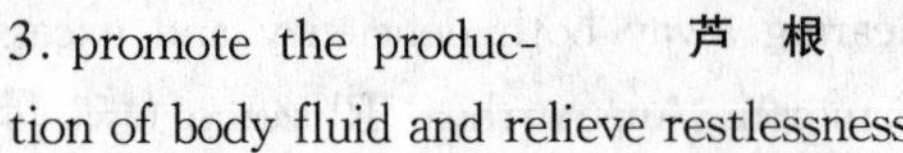

芦 根

Meridian tropism: lung, stomach

Functions: 1. clear away heat and expel pathogen in the exterior

2. clear away stomach-heat and arrest vomiting

3. promote the production of body fluid and relieve restlessness

4. clear away lung-heat and discharge pus

5. induce diuresis for treating stranguria syndrome

6. promote eruption

Indications:

1. exogenous wind-heat——cough, pharyngitis with ache

2. gastropyretic vomiting and adverse rising——vomiting, nausea from pyretic damage of stomach

3. pyreticosis damage of body fluid——thirst with dysphoric fever, sausarism slight body-fluid

4. cough with lung heat——yellow sticky sputum or cough vomiting pus sputum with stinking odor, high fever, dry mouth and thirst

5. pyrepic stranguria——scanty dark urine and painful urination

6. measles without relieving superficies.

Dosage: 15～30g

Combinations:

1. add Mulberry Leaf (桑叶, Sangye)——anemopyretic cold

2. add Bamboo Shavings (竹茹, Zhuru)——gastropyretic vomiting and adverse rising

3. add Dwarf Lilyturf Root (麦门冬, Maimendong)——pyreticosis consumption of body-fluid, thirst and dysphoria

4. add Apricot Seed (杏仁, Xingren) and Loquat Leaf (枇杷叶, Pipaye)——cough of lung heat with yellow sticky sputum

5. add Heartleaf Houttuynia Herb (鱼腥草, Yuxingcao), Coix Seed (薏苡仁, Yiyiren) Snakegourd Root (天花粉, Tianhuafen), Chinese Waxgourd Seed (冬瓜仁, Dongguaren)——pulmonary abscess

6. add Lalang Grass Rhizome (白茅根, Baimaogen)——the pyrepic stranguria or pharyngalgia

7. add Lobed Kudzuvine Root (葛根, Gegen)——promote eruption.

8. add Job's tears and Snakegourd Root (天花粉, Tianhuafen)——pulmonary abscess.

Prescription: Rhizoma Phragmitis Decoction (苇茎汤, Weijing Tang)

Notes: This drug promotes the production of body fluid, and it hasn't a disadvantage of keeping evil, so it is more suitable than other nourishing yin drugs for damage of body fluid and febrile disease in early stage. This drug also can remove heat from the urine, therefore it is often used for pyretic stranguria as well.

Reed Rhizome (芦根, Lugen) and Common Anemarrhea Rhizome (知母, Zhimu) can clear away heat of lung-stomach. They are used for dysphoric fever and thirst syndrome of excessive heat in lung-stomach. Their differences are: Common Anemarrhea Rhizome (知母, Zhimu) purges asthenic heat of the kidney parlyc. It can treat hectic fever, night sweating, and diabetes mellitus of asthenic yin causing excessive pyrexia. Reed Rhizome (芦根, Lugen) has a nature of releasing and relieving, it is usually used to promote eruption and it can treat carbuncle with drainage of pus. It is said in *Annotation on Shennong's Herbal Classic* (《本草经疏》, Bencaojingshu) that: "Reed Rhizome (芦根, Lugen) has tastes sweet, cold and non-toxic, sweet can nourishing stomach and harmonizing the middle, cold can reducing heat and removing fire, heat has been reduced and stomach has been harmonized, so body-fluid has been dredged and thirst-slaking." Reed Rhizome (芦根, Lugen) can calm the stomach harmonizing the middle. Without Common Anemarrhea Rhizome (知母, Zhimu) one has anxiety from a bitter cold obstructed stomach.

4. 天花粉, Tianhuafen

English name: Snakegourd Root

Pharmaceutical name: Radix Thichosanthis

Botanical name: Trichosanthes kirilowii Maxim.

Properties and tastes: bitter, slightly sweet, sour, and cold

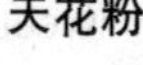

天花粉

Meridian tropism: lung, stomach

Functions:

1. promote the production of body fluid to relieve thirst and quench thirst
2. clear away lung-heat and moisten dryness
3. subdue swelling and discharge pus
4. inhibit the growth of fumor in Langhan's layer

Indications:

1. pyreticosis consumption of body-bluid——that dry mouth, dry tongue, dysphoria
2. the diabetes——thirst, requiring more fluids
3. cough of lung heat——cough with sticky sputum or dry cough with slight sputum and hemoptysis
4. Swelling pyocutaneous disease ulcerative carbuncle——excessive noxious heat, red swelling hot pain

Dosage: 9～15g.

Contraindication: Pregnant women must not use this drug, its corrigent is rhizome of Chinese monkshood. The person with asthenia cold of spleen and stomach must use it carefully.

Combinations: 1. add Reed Rhizome (芦根, Lugen)——dry mouth, thirst, dysphoria of heat consuming body fluid

2. add Common Anemarrhea Rhizome (知母, Zhimu)——diabetes and morbid thirst of pyreticosis, consumption of body fluid

3. add Tendrilleaf Fritillary Bulb (贝母, Beimu)——phlegmatic and hot cough, expectoration is sticky sputum, difficulty in coughing up phlegm, sore throat and swelling

4. add Honeysuckle Flower (金银花, Jinyinhua)——swelling-poison of skin and external disease

5. add Cochinchinese Asparagus Root (天门冬, Tianmendong) and Dwarf Lilyturf Root (麦门冬, Maimendong)——cough with lung dryness, light sputum and difficulty in coughing up phlegm

Prescription: Fairy Decoction for Treating Cutancous Infections (仙方活命饮, Xianfanghuoming Yin).

Notes: This drug is good at helping produce saliva and quenches thirst, it can reduce swelling and discherging pus, and it is an important drug for treating diabetes. It is the drug used most often for treating carbuncle swelling and wound poison. It is said in *Collected Decoction of Herbals* (《本草汇言》, Bencaohuiyan): "Snakegourd Root (天花粉, Tianhuafen) is sweet and cold in nature, it is good at relieving thirst, it treats asthenic thirst by tonic, it treats fire thirst by cool-natured drugs, it treats stagnant thirst by qi-layer drugs, it treats morbid thirst by blood-layer drugs, it is an important drug for treating thirst."

Snakegourd Root(天花粉, Tianhuafen) and Reed Rhizome(芦根, Lugen) can clear away heat of the lung and stomach and nourish yin to help produce saliva. Therefore they are often used together for treating pyrelicosis damage of body fluid, thirst with poor body fluid and cough with lung heat etc. But Snakegourd Root(天花粉, Tianhuafen) has a less effect than Reed Rhizome (芦根, Lugen), but it has better ability to nourish yin and help produce saliva. It has the effect of detoxication, it promotes circulation, detumescentifies, and is used for swelling-poison of the skin and external diseases. Reed Rhizome(芦根, Lugen) has a great ability to clear away heat of the lung-stomach in qi-stage, and may be releasing and relieving the pyretic pathogenic factor. It is used for exogenous seasonal febrile disease in its early stages. It is also used to treat pulmonary abscess because it has the function of removing pus.

Snakegourd Root(天花粉, Tianhuafen) is the root of Snakegourd with fruit of Mongolian sankegourd, peel of Mongolian sankegourd and seed of Mongolian sankegourd can both be used as drugs, which are cool descending and slippery humidifying. It is often used for phlegm fire, excess heat syndrome and swelling with stagnated heat syndrome. They have every special feature. Snakegourd Root(天花粉, Tianhuafen) has nature of sweet, bitter, sour and cold. It is good at helping produce saliva and slake thirst, falling fire and moistening dryness. Sthenia of Mongolian sankegourd has nature of sweet bitter cold, it opens pulmonary thoracic obstruction from above, and it purges pyretic retention of the large intestine from below. The peel and seed of the Mongolian sankegourd all belong to sweet-cold drug, its peel is good at relieving the thorax and lung. Its seed is good at removing stomach obstruction and relaxing the bowels.

5. 竹叶, Zhuye

English name: Bamboo Leaf

Pharmaceutical name: Folium Phyllostachydis Henonis

Botanical name: Phyllostachys nigra(Lodd. ex Lindl.) Munro var. Henonis (Mitf.) Stapf ex Rendle

竹叶

Properties and tastes: pungent, sweet, and cold

Meridian tropism: heart, lung, and stomach

Functions: 1. clear away heat and relieve restlessness

2. relieve the exterior syndrome with drugs pungent in flavor and cool in nature

3. promote the production of body fluid to relieve thirst

4. reduce diuresis

Indications: 1. heat attacking pericardium syndrome—it may be an effective drug when seasonal febrile disease has appeared with coma and delirium

2. exogenous wind-weed syndrome—aversion to cold, dysphoric, thirst and reddish tongue, it is also used to treat infantile wind-weed convulsive epilepsy

3. pyreticosis later stage, residual heat isn't cleared away, dysphoria and insomnia

4. it is an effective drug for infections of urinary system

5. mouth and tongue with an infection or a wound

Dosage: 6～15g.

Combinations: 1. add Honeysuckle Flower(金银花, Jinyinhua) and Weeping Forsythia Capsule(连翘, Lianqiao)——wind-weed superficial syndrome

2. add Gypsum(生石膏, Shengshigao) and Dwarf Lilyturf Root(麦门冬, Maimendong)——pyreticosis in its late stage with residual heat

3. add Weeping Forsythia Capsule(连翘, Lianqiao) and Figwort Root(玄参, Xuanshen)——that heat attacking pericardium syndrome

4. add Akebia Stem(木通, Mutong) and Rehmannia Dried Root(生地黄, Shengdihuang)——mouth and tongue with an infection or wound

5. add Plantain Seed(车前子, Cheqianzi) and Akebia Stem(木通, Mutong)——infection of the urinary system

6. add Gambirplant Hooked Stem and Branch(钩藤, Gouteng) and Cicada Slough (蝉蜕, Chantui)——the infantile wind-weed convulsive epilepsy, fever

7. add Hindu Lotus Petiole (荷梗, Hegeng)——eliminate summer-heat and dampness, relieve the thorax and diaphragm, relieve flatulence

Prescriptions: 1. Powder for Dark Urine(导赤散, Daochi San).

2. Decoction of Bamboo Leaf and Gypsum Combination (竹叶石膏汤, ZhuyeshigaoTang)

Notes: Bamboo Leaf(竹叶, Zhuye) has a delicate fragrance and acts on the heart meridian. It is bitter in taste and can clear away heat, (it is good at clearing away pyretic pathogenic factor of heart-lung in Upperjiao.) Bamboo Leaf(竹叶, Zhuye) can be used for diabetes of summer-heat, phlegmopyrexia in the thorax, deficient restlessness of exogenous febrile disease, hiccup and dyspnea syndrome. Li Dongyuan(李东垣) said that this drug" has two fanctions: removing dysphoric of new or old pathogenic wind, relieving dyspnea excessive qi." *Seeking Truth of Herbals* (《本草求真》, Bencaoqiuzhen) discusses it in detail, for Bamboo Leaf(竹叶, Zhuye) Bamboo Leaf (竹叶, Zhuye) was recorded consistently in books that it can cool the heart and relieve the spleen, remove sputum and quench the thirst. It is a drug to treat the upper energizer wind pathogen and dysphoric fever, hiccup and dyspnea, vomiting, hiccup and spitting blood, all apoplectic convulsive epilepsy etc. (What is nothing but because its floating can expel upper, acid can disperse superficial exopthogens, sweet can relieve spleen, slightly cold can attack heart, cold can treat heat. They all belong to clearing drugs, with Gypsum(石膏, Shigao) together, it can relieve gastric heat and without leading to dysphoria)

6. 栀子, Zhizi

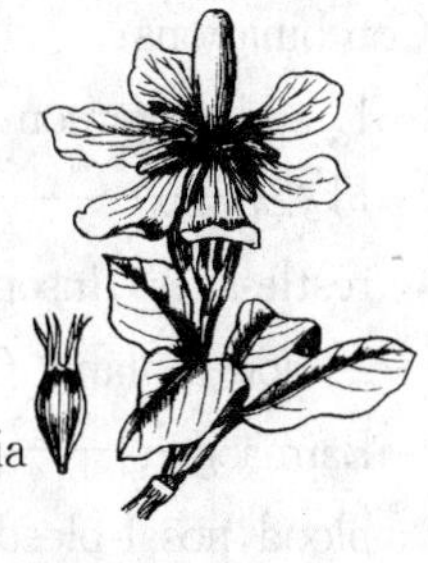

English name: Cape Jasmine Fruit

Pharmaceutical name: Fructus Gardeniae Jasminoidis

Botanical name: Gardenia jasminoides Ellis

栀子

Properties and tastes: bitter, cold

Meridian tropism: heart, lung, stomach, and Sanjiao

Functions: 1. clear away heat and eliminate

dampness

2. eliminate pathogenic fire and relieve restlessness

3. remove pathogenic heat from blood and toxic substance from the body

4. relieve inflammation and promote the function of the gall bladder

5. tranquilizer

6. reduce blood pressure

7. external use for stopping pain

Indications: 1. pyretic pathogenic factor full in Sanjiao——high fever, dysphoria, mental depression, restlessness, even coma and delirium

2. hepatochlic hygropyrexia——the maundice, fever and scanty dark urine

3. hemopyrexia syndrome——the hemoptysis, haematemesis, non-traumatic hemorrhage, hematuria

4. skin infection——include burn and scald, furuncle and carbuncle, acne, erysipelas

5. swelling and pain of traumatic injury——grind into powder and then mix the powder with wine before applying it to the affected part.

Dosage: 3～9g.

Contraindication: Do not use in the case of spleen deficiency and poor appetite.

Combinations:

1. add Common Anemarrhea Rhizome(知母, Zhimu)——excessive heat and deficient restlessness, insomni, thirst, red tougue

2. add Lalang Grass Rhizome(白茅根, Baimaogen)——pyretic dysentery, spitting blood, nosal-bleeding, hematuria

3. add Juice of Fresh Ginger(生姜汁, Shengjiangzhi)——gastric abscess belonging to heat

4. add Tumeric Rhizome (姜黄, Jianghuang)——accumulation of toxic heat withstagnation of liver and gall bladder leading to fever, bitter taste in the mouth, hypochondriac pain and disease of liver-gall bladder like cholecystitis, choleithiasis, hepatitis etc.

5. add Chinese Corktree Bark(黄柏, Huangbai)——body and eyes become yellow. The color is bright like tangerine's yang jaundice. Intermittent fever, polydipsia thirst, scanty dark urine, red tongue with yellowish coating

6. add Ural Licorice Root Tip(甘草梢, Gancaoshao)——pyelonephritis and urethritis lead to dysuria

7. add Chrysanthemum Flower(菊花, Juhua)——acute conjunctivitis

8. add Tree Peony Bark(牡丹皮, Mudanpi)——osteopyrexia and fever/hectic fever and tidal fever, daytime sweating and night sweating of hepatic stagnation and blood deficiency

9. add Prepared Soybean(淡豆豉, Dandouchi)——pyretic depression dysphoria

10. add Officinal Magnolia Bark(厚朴, Houpo) and Immature Bitter Orange(枳实, Zhishi)——middle energizer hygropyretic flatulenc

11. add Talc(滑石, Huashi)——bloody stranguria and anuresis

12. add Chinese Thorowax Root(柴胡, Chaihu) and White Peony Root(白芍药, Baishaoyao)——pyrostagnant of liver and gall bladder

13. add Rehmannia Dried Root(生地黄, Shengdihuang) and Tree Peony Bark(牡丹皮, Mudanpi)——pyro-stagnated bleeding

14. add Spine Date Seed(酸枣仁, Suanzaoren)——insomnia and dreamful sleep, panasthenic syndrome

Prescriptions: 1. Decoction of Capejasmine and

Fermented Soybean (栀子豉汤, Zhizichi Tang).

2. Decoction of Artemisae Scopariae(茵陈蒿汤, Yinchenhao Tang).

3. Xiaoyao Powder adding Cortex Moutan Radicis and Fructus Gardeniae(丹栀逍遥散, Danzhixiaoyao San).

Notes: This drug is a extremely bitter cold agent, the nature "bending and falling/decrease by bend", part time treating pathogenic fire of the abdominal mass. This drug removes heat and dispels dampness, so it is the first choice for damp heat in triple energizer. Raw cape-jasmine is good at removing heat and purging fire. It has the effect of eliminating stasis to subdue swelling after drug levitation with wine and vinegar used externally. It mainly treats traumatic swelling-pain, reddish complexion, Roscoe. Fried Cape Jasmine Fruit(栀子, Zhizi) and charcoal of Cape Jasmine Fruit(栀子, Zhizi) are often used to stop bleeding. Seed of Cape Jasmine Fruit(栀子, Zhizi) is good at clearing away heart heat and is used mainly to treat intermittent heat of uterus. Peel of Cape Jasmine Fruit (栀子, Zhizi) part time treat superficial heat. It is said in *Records of the Discerning of Herbals* (《本草思辨录》, Bencaosibianlu): "Cape Jasmine Fruit (栀子, Zhizi) can alleviate mental depression but it can't dissipate mass. It can't descend adverse qi, so abdominal fullness with dry stool, exogenous fever of lung disease has cough and asthma. These symptoms cannot be treated with this drug." It also points out the difference between Cape Jasmine Fruit (栀子, Zhizi) and Rhubarb (大黄, Dahuang), Baikal Skullcap Root (黄芩, Huangqin).

7. 夏枯草, Xiakucao

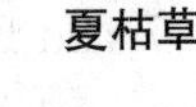

夏枯草

English name: Common Selfheal Fruit-spike

Pharmaceutical name: Spica Prunellae Vulgaris

Botanical name: Prunella vulgaris L.

Properties and tastes: bitter, pungent, cold

Meridian tropism: liver, gallbladder

Functions:

1. clear away liver-fire
2. disperse accumulated pathogens
3. reduce blood pressure
4. prevent cancer(tumor)

Indications:

1. conjunctival congestion swelling-pain and ophthal malgia——photophobia lacrimation lachrymation tears, headache, vertigo and so on. Syndrome belongs to hyperpyrexia of liver or hyper activity of liver yang
2. hypertension——belongs to hyperheaptic that is dizziness, headache, giddiness
3. scrofula and goiter——like crewels, lymphnoditis, lymphadenoma, thyroma
4. pulmonary tuberculosis(TB)

Dosage: 9～15g.

Combinations:

1. add Twotooth Achyranthes Root(牛膝, Niuxi) and Chinese Gentian Root(龙胆草, Longdancao)——the hyperheaptic, vertigo
2. add Abalone Shell(石决明, Shijueming) and Cassia Seed(决明子, Juemingzi)——glaucoma and ophthal malgia
3. add Chrysanthemum Flower (菊花, Juhua) and Cicada Slough (蝉蜕, Chantui)——acute conjunctivitis, epidemic keratitis, conjunctival congestion with swelling-pain

4. add Figwort Root(玄参, Xuanshen) and Oyster Shell(牡蛎, Muli)——crewels, lymphnoditis, lymphadenoma, thyroma
5. add Chinese Date(大枣, Dazao)——acute choleplania, catarrhal jaundice/infective hepatitis
6. add Motherwort Herb (茺蔚子, Chongweizi)——hypertension, cerebral arteriosclerosis
7. add Pinellia Rhizome(半夏, Banxia)——lose sleep, panasthenia

Notes: This drug is sour and can come to stasis. It is bitter cold and can expel heat. It is an important drug for removing liver heat and removing obstruction, therefore it treats diseases of the liver meridian such as eye diseases due to liver-fire, or vertigo of hepatic yang, or tumour due to liver depressed and phlegm curdled. In recent years, it is mostly used for hypertension and tumour. Research has shown that: Common Selfheal Fruit-spike(夏枯草, Xiakucao) has the function of reducing blood pressure, anti tumourigenesis, and is an antibacterial agent. It has a special function as an anti tubercle bacillus. So it is also used to treat crewels. This drug may treat thyroma that it stews with crucian together.

It is recorded in *Compendium of Materia Medica* (《本草纲目》, Bencaogangmu): Common Selfheal Fruit-spike (夏枯草, Xiakucao) has the magical effect on treating pain of eye balls which is getting worse at night. It also takes effect when the patient becomes more serious after he is given other bitter and cold drugs.

Appendix: Other Drugs For Clearing Heat and Purging Fire

Drug Name	Properties and Tastes	Meridian tropism	functions	Indications	Dosage and usage	Contraindication
Mirabilita Crystal(寒水石, Hanshuishi)	salty, cold	Stomach, kidney	Remove heat and purge fire.	Used similarly to Gypsum (石膏, Shigao), but its power is weaker than Gypsum (石膏, Shigao).	9～15g	Asthenia-cold of spleen and stomach forbid its use
Common Dayflower Herb (鸭跖草, Yazhicao)	sweet, bitter and cold	Lung, stomach, urinary bladder	Expel toxin, clear heat. promote diuresis for stranguria.	Influenza, fever, sore throat and swelling, carbuncle swelling and wound poison, pyrepic stranguria, hydroncus, it is also used to treat poisonous snake with Chinese Lobelia(半边莲, Banbianlian).	15～30g	
Buerger Pipewort Flower(谷精草, Gujingcao)	sweet, medium	Liver, stomach	Dispel wind and heat, improve acuity of vision and remove nebula.	Conjunctival congestion with swelling and pain, photophibia over-tear punctate keratitis, anemopyretic headache, toothache, pharyngal may use it too.	6～9g	

Drug Name	Properties and Tastes	Meridian tropism	functions	Indications	Dosage and usage	Contraindication
Pale Butterflybush Flower(密蒙花, Mimenghua)	sweet, slightly cold	Liver	Clear away liver fire, improve eyesight, deduce nebula.	It treats eye disease with Buerger Pipewort Flower (谷精草, Gujingcao)	6～9g	
Feather Cockscomb Seed(青葙子, Qingxiangzi)	bitter, slightly cold	Liver	Clear away liver fire and purge fire, improve acuity of vision and remove nebula.	Cojunctival congestion with swelling and pain, punctate keratitis, hypertension, hyperheaptic yang, anemopyretic headache.	6～15g	Those with glaucoma and mydriasis must be careful when using it.
Watermelon (西瓜, Xigua)	sweet, cold	Heart, stomach, urinary bladder	Eliminate summer-heat by cooling, quenching thirst, diuresis.	Disease of summer heat, pyreticosis damage of body fluid, dysuria.	9～30g Eating properly	
Watermelon Pericarp(西瓜皮, Xiguapi)	sweet, cold	Heart, stomach, urinary bladder	As well as watermelon.	As well as watermelon	9～30g	
Watermelon Frost (西瓜霜, Xiguashuang)	salty, cold		Remove heat to detumescentify	Sore throat with swelling. aphtha, ulcerative gingivitis.	1～2g. levigation, laryngeal insfflation of drug power.	

Section 2
Heat-clearing and Dampness-drying drugs

1. 黄芩, Huangqin

English name: Baikal Skullcap Root

Pharmaceutical name: Radix Scutellariae Baicalensis

Botanical name: Scutellaria baicalensis Georgi

Properties and tastes: bitter, cold

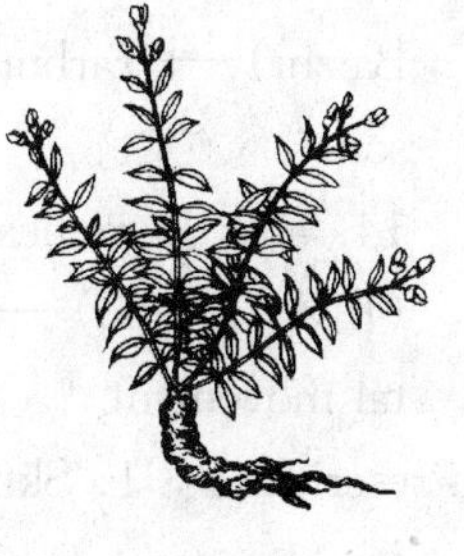
黄 芩

Meridian tropism: lung, stomach, and large intestine

Functions: 1. clear away heat and eliminate dampness

2. eliminate pathogenic fire and detoxicate

3. arrest bleeding

4. miscarriage prevention

5. function as broad spectrum antibiotic

6. resist inflammation and allergic reaction

7. reduce blood pressure

8. tranquilize

Indications: 1. damp heat syndrome——damp thermosis syndrome, choleplania, diarrhea, pyretic stranguria

2. the excess pyrosyndrome in qi-layer——pyreticosis with high fever, polydipsia, yellowish fur, and rapid pulse

3. cough due to lung heat——fever, cough with yellowish sputum, slippery-rapid pulse

4. blood-heat bleeding syndrome——due to excessive interior heat hematochezia, metrorrhagia, non-traumatic hemorrhage, bedpan, metrorrhagia

5. external ulcer, internal carbuncle and various toxic-heat syndromes

6. excessive fetal movement caused by heat

Dosage: 3～9g.

Contraindication: This drug, cold in nature and bitter in taste, can damage qi. Those suffering from poor appetite and loose stool due to deficiency-cold in stomach and spleen must be prohibited in use of the drug.

Combinations:

1. add Largehead Atractylodes Rhizome(白术, Baizhu)——excessive fetal movement due to heat

2. add White Mulberry Root-bark(桑白皮, Sangbaipi)——cough with lung heat and the pulmonary abscess

3. add Cochinchinese Asparagus Root(天门冬, Tianmendong)——dry cough with slight sputum, dry pharynx, aphasia due to lung asthenia with dryness heat, lung heat leading to damage. Or upper diabetes mellitus syndrome with thirst and oliguria of yin asthenia of lung and kidney. Or pus sputum has been reduced in the pulmonary abscess later stage, but normal climate has been damaged, residual heat is raging

4. add Janpanese Pagodatree Flower(槐花, Huaihua)——heat damaging of blood vessel led to bloody defecation, hemorrhoids bleeding and metrorrhagia. It treats high blood pressure.

5. add Chrysanthemum Flower(菊花, Juhua)——hyper activity of yang of liver led to headache, conjunctiva congestion, bitter tastes in the of mouth, reddish complexion, dysphoria

6. add White Peony Root(白芍药, Baishaoyao)——dysenteric abdomen

7. add Coptis Rhizome(黄连, Huanglia n)—— reddish complexion with swelling-pain, vomiting with gastric cavity mass, terrified palpitation without sleep

8. add Pinellia Rhizome(半夏, Banxia)——cough with yellowish sputum

9. add Cape Jasmine Fruit(栀子, Zhizi)——hematemesis, non-traumatic hemorrhage

10. add Talc(滑石, Huashi) and Round Cardamom Seed(白豆蔻, Baidoukou)——damp-warm fever, Chest distress, greasy tongue coating

11. add Cape Jasmine Fruit(栀子, Zhizi) and Capillary Wormwood Herb(茵陈蒿, Yinchenhao)——damp-heat with yellowish body.

12. add and Gypsum(生石膏, Shengshigao)——the excess pyrosyndrome in qi-stage

13. add Snakegourd Root(天花粉, Tianhuafen) and Dahurian Angelica Root(白芷, Baizhi)——carbuncle swelling wound poison

14. add Largehead Atractylodes Rhizome (白术, Baizhu)——fetal fever, excessive fetal movement

Prescriptions: 1. Skutellaria Decoction(黄芩汤, Huangqin Tang).

2. Minor Decoction of Bupleurum(小柴胡汤, Xiaochaihu Tang).

Notes: Baikal Skullcap Root(黄芩, Huangqin) has the function of clearing away heat and drying dampness by bitter and cold. It is an important drug for clearing and purging the excess pyrosyndrome in qi-stage. It is good at purging lung-heat. Modern clinical research and pharmacodynamics have shown: Baikal Skullcap Root(黄芩, Huangqin) can reduce fever, resist inflammation and allergies. It has a wide antimicrobial spectrum, it is used for acute respiratory infection in children, chronic bronchitis, acute bacillary dysentery, leptospirosis, infective hepatitis, nephritis, and pyelonephritis. Another Baikal Skullcap Root(黄芩, Huangqin) has the function of reducing blood pressure, promoting urination, reducing blood lipids, reducing blood sugar, regulating function of the gall bladder and relieving spasm, and tranquilizing. Therefore it is used for high blood pressure, high blood lipids, diabetes mellitus and so on in combination with other herbs.

Baikal Skullcap Root(黄芩, Huangqin) has a different effect because of its different preparation. Dried Baikal Skullcap Root(黄芩, Huangqin) is used more for clearing away heat. Parched Baikal Skullcap Root(黄芩, Huangqin) anti-abortion is most frequently steeped in wine. when clearing away heat Upper-jiao it may be used with wine of Baikal Skullcap Root(黄芩, Huangqin) and for stopping blood, most use the stir-fry charcoal methed. *Compendium of Materia Medica* (《本草纲目》, Bencaogangmu) said:" When Baikal Skullcap Root(黄芩, Huangqin) meet with wine it floats up and goes up, it combined Juice of Pig Bladder (猪胆汁, Zhudanzhi) it can remove heat of liver and gall bladder; it can reduce cold and heat with Chinese Thorowax Root(柴胡, Chaihu); it treats diarrhea with White Peony Root(白芍药, Baishaoyao); it purges the lung-heat with White Mulberry Rootbark(桑白皮, Sangbaipi), it has the function of anti-abortion with Largehead Atractylodes Rhizome(白术, Baizhu)." But Annotated and *Identified Shennong's Herb Classic* (《本经疏证》, Benjingshuzheng) said: Baikal Skullcap Root(黄芩, Huangqin) helps Chinese Thorowax Root(柴胡, Chaihu) to clear away the heat in qi-stage; it helps White Peony Root (白芍药, Baishaoyao) to expel heat of the blood; it helps Coptis Rhizome(黄连, Huanglian) to reduce dampness producing heat. "What are mentioned above can be referred.

2. 黄连, Huanglian

English name: Coptis Rhizome

Pharmaceutical name: Rhizoma Coptidis

Botanical name: Coptis chinesnis Franch., C. Deltoidea C. Y. Cheng, C. Omeiensis (Chen) C. Y. Cheng, or C. Teetoides C. Y. Cheng

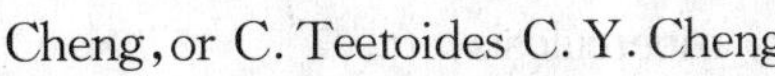

黄 连

Properties and tastes: bitter, cold.

Meridian tropism: heart, liver, stomach, large intestine.

Functions: 1. clear away heat and eliminate dampness

2. eliminate pathogenic fire and detoxication

3. promot digestion(little)

4. reduce fever

5. reduce blood pressure

6. resist microongnism and protozoon

7. normalize function of the gallbadder

8. calm the mind

Indications:

1. pyreticosis——high fever, restlessness, even coma and delirium belong to excessive heat of heart and stomach
2. diarrhea dysentery——the lapaxis bad smell, anus scorching hot and tenesmus belong to intestinal accumulation of damp-heat pathogen.
3. vomiting with gastric heat, toothache with gastric heat
4. thoracic retention syndrome——epigastric fullness with tender pain due to stagnant phlegm and heat
5. insomnia with cardiac heat
6. carbuncle swelling wound poison, furunculosis entering, swelling-pain of ear and eye——local redness, swelling, heat, pain belong to stagnant toxic heat
7. diabetes mellitus——polyrexia, polydipsia over drinking belongs to middle stage of diabetes mellitus of excessive gastric heat
8. high blood pressure——essential hypertension, renal hypertension
9. arythmia——room-rapidity arythmia
10. syndrome——dysphoria, insomnia, "short fuse", even mania
11. chronic cholecystitis, otitis media, pulmonary tuberculosis, etc.
12. burn and eczema (for external use)

Dosage: 3～9g. Proper amount for external use.

Contraindication: This drug is very bitter and very cold in nature, it easily damages the stomach by overdosage or taking for a long time. Those suffering from stomach-cold and diarrhea due to spleen deficiency must be prohibited in use of the drug.

Combinations:

1. add Baikal Skullcap Root (黄芩, Huangqin) and Cape Jasmine Fruit (栀子, Zhizi)——pyreticosis restlessness, coma, hyperactivity of cardiac fire or mania
2. add Baikal Skullcap Root (黄芩, Huangqin) and Rhubarb (大黄, Dahuang)——hematochezia, non-traumatic hemorrhage of gastric heat
3. add Baikal Skullcap Root (黄芩, Huangqin) and Lobed Kudzuvine Root (葛根, Gegen)——damp-heat diarrhea
4. add Common Aucklandia Root (木香, Muxiang)——dysentery, tenesmus
5. add Fresh Ginger (生姜, Shengjiang) and Bamboo Shavings (竹茹, Zhuru)——Vomiting with gastric heat
6. add Ass-hide Glue (阿胶, Ejiao)——dysphoria, loss sleep/insomnia belong to cardiac and renal disharmony. It also treats dyspeptic diarrhea pus and blood.
7. add Red Peony Root (赤芍药, Chishaoyao) and Tree Peony Bark (牡丹皮, Mudanpi)——skin and external disease with furuncle
8. add Common Anemarrhea Rhizome (知母, Zhimu)——diabetes mellitus
9. add Medicinal Evodia Root (吴茱萸, Wuzhuyu)——gastropyretic acid regurgitation.
10. add Cinnabar (朱砂, Zhusha)——dysphoria, loss of sleep, insomnia belong to hyperactivity of cardiac fire
11. add Tumeric Root-tuber (郁金, Yujin)——chronic cholecystitis
12. add Gambirplant Hooked Stem and Branch (钩藤, Gouteng)——high blood pressure
13. add Rhubarb (大黄, Dahuang) and Garden Burnet Root (地榆, Diyu)——treat burn and scalding for external use
14. add Shunk Bugbane Rhizome (升麻, Shengma)——toothache with gastric heat,

gingival swelling and ache

15. add Dried Ginger(干姜, Ganjiang)——cold heat complex, epigastric fullness

16. add Cassia Bark(肉桂, Rougui)——cardionephric disharmony, insomnia severe palpitation

Prescriptions: 1. Decoction of Puerariae, Scutellariae and Coptidis(葛根芩连汤, Gegenqinlian Tang).

2. Antidotal Decoction of Coptis(黄连解毒汤, Huanglianjiedu Tang).

3. Zuojin Bolus(左金丸, Zuojin Wan).

Notes: Coptis Rhizome(黄连, Huanglian) is bitter in taste and cold in nature. It is good at purging heart heat and may be used for various stagnant toxic-heat syndromes. Li Shizhen(李时珍) called it"the main drug for treating heat."Modern research has shown: Coptis Rhizome(黄连, Huanglian) has the function of resistance of microbe and protozoon of wide spectrum. There is a curative effect for bacillary dysentery, acute gastritis, acute enteritis, cholera, exogenous febrile disease, chronic cholecystitis of alimentary canal infection, and diphtheria, bpertussis, pulmonary tuberculosis, tuberculosis pleuritis, bronchitis, pneumonia, pumlonary abscess of respiratory infection, and otitis media, otitis externa, forntal sinus, chronic rhinitis, acute and chronic amygdalitis, External ophthalmia or the five sense organs infections, and surgical infection, general infection, another causative agent infection, like amebic dysentery, haustra coli ciliates disease, prevention and cure bovillae. *The Pearl Bag* (《珍珠囊》, Zhenzhunang) said: "Coptis Rhizome(黄连, Huanglian) has six functions: first is to clear away heart-heat, second to reduce heat in Middle-jiao, third is to treat skin diseases, fourth is to expel wind-dampness evil, fifth is to treat sudden redness of eyes, sixth is to stop bleeding of the stomach."

Coptis Rhizome(黄连, Huanglian), bitter in taste and cold in nature, can purge all types of damp-heat. This very bitter and dry drug can not be used for those with thick yellowish fur or greasy fur on the tongue. Ancients were quite careful when using Coptis Rhizome(黄连, Huanglian). As it is said in *Compendium of Materia Medica* (《本草纲目》, Bencaogangmu): Coptis Rhizome(黄连, Huanglian) is a key drug of treating eyes. Ancient prescriptions for treating dysentery were Pill of Aucklandia and Coptis(香连丸, Xianglian Wan), which consists of Coptis Rhizome(黄连, Huanglian) and Common Aucklandia Root(木香, Muxiang); Powder of Ginger and Coptis(姜连散, Jianglian San) consists of Dried Ginger (干姜, Ganjiang) and Coptis Rhizome(黄连, Huanglian); Pill of Biantong(变通丸, Biantong Wang) consists of Coptis Rhizome (黄连, Huanglian) and Medicinal Evodia Root(吴茱萸, Wuzhuyu), Powder of Rhizoma Carcumae Longae(姜黄散, Jianghuang San), it consists of Coptis Rhizome(黄连, Huanglian) and fresh Ginger. Ancient prescriptions treat diabetes mellitus by wine steaming Coptis Rhizome(黄连, Huanglian), they treat summer-heat by wine boiling Coptis Rhizome(黄连, Huanglian), they treat hematockezia by Coptis Rhizome(黄连, Huanglian) and garlic, they treat liver heat by Coptis Rhizome(黄连, Huanglian) and Medicinal Evodia Root(吴茱萸, Wuzhuyu) aphtha can be treated by Coptis Rhizome(黄连, Huanglian) and Manchurian Wildginger Herb(细辛, Xixin), one is cold, the other hot, one belongs to yin, the other yang. The principle is to use drugs of cold nature to treat pseudo-hot syndrome, and vice versa.

3. 黄柏, Huangbai

English name: Chinese Corktree Bark

Pharmaceutical name: Cortex Phellodendri

Botanical name: Phellodendron amurense Rupr. Or P. Chinense Schneid

黄 柏

Properties and tastes: bitter, cold

Meridian tropism: kidney, urinary bladder, large intestine

Functions: 1. clear away heat and eliminate dampness

2. eliminate pathogenic fire and detoxication

3. clear away deficiency heat

4. broad-spectrum antibiotic

5. control HBsAg

6. reduce blood pressure

7. promote the secretion of bile

Indications: 1. endoretention of damp heat syndrome——dysentery, choleplania, leukorrhagia, pyretic stranguria and hygropyretic flaccidity etc.

2. stagnant toxic heat——the skin and external disease, furuncle, eczema, herpes zoster. It is also used to treat burn.

3. fever with yin asthenia——osteopyrexia and fever/hectic fever, night sweating, emission

4. high blood pressure——chronic renal hypertension

Dosage: 3～9g.

Contraindication: This drug is very bitter in taste and very cold in nature. It easily damages stomach-qi. Those suffering from insufficiency of the spleen-yang must be prohibited in use of the drug.

Combinations: 1. add Chinese Pulsatiall Root (白头翁, Baitouweng) and Coptis Rhizome (黄连, Huanglian)——hygropyretic dysentery

2. add Cape Jasmine Fruit (栀子, Zhizi) and Rhubarb (大黄, Dahuang)——jaundice with damp-heat pathogen

3. add Plantain Seed (车前子, Cheqianzi) and Ginkgo Seed (白果, Baiguo)——hygropyretic leukorrhagia

4. add Bamboo Leaf (竹叶, Zhuye) and Akebia Stem (木通, Mutong)——pyretic stranguria

5. add Fineleaf Schizomepeta Herb (荆芥, Jingjie) and Lightyellow Sophora Root (苦参, Kushen)——the edema

6. add Coptis Rhizome (黄连, Huanglian) and Cape Jasmine Fruit (栀子, Zhizi)——the skin and external disease and furuncle

7. add Common Anemarrhea Rhizome (知母, Zhimu)——emission, night sweating due to yin deficiency and excessive fire. It also treats priapism of the man and aphrodisia of the woman

8. add Tortoise Shell and Plastrom (龟板, Guiban)——the hypertension

9. add Swordlike Atractylodes Rhizome (苍术, Cangzhu)——the hygropyretic flaccidity, moist ulcer, leukorrhagia of the woman, articulation red swelling heat pain. It also treats nodositas erythema

Prescriptions: 1. Decoction of Capejasmine and Phellodendron (栀子柏皮汤, Zhizibaipi Tang).

2. Bolus of Rhizoma Anemarrhenae, Cortex Phollodendri and Rhizoma Rehmanniae (知柏地黄丸, Zhibaidihuang Wan).

Notes: Chinese Corktree Bark (黄柏, Huangbai) treats fever due to yin-deficiency, night sweat, emission etc. Its aim is to invigorate by means of purging (i.e., clear away fire in order to keep yin). It has no function of nourishing yin and replenishing the kidney. Unripe Chinese Corktree Bark (黄柏, Huangbai) has a good effect on reducing heat. Fried Chinese Corktree Bark (黄柏, Huangbai) salt may improve the effect of purging heat of the kidney. In the clinic, Chinese Corktree Bark (黄柏, Huangbai) is always used with Common Anemarrhea Rhizome (知母, Zhimu) and Swordlike Atractylodes Rhizome (苍术, Cangzhu). Zhu Zhenheng (朱震亨) said: "Chinese Corktree Bark (黄柏, Huangbai) can nourish yin and fall fire with Common Anemarrhea Rhizome (知母, Zhimu), it can expel dampness and remove heat with Swordlike Atractylodes Rhizome (苍术, Cangzhu)."

Modern research shows that Chinese Corktree Bark (黄柏, Huangbai) can restrain various coccidia and many kinds of bacillus and fungus. So this drug is used to treat bacillary dysentery and enteritis in the clinic.

Chinese Corktree Bark (黄柏, Huangbai), Baikal Skullcap Root (黄芩, Huangqin) and Coptis Rhizome (黄连, Huanglian) are bitter in taste cold in nature, they can clear away damp-dryness and detoxicate. However Chinese Corktree Bark (黄柏, Huangbai) is good at purging kidney fire, reducing deficiency heat and expelling dampness-heat in the Lower-jiao. Baikal Skullcap Root (黄芩, Huangqin) is good at clearing away lung-heat and preventing abortion. Coptis Rhizome (黄连, Huanglian) is good at clearing away heart heat and relieving restlessness, and it can stop vomiting by clearing away stomach heat. In a word, Baikal Skullcap Root (黄芩, Huangqin) is good attreating diseases in the Upper-jiao, Coptis Rhizome (黄连, Huanglian) is good at treating diseases in the Middle-jiao, Chinese Corktree Bark (黄柏, Huangbai) is good at treating diseases in the Lower-jiao, but they are often used in combination.

4. 龙胆草, Longdancao

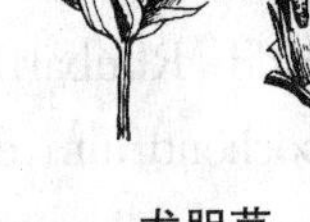
龙胆草

English name: Chinese Gentian Root

Pharmaceutical name: Radix Gentianae Scabrae

Botanical name: Gentiana scabra Bge. In Manchuria G. Triflora Pall. Is used instead

Properties and tastes: bitter, cold

Meridian tropism: liver, gall bladder, stomach

Functions: 1. clear away heat and eliminate dampness

2. eliminate pathogen in the liver and arrest convulsion

3. strengthen the stomach with the drug of bitter in taste

4. normalize the function of the gallbladder

5. reduce blood pressure and tranquilize

6. resist inflammation

7. resist bacteria

Indications: 1. damp heat syndrome——damp-heat pudendal swelling, pruritus vuluae, leukorrhagia, eczema

2. excessive heat generting wind syndrome——excessive heat of the liver meridian, excessive heat generating wind leading to high fever, convulsion, spasm of hands and feet

3. the excess pyrosyndrome of liver and gall bladder——hypochondrium, headache, bit-

ter taste in the mouth, conjunctiva congestion, deafness, high blood pressure etc.

4. unresolved hepatitis and chronic hepatitis

5. acute conjunctivitis

Dosage: 6 ~ 9g. Proper amount for external use.

Contraindication: Those suffering from insufficiency of spleen-yang are unsuitable for use of the drug.

Combinations: 1. add Abalone Shell(石决明, Shijueming)——dizziness and blurred vision, conjunctival congestion with swelling ache, convulsive disease, convulsion of hands and feet

2. add Rhubarb (大黄, Dahuang)——hypochondrium, deafness, bitter taste in the mouth, conjunctiva congestion, pudendal, hygropyretic dysentery, scrotitis swelling, constipation, hematochezia, non-traumatic hemorrhage, mania etc.

3. add Capillary Wormwood Herb(茵陈蒿, Yinchenhao) and Tumeric Root-tuber (郁金, Yujin)——damp-heat with yellowish body and damp-heat of liver-gall bladder lead to fullness in chest and hypochondrium, bitter taste in the mouth

4. add Lightyellow Sophora Root (苦参, Kushen) and Great Burdock Achene (牛蒡子, Niubangzi)——skin and external disease of damp-heat, genital puritus, skin scabies and tinea

5. add Gambirplant Hooked Stem and Branch(钩藤, Gouteng) and Tall Gastrodia Rhizome(天麻, Tianma)——hepatopyretic convulsion

6. add Cow—bezoar (牛黄, Niuhuang) and Gambirplant Hooked Stem and Branch (钩藤, Gouteng)——excessive heat of liver meridian, high fever convulsive disease, convulsion of hands and feet

7. add Akebia Stem(木通, Mutong), Plantain Seed(车前子, Cheqianzi) and Japanese Climbing Fern Spores (海金沙, Haijinsha)——urethritis, cystitis

8. add Coastal Glehnia Root, and Fourleaf Ladybell Root(沙参, Shashen), Dwarf Lilyturf Root(麦门冬, Maimendong) and Dendrobium Herb (石斛, Shihu)——gastric mucosa prolapse and chronic gastritis lead to dry mouth, tongue without fur, inappetence, postcibal epigastric distention

9. add Chinese Corktree Bark(黄柏, Huangbai), Talc(滑石, Huashi) and Plantain Seed (车前子, Cheqianzi)——hot urination, leukorrhagia, eczema.

Prescription: Bolus of Radix Gentianae for Purging Liver-Fire (龙胆泻肝汤, Longdanxiegan Tang).

Notes: Chinese Gentian Root(龙胆草, Longdancao) is very bitter in taste and very cold in nature, its function is similar to that of Baikal Skullcap Root(黄芩, Huangqin) and Coptis Rhizome (黄连, Huanglian). But Chinese Gentian Root(龙胆草, Longdancao) is used primarily to clear away fire of the liver and gall bladder, it mainly treats ophthalmalgia, neck pain, hypochondric pain, and convulsion belonging to excessive heat of the liver meridian. Chinese Gentian Root (龙胆草, Longdancao) and Baikal Skullcap Root(黄芩, Huangqin) all can clear away damp-heat in the Lower-jiao, but Chinese Gentian Root(龙胆草, Longdancao) is good at pursing the access heat of liver and gall bladder, Baikal Skullcap Root (黄芩, Huangqin) purges fire of deficiency type in the kidney to reduce deficiency heat.

5. 苦参, Kushen

English name: Lightyellow Sophora Root

Pharmaceutical name: Radix Sophorae Flavescentis

Botanical name: Sophora flavescens Ait

Properties and tastes: bitter, cold

Meridian tropism: heart, liver, stomach, large intestine, urinary bladder

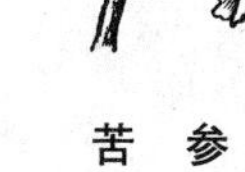

苦 参

Functions: 1. clear away heat and eliminate dampness

2. expel wind and kill pest

3. reduce diuresis

4. resist arrhythmia and protect

5. reduce blood-fat

6. subdue asthma and expel phlegm

7. prevent leukopenia and resist radiation

8. resist bacteria, inflammation, and hypersensitivity and stop pain

9. resist tumor

Indications: 1. damp-heat syndrome——pudendal, dysentery, leukorrhagia, genital puritus, nocturnal emission, spermatorrhea

2. skin disease——skin itching, acne pustulosa, nettle-rash, psoriasis, skin scabies and tinea, leprosy, and etc.

3. stranguria——endoretention of damp heat, dysuria, burning sensation and pain of urination

Dosage: 3～9g.

Contraindication: This drug is bitter in taste and cold in nature. Those suffering from insufficiency of the spleen-yang must be prohibited in use of the drug. *Herbals for Easy Approaching* (《本草便读》, Bencaobiandu) said that after over-eating this drug, the patient feels heavy of the lumbar and can not go and stand, because it has over descending properties, it easily damages kidney and bone. You should use it carefully it in the clinic.

Combinations:

1. add Chinese Angelica Root(当归, Danggui)——seborrhea, acne pustulosa

2. add Dried Alum (枯矾, Kufan)——it treats skin tinea by making ointment for external use

3. add Chrysanthemum Flower (菊花, Juhua)——eye disease with over tear

4. add Janpanese Pagodatree Flower(槐花, Huaihua)——bedpan and hygropyretic dysentery

5. add Chaulmoogratree Seed (大风子, Dafengzi) and Siberian Cocklebur Fruit(苍耳子, Cangerzi)——it treats leprosy by soaking in wine before eating

6. add Ephedra(麻黄, Mahuang)——general prurigo

7. add Coptis Rhizome (黄连, Huanglian)——dysentery

8. add Chinese Corktree Bark(黄柏, Huangbai) and Common Cnidium Fruit(蛇床子, Shechuangzi)——yellowish sticky leukorrhagia, genital puritus

9. add Tuckahoe(茯苓, Fuling)——dysuria, edema with damp-heat

10. add Chinese Corktree Bark (黄柏, Huangbai) and Plantain Seed (车前子, Cheqianzi)——hot urination, leukorrhagia, eczema

Prescription: Powder for Dispersing Wind-Evil (消风散, Xiaofeng San)

Notes: Lightyellow Sophora Root (苦参, Kushen) has a bitter taste and is cold in nature. It has the function of descending and reducing fever, clearing away heat and drying dampness, killing parasites to relieve itching. The effect is as good as that of Baikal Skullcap Root (黄芩, Huangqin), Coptis Rhizome (黄连, Huanglian), cotktree. But Lightyellow Sophora Root(苦参, Kushen)is extremely bitter, the dry property is strongest, so it can kill parasites from damp-heat, its effect is stronger than that of Baikal Skullcap Root(黄芩, Huangqin), Coptis Rhizome(黄连, Huanglian). Therefore the ancients said: "if the disease is not due to excessive damp-heat in the Lower-jiao, the drug can not be used." But leprosy can be cured by using a large dosage of Lightyellow Sophora Root(苦参, Kushen).

section 3

Heat-clearing and Toxin-expelling Drugs

1. 金银花, Jinyinhua

English name: Honeysuckle Flower

Pharmaceutical name: Flos Lonicerae Japonicae

Botanical name: Lonicera japonica Thunb. L. Hypoglauca Miq., L. Confusa DC., and L. Similis Hemsl. Are used instead in different parts of China

金银花

Properties and tastes: sweet, cold

Meridian tropism: lung, stomach, and large intestine

Functions: 1. clear away heat-toxin

2. expel pathogenic factors from the exterior

3. resist bateria

4. resist inflammation

Indications: 1. exogenous febrile disease——exogenous wind-heat, summer-heat, febrile disease, pathogen exists in wei-layer, it is also used to each stage that pathogen lives in qi-stage, pathogen lives in ying-layer, pathogen lives in blood-layer

2. wound carbuncle with furuncle

3. vusceral carbuncle, like intestinal abscess, pulmonary abscess etc.

4. hygropyretic dysentery——tenesmus, dyspeptic pus and blood

Dosage: 9～15g. 30～60g may be used for the patients with excessive heat-toxin.

Combinations: 1. add Fineleaf Schizomepeta Herb(荆芥, Jingjie) and Weeping Forsythia Capsule(连翘, Lianqiao)——wind-weed superficial syndrome and carbuncle swelling, furuncle, skin and external disease etc.

2. add Licorice Root(甘草, Gancao)——amygdalitis, tharyngitis, enteritis, dysentery of bacteria

3. add Gypsum(石膏, Shigao) and Common Anemarrhea Rhizome(知母, Zhimu)——seasonal febrile disease heat entering qi-layer

4. add Tree Peony Bark(牡丹皮, Mudanpi) and Rehmannia Dried Root(生地黄, Shengdihuang)——seasonal febrile disease heat entering ying-layer and blood-layer

5. add Dandelion(蒲公英, Pugongying) and Tokyo Violet Herb(紫花地丁, Zihuadiding)——acute mammitis, vusceral carbuncle

6. add Figwort Root(玄参, Xuanshen)——gangrenosis, angitis

7. add Coptis Rhizome(黄连, Huanglian) and Chinese Pulsatiall Root(白头翁, Baitouweng)——hygropyretic dysentery

8. add Hindu Lotus Leaf(荷叶, Heye)——summer-heat syndrome

Prescriptions: 1. Powder of Lonicerae and Forsythiae(银翘散, Yinqiao San).

2. Fairy Decoction for Treating Cutancous Infections(仙方活命饮, Xianfanghuoming Yin).

Notes: Honeysuckle Flower(金银花, Jinyinhua)is widely used to treat various hygropyretic syndromes. It is sweet in taste, cold in nature and nonpoisonous. Heavy toxic heat can be treated by adding more Honeysuckle Flower(金银花, Jinyinhua). *Essentials of Materia Medica* (《本草备要》, Bencaobeiyao)said:" It is the best drug for carbuncle and cellulitis." Modern research proved Honeysuckle Flower(金银花, Jinyinhua) can restrain bacteria, virus and fungus. And it has better effect on reducing fever. *Complete Works of Jingyue* (《景岳全书》, Jingyuequanshu) said:" Honeysuckle is good at detoxicating, so it is an important drug for treating carbuncle or abscess, swelling toxic, wound tinea, syphilitic, wind-damp etc. It can resolve pathogenic factors of external disease when they have made, it can make ulcer drain away when it has made."

[Add]: 忍冬藤, Rendongteng

English name: Honeysuckle Stem

Pharmaceutical name: Caulis Lonicerae

Botanical name: Lonicera japonica Thunb.

Properties and tastes: sweet, cold

忍冬藤

Meridian tropism: lung, stomach, large intestine

Functions: 1. clear away heat-toxin

2. expel wind-dampness, dredge the meridian, alleviate arthralgia syndrome

Indications: 1. carbuncle swelling wound poison

2. rheumatic fever arthralgia——articulation reddish swelling, pain, flexion and extension unfavorable

3. skin itching

Dosage: 9～13g.

Combinations: 1. add Mulberry Twig(桑枝, Sangzhi)——articulation pain, Rheumatic arthralgia

2. add Licorice Root(甘草, Gancao)——various carbuncle or agscess

3. add Heartleaf Houttuynia Herb(鱼腥草, Yuxingcao)——prevent and treat common cold

4. add Suberect Satholobus Stem(鸡血藤, Jixueteng)——rheumatic arthritis

Notes: This drug and Honeysuckle Flower(金银花, Jinyinhua) are cormophyte and bud of the same plant. Its properties, tastes and functions are the same as those of Honeysuckle Flower(金银花, Jinyinhua). It is used to treat carbuncle swelling wound poison. This drug also can remove wind-damp-heat of meridians and collaterals to stop arthralgia pain, so it is used for Rheumatic fever arthralgia, articulation reddish swelling and pain.

2. 连翘, Lianqiao

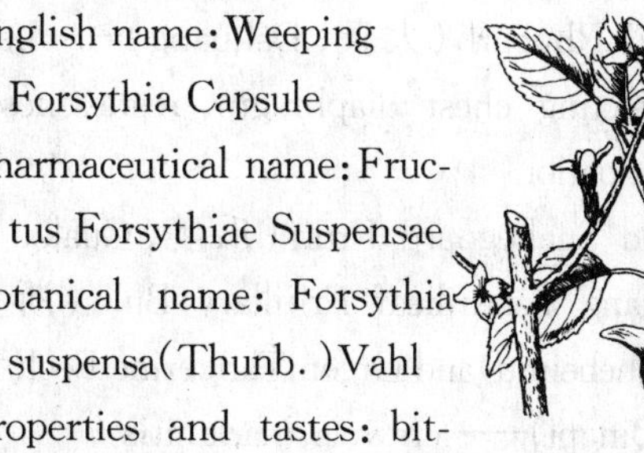

English name: Weeping Forsythia Capsule

Pharmaceutical name: Fructus Forsythiae Suspensae

Botanical name: Forsythia suspensa(Thunb.)Vahl

Properties and tastes: bitter, slightly cold

连 翘

Meridian tropism: lung, heart, gall bladder

Functions: 1. clear away heat-toxin

2. treat boils and resolve masses

3. control influenza virus

4. resist bacteria

5. reduce diuresis.

6. resist hepatic injury

7. relieve vomitting

Indications: 1. wind-heat cold or febrile disease early stage——aversion to cold, high fever, thirst, pharyngalgia etc.

2. heat attacking pericardium syndrome——high fever, restlessness, coma and delirium

3. carbuncle swelling wound poison——various suppurate infection, include crewels, mammitis, powder, vusceral carbuncle

4. acute nephritis, nephrotic tuberculosis

5. purpura

Dosage: 6～15g.

Combinatins: 1. add Fineleaf Schizomepeta Herb(荆芥, Jingjie) and Wild Mint(薄荷, Bohe)——wind-heat cold

2. add Buffalo Horn(水牛角, Shuiniujiao) and Lotus Seed(莲子, Lianzi)——high fever, restlessness, coma and delirium belong to heat attacking pericardium syndrome

3. add Red Peony Root(赤芍药, Chishaoyao), Tree Peony Bark(牡丹皮, Mudanpi) and Indigowoad Leaf(大青叶, Daqingye)——hot blood eruptive

4. add Baikal Skullcap Root(黄芩, Huangqin), Cape Jasmine Fruit(栀子, Zhizi) and Rhubarb(大黄, Dahuang)——heat obstructing chest diaphragm, restlessness, Constipation

5. add Snakegourd Fruit(瓜蒌, Gualou), Zhejiang Tendrilleaf Fritillary Bulb(浙贝母, Zhebeimu) and Green Tangerine Peel(青皮, Qingpi)——crewels, mammitis

6. add, Honeysuckle Flower(金银花, Jinyinhua) Tokyo Violet Herb(紫花地丁, Zihuadiding) and Dandelion(蒲公英, Pugongying)——skin and external disease, erysipelas, fever of acute communicable disease

7. add Ephedra(麻黄, Mahuang), Red Peony Root(赤芍药, Chishaoyao) and Licorice Root(甘草, Gancao)——anaphylactoid purpura

8. add Figwort Root(玄参, Xuanshen), Indigwoad Root(板蓝根, Banlangen) and Rehmannia Dried Root(生地黄, Shengdihuang)——swelling toxin of throat

9. add Honeysuckle Stem(忍冬藤, Rendongteng)——carbuncle swelling wound poison

10. add Great Burdock Achene(牛蒡子, Niubangzi)——reddish swelling of the throat, excessive heat toxin, mumps swelling toxic, wind-heat eczema

11. add Akebia Stem(木通, Mutong)——urinary system

12. add Chinese Corktree Bark(黄柏, Huangbai) and Licorice Root(甘草, Gancao)——mouth and tongue wounds

Prescription: Antiphlogistic Powder with Forsythia Fruit(连翘败毒散, Lianqiaobaidu San)

Notes: Weeping Forsythia Capsule(连翘, Lianqiao) can clear away heat and expel toxin and it is the best drug for treating ulcer. Its function is the same as that of Honeysuckle Flower(金银花, Jinyinhua). So the two drugs are used in combination. This drug enters the heart meridian, it is good at clearing away heart heat and purging intense heat, so it is good at treating heat-attacking pericardium leading to coma and delirium. The Honeysuckle Flower(金银花, Jinyinhua) is good at wind-heat and diaphoretic relieving superficies, and can remove heat from the blood and relieve dysentery.

Records of Traditional Chinese and Western Medicine in Combination (《医学衷中参西录》, Yixuezhongzhongcanxilu) said: it has the function of dispelling and dredging qi-blood, treating blood stasis and qi stagnation of twelve meridians for the patient susceptible to ulcer. It can expel pathogenic factors from the exterior, clear away heat and dispel wind, treat wind-dampness. It can also expel toxins and it is an important drug that promotes eruption. Its nature is slightly cold and ascending, so it is also good at treating head and eye diseases. It mainly treats headache, ophthalmalgia, toothache, nasosinusitis, or rhinorrhea leading to nasal sinusitis.

Another seed of Weeping Forsythia Capsule (连翘, Lianqiao) is called plumula nelumbini, its effect of clearing away heat and expelling toxin is similar with that of Weeping Forsythia Capsule (连翘, Lianqiao). It is used for exogenous febrile disease evil entering heart ying-layer synease.

3. 蒲公英, Pugongying

English name: Dandelion

Pharmaceutican name: Herba Taraxaci Mongolici cum Radice

Botanican name: Taraxacum mongolicum Hand-Mazz

蒲公英

Properties and tastes: bitter, sweet, and cold

Meridian tropism: liver, stomach

Functions: 1. clear away heat-toxin
2. relieve stranguria by diuresis
3. normalize the function of the gallbadder

Indications: 1. acute infection of the upper respiratory tract, amygdalitis, tharyngitis acute mammitis
2. carbuncle swelling wound poison and vusceral carbuncle
3. cholecystitis
4. gastritis, appendicitis and alimentary canal ulcer
5. pyelonephritis

Dosage: 9 ~ 30g, proper amount for external use.

Contraindication: Over dosage may lead to mild diarrhea. Those with splenasthenic loose stool should not use this drug.

Combinations: 1. add Tokyo Violet Herb(紫花地丁, Zihuadiding), Perilla Leaf (紫苏, Zisu) and Indigowoad Leaf (大青叶, Daqingye)——infection of the upper respiratory tract, amygdalitis, tharyngitis
2. add Honeysuckle Flower(金银花, Jinyinhua), Weeping Forsythia Capsule (连翘, Lianqiao) and Snakegourd Root (天花粉, Tianhuafen)——acute mammitis
3. add Chrysanthemum Flower (菊花, Juhua)——decoct drug for oral taking, use second decocting fumigation and ocular wash method, it can treat simple conjunctivitis, hordeolum
4. add Japanese Climbing Fern Spores(海金沙, Haijinsha) and Tumeric Root-tuber (郁金, Yujin)——acute cholecystitis
5. add Capillary Wormwood Herb(茵陈蒿, Yinchenhao) and Asiatic Plantain Herb (车前草, Cheqiancao)——jaundice hepatitis
6. add Rhubarb (大黄, Dahuang) and Tree Peony Bark (牡丹皮, Mudanpi)——appendicitis
7. add Honeysuckle Flower(金银花, Jinyinhua) and Tree Peony Bark(牡丹皮, Mudanpi)——pyelonephritis

8. add Heartleaf Houttuynia Herb(鱼腥草, Yuxingcao) and Reed Rhizome(芦根, Lugen)——pulmonary absdess, purulent sputum

9. add Indigwoad Root(板蓝根, Banlangen) and Figwort Root(玄参, Xuanshen)——sore throat with swelling

10. add Dried Ginger(干姜, Ganjiang)——gastritis, hyperchlorhydria

Prescription: Antiphlogistic Decoction of Five Drugs(五味消毒饮, Wuweixiaodu Yin).

Notes: Zhu Zhengheng(朱震亨) says Dandelion(蒲公英, Pugongying)"has a wonderful effect on removing heat-toxin and clearing away swelling." It may be used for infectious disease. Modern research has shown Chinese Corktree Bark(黄柏, Huangbai) can remarkably restrain golden staphylococcus, hemolytic streptococcus and catarrhcoccus. It also improves body immunity.

In addition, nipple belongs to liver, breast belongs to stomach. Zhu Zhengheng(朱震亨) says it acts on liver and stomach meridious, clearing away heat and expelling toxin. It may treat mammary abseass and mastocarcinome for external and oral use.

4. 紫花地丁, Zihuadiding

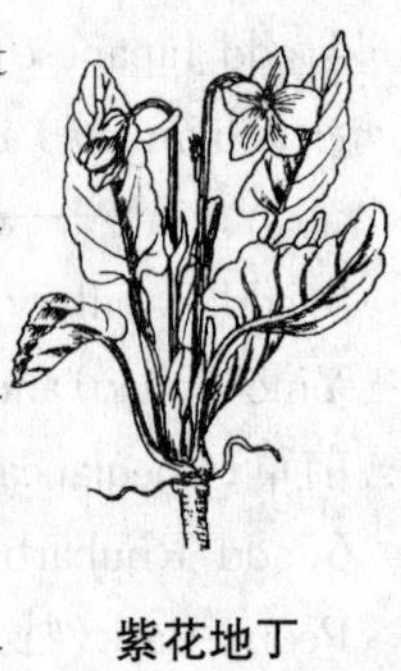

English name: Tokyo Violet Herb

Pharmaceutical name: Herba Violae cum Radice

Botanical name: Viola yedonensis Mak. or Viola japonica Langsd

紫花地丁

Properties and tastes: bitter, pungent, cold

Meridian tropism: heart, liver

Functions: 1. clear away heat and toxic substances

2. resist bacteria

Indications: 1. skin and external disease——fire-toxin, furuncle, mammary abseass, intestinal abseass, erysipelas

2. conjunctival congestion with swelling pain due to liver-heat

3. enteritis, dysentery

4. jaundice

5. scarlet fever

Dosage: 9~15g.

Contraindication: Those suffering from skin and external diseases belonging to yin syndrome, which must be prohibited in use of the drug.

Combinations: 1. add Chrysanthemum Flower (菊花, Juhua) and Weeping Forsythia Capsule(连翘, Lianqiao)——carbuncle and furuncle

2. add Dandelion(蒲公英, Pugongying)——mammary abseass, intestinal abseass, furuncle, carbuncle swelling, damp-heat yellowish body, urinary tract infection and so on, all kinds of inflammation

3. add Honey(蜂蜜, Fengmi)——hepatic heat epistaxis in children

4. add Dandelion(蒲公英, Pugongying) and Capillary Wormwood Herb(茵陈蒿, Yinchenhao) Artemisia capillaris——jaundice.

5. add Chinese Sage Herb(紫参, Zishen), Asiatic Plantain Herb(车前草, Cheqiancao) and Japanese Climbing Fern Spores(海金沙, Haijinsha)——prostatitis

6. add Dandelion(蒲公英, Pugongying) and Honeysuckle Flower(金银花, Jinyinhua)——body's head, face and back furuncle

7. add Honeysuckle Flower(金银花, Jinyinhua), Manyleaf Paris Rhizome(蚤休, Zaoxiu) and Red Peony Root(赤芍药,

Chishaoyao)——virulent fire furuncle, mammary abseass, intestinal abseass, erysipelas

8. add Dandelion(蒲公英, Pugongying), Figwort Root(玄参, Xuanshen) and Red Peony Root(赤芍药, Chishaoyao)——scarlet fever

9. add Sargentoglory Vine Stem(红藤, Hongteng) and Baikal Skullcap Root(黄芩, Huangqin)——enteritis, dysentery

10. add Chrysanthemum Flower(菊花, Juhua) and Common Selfheal Fruit-spike(夏枯草, Xiakucao)——Reddish complexion with swelling-pain of hepatic heat

Notes: This drug is an important drug for treating furuncle. It has a curative effect when used alone. It can be freshly pressed into juice for oral use. Snake-bite can be treated with its residue for external use.

Tokyo Violet Herb(紫花地丁, Zihuadiding) and Dandelion(蒲公英, Pugongying) are all bitter in taste, cold in nature and have the functions of clearing away heat and expelling toxin. They are commonly used for treating ulcer carbuncle and swelling. They are often used together. But as Tokyo Violet Herb(紫花地丁, Zihuadiding) has an acid taste, it can remove blood stasis, it is good at treating malignant boils, and relieving snake poison. Dandelion(蒲公英, Pugongying) has a sweet taste and slippery properties, it can remove obstruction of orifices, it is good at treating acute mastitis. Modern pharmacodynamics research proved that they can resist bateria, protect liver and restrain cancer.

5. 大青叶, Daqingye

English name: Indigowoad Leaf

Pharmaceutical name: Foliun Isatidis

Botanical name: Isatis tinctoria L., I. indigota Fort., B aphicacanthus cusia (Nees) Bremek., Clerodendron cyrtophyllum Turcz., or Polygonum tinctorium Ait.

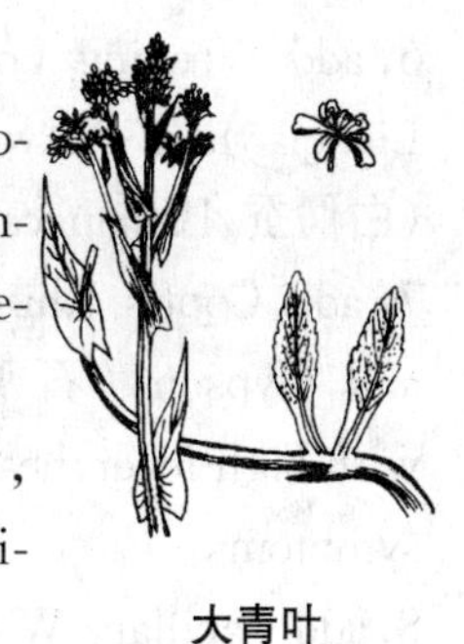

大青叶

Properties and tastes: bitter, extremely cold

Meridian tropism: heart, lung, and stomach

Functions: 1. clear away heat and toxic material

2. remove pathogenic heat from blood and ecchymoses

3. resist bateria and virus

4. reduce fever and resist inflammation

Indications: 1. epidcmic febrile disease in blood-stage——eruption, high fever, restlessness, and coma due to heat-toxin of epidemic febrile disease entering blood-stage

2. erysipelas, aphtha, sore throat with swelling

3. measles

4. mumps

5. communicable hepatitis

Dosage: 9～15g, for external use.

Contraindication: Do not use with patirents in the case of deficiency cold of the spleen and stomach.

Combinations: 1. add Gypsum(生石膏, Shengshigao)——high fever, headache

2. add Honeysuckle Flower(金银花, Jinyinhua)——furuncle, erysipelas, mumps

3. add Dan-shen Root(丹参, Danshen)——jaundice, nonjaundice hepatitis, cholecystitis

4. add Tonkin Sophora Root(山豆根, Shandougen) and Blackberrylily Rhizome(射干, Shegan)——laryngalgia swelling pain

5. add Indigwoad Root(板蓝根, Banlangen) and Fineleaf Schizomepeta Herb(荆芥, Jingjie)——encephalitis B.

6. add Weeping Forsythia Capsule(连翘, Lianqiao) and Silkworm with Batrytis Larva (白僵蚕, Baijiangcan)——mumps

7. add Coptis Rhizome(黄连, Huanglian) and Gypsum(石膏, Shigao)——measles with high fever, headache, obvious poisoning symptoms

8. add Capillary Wormwood Herb(茵陈蒿, Yinchenhao)——damp-heat jaundice

9. add Shunk Bugbane Rhizome(升麻, Shengma) skunk bugbare and Figwort Root (玄参, Xuanshen)——treating aphtha

Notes: Indigowoad Leaf(大青叶, Daqingye) has the function of clearing away heat and expelling toxins and removing heat from the blood and removing ecchymosis. It mainly treats encephalitis B, epidemic encephalitis B, influenza with high fever, enteritis, dysentery, jaundice, toothache, epistaxis, sore throat with swelling, etc. Therefore, Indigowoad Leaf(大青叶, Daqingye) treats all diseases due to heat with pathogenic factors.

Indigowoad Leaf(大青叶, Daqingye) is often used in clinical paediatrics as well. As it is said in *Origin of Shennong's Herbal Classic* (《本经逢源》, Benjingfengyuan): Indigowoad Leaf(大青叶, Daqingye) can purge excessive heat of the liver and gall bladder, and remove pathogenic heat of the heart and stomach. So it is an important drug for infantile maluntrition with fever and erysipelas.

6. 板蓝根, Banlangen

English name: Indigwoad Root

Pharmaceutical name: Radix Isatidis

Botanical name: Isatis tinctoria L.

Properties and tastes: bitter, cold

Meridian tropism: heart, stomach

Functions: 1. clear away heat and toxic material

2. remove pathogenic heat from blood and relieve sore throat

3. resist virus

4. resist bateria

板蓝根

Indications: 1. exogenous febrile disease pyrosyndrome involving qi-stage and blood-stage——high fever, sore throat, eruption, restlessness, coma etc.

2. serum hepatitis and epidemic encephalitis

3. influenza

4. hepatitis

5. mumps

6. viral skin disease

7. acute conjunctivitis

Dosage: 9~15g.

Combinations: 1. add Capillary Wormwood Herb(茵陈蒿, Yinchenhao) and Cape Jasmine Fruit(栀子, Zhizi)——catarrhal jaundice

2. add Indigowoad Leaf(大青叶, Daqingye)——sore throat with swelling, exogenous febrile disease eruptive.

3. add Figwort Root(玄参, Xuanshen) and Great Burdock Achene(牛蒡子, Niubangzi)——mumps, sore throat with swelling

4. add Honeysuckle Flower(金银花, Jinyinhua) and Fineleaf Schizomepeta Herb(荆芥, Jingjie)——influenza

5. add Gypsum(石膏, Shigao) and Common Anemarrhea Rhizome(知母, Zhimu)——meningococal meningitis, epidemic encephalitis B.

Prescription: Universal Relief Decoction for Disinfection(普济消毒饮, Pujixiaodu Yin).

Notes: Indigwoad Root(板蓝根, Banlangen) and Indigowoad Leaf(大青叶, Daqingye) are the root and leaf of the same plant. They have the function of clearing away heat and expelling toxins and removing heat from the blood. But Indigwoad Root(板蓝根, Banlangen)is good at expelling toxins and scattering blockage, Indigowoad Leaf(大青叶, Daqingye) flower is good at removing heat from the blood and removing ecchymosis. In modern times they are used for various infectious diseases, especially diseases due to viral infection, such as encephalitis B, jaundice, varicella, mumps, herpes simples, herpes zoster, pityriasis rosea, plane warts, and etc.

7. 牛黄, Niuhuang

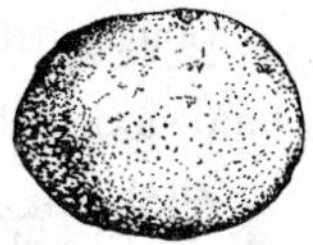

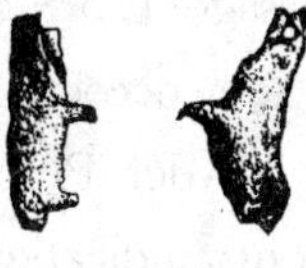

牛 黄

English name: Cow-bezoar

Pharmaceutical name: Calculus Bovis

Botanical name: Bos taurus domesticus Gmelin

Properties and tastes: bitter, cool

Meridian tropism: liver, heart

Functions: 1. clear away heart-fire and eliminate phlegm to restore the consciousness
2. clear away heat-toxin
3. tranquilize the mind and arrest cough
4. excite respiration, strengtnen the function of heart, reduce blood pressure
5. regulate function of the gallbladder
6. promote hematopoietic
7. relieve cough and asthma

Indications: 1. febrile disease, coma——high fever, restlessness, coma, eruption due to heat attacking ying-layer and blood-layer
2. apoplexy, convulsive disease, epilepsy——phlegm-fire confusing the heart
3. sore throat with swelling, ulceration, aphtha with tongue, carbuncle or agscess, furunculosis——belong to stagnated heat toxin
4. infection of the upper respiratory tract, influenza, bronchial pneumonia——cough, more yellowish phlegm belong to phlegm-fire obstrucing lung
5. catarrhal jaundice——it has the function of reducing glutamic-pyruvic transaminase
6. influenza fever, amygdalitis, neurosrgery, rheumatic arthritis

Dosage: 0.2～0.5g, the drug doesn't enter decoction, it only enter pill and powder.

Contraindication: Pregnant women must be cautious in use of the drug. Those not suffering from excessive heat are prohibited in use of it.

Combinations: 1. add Mush (麝香, Shexiang)——febrile disease, coma
2. add Buffalo Horn (水牛角, Shuiniujiao)——exogenous febrile disease, disturbance of mind by heat, unconsciousness and delirium, high fever
3. add Coptis Rhizome(黄连, Huanglian) and Cape Jasmine Fruit(栀子, Zhizi)——high fever, restlessness, skin and external disease, jaundice
4. add Arisaema With Bile(胆南星, Dannanxing) and Scorpion(全蝎, Quanxie)——high fever convulsion in children
5. add Olibanum, Frankincense(乳香, Ruxiang) and Myrrh(没药, Moyao)——crewels, breast cancer
6. add Silkworm with Batrytis Larva(白僵蚕, Baijiangcan), Centipede(蜈蚣, Wugong) and Tabasheer (天竺黄, Tianzhuhuang)——apoplexy phlegm syncope coma, acute infantile convulsion and chronic infantile convulsions in children, epilepsy
7. add Cinnabar(朱砂, Zhusha)——restless sleep in children, alienated
8. add Tendrilleaf Fritillary Bulb (贝母,

Beimu)and Bamboo Juice(竹沥,Zhuli)——pneumonia cough with asthma,coma,eruption

Prescriptions: 1. Cow-bezoare Sedative Bolus (牛黄清心丸,Niuhuangqingxin Wan).

2. Bezoare Pill for Resurrection(安宫牛黄丸,Angongniuhuang Wan).

Notes: Cow-bezoar(牛黄,Niuhuang) has the function of clearing away heat, expelling toxins, expelling phlegm, and stopping convulsion and inducing resuscitation by clearing away heat. Its effect in inducing resuscitation is less effective than that of Mush(麝香,Shexiang), so it is used for coma due to heat-phlegm in combination with Mush(麝香,Shexiang).

Cow-bezoar(牛黄,Niuhuang) has the function of clearing away heat and inducing resuscitation, so *Shennong's Herbal Classic* (《神农本草经》,Shennongbencaojing) said "it mainly treats convulsion and epilepsy due to cold or heat, or serious spasm due to excessive heat."

Cow-bezoar(牛黄,Niuhuang) is the gall stone of cattle, so it is rare but expensive. At present, synthetic Cow-bezoar(牛黄,Niuhuang) has also been used besides natural Cow-bezoar(牛黄,Niuhuang). Synthetic Cow-bezoar(牛黄,Niuhuang) is salvaged from bile of a cattle or a pig. It is reported that the curative effect is similar.

8. 熊胆, Xiongdan

English name: Bear Gall

Pharmaceutical naem: Fel Ursi

Properties and tastes: bitter, cold

Meridian tropism: liver, gall bladder, heart

Functions: 1. clear away heat and detoxicate

2. stop contracture

3. improve eyesight

4. benefit the gallnladder, dissolve the stones in the gallbladder

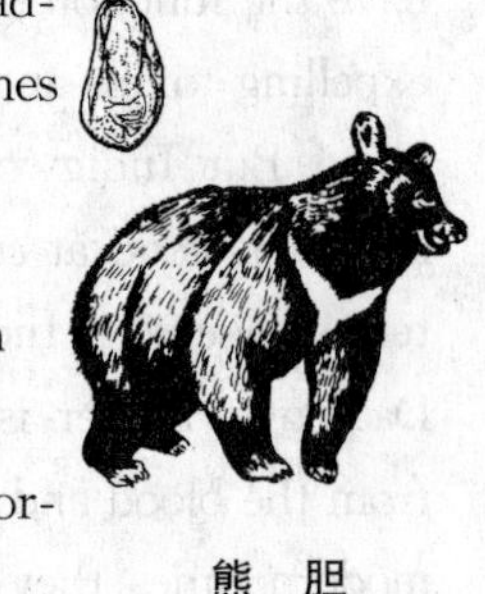

熊胆

Indications: 1. skin and external diseases with swelling due to pathogenic heat, hemorrhoids with swelling pain, sore throat. (For external use more)

2. endogenous liver wind syndrome——epilepsy with spasm, acute infantile convulsion, epilepsy, eclampsia, and also high blood pressure

3. conjunctivitis due to liver-heat, conjunctival congestion with swelling pain, photophobia with tearing, for both external use and oral medication

4. cholecystalgia, jaundice hepatitis

Dosage: 1.5~2.5g, the drug is unsuitably put into decoction, it is only put into pills and powder. Proper amount for external use.

Contraindication: Do not use in the case of deficiency syndrome.

Combinations: 1. add Cinnabar(朱砂,Zhusha)——convulsion. epilepsy

2. add Tumeric Root-tuber(郁金,Yujin)——cholelithiasis, epilepsy

3. add Bamboo Juice(竹沥,Zhuli)——infantile convulsion

Notes: This drug is bitter in taste, or slightly cold and humidifying in nature. So it reduces heat to improve eyesight, it also effectively treats chronic suppurative otitis media hemorrhoid, and toothache for external use. Research has shown that Bear Gall(熊胆,xiongdan) has the effect of detoxicating, antibiosis, anti-inflammatory, antianaphylaxis, relieving cough, eliminating phlegm, relieving asthma, aiding digestion, and reducing blood pressure.

9. 土茯苓, Tufuling

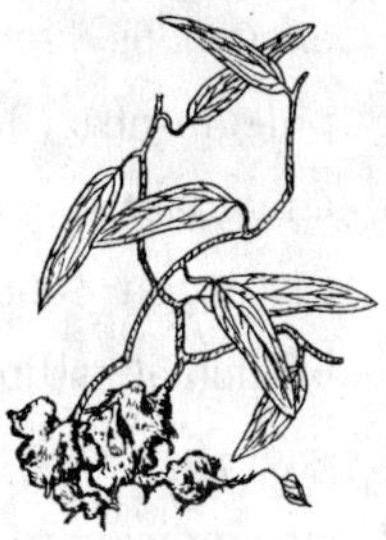

English name: Glabrous Greenbrier Rhizome

Pharmaceutical name: Rhizoma Smilacis Glabrae

Botanical name: Simlax glabra Roxb.

Properties and tastes: sweet, tastesless, and medium.

土茯苓

Meridian tropism: liver, stomach.

Functions: 1. clear away heat-toxin
2. eliminate dampness
3. relieve rigidity of joints

Indications: 1. syphilis
2. heat toxic carbuncle
3. pyretic stranguria

Dosage: 15～60g.

Contraindication: Do not drink tea during administration.

Combinations: 1. add Honeysuckle Flower(金银花, Jinyinhua), Densefruit Pittany Rootbark(白鲜皮, Baixianpi), and Licorice Root (甘草, Gancao)——syphilis
2. add Honeysuckle Flower(金银花, Jinyinhua), Weeping Forsythia Capsule (连翘, Lianqiao) and Dandelion(蒲公英, Pugongying)——heat toxic carbuncle
3. add Akebia Stem (木通, Mutong), Dandelion(蒲公英, Pugongying) and Common Knotgrass Herb(萹蓄, Bianxu)——pyretic stranguria
4. add Lightyellow Sophora Root (苦参, Kushen) and Belvedere Fruit (地肤子, Difuzi)——psoriasis

Notes: Rhizome Smilacis Glabrae(土茯苓, Tufuling) is sweet and tastesless. It has the function of removing dampness to expel heat and concurrenthy detoxicating, it is good at treating malignant boils, and syphilis. In recent years, it has been used to treat leptospirosis in clinics. It is reported that it has some curative effect.

Li Shizhen (李时珍) said: "Glabrous Greenbrier Rhizome(土茯苓, Tufuling) can invigorate the spleen and stomach, strengthen muscles and bones, expel wind-dampness evil, benefit joints, and relieve diarrhea. It treats spasm, ostealgia, malignant boil and carbuncle with swelling. It can detoxicate mercurialism and cennabar."

10. 鱼腥草, Yuxingcao

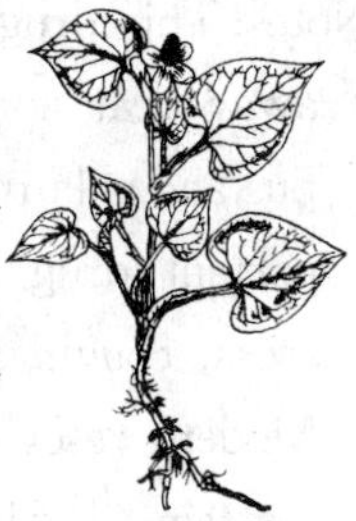

English name: Heartleaf Houttuynia Herb

Pharmaceutical name: Herba Houttuyniae Cordatae

Botanical name: Houttuynia cordata Thunb

Properties and tastes: pungent, slightly cold

鱼腥草

Meridian tropism: lung

Functions: 1. clear away heat-toxin
2. discharge pus and treat boils
3. induce diuresis for treating stranguria syndrome

Indications: 1. respiratory tract infection——bronchial pneumonia, lobar pneumonia, pulmonary abscess, infection of the upper respiratory tract, chronic bronchitis
2. pyretic stranguria
3. heat toxic skin and external disease

Dosage: 15～30g, proper amount for external use

Combinations: 1. Add Balloonflower Root (桔梗, Jiegeng)——pulmonary abscess, consumptive pneumonia, cough and vomiting of pus-blood
2. add Tokyo Violet Herb (紫花地丁, Zihuadiding)——chickenpox.

3. add Coptis Rhizome (黄连, Huanglian) and Chinese Corktree Bark (黄柏, Huangbai)——damp-heat diarrhea

4. add Honeysuckle Flower(金银花, Jinyinhua) and Dandelion (蒲公英, Pugongyin g)—— damp-heat wound carbuncle swelling poison

5. add Asiatic Plantain Herb (车前草, Cheqiancao) and Lalang Grass Rhizome(白茅根, Baimaogen)——pyretic stranguria

6. add Baikal Skullcap Root (黄芩, Huangqin) and Mulberry Leaf (桑叶, Sangye)——cough with lung heat

Notes: This drug has the function of clearing away heat and expelling toxin, evacuating pus and ablating boils. Therefore it is an important drug for treating pulmonary abscess, cough and vomiting of pus-blood. Modern research has shown it remarkably restrains golden staphylococcus, white staphylococcus, hemolytic streptococcus and catarrhcoccus and many other kinds of bacteria. So the drug is used for infection of the upper respiratory tract, urinary tract and enteropathy infection, derma infection, pelvic peritionitis and various infectious diseases.

11. 射干, Shegan

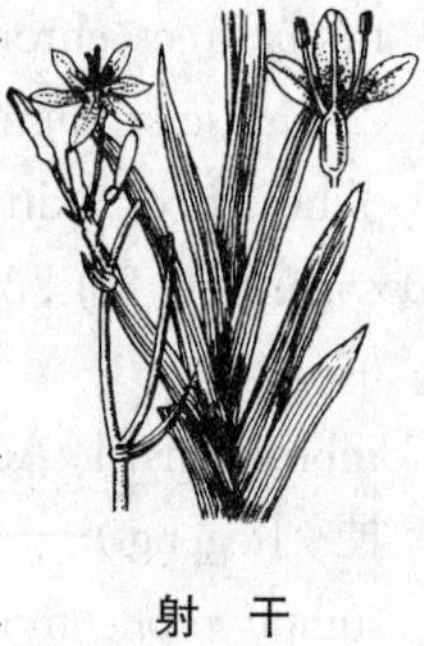

English name: Blackberrylily Rhizome

Pharmaceutical name: Rhizoma Belamcandae Chinensis

Botanical name: Belamcanda chinensis(L.)DC.

射 干

Properties and tastes: bitter, cold.

Meridian tropism: lung.

Functions: 1. clear away heat-toxin

2. expel phlegm and relieve sore throat

Indications: 1. sore throat with swelling——exogenous febrile disease or excessive phlegm-heat, like acute pharyngitis, acute amygdalitis

2. cough and asthma——bronchitis or bronchial asthma

Dosage: 6~9g.

Contraindication: Do not use with pregnant women, or use it cautiously.

Combinations: 1. add Baikal Skullcap Root(黄芩, Huangqin)——sore throat with swelling, pulmonary abscess

2. add Apricot Seed (杏仁, Xingren)——cough with lung heat, sore throat with swelling, vomiting sputum

3. add Ephedra(麻黄, Mahuang)——phlegmatic retention, cough and asthma, wheezy phlegm

4. add Cape Jasmine Fruit(栀子, Zhizi)——sore throat with swelling

5. add Giant Knotweed Rhizome (虎杖, Huzhang) and Juice of Pig Bladder(猪胆汁, Zhudanzhi)——hepatic coma

6. add Weeping Forsythia Capsule (连翘, Lianqiao) and Common Selfheal Fruit-spike (夏枯草, Xiakucao)——crewels.

7. add Ephedra (麻黄, Mahuang), Manchurian Wildginger Herb(细辛, Xixin) and Fresh Ginger (生姜, Shengjiang)——cold phlegmatic asthma, wheezy phlegm

8. add Ephedra (麻黄, Mahuang), Pepperweed Seed or Flixweed Tansymustard Seed (葶苈子, Tinglizi) and Chinese Date(大枣, Dazao)——phlegmatic cough and asthma, excessive phlegm

9. add Dutchmanspipe Fruit (马兜铃, Madouling)——cough with lung heat, excessive phlegm

Notes: Blackberrylily Rhizome(射干, Shegan)

has the function of checking upward adverse flow of qi and expelling phlegm, removing obstruction and purging fire, it is used for respiratory system infection. So Li Shizhen (李时珍) said: "Blackberrylily Rhizome(射干, Shegan) can purge fire, so it is an important drug of treating laryngalgia and pharyngalgia in ancient prescriptions." In addition, the drug has the function of ablating tumors, removing malaria, and restoring menstruation, which was recorded in ancient prescriptions. In recent years, affected parts can be washed with single hot decoction of Blackberrylily Rhizome(射干, Shegan).

12. 山豆根, Shandougen

English name: Tonkin Sophora Root

Pharmaceutical name: Radix Sophorae Subprostratae

Botanical name: Sophora subprostrata Chun et T. Chen

山豆根

Properties and tastes: bitter, cold

Meridian tropism: lung

Functions: 1. clear away heat-toxin
2. relieve sore throat
3. subdue swelling and relieve pain
4. restrain tumors
5. elevate rohite blood cell
6. resist arrhythmia

Indications: 1. sore throat with swelling from stagnant excessive heat-toxin
2. damp-heat jaundice
3. wound carbuncle with swelling poison
4. cough with lung heat
5. cancer
6. hypoleucocytosis

Dosage: 6～9g. It is reported that over eating may lead to toxicity and side effects. The main symptoms are headache, dizziness, nausea, vomiting, and acratia. Some People manifest as convulsion, abdominalgia, diarrhea, limbs tremor, severe palpitation etc.

Contraindication: This drug is bitter and cold and should not be used in cases of gastric cold, poor appetite, and loose stool.

Combinations: 1. add Great Burdock Achene (牛蒡子, Niubangzi) and Blackberrylily Rhizome (射干, Shegan)——sore throat with swelling, cough with lung heat
2. add Lalang Grass Rhizome (白茅根, Baimaogen)——toothache with swelling
3. add Heartleaf Houttuynia Herb(鱼腥草, Yuxingcao) and long-noded pit viper——lung cancer in early stage
4. add Capillary Wormwood Herb(茵陈蒿, Yinchenhao), Cape Jasmine Fruit (栀子, Zhizi) and Rhubarb (大黄, Dahuang)——damp-heat jaundice
5. add weep forsythia and Honeysuckle Flower(金银花, Jinyinhua)——wound carbuncle with swelling poison
6. add Lightyellow Sophora Root (苦参, Kushen)——hypoleucocytosis. It is also used for various arythmia

Notes: Tonkin Sophora Root (山豆根, Shandougen) has the function of clearing away heat and expelling toxic materials. It is an important drug for treating sore throat with swelling caused by excessive heat. *Illustrated Materia Medica* (《图经本草》, Bencaotujing) said "people at that time held it in the mouth that is cut in a unit of length, it is effective to relieve sore throat with swelling. It is thus clear that it is used widely." Modern research has shown that this drug not only remarkably restrains shigella dysenteriae, proteus, colibacillus, and golden staphylococcus but also has the effect of anticancer. So the drug is used to treat lung cancer, throat cancer, and bladder cancer.

Blackberrylily Rhizome (射干, Shegan) and Tonkin Sophora Root (山豆根, Shandougen) have the functions of clearing away heat and expelling toxic materials. It is the drug for treating sore throat with swelling due to noxious heat. But Blackberrylily Rhizome (射干, Shegan) also has the effect of promoting circulation of blood, expelling phlegm, and scattering blockage. It is used to treat sore throat with swelling due to accumulation or phlegm and heat. It also can relieve asthma and cough. Tonkin Sophora Root (山豆根, Shandougen) is very bitter in taste and very cold in nature. It is good at treating sore throat with swelling and toothache with swelling due to excessive heat.

13. 马勃, Mabo

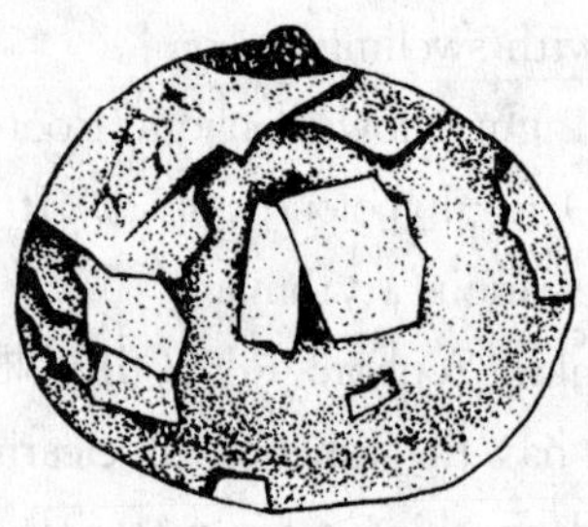

马 勃

English name: Puff-ball

Pharmaceutical name: Frucificatio Lasiosphaerae

Botanical name: Lasiosphaera fenslii Reich. or L. Nipponica (Kawam.) Y. Kobayashi

Properties and tastes: pungent, medium

Meridian tropism: lung

Functions: 1. clear away lung heat

2. relieve sore throat

3. arrest bleeding

Indications: 1. cough due to lung heat

2. sore throat

3. hematemesis, epistaxis due to heat in blood, bleeding in the mouth, bleeding after tooth extraction. (Oral taking or external use)

Dosage: 3～6g; proper dosage for external use.

Combinations: 1. add Baikal Skullcap Root (黄芩, Huangqin)——cough due to lung heat

2. add Figwort Root (玄参, Xuanshen), Indigwoad Root (板蓝根, Banlangen)——sore throat

3. add Mirabilite (芒硝, Mangxiao), Blackberrylily Rhizome (射干, Shegan), Shunk Bugbane Rhizome (升麻, Shengma)——sore throat, aphagia

4. add Rehmannia Dried Root (生地黄, Shengdihuang), Tree Peony Bark (牡丹皮, Mudanpi)——hematemesis, epistaxis due to heat in blood

Prescription: Universal Relief Decoction for Disinfection (普济消毒饮, Pujixiaodu Yin)

Notes: It is sour in taste and light in nature. It has the functions of dispersing the stagnated heat in lung meridian, especially soothing the throat, detoxifying and relieving swelling. It is the commonly used herb for treating sore throat, cough and hoarseness of voice due to wind-heat. It can be used as oral medicine or prepared into powder for blowing use.

Puff-ball (马勃, Mabo), Tonkin Sophora Root (山豆根, Shandougen), Blackberrylily Rhizome (射干, Shegan) are all the herbs for clearing heat and toxins for sore throat. The difference is that Puff-ball (马勃, Mabo) is light and dipersing and good at treating sore throat due to wind-heat; Tonkin Sophora

Root(山豆根, Shandougen) is very bitter and cold and good for sore throat and swelling and pain caused by excessive toxic-fire. Besides descending fire and detoxifying, Blackberrylily Rhizome(射干, Shegan) also can promote blood circulation, eliminate phlegm and remove stasis for sore throat by stagnation of phlegm and fire.

14. 马齿苋, Machixian

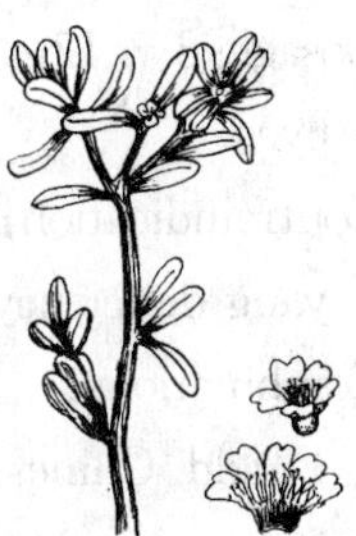

马齿苋

English name: Purslane Herb

Pharmaceutical name: Radix Sophorae Subprostratae

Botanical name: Sophora subprostrata Chun et T. Chen

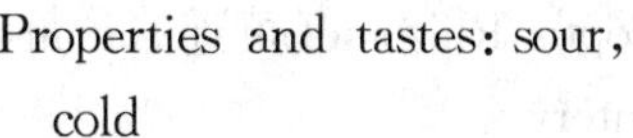

Properties and tastes: sour, cold

Meridian tropism: large intestine, liver

Functions: 1. clear away heat-toxin
2. cool blood for hemostasis
3. relieve stranguria by diuresis
4. resist bacteria

Indications: 1. diarrhea due to damp and heat
2. dysentery due to damp and heat
3. leukorrhagia with reddish discharge
4. carbuncle and boil due to evil fire and toxin
5. stranguria caused by evil heat and hematuria
6. uterine bleeding due to blood heat

Dosage: 30 ~ 60g, proper dosage for external use.

Combinations: 1. add Baikal Skullcap Root(黄芩, Huangqin), Coptis Rhizome(黄连, Huanglian)——diarrhea due to damp and heat
2. add Largeleaf Chinese Ash Bark(秦皮, Qinpi), Chinese Pulsatiall Root(白头翁, Baitouweng)——dysentery
3. add Glabrous Greenbrier Rhizome(土茯苓, Tufuling)——leukorrhagia with reddish discharge
4. add Honeysuckle Flower(金银花, Jinyinhua)——carbuncle and boil with evil fire and toxin
5. add Akebia Stem(木通, Mutong), Plantain Seed(车前子, Cheqianzi)——stranguria caused by evil heat
6. add Lalang Grass Rhizome(白茅根, Baimaogen), Motherwort Herb(益母草, Yimucao)——hematuria

Notes: It is an important herb for treating bacillary desentery. The effect of the fresh herb is the best. The application of Purslane Herb(马齿苋, Machixian) was developed in these years, including the treatment of whooping cough, pulmonary tuberculosis, pyogenic diseases. It can be used as a vegetable with safety in large quantity.

15. 白头翁, Baitouweng

白头翁

English name: Chinese Pulsatilla Root

Pharmaceutical name: Radix Pulsatillae Chinensis

Botanical name: Pulsatilla chinensis(Bge.)Reg.

Properties and tastes: bitter, cold

Meridian tropism: large intestine

Functions: 1. clear away heat-toxin
2. eliminate pathogenic heat from blood to cure dysentery

Indication: dysentery due to damp and heat, dysentery with pus and blood, and the important herb for treating amebic dysentery.

Dosage: 6~15g or 30g for maximal dosage.

Combinations:
1. add Chinese Corktree Bark(黄柏, Huang-

bai)——dysentery with pus and blood, abdominal pain, tunesmus. Such as acute bacillary dysentery, toxic dysentery

2. add Coptis Rhizome(黄连, Huanglian), Largeleaf Chinese Ash Bark(秦皮, Qinpi)——amebic dysentery

3. add Dang-shen Root(党参, Dangshen), Largehead Atractylodes Rhizome(白术, Baizhu)——vital qi is damaged by chronic dysentry

4. add Ass-hide Glue(阿胶, Ejiao), Licorice Root(甘草, Gancao) - dysentery due to blood deficiency, postpartum dysentery

Notes: Chinese Pulsatiall Root(白头翁, Baitouweng) is an important herb for dysentery. Modern research has shown that it has an inhibiting effect to bacillus dysenteriae and ameba protozoon. It is mainly used for acute and chronic dysentery, and amebic dysentery. The Chinese Pulsatiall Root(白头翁, Baitouweng) extract and powder can kill trchomonas vaginalis and have an inhibiting effect to staphylococcus, bacillus subtilis, virus influenzae and some fungus in different degree.

16. 秦皮, Qinpi

English name: Largeleaf Chinese Ash Bark

Pharmaceutical name: Cortex Fraxini

Botanical name: Franxinus rhyncholphylla Hance., F. Bungeana DC., of F. Paxiana Lingelsh

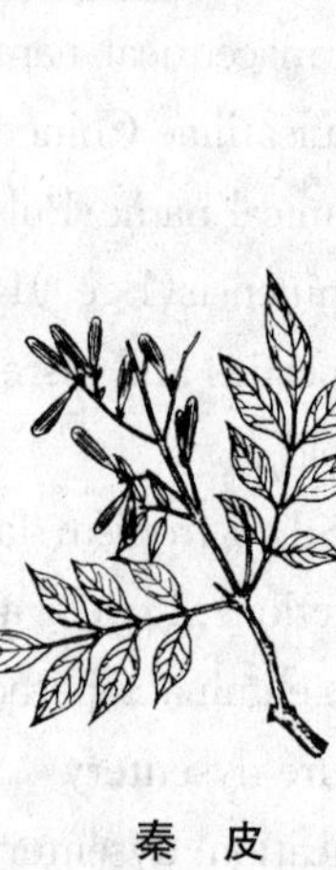

秦 皮

Properties and tastes: bitter, cold

Meridian tropism: liver, gall bladder, large intestine

Functions: 1. clear away haet-toxin

2. remove heat from the liver to improve acuity of eye sight

3. stop pain

4. inhibit smooth muscle

Indications: 1. dysentery due to evil heat and toxin, diarrhea with bloody stool, tenesmus

2. eyes disases——redness of eye, swelling and pain, cataract due to heat of liver qi stganation

3. leukorrhagia due to damp-heat evil of liver and gall bladder attacking the Lower-jiao

Dosage: 3～12g, or external use for washing eyes.

Contraindication: Do not use in the case of yang deficiency of spleen and stomach.

Combinations:

1. add Chinese Pulsatiall Root(白头翁, Baitouweng), Coptis Rhizome(黄连, Huanglian)——dysentery

2. add Coptis Rhizome(黄连, Huanglian), Bamboo Leaf(竹叶, Zhuye)——eye diseases due to stagnation of heat in the liver meridian

3. add Lightyellow Sophora Root(苦参, Kushen), Chinese Gentian Root(龙胆草, Longdancao)——leukorrhagia due to damp-heat

Notes: It is the herb for clearing heat and fire and drying dampness with astringent nature, and used for dysentery and leukorrhagia due to damp-heat. It acts on the liver meridian and has the effect of clearing heat in the liver and gall bladder, brightening eyes. So it is also the commonly used herb for redness, swelling and pain of eyes due to stagnation of heat in the liver meridian.

Largeleaf Chinese Ash Bark(秦皮, Qinpi) and Coptis Rhizome(黄连, Huanglian) can be used together due to their common effect of treating redness and swelling pain of eyes and dysentery caused by damp-heat.

But Coptis Rhizome(黄连,Huanglian) has strong effect of clearing heat with bitter tastes and cold nature, and is good at clearing heart fire to stop vomiting; Largeleaf Chinese Ash Bark(秦皮,Qinpi) is astringent in nature and used for leukorrhagia due to damp-heat.

17. 败酱草, Baijiangcao

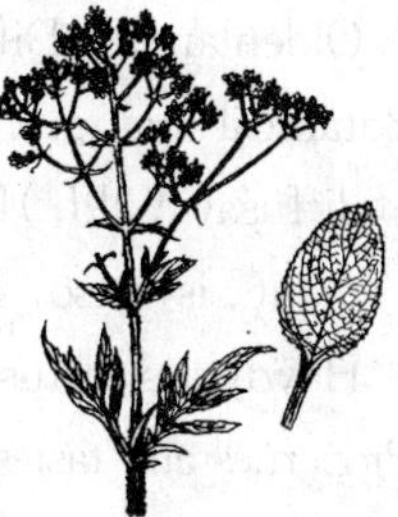
败酱草

English name: Whiteflower Patrinia Herb

Pharmaceutical name: Herba Whiteflower Patrinia Herb(败酱草, Baijiangcao)

Botanical name: Patrinia scabiosaefolia Fisch. or Patrinia villosa Juss. are the plants used in Sichuan and central China for this herb. In northern China the plants most often used are Sonchus arvensis L. Or S. Brachyotus DC. While in southern China Thiaspi arvense L. Is used.

Properties and tastes: pungent, bitter, and slightly cold

Meridian tropism: stomach, large intestine, liver

Functions: 1. clear away heat-toxin

2. discharge pus and treat boils

3. remove blood stasis for alleviating pain

Indications: 1. carbuncle of internal organ——appendicitis with pus, or appendicitis without pus, high fever, purulent and bloody sputum due to lung carbuncle

2. pain of the chest and abdomen, dysmenorrhea, postpartum abdominal pain due to qi stagnation and blood stasis

3. common cold, influenza-fever and chills, soreness and general pain of the body

4. redness, swelling and pin of the eyes due to liver heat

Dosage: 6 ~ 15g. Proper dosage for external use.

Contraindication: Over dosage may cause dizziness, vomiting and temporary decrease of blood cells.

Combinations:

1. add Red Peony Root (赤芍药, Chishaoyao)——abdominal pain due to postpartum blood stasis and heat, the early stage of appendicitis without pus but with masses

2. add Coix Seed(薏苡仁, Yiyiren)——appendicitis with pus, no fever

3. add Honeysuckle Flower(金银花, Jinyinhua)——abdominal pain and fever due to appendicitis, chest pain, postpartum abdominal pain, redness, swelling and pain of eyes

4. add Chinese Pulsatiall Root (白头翁, Baitouweng)——dysentery with pus, fever, tenesmus

5. add Tokyo Violet Herb(紫花地丁, Zihuadiding)——carbuncle and boil

6. add Heartleaf Houttuynia Herb(鱼腥草, Yuxingcao), Balloonflower Root (桔梗, Jiegeng)——purulent and bloody sputum due to lung carbuncle

7. add Chinese Angelica Root(当归, Danggui), Frankincense (乳香, Ruxiang)——heart and abdominal pain due to heat in blood and blood stasis

8. add Fineleaf Schizomepeta Herb(荆芥, Jingjie), Puncturevine Caltrap Fruit(白蒺藜, Baijili)——redness and pain of eyes, pterygium

9. add Indigwoad Root(板蓝根, Banlangen), Tonkin Sophora Root(山豆根, Shandougen)——acute pharyngitis

Notes: It is an important herb for clearing heat-toxin, excreting pus, and removing stasis. It is good at dispersing stagnation of heat in blood, and has the obvious effect for pulmonary abscess, and appendicitis. Both Whiteflower Patrinia Herb (败酱草, Baijiangcao) and Coix Seed (薏苡仁, Yiyiren) can be used to treat appendicitis and pulmonary abscess, but the former is good at clearing heat and eliminating blood stasis, while the latter is good at excreting pus and eliminating phlegm for the case with pus.

18. 红藤, Hongteng

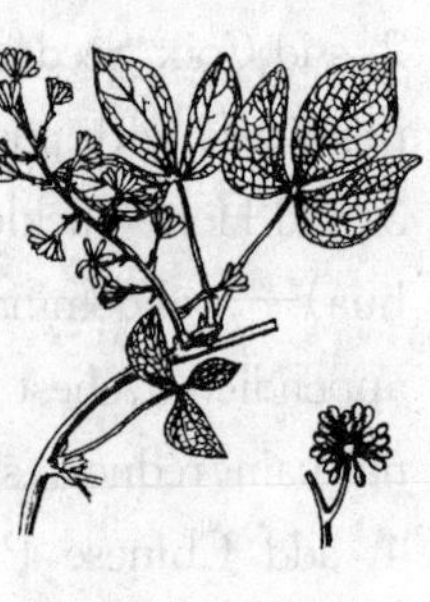

English name: Sargentoglory Vine Stem

Pharmaceutical name:

Botanical name: Sargentodoxa cuneata Rend. Et Wils (Lardizabalaceae)

Properties and tastes: bitter, medium

红 藤

Meridian tropism: large intestine

Functions: 1. clear away heat-toxin

2. remove blood stasis for alleviating pain

3. anti-bacterium

4. anti-thrombosis

Indications: 1. appendicitis——abdominal pain due to appendicitis

2. carbuncle and boil

3. pain syndromes-arthritis, pain due to injury, abdominal pain of women due to blood stasis

Dosage: 9～15g or 30g for maximal dosage.

Combinations: 1. add Whiteflower Patrinia Herb (败酱草, Baijiangcao)——appendicitis

2. add Weeping Forsythia Capsule (连翘, Lianqiao)——carbuncle and boil

3. add Red Peony Root (赤芍药, Chishaoyao)——pain syndromes

Notes: Sargentoglory Vine Stem (红藤, Hongteng) can be used to clear heat-toxin and promote blood circulation, it is good for appendicitis, as well as lower abdominal pain of women due to blood stasis, such as pelvic inflammation, adnexitis, endometriosis.

19. 白花蛇舌草, Baihuasheshecao

English name: Spreading Hedyotis Herb

Pharmaceutical name: Herba Oldenlandiae Diffusae

Botanical name: Oldenlandia diffusa (Willd.) Roxb. This plant is also known as Heydyotis diffusa.

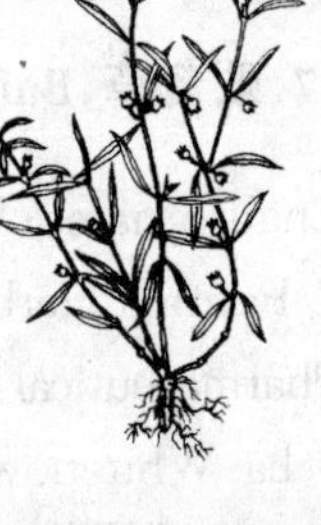

白花蛇舌草

Properties and tastes: slightly bitter, sweet, cold

Meridian tropism: stomach, large intestine, and small intestine

Functions: 1. clear away heat-toxin

2. relieve stranguria by diuresis

3. anticancer

Indications: 1. simple acute appendicitis, minor localized peritonitis

2. pelvic inflammation, inflammation of urinary system

3. mumps

4. hepatitis, inflammation of biliary tract

5. cancer——gastric cancer, esophagus cancer, rectum cancer, etc.

Dosage: 15～60g.

Contraindication: Use cautiously with pregnant women.

Combinations: 1. add Indian Chrysanthemum Flower (野菊花, Yejuhua), Tree Peony Bark (牡丹皮, Mudanpi)——simple acute appendicitis

2. add Chinese Angelica Root (当归, Danggui)——pelvic inflammation

3. add Lalang Grass Rhizome (白茅根, Baimaogen), Plantain Seed (车前子, Cheqianzi)——infant nephritis

4. add Indigwoad Root(板蓝根, Banlangen)——mumps
5. add Tonkin Sophora Root(山豆根, Shandougen)——hepatitis, inflammation of biliary tract
6. add Lalang Grass Rhizome(白茅根, Baimaogen)——gastric cancer
7. add Lightyellow Sophora Root(苦参, Kushen)——rectum cancer

Notes: It has the function of clearing heat-toxin and is used for carbuncle, boil, sore throat, and ophidism in the traditional way. Modern research has shown that the herb has the effect of anti-tumor, and mainly used for gastric cancer, esophagus cancer, rectum cancer and so on.

20. 白鲜皮, Baixianpi

English name: Densefruit Pittany Root-bark

Pharmaceutical name: Cortex Dictamni Dasycarpi Radicis

Botanical name: Dictamnus dasycarpus Turcz.

白鲜皮

Properties and tastes: bitter, cold

Meridian tropism: spleen, stomach

Functions: 1. eliminate fire and detoxicate
2. clear away heat and eliminate dampness
3. dispel wind to relieve itching
4. antifungus

Indications: 1. boil and eruptions due to damp-heat——damp skin ulcer with purulent, eczema, wind rash, itch of skin
2. jaundice due to damp-heat
3. arthritis due to damp-heat
4. neurodermatitis, vulvitis, vaginitis

Dosage: 6～9g.

Contraindication: It is not used for deficiency cold syndromes.

Combinations:
1. add Lightyellow Sophora Root(苦参, Kushen), Swordlike Atractylodes Rhizome(苍术, Cangzhu)——boil and eruptions due to damp-heat
2. add Capillary Wormwood Herb(茵陈蒿, Yinchenhao), Cape Jasmine Fruit(栀子, Zhizi)——jaundice due to damp-heat
3. add Fourstamen Stephania Root(防己, Fangji), Coix Seed(薏苡仁, Yiyiren)——arthritis due to damp-heat

Notes: It is good at eliminating wind-dampness in the skin and expelling damp-heat in the Lower-jiao, and also soothing the blood vessels and joints. It is effective for wind-bi syndrome and damp-bi syndrome. So Dr. Li Shizhen(李时珍) described Densefruit Pittany Root-bark(白鲜皮, Baixianpi) an important herb for all kinds of jaundice and wind-bi syndrome. It is not limited to external diseases.

Lightyellow Sophora Root(苦参, Kushen) and Densefruit Pittany Root-bark(白鲜皮, Baixianpi) have the functions of clearing damp-heat in the Lower-jiao and skin, inducing diuresis. They are used for eczema, damp carbuncle, jaundice, and leukorrhagia. Lightyellow Sophora Root(苦参, Kushen) has the functions of expelling wind and pesticide for treating itching of skin, leukorrhagia, and itch in the vulvae; Densefruit Pittany Root-bark(白鲜皮, Baixianpi) acts on the muscle and promotes blood circulation and smooths the joints. It is suitable for wind-bi syndrome and damp-bi syndrome accompanied with fever.

21. 半枝莲, Banzhilian

English name: Barbed Skullcap Herb

Pharmaceutical name: Herba Scutellariae Barbatae

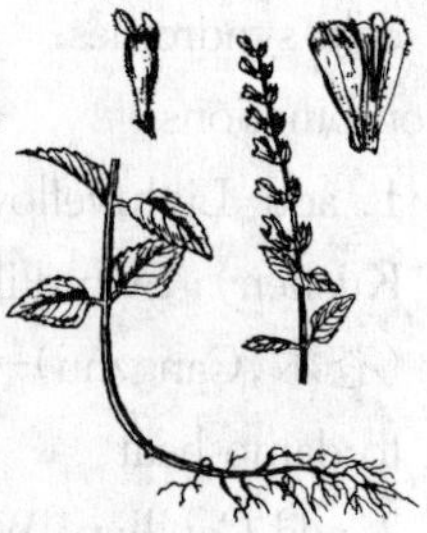

Botanical name: Scutellaria barbata D. Don

Properties and tastes: slightly bitter, cool

半枝莲

Meridian tropism: liver, lung, and stomach

Functions: 1. clear away heat-toxin

2. induce diuresis to remove edema

3. disspate blood stasis and alleviate pain

4. arrest bleeding

5. anticancer

Indications: 1. carbuncle and boil due to evil heat and toxic, poisonous snake bite

2. pain and swelling with blood stasis due to wound

3. lung carbuncle

4. cancer——such as the early stage of lung cancer, liver cancer, rectum cancer, nasopharyngeal carcinoma

5. lymphatic gland inflammation, scrofula

6. hepatitis hepatomegaly, ascites of cirrhosis

7. pharyngitid and tonsillitis

8. hematemesis, epistaxis, hematuria and dysentery with blood

Dosage: 9~30g.

Contraindication: Use it cautiously in the case of gravida. Do not use in the case of blood deficiency.

Combinations: 1. add Honeysuckle Flower (金银花, Jinyinhua), Dandelion (蒲公英, Pugongying)——carbuncle and boil due to evil heat and toxin

2. add Tokyo Violet Herb (紫花地丁, Zihuadiding)——poisonous snake bite

3. add Heartleaf Houttuynia Herb (鱼腥草, Yuxingcao)——lung carbunle

4. add Snakegourd Root (天花粉, Tianhuafen), Blackberrylily Rhizome (射干, Shegan)——lung cancer

5. add Spreading Hedyotis Herb (白花蛇舌草, Baihuasheshecao), Dandelion (蒲公英, Pugongying)——gastrointestinal cancer

6. add Zedoray (莪术, Ezhu), Oyster Shell (牡蛎, Muli)——ascites of cirrhosis

Notes: It was used for ophidism, carbuncles and boils originally. In recent years it has been used mainly for ascites of cirrhosis and cancers.

22. 鸦胆子, Yadanzi

English name: Java Brucea Fruit

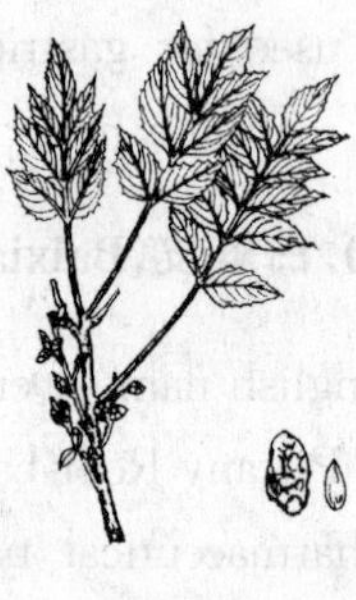

Pharmaceutical name: Fructus Brucae Javanicae

Botanical name: Brucea javanica (L.) Merr.

Properties and tastes: bitter, cold, and poisonous

鸦胆子

Meridian tropism: Large intestine, liver

Functions: 1. clear away heat-toxin

2. prevent the attack of malaria

3. anticancer

4. decay vegetation

Indications: 1. malaria——tertian fever or quartan (it can be used in capsule form)

2. dysentery——amebic dysentery, bacillary dysentery

3. cancer——rectum cancer, mammary gland cancer

4. external use to corrosive vegetation-verruca vulgaris, corn, also used for flat wart

Dosage: 10~30 (about 1.5~3g), it is usually used alone and not suitable for decoction.

Contraindication: It is bitter in taste and easy to stimulate the stomach and intestine, and may harm the liver and kidney. So stop administration as soon as the disease is recovered. Do not use in the case of dysfunction of the liver and kidney.

Notes: Java Brucea Fruit(鸦胆子, Yadanzi) is bitter in taste and toxic in property, and is not used unless it is necessary. But Dr. Zhang Xichun(张锡纯) was experienced in use of Java Brucea Fruit(鸦胆子, Yadanzi) and called it "an important herb for cooling blood and detoxifying and good for dysentery with bloody stools, hematuria and bloody stools due to heat in xue-fen and intestine".

In addition, attention should be paid to the use of Java Brucea Fruit (鸦胆子, Yadanzi).

Appendix: Other Herbs For Clearing Heat And Removing Toxins

Name	Properties and tastes	Meridian tropism	Functions	Indications	Dosage	Contra-indications
Natural Indigo (青黛, Qingdai)	salty, cold	Liver, lung, stomach	Clear away heat and toxic materials, remove sheat from the blood and relieve homatoma, functions as anti-cancer and antibacteriai	Infantile convulsion due to liver heat, cough due to lung heat, eczema and aphtha, eruption due to heat and toxic, hematemesis, epistaxis due to blood heat, carbuncle, parotitis, chronic granulocytic anemia	1.5～3g in pills, or proper amount for external use.	Carefully with stomach cold. May induce a gastrointestinal reaction, dysfunction of the liver and descending of blood platelets
Common Andrographis Herb(穿心莲, Chuanxinlian)	bitter, cold	Lung, stomach, large intestine, small intestine	Promote circulation and relieve toxins, dispel dampness stop dysentery, anti-inflammation and relieve fever	Early stage of febrile diseases, common cold of wind heat type, influenza, rhinitis, nasal sinusitis, cough due to lung heat, carbuncle and boil, poisonous snake bite, dysentery of damp and heat, heat-type stranguria, eczema, pelvic inflammation, chronic epitheliioma	6～12g	May injure the stomach due to its bitter and cold nature, not for large dosage and long term use
Manyleaf Paris Rhizome (蚤休, Zaoxiu)	bitter, slightly cold, slightly toxic	Liver	Promote circulation and relieve toxicity, detumescentify and stop pain, calm wind-syndrome and convulsion, antibacterium, contract womb	Carbuncle and boil, swelling and pain due to wound, poisonous snake bite, convulsion due to liver heat, metrorrhagia	6～9g	Carefully with deficient syndrome and pregnant women

Name	Properties and tastes	Meridian tropism	Functions	Indications	Dosage	Contra-indications
Chinese Lobelia Herb(半边莲, Banbianlian)	acrid, cold	Heart, small intestine, lung	Clear heat and toxin, induce diuresis to relieve edema, activate respiration, soothe gall bladder, lower blood pressure, stop bleeding, anti-snake poison	Poison snake bite, edema, tympanites, late stage of schistosomial cirrhosis	9～18g.	Use carefully for deficient syndrome
Stringy Stonecrop Herb(垂盆草, Chuipencao)	sweet, tasteless, slightly sour, cool	Liver, gall bladder, small intestine	Clear heat, and toxin, eliminate dampness to relieve jaundice, descend transaminase, protect the liver, inhibit bacterium and immunity of cells	Damp-heat type jaundice, poisonous snake bite, scald, sore throat, carbuncle	9～30g	
Japanese Ampelopsis Root(白蔹, Bailian)	bitter, acid, slightly cold	Heart, stomach, liver	Clear heat, heal carbuncle, promote regeneration of tissues	Carbuncle, swelling, scald, acute and chronic bacillary dysentery	9～6g	Incompatible with Sichuan Aconite Root（乌头, Wutou）
Uniflower Swisscentaury Root(漏芦, Loulu)	bitter, cold	stomach	Clear heat and toxin, eliminate mastitis, promote milk, reduce blood fat, antiarteriosclerosis, anti-aging	Carbuncle, swelling and pain, mastitis, insufficient lactation	6～12g	
Appendiculate Cremastra Pseudobulb（山慈姑, Shancigu）	acid, cold, slightly toxic	Liver and stomach	Clear heat and toxins, eliminate carbuncle and disperse stagnation	Furuncle, carbuncle, sore, swelling, scrofula	3～6g	
Rhizome of Wild Buckwheat（野荞麦, Yeqiaomai）	bitter and medium	Lung, spleen, stomach	Clear heat and toxin, eliminate phlegm and soothe throat, strengthen the stomach and promote digestion	Cough and sore throat and pulmonary abscess due to lung heat, scrofula, boil, dysentery, poison snake bite, malnutrition, emaciation,	15～30g	
Green Gram Seed(绿豆, Lüdou)	sweet, cold	Heart, stomach	Clear heat and toxin, relieve summer-heat and thirst	Detoxifying poison of Croton Seed（巴豆, Badou）and Prepared Daughter Root of Common Monkshood（附子, Fuzi）, carbuncle, boil, thirst due to summer-heat	15～30g, proper for external use	

Name	Properties and tastes	Meridian tropism	Functions	Indications	Dosage	Contra-indications
Nudicaulous Grounsel Herb (紫背天葵, Zibeitiankui)	sweet, bitter, cold	Liver, spleen, bladder	Clear heat and toxin, relieve swelling and stagnation	Carbuncle, boil, poison snake bite, scrofula, cancer	3～9g	
Franchet Groundcherry Calyx or Fruit (锦灯笼, Jindenglong)	sour, medium	Heart, lung bladder	Clear heat and toxin, soothe throat and eliminate phlegm	Sore throat, cough due to lung heat	6～12g	
Olive (橄榄, Ganlan)	sweet, sour, medium	Lung,	Clear heat and toxin, soothe throat and eliminate phlegm	Sore throat, cough due to lung heat, dispel the effect of alcohol	6～15g	

Section 4
Heat-clearing Drugs in Blood Stage

1. 水牛角, Shuiniujiao

English name: Buffalo Horn

Pharmaceutical name: Cornu Bubali

Botanical name: Bubalus bubalis Linnaeus

Properties and tastes: bitter, salty, and cold

Meridian tropism: heart, liver

水牛角

Functions: 1. cool blood for hemostasis

2. remove toxic substance and dissipate rashes

3. tranquilize and arrest convulsion

4. cardiac tonic

5. anticonvulsant

6. anti-inflamation and anti-infection

7. gonadotropic function

Indications: 1. hemorrhage——hematemesis, epistaxis due to attack of blood heat

2. febrile diseases——high fever, loss of consciousness, delirium, eruption and dark eruption due to excess of toxin heat

3. thrombocytopenic purpura

4. encephalitis B

5. schizophrenia

Dosage: 6～15 g, ground into pieces and decoct first. Prepared into powder for oral taking with water, 1～3g per time.

Contraindication: Use it cautiously in the case of gravida.

Combinations: 1. add Rehmannia Dried Root (生地黄, Shengdihuang), Tree Peony Bark (牡丹皮, Mudanpi), Red Peony Root (赤芍药, Chishaoyao)——hematemesis due to attack of blood heat

2. add Honeysuckle Flower (金银花, Jinyinhua), Figwort Root (玄参, Xuanshen), Coptis Rhizome (黄连, Huanglian)——The Ying-blood system being attacked by evil heat of febrile diseases, high fever, restlessness, thirst, insomnia, loss of consciousness, delirium, skin eruptions, convulsion, tremor

3. add Antelope Horn (羚羊角, Lingyangjiao),

Cow-bezoar (牛 黄, Niuhuang)——high fever, restlessness, convulsion, of infantile convulsion

4. add Indigowood Leaf (大青叶, Daqingye), Figwort Root (玄参, Xuanshen), Gypsum (石膏, Shigao)——fever due to febrile diseases, skin eruptions

Prescription: Decoction of Rhinoceros Horn and Rehmannia (犀角地黄汤, Xijiao Dihuang Tang)

Notes: Buffalo Horn (水牛角, Shuiniujiao) is bitter and salty in taste and cold in nature, its function is similar to that of Asiatic Rhinoceros Horn (犀角, Xijiao). It has the functions of clearing heat, cooling blood, and removing toxins. As Asiatic Rhinoceros Horn (犀角, Xijiao) is forbidden to be used, Buffalo Horn (水牛角, Shuiniujiao) is used instead of Asiatic Rhinoceros Horn (犀角, Xijiao). The dosage of Buffalo Horn (水牛角, Shuiniujiao) should be increased because of its weak function, the common dosage of Buffalo Horn (水牛角, Shuiniujiao) is 8～10 times of Asiatic Rhinoceros Horn (犀角, Xijiao). Recently, it is often used for headache in febrile diseases, high fever, coma, eruption, epistaxis, hematemesis, infantile convulsion, sore throat, fiu, encephalitis B.

2. 生地黄, Shengdihuang

English name: Rehmannia Dried Root

Pharmaceutical name: Radix Rehmanniae Glutinosae

Botanical name: Rehmannia glutinosa (Gaertn.) Libosch. Or R. Glutinosa Libosch. F

生地黄

Properties and tastes: sweet, bitter, and cold

Meridian tropism: heart, liver, kidney

Functions: 1. clear away heat and nourish yin

2. cool blood for hemostasis

3. promote the production of body fluid and quench thirst

4. cardiac tonic, promote urination

5. reduce blood suger

Indications: 1. the Ying-blood system being attacked by evil heat of febrile diseases——fever, dry mouth, red tongue or loss of consciousness, skin eruptions

2. attack of blood by heat——hematemesis, epistaxis, hematuria, uterine bleeding

3. lack of body fluid——steaming bone consumptive fever, fever in chronic consumptive diseases, constipation, dry cough, feverish sensation in the five centers

4. diabetes

5. urticaria, eczema, neurodermatitis due to blood heat or blood deficiency

Dosage: 9～30g. Double dosage is used if the herb is fresh.

Contraindication: Use it cautiously in the case of gravida due to deficiency cold, or qi and blood deficiency, loose bowels due to stomach and intestine deficiency.

Combinations: 1. add Red Peony Root (赤芍药, Chishaoyao)——hematuria due to attack of blood heat

2. add Common Cephalanoplos Herb (小蓟, Xiaoji)——excess of heat evil in the Ying-blood system, skin eruptions, vomit blood, dry lips, crimson tongue

3. add Lalang Grass Rhizome (白茅根, Baimaogen)——the Ying-blood system being attacked by evil heat, fever, crimson tongue, skin eruptions, haematemesis and epistaxis

4. add Rhubarb (大黄, Dahuang)——flaring up of excess fire in the heart and stomach, vomiting blood, epistaxis

5. add Akebia Stem(木通, Mutong)——aphtha, oliguria with reddish urine and hematuria
6. add Figwort Root(元参, Xuanshen), Dwarf Lilyturf Root(麦门冬, Maimendong)——impairment of yin by heat evil, constipation due to lack of body fluid
7. add Membranous Milkvetch Root(黄芪, Huangqi), Snakegourd Root(天花粉, Tianhuafen), Lobed Kudzuvine Root(葛根, Gegen)——diabetes
8. add Japanese Pagodatree Fruit(槐角, Huaijiao) Garden Burnet Root(地榆, Diyu)——hemorrhoid
9. add Turtle Carapace(鳖甲, Biejia), Chinese Wolfberry Root-bark(地骨皮, Digupi)——fever in chronic consumptive diseases due to yin deficiency
10. add Licorice Root(甘草, Gancao), Tonkin Sophora Root(山豆根, Shandougen)——chronic pharyngitis
11. add Densefruit Pittany Root-bark(白鲜皮, Baixianpi), Divaricate Saposhnikovia Root(防风, Fangfeng)——urticaria, eczema, psoriasis
12. add Lily Bulb(百合, Baihe)——trance, bulbus lilii syndrome
13. add Manchurian Wildginger Herb(细辛, Xixin)——headache, toothache due to flaring up of deficiency fire

Prescriptions: 1. Decoction for Clearing Away Heat Evil in Yingfen(清营汤, Qingying Tang)
2. Increasing Fluid Decoction(增液汤, Zengye Tang)

Notes: Rehmannia Dried Root(生地黄, Shengdihuang) is sweet in taste and cold in nature. It can be used to clear heat and cool blood, also nourish yin. So it is a commonly used herb for heat invading the Ying-xue system and yin damage in late stage in seasonal febrile disease. Due to its function of nourishing yin and inducing production of body fluid, it is commonly used for diabetes, as well as tidal fever due to yin deficiency in chronic diseases. It is said in *Shennong's Herbal Classic* (《神农本草经》, Shennongbencaojing): Rehmannia Dried Root(生地黄, Shengdihuang) has the function of relieving Bi syndrome due to blood stasis, so it is used to treat rheumatic and rheumatoid arthritis.

Rehmannia Dried Root(地黄, Shengdihuang) was not divided into Rehmannia Dried Root(生地黄, Shengdihuang) and Prepared Rhizome of Adhesive Rehmannia (熟地黄, Shoudihuang) before the Song Dynasty. Rehmannia Dried Root(生地黄, Shengdihuang) has the functions of clearing heat and nourishing yin and primarily used to treat hematemesis, epistaxis, and diabetes due to yin damage in febrile diseases. After a long period of steaming and sun-curing, prepared Rhizome of Adhesive Rehmannia(熟地黄, Shoudihuang) is sweet in taste and warm in nature. It is mainly used for nourishing yin and blood, tonifying the kidney and liver.

3. 玄参, Xuanshen

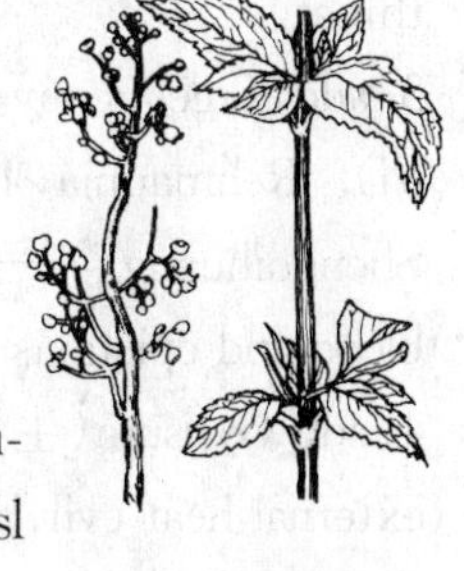
玄参

English name: Figwort Root
Pharmaceutical name: Radix Scrophulariae Ningpoensis
Botanical name: Scrophularia ningpoensis Hemsl
Properties and tastes: bitter, sweet, salty, and cold
Meridian tropism: lung, stomach, and kidney

Functions: 1. clear away heat-toxin
2. cool blood and remove ecchymoses
3. nourish yin to lower pathogenic fire
4. remove obstruction and treat boils
5. reduce blood suger

Indications: 1. ying stage being attacked by evil heat of febrile diseases——fever, dry mouth, deep red tongue, loss of consciousness, delirium, skin eruptions
2. cough due to dryness of the lung——dry cough due to yin deficiency, night sweating, tidal fever
3. sore throat——it is suitable to the early stage of wind-heat and seasonal febrile diseases. Such as diphtheria
4. carbuncle——commonly used for thromboangitis, acute mastitis
5. scrofula——tuaberculouslymphadenitis, goiter

Dosage: 9～15g

Contraindication: It is cold in nature and tends to stagnate so that it is not suitable for yang deficiency of spleen and stomach, fullness of chest, or poor appetite.

Combinations: 1. add Wild Mint(薄荷, Bohe), Great Burdock Achene(牛蒡子, Niubangzi)——external wind and heat
2. add Shunk Bugbane Rhizome(升麻, Shengma), Licorice Root(甘草, Gancao)——eruptions due to heat evil, sore throat
3. add Tree Peony Bark(牡丹皮, Mudanpi), Rehmannia Dried Root(生地黄, Shengdihuang)——erysipelas, vomiting blood and epistaxis due to febrile disease
4. add Gypsum(生石膏, Shengshigao)——external heat evil, high fever, thirst
5. add Indigwoad Root(板蓝根, Banlangen)——sore throat, dry mouth, red tongue, thin rapid pulse due to yin deficiency and five excess
6. add Great Burdock Achene(牛蒡子, Niubangzi), Balloonflower Root(桔梗, Jiegeng)——sore throat, acute tonsillitis and pharyngolaryngitis
7. add Rehmannia Dried Root(生地黄, Shengdihuang), Dwarf Lilyturf Root(麦门冬, Maimendong)——constipation in the late stage of the febrile diseases
8. add Honeysuckle Flower(金银花, Jinyinhua), Chinese Angelica Root(当归, Danggui)——thromboangiitis obliterans
9. add Tendrilleaf Fritillary Bulb(贝母, Beimu), Lily Bulb(百合, Baihe)——yin deficiency and dryness of the lung, cough with little sputum, hemoptysis, tidal fever
10. add Honeysuckle Flower(金银花, Jinyinhua), Dandelion(蒲公英, Pugongying)——carbuncle, acute mastitis
11. add Oyster Shell(牡蛎, Muli), Tendrilleaf Fritillary Bulb(贝母, Beimu)——tuberculous lymphadenitis, goiter, scrofula
12. add Gypsum(生石膏, Shengshigao), Dang-Shen Root(党参, Dangshen)——yin exhausted by exopathgenic heat, dry tongue, sweet taste in the mouth, auorexia

Prescriptions: 1. Decoction for Clearing Away Heat Evil in Yingfen(清营汤, Qingying Tang)
2. Decoction for Nourishing Yin and Clearing Lung-heat(养阴清肺汤, Yangyinqingfei Tang)

Notes: Figwort Root(玄参, Xuanshen) is bitter, sweet and salty in taste and cold in nature. It can be used to clear heat and detoxify, and nourish yin to descend deficient fire. It also has the functions of nourishing yin and inducing production of body fluid. So it is widely used in different stages of febrile disease. It is often used with Rehmannia

Dried Root(生地黄,Shengdihuang) for seasonal febrile diseases. Rehmannia Dried Root (生地黄,Shengdihuang) is good at cooling blood to stop bleeding for hematemesis and epistaxis, hematuria, metrorrhagia due to heat in blood. Figwort Root(玄参,Xuanshen) is good at detoxifying and removing stagnation for sore throat, carbuncle, and scrofular due to heat stagnation, as well as eruption caused by warm-toxins.

There are descriptions in ancient books: Figwort Root(玄参,Xuanshen) can relieve sore throat and clear fire without root. It has the function of tonifying in reducing and nourishing in clearing, so that it can be used for both deficiency and excess.

4. 牡丹皮, Mudanpi

English name: Tree Peony Bark

Pharmaceutical name: Cortex Moutan Radicis

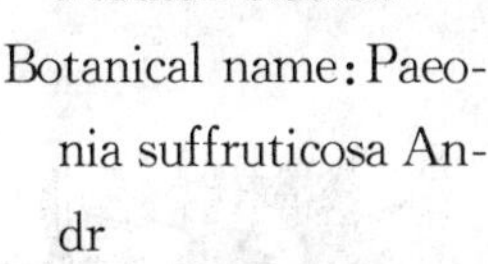

Botanical name: Paeonia suffruticosa Andr

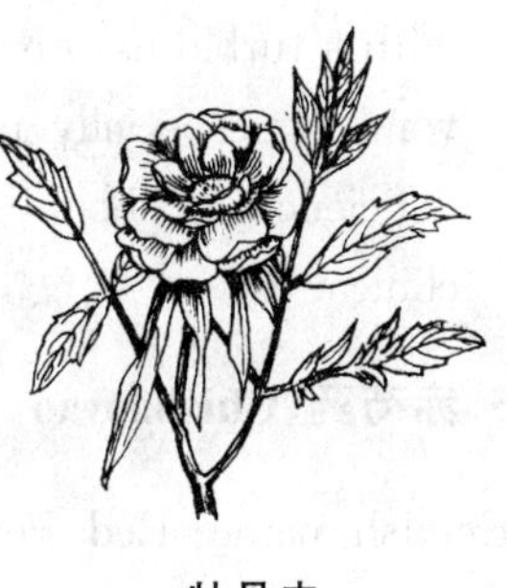

牡丹皮

Properties and tastes: bitter, pungent, and slightly cold

Meridian tropism: heart, lung, kidney

Functions: 1. clear away heat and cool blood

2. activate blood circulation to dissipate blood stasis

3. treat boils and detoxicate

4. lower blood pressure

5. broad antibiosis

Indications: 1. the blood system being attacked by evil heat of febrile diseases——Fever, hematemesis, epistaxis, eruptions, loss consciousness

2. Yin-fen(阴分) being attacked by evil heat of the end stage of febrile diseases, fever in the night, or no sweating and hectic fever due to yin deficiency

3. amenorrhea due to blood stagnation, dysmenorrhea, mass in the abdomen of women due to blood stasis

4. preceded menstrual cycle, fever before menstruation, or blood heat

5. carbuncle and sores, intestine carbuncle appendicitis

6. swelling and pain by blood stasis due to sprain and damage

7. hypertension——vertigo, delirium due to fire of liver qi stagnation and hyperactivity of liver yang

Dosage: 6～12g. It can be decocted or prepared into pills and powder. The raw one is suitable to clear heat and cool blood; the one baked with wine promotes blood circulation and removes stasis; the charred one stops bleeding.

Contraindication: It is not suitable for the case of blood deficiency with cold, pregnant women, menorrhagia.

Combinations: 1. add Dan-shen Root(丹参, Danshen)——the syndrome of heat in blood stage, or eruption due to heat-toxin, irregular menstruation, due to blood stasis, postpartum, fever due to yin deficiency, Bi syndrome due to heat

2. add Red Peony Root(赤芍药, Chishaoyao)——bleeding syndrome due to heat

3. add Cape Jasmine Fruit(栀子,Zhizi)——red face, dry mouth, restlessness due to liver fire

4. add Rehmannia Dried Root(生地黄, Shengdihuang) and Buffalo Horn(水牛角, Shuiniujiao)——eruption, hematemesis, epistaxis due to heat in the blood

5. add Rhubarb(大黄, Dahuang)——appendicitis

6. add Chinese Wolfberry Root-bark(地骨皮, Digupi)——hectic fever and flushed cheeks due to yin deficiency and blood heat

7. add Cassia Twig(桂枝,Guizhi)and Peach Seed(桃仁, Taoren)——amenorrhea, dysmenorrhea, hysteromyoma due to blood stasis

8. add Red Peony Root (赤芍药, Chishaoyao), Weeping Forsythia Capsule (连翘,Lianqiao) and Cicada Slough(蝉蜕, Chantui)——acute urticaria

Prescriptions: 1. Rhubarb and Peony Decoction (大黄牡丹皮汤,Dahuangmudanpi Tang)

2. Xiaoyao Powder adding Cortex Moutan Radicis and Fructus Gardeniae(丹栀逍遥散,Danzhixiaoyao San)

Notes: Tree Peony Bark(牡丹皮, Mudanpi) has the function of both cooling blood and promoting blood circulation with sour taste and fragrant flavor. It is suitable for blood stasis and bleeding due to heat leading to blood stasis in the course of epidemic diseases and can be used together with Red Peony Root(赤芍药, Chishaoyao). It is also commonly used to treat irregular menstruation, metorrhagia, and pelvic inflammation due to blood stasis caused by heat, as well as stranguria, dysentery, abdominal pain. Tree Peony Bark(牡丹皮, Mudanpi) also can clear defiient fire and heat in the liver, disperse stagnated heat, anti-inflammation and stop pain, so it can be used in all the stages of febrile disease. It is not applicable when heat is superficial.

Both Tree Peony Bark(牡丹皮, Mudanpi) and Rehmannia Dried Root(生地黄, Shengdihuang) can be used for deficient fever, Rehmannia Dried Root(生地黄, Shengdihuang) is mainly for nourishing yin with sweet tastes and cold nature and it can clear heat by nourishing yin; Tree Peony Bark(牡丹皮, Mudanpi) is for clearing and dispersing heat with sour tastes and it can clear heat to recover yin.

Tree Peony Bark(牡丹皮, Mudanpi) and Cassia Twig(桂枝, Guizhi) are all attributed to the heart meridian and used for removing stasis in blood vessels. Guzhi is warm in nature and good at warming the meridian to remove cold stagnation; Tree Peony Bark (牡丹皮, Mudanpi) is cold in nature and good at removing heat stagnation in meridians.

In *Chong Qing Tang Jottings* (《重庆堂随笔》, Chongqingtangsuibi), it is said: Tree Peony Bark(牡丹皮, Mudanpi) is fragrant with a turbid nature and it is used to induce vomiting especially in the case of stomach deficiency. It should be given attention for clinical use.

5. 赤芍药, Chishaoyao

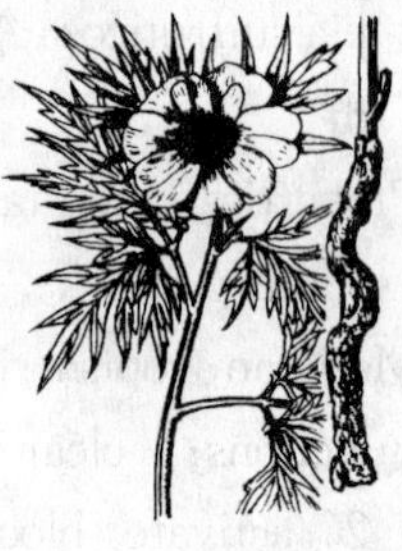

赤芍药

English name: Red Peony Root

Pharmaceutical name: Radix Paeoniae Rubra

Botabical name: Paeonia lactiflora Pall. Or Paeonia veitchii Lynch

Properties and tastes: bitter, slightly cold

Meridian tropism: liver

Functions: 1. clear away heat and cool blood

2. remove blood stasis to alleviate pain

3. relieve swelling and treat boils

4. relieve muscular spasm

5. sedation, anticonvulsation

6. antibiosis

7. dilate coronary artery and increase the ability to myocardial tolerance oxygen defect

Indications: 1. blood stage syndrome in seasonal febrile diseases——fever, eruption, hematemesis, epistaxis due to heat in blood

2. menstrual diseases——amenorrhea, dysmenorrhea due to blood stasis

3. external injury and wound with blood stasis, swelling and pain in local region

4. carbuncle, redness, swelling and pain of eyes

5. heat type stranguria and stranguria complicated with hematuria——frequent, rapid and painful urination, hematuria

6. dysentery——dysentery with purulent and bloody stools, abdominal pain, tenesmus

7. coronary heart disease, pulmonary heart disease

8. acute cerebral thrombosis

Dosage: 6～15g.

Contraindication: It is forbidden in cases of amenorrhea due to yang deficiency. It is incompatible with Black False Bellebore (藜芦, Lilu).

Combinations:

1. add Licorice Root (甘草, Gancao)——abdominal pain and contraction and weakness of the lower limbs due to incooperation of the liver and spleen, or headache due to blood deficiency

2. add Peach Seed (桃仁, Taoren) and Szechwan Lovage Rhizome (川芎, Chuanxion g)——abdominal masses, amenorrhea, abdominal pain due to blood stasis, pain caused by external injury, carbuncle and cellulitis

3. add Nutgrass Galingale Rhizome (香附, Xiangfu)——abdominal pain, hypochondriac pain, dysmenorrhea due to stagnation of qi and blood stasis

4. add Rehmannia Dried Root (生地黄, Shengdihuang) and Tree Peony Bark (牡丹皮, Mudanpi)——syndrome of heat in Ying-xue system in seasonal febrile diseases

5. add Wild Mint (薄荷, Bohe) and Chrysanthemum Flower (菊花, Juhua)——acute conjunctivitis, redness, swelling and pain of eyes

6. add Dandelion (蒲公英, Pugongying) and Whiteflower Patrinia Herb (败酱草, Baijiangcao)——chronic prostatitis

7. add Chinese Angelica Root (当归, Danggui) and Weeping Forsythia Capsule (连翘, Lianqiao)——swelling and pain of carbuncle and sore

8. add Szechwan Lovage Rhizome (川芎, Chuanxiong) and Safflower (红花, Honghua)——coronary heart disease and angina pectoris

9. add Dan-shen Root (丹参, Danshen) and Peach Seed (桃仁, Taoren)——blood stasis and pain in local region due to external injury

10. add Chinese Corktree Bark (黄柏, Huangbai)——dysentery

11. add Plantain Seed (车前子, Cheqianzi)——stranguria

12. add Szechwan Lovage Rhizome (川芎, Chuanxiong), Dahurian Angelica Root (白芷, Baizhi) and Rhizome or Root of Forbes Notopterygium (羌活, Qianghuo)——headache due to blood stasis in sequela of cerebral concussion.

Prescriptions: 1. Decoction of Rhinoceros Horn and Rehmannia (犀角地黄汤, Xijiao Dihuang Tang)

2. Decoction for Removing Blood Stasis in Chest (血府逐瘀汤, Xuefuzhuyu Tang)

Notes: Both Red Peony Root (赤芍药, Chishaoyao) and Tree Peony Bark (牡丹皮,

Mudanpi) have the functions of cooling and promoting circulation of blood. Tree Peony Bark(牡丹皮, Mudanpi) is good at cooling blood and relieving deficient fire and is used for the syndrome of both heat in blood stage and internal heat caused by yin deficiency; Red Peony Root (赤芍药, Chishaoyao) is good at promoting blood circulation to remove stasis and relieving pain. It is used not only for pain syndrome due to blood stasis but also stranguria, dysentery and abdominal pain.

It is indicated in *Seeking Truth of Herbals* (《本草求真》, Bencaoqiuzhen): the function of Red Peony Root (赤芍药, Chishaoyao) is similar to that of baishao, but bai (white color) has the role of astringing yin and nourishing Ying and chi (red color) has the role of dispersing pathogenic factors to promote blood circulation. So that White Peony Root (白芍药, Baishaoyao) can regulate liver qi as well as nourish spleen and stomach; Red Peony Root (赤芍药, Chishaoyao) can cool blood and activite blood stasis, treating abdominal hard masses, pain, amenorrhea and redness of eyes.

6. 紫草, Zicao

English name: Root of Sinkiang Arnebia

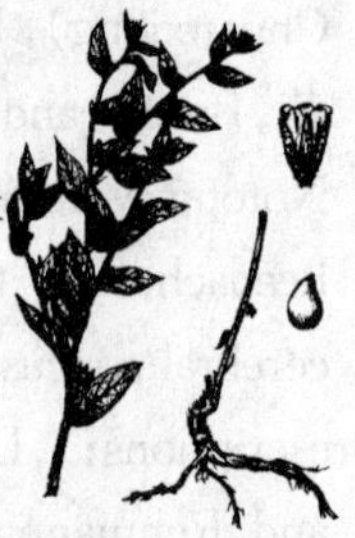

Pharmaceutical name: Radix Lithospermi seu Arnebiae

Botanical name: Lithospermum erythrorhizon Sieb. Et Zucc. Or Arnebia euchroma (Royle) Johnst. In some parts of China Onosma paniculatum Bru. Et Franch. Is used instead.

紫 草

Properties and tastes: sweet, cold

Meridian tropism: heart, liver

Functions: 1. clear away heat and cool blood
2. activate blood circulation and relieve swelling
3. decoxicate and promote eruption
4. anti-bacterium
5. anti-tumor
6. contraception

Indications: 1. eruption in warm-heat syndrome——unsmooth dispersing of eruption or that with dull color due to heat-toxin
2. hives——unsmooth dispersing of hives with dull color and sore throat
3. carbuncle and sore, eczema, itching in vulva
4. scald

Dosage: 3 ~ 9g. Soaked in oil or prepared in paste for external use.

Contraindication: Do not use it in the case of diarrhea due to spleen deficiency.

Combinations:

1. add Licorice Root (甘草, Gancao)——prevention of measles
2. add Indigowoad Leaf (大青叶, Daqingye)——dense eruptions with dark color due to excessive heat-toxin in seasonal febrile disease
3. add Chinese Corktree Bark (黄柏, Huangbai)——external use for carbuncle, furuncle, sore, eczema, scald
4. add Red Peony Root (赤芍药, Chishaoyao) and Cicada Slough (蝉蜕, Chantui)——unsmooth dispersing of eruptions with dull color
5. add Cuttle Bone (海螵蛸, Haipiaoxiao) and India Madder Root (茜草, Qiancao)——thrombocytopenic purpura
6. add Dahurian Angelica Root (白芷, Baizhi) and Chinese Angelica Root (当归, Danggui)——prepared into paste for external use to treat unhealed carbuncles due to

toxins

Notes: This herb has the functions of cooling and promoting circulation of blood and is good at removing toxic material and dispersing eruption. It is mainly used for measles, eruption in warm syndrome, acute and chronic hepatitis, carbuncle, eczema, cervical erosion, itching of vulvae, as well as scald. The modern pharmacological experiment has proved that Groomewell Root of Sinkiang Arnebia(紫草, Zicao) has the actions of contraception, anti-bacterium, anti-inflammation, anti-tumor, inhibiting virus, etc. It is said in *Proper Sense of Herbal Medicine* (《本草真义》, Bencaozhenyi): Groomewell Root of Sinkiang Arnebia(紫草, Zicao) can be used for all kinds of carbuncles due to excessive heat in blood stage, as well as bleeding syndrome due to excessive heat in blood, dysentery with blood, hemorrhoids, hematuria, and stranguria with bloody urine belonging to excessive type.

Section 5
Fever-reducing Drugs

1. 青蒿, Qinghao

English name: Sweet Wormwood

Pharmaceutical name: Herba Artemisiae Apiaceae

Botanical name: Artemeisia apiacea Hance

Properties and tastes: bitter, pungent, and cold

青 蒿

Meridian tropism: liver, gall bladder

Functions: 1. reduce the deficient fever

2. cool blood and clear away haet

3. expel summer-heat

4. prevent the attack of malaria

5. antibechic, expectorant, antiasthmatic

Indications: 1. fever due to yin deficiency——low fever, night sweating, hectic fever, and feverish sensation in the five centers due to chronic and consumptive diseases

2. the late stage of febrile diseases——warm and heat evil in yin-fen, fever during night, fever relieve with out sweating, or continues low fever

Dosage: 3 ~ 9g, it can not be decocted for a long time. The dosage for anti-marlaria is 20 ~ 40g.

Contraindication: Use it cautiously in the case of diarrhea and profuse sweat.

Combinations: 1. add Chinese Wolfberry Rootbark(地骨皮, Digupi)——steaming bone consumptive fever due to yin deficiency

2. add Turtle Carapace(鳖甲, Biejia)——deep-lying heat in yin-fen, night fever abating at dawn, abatement of fever, without sweating, steaming bone tidal fever due to yin deficiency, red tongue with less coating, low fever

3. add Hyacinth Bean (白扁豆, Baibiandou)——fever and vomiting due to external summer-heat

4. add Honeysuckle Flower(金银花, Jinyinhua)——fever in common cold

5. add Asiatic Plantain Herb (车前草, Cheqiancao)——diarrhea in children due to summer heat, scanty with reddish urine

6. add Membranous Milkvetch Root(黄芪, Huangqi)——damp-heat in shaoyang, alternating cold and heat, severve heat and mild cold, yellow and greasy coating

7. add Wild Mint(薄荷, Bohe)——fever without sweat, fullness in the chest, dizziness

8. add Antifebrile Dichroa Root(常山, Changshan)——malaria

9. add Chinese Clematis Root(威灵仙, Weilingxian)——benedict's filariasis

10. add Shunk Bugbane Rhizome(升麻, Shengma), Turtle Carapace(鳖甲, Biejia)——purpura

Prescriptions: 1. Sweet Wormwood and Scutellaria for Clearing Away Heat from Gallbladder(蒿芩清胆汤, Haoqinqingdan Tang)

2. Decoction of Sweet Wormwood and Turtle Shell(青蒿鳖甲汤, Qinghaobiejia Tang)

Notes: Ancient people thought Sweet Wormwood(青蒿, Qinghao) was a good herb for hectic fever. It has the function of anti-malaria, not only for controlling fever but also inhibiting the development of malarial parasites. It can be used singly in large doses (20～40g). Sweet Wormwood(青蒿, Qinghao) has fragrant flavor and without side effects in damaging the stomach and spleen as other bitter and cold herbs.

Sweet Wormwood(青蒿, Qinghao) and Chinese Thorowax Root(柴胡, Chaihu) act on the liver and gall bladder meridians and are good at treating alternate heat and cold of malaria. But Chinese Thorowax Root(柴胡, Chaihu) is good at dispersing the liver qi stagnation. It has the nature of ascending and dispersing and can lift up clear yang qi. It tends to damage yin. Sweet Wormwood (青蒿, Qinghao) is cool in nature and has fragrant flavor, it can clear summer heat and eliminate dampness without damaging yin, so it is often used for fever due to warm-heat and summer heat or hectic fever due to yin deficiency. It does not have the action of lifting up yang qi.

2. 地骨皮, Digupi

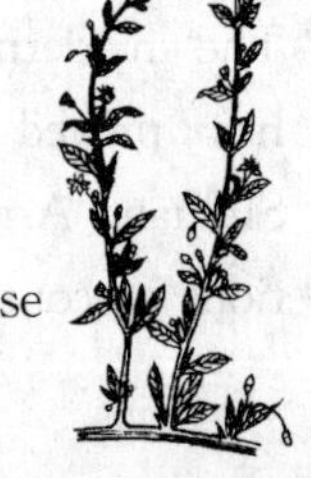
地骨皮

English name: Chinese Wolfberry Root-bark

Pharmaceutical name: Cortex Lycii Chinensis Radicis

Botanical name: Lycium chinense Mill.

Properties and tastes: sweet, tasteless and cold

Meridian tropism: lung, kidney

Functions: 1. cool blood and reduce the hectic fever due to yin deficiency

2. clear away lung-heat

3. reduce blood sugar

4. lower blood fat

5. reduce blood pressure

6. excite uterine

Indications: 1. blood heat due to yin deficiency——feverish sensation in five centers, hectic and tidal fever, night sweating

2. cough and asthma due to heat in the lung——high fever, cough and rapid respiration, yellow and sticky phlegm

3. bleeding due to blood heat——hematemesis, epistaxis, uterine bleeding

4. diabetes——thirst, diuresis

5. hypertension

6. toothache due to deficient fire——toothache especially during night, accompanied with fever in chronic consumptive diseases, night sweating, thirst, and restlessness

Dosage: 6～15g.

Contraindication: It is not advisable in the case of fever in external syndrome due to wind-cold and loose stool due to deficiency of the spleen.

Combinations: 1. add Sweet Wormwood (青蒿, Qinghao), Common Anemarrhea Rhizome (知母, Zhimu)——fever due to yin deficiency

2. add White Mulberry Root-bark (桑白皮, Sangbaipi)——cough due to lung heat and edema in acute nephritis

3. add Lalang Grass Rhizome (白茅根, Baimaogen) and Chinese Arborvitae Leafy Twig (侧柏叶, Cebaiye)——hematemesis, epistaxis, hematuria due to heat in blood

4. add Coptis Rhizome (黄连, Huanglian)——diabetes, hypertension

5. add Rehmannia Dried Root (生地黄, Shengdihuang)——toothache due to deficiency fire

6. add Oriental Waterplantain Rhizome (泽泻, Zexie)——hypertension due to blood heat and hyperactivity of the liver yang

Prescription: Powder for Expelling Lung Heat (泻白散, Xiebai San)

Notes: Chinese Wolfberry Root-bark (地骨皮, Digupi) is sweet and bitter in taste and cold in nature, it has the functions of clearing heat and cooling blood. It can be used for both clearing deficient and excessive heat, such as hectic fever due to consumed disease, cough due to heat in the lung, epistaxis, hematemesis, hematuria, and diabetes. Modern research proved that Chinese Wolfberry Root-bark (地骨皮, Digupi) has the actions of descending blood sugar and blood fat, and lowering blood pressure, so it also can be used to treat diabetes and hypertension clinically.

Both Chinese Wolfberry Root-bark (地骨皮, Digupi) and Tree Peony Bark (牡丹皮, Mudanpi) have the functions of cooling blood and relieving fever and is used for fever due to yin deficiency. Chinese Wolfberry Root-bark (地骨皮, Digupi) can be used to clear lung heat; Tree Peony Bark (牡丹皮, Mudanpi) is used to clear liver heat and heat in blood stage, also promote blood circulation to remove stasis. So there is the description in *Seeking Truth of Herbals* (《本草求真》, Bencaoqiuzhen): although both Chinese Wolfberry Root-bark (地骨皮, Digupi) and Tree Peony Bark (牡丹皮, Mudanpi) are used for hectic fever, Tree Peony Bark (牡丹皮, Mudanpi) is sour in taste and used for hectic fever without sweat, Chinese Wolfberry Root-bark (地骨皮, Digupi) is sweet in taste and used for hectic fever with sweating.

3. 白薇, Baiwei

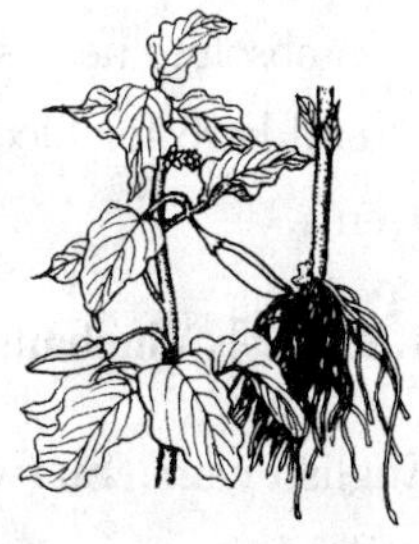
白 薇

English name: Blackend Swallowwort Root

Pharmaceutical name: Radix Cynanchi

Botanical name: Cynanchum atratum Bge. Or C. Versicolor Bge.

Properties and tastes: sweet, salty, and cold

Meridian tropism: stomach, liver

Functions: 1. clear away heat and cool blood

2. relieve stranguria by diuresis

Indications: 1. fever due to yin deficiency——the late stage of the febrile diseases, heat evil attacking ying stage and blood stage, or latent heat, or fever due to yin and blood deficiency. It is manifested as a continuous low fever

2. fever due to external evil——chilliness, fever, thin pules due to deficient yin with external evil

Dosage: 6～12g.

Combinations:

1. add Chinese Wolfberry Root-bark(地骨皮,Digupi)——hectic fever, steaming-bone night sweating

2. add Wild Mint(薄荷,Bohe)——blood deficiency with external syndrome

Notes: Blackend Swallowwort Root(白薇,Baiwei, Weirui in ancient time) is salty, bitter in taste and cold without dry nature. It is used for both deficient and excessive heat syndromes. So It is indicated in *Proper Sense of Herbal Medicine* (《本草真义》, Bencaozhenyi) that: for the cases of yin deficiency with heat, spontaneous sweating and night sweating, damage of body fluid due to chronic malaria, yin fluid damage with lasting heat in late stage of febrile diseases, it is an absolute necessary herb. It is a commonly used herb for blood heat syndrome of women.

4. 银柴胡, Yinchaihu

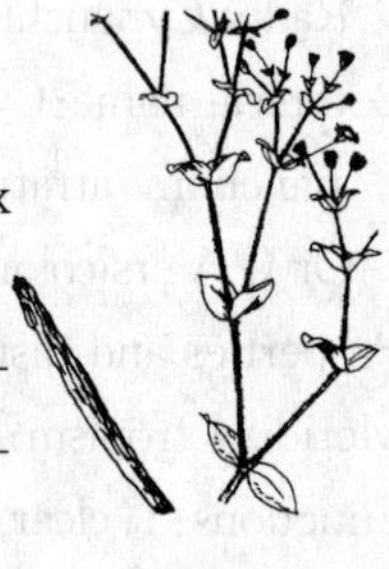

English name: Starwort Root

Pharmaceutical name: Radix Stellariae Dichotomae

Botanical name: Stellaria dichotoma L. Var. Lanceolata Bge.

银柴胡

Properties and tastes: sweet, slightly, and cold

Meridian tropism: liver, stomach

Functions: 1. relieve asthenic fever

2. dispel fever with infantile malnutrition

Indications: 1. fever due to yin deficiency——fever due to consumptive disease, night sweating

2. fever due to infant parasitosis——abdominal distension, emaciation, thirst, redness of eyes, and other symptoms in malnutrition involving the liver

Dosage: 3～9g for decoction, or prepared into pills and powder.

Contraindication: Do not use it in the case of external syndrome due to wind-cold, blood deficiency without fever.

Combinations:

1. add Sweet Wormwood(青蒿,Qinghao), Chinese Wolfberry Root-bark(地骨皮,Digupi) and Turtle Carapace(鳖甲,Biejia)——fever due to yin deficiency

2. add Cape Jasmine Fruit(栀子,Zhizi), Dan-shen Root(丹参,Danshen), Baikal Skullcap Root(黄芩,Huangqin)——infantile fever due to parasitosis

Notes: Starwort Root(银柴胡,Yinchaihu) is sweet in taste and cool in nature, it can clear heat without damaging the stomach and nourish yin. It is commonly used to treat hectic fever due to yin deficiency and fever due to malnutrition of an infant.

Starwort Root(银柴胡,Yinchaihu) and Chinese Thorowax Root(柴胡,Chaihu) have the function of clearing heat. Starwort Root(银柴胡,Yinchaihu) is good at cooling blood, relieving hectic fever due to yin deficiency and malnutrition. Chinese Thorowax Root(柴胡,Chaihu) is good at regulating shaoyang to relieve heat and is used for alternate fever and cold due to pathogenic factor in shaoyang and malaria. It has the functions of ascending and dispersing, not for hectic fever and malnutrition.

5. 胡黄连, Huhuanglian

English name: Figwortflower Picrorhiza Rhizome

Pharmaceutical name: Rhizoma Picrorrhizae

Botanical name: Picrorrhiza kurrooa Royle ex Benth. or P. Scrophulariaeflora Pennell

Properties and tastes: bitter, cold

Meridian tropism: heart, liver, kidney, large intestine

Functions: 1. relieve asthenic fever, dispel fever with infantile malnutrition

2. clear away heat and eliminate dampness

胡黄连

Indications: 1. fever due to yin deficiency——hectic and tidal fever, night sweating

2. infantile fever due to malnutrition——chronic fever, abdominal distension, emaciation, poor appetite, diarrhea

3. clearing heat and drying dampness——dysentery and diarrhea due to damp-heat, pain and swelling of hemorrhoids

Dosage: 3～9g.

Contraindication: Use it cautiously in the case of deficiency cold in the spleen and stomach.

Combinations:

1. add Starwort Root (银柴胡, Yinchaihu)——hectic and tidal fever

2. add Largehead Atractylodes Rhizome (白术, Baizhu)——infantile fever due to malnutrition

3. add Smoked Plum (乌梅, Wumei)——dysentery with bloody stools

4. add Chicken Liver (鸡肝, Jigan)——infantile keratitis

5. add Chinese Angelica Root (当归, Danggui) and Szechwan Lovage Rhizome (川芎, Chuanxiong)——heat stagnantion in blood stage

Notes: The functions of Figwortflower Picrorhiza Rhizome (胡黄连, Huhuanglian) are similar to that of Coptis Rhizome (黄连, Huanglian). It can be used for clearing heat, drying dampness and detoxifying. But the functions of Figwortflower Picrorhiza Rhizome (胡黄连, Huhuanglian) is weaker than that of Coptis Rhizome (黄连, Huanglian), and the function of relieving hectic fever and malnutrition is stronger than the Starwort Root (银柴胡, Yinchaihu). Mr. Zhang Bingcheng (张秉承) said the main function of Figwortflower Picrorhiza Rhizome (胡黄连, Huhuanglian) is clearing damp-heat, besides relieving hectic fever; the relation between Coptis Rhizome (黄连, Huanglian) and Figwortflower Picrorhiza Rhizome (胡黄连, Huhuanglian) is the same as Chinese Thorowax Root (柴胡, Chaihu) and Starwort Root (银柴胡, Yinchaihu). The only difference between the two drugs is stronger or weaker in their action.

Chapter 5
Drugs for Warming the Interior

Definition: These herbs, pungent in taste and hot in nature, are for warming the interior applied to the interior cold syndrome.

Functions: These drugs can warm the Middle-jiao, invigorate the spleen and stomach, dispel cold, and alleviate pain. Some of them may invigorate yang or recuperate the depleted yang.

Indications: These drugs are applied to the interior cold syndrome, which includes three types:

Exterior pathogenic cold invading the Middle-jiao: exterior pathogenic cold invades the interior of the body and obstructs yang qi of the spleen and stomach, causing a cold sensation and pain in the gastric and abdominal area, vomiting and diarrhea.

Interior cold due to yang deficiency: interior cold is excessive while yang qi is deficient, causing aversion to cold and cold sensation in the limbs, pale complexion, profuse clear urine, pale tongue and white coating, and deep and thin pulse.

Yang exhaustion: profuse sweating, cold sensation in the limbs and a faint pulse which is barely perceptible.

Classification: These herbs are usually classified into two categories, herbs for warming the Spleen yang and herbs for warming the kidney yang. The latter also has the function of warming the Spleen yang.

Cautions: These drugs are pungent, hot and dry in property, causing injury of body fluid when being used improperly. Therefore they should not be applied to heat and yin deficiency syndromes. Being pungent and hot, these drugs are prone to cause bleeding. Thus they should be used carefully for pregnant women.

1. 附子, Fuzi

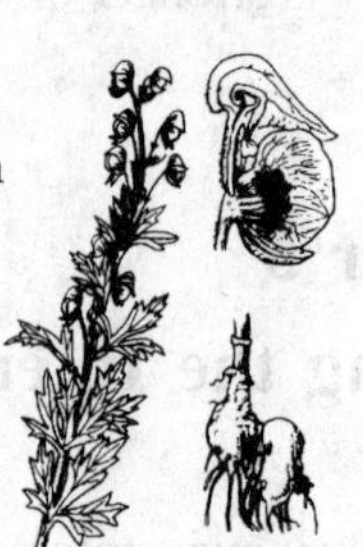

附 子

English name: Prepared Daughter Root of Common Monkshood

Pharmaceutical name: Radix Aconiti Carmichaeli Praeparata

Botanical name: Aconite carmichaeli Debx.

Properties and tastes: pungent, hot, poisonous

Meridian tropism: kidney, heart, and spleen

Functions: 1. recuperate depleted yang and rescue the patient from collapse

2. supplement fire of the Gate of life and restore yang

3. expel cold to relieve pain

4. invigorate yang to release the external syndrome

5. strengthen the function of heart

6. have excitation to pituitary adrenal cortex

Indications: 1. yang exhaustion syndrome——dripping cold sweat, extreme cold of the limbs, and a faint pulse, which is about to disappear. This is equivalent to shock in modern medicine.

2. insufficiency of the kidney yang, decline of the fire from the Gate of life——aversion to cold, cold limbs, soreness of the loins and knees, impotence and frequent urination

3. yin cold in the interior syndrome, inactivity of the spleen yang——abdominal cold and pain, and chronic diarrhea with loose stools

4. edema due to deficiency of yang——edema in the face and whole body, especially severe edema below the waist accompanied by soreness and a heavy sensation in the back, lumbago, lack of urine, palpitation, and shortness of breath. This is equivalent to cardianeuria

5. arthralgia due to wind-cold-dampness pathogen——Bi-syndrome, arthralgia and swelling of the extremities, difficulty in flexing and extending

6. external syndrome due to deficiency of yang——aversion to cold and fever, anhidrosis, a deep pulse

7. jaundice of insufficiency cold type——jaundice complicated by deficiency of spleen, syndrome

8. obstruction and pain in the chest

Dosage: 3～15g. Decoct it with water for 30～60 minutes.

Contraindication: Contraindicated in patients with interior heat caused by deficiency of yin and pregnant women. Incompatible with Pinellia Rhizome (半夏, Banxia), Snakegourd Fruit(瓜蒌, Gualou), Tendrilleaf Fritillary Bulb(贝母, Beimu), Root of Japanese Ampelopsis(白蔹, Bailian), Bletilla Rhizome(白及, Baiji).

Combinations: 1. add Ginseng (人参, Renshen)——yang exhaustion syndrome. Dripping cold sweat, extreme cold of the limbs, collapse syndrome of exhaustion of vital energy and a faint pulse which is about to disappear. This is caused by serious and chronic diseases, loss of blood, heart disease

2. add Membranous Milkvetch Root(黄芪, Huangqi)——superficial-loose syndrome due to deficiency of yang, continious perspiration

3. add Cassia Twig (桂枝, Guizhi)——arthralgia due to wind-cold-dampness pathogen, BI syndrome

4. add Tuckahoe(茯苓, Fuling)——edema due to yang deficiency, urine retention, heavy sensation in the extremities, edema of limbs, and palpatation

5. add Dried Ginger(干姜, Ganjiang)——this combination can improve the power of recuperating the depleted yang and rescuing the patient from collapse, which can be used in yang exhaustion, syndrome and cold pain in the epigastrium

6. add Prepared Rhizome of Adhesive Rehmannia(熟地黄, Shoudihuang)——insufficiency of the kidney yang, decline of the fire from the vital gate

7. add Largehead Atractylodes Rhizome(白术, Baizhu)——deficiency of spleen yang syndrome or conjoint invasion of the body wetness evils, general arthralgia and myalgia

8. add Capillary Wormwood Herb(茵陈蒿, Yinchenhao)——cold of insufficiency type jaundice

9. add Ginseng (人参, Renshen), Dwarf Lilyturf Root(麦门冬, Maimendong), Chinese Magnoliavine(五味子, Wuweizi)——shock.

10. add Rhizome or Root of Forbes Notopterygium(羌活, Qianghuo), Divaricate Saposhnikovia Root(防风, Fangfeng)——yang deficiency type of exopathic disease or wind-cold-damp arthralgia due to wind-cold-dampness pathogen, BI syndrome

11. add Rhuburb(大黄, Dahuang)——constipation due to yang deficiency

12. add Coptis Rhizome(黄连, Huanglian), Baikal Skullcap Root(黄芩, Huangqin)——feeling of fullness and oppression in the chest and upper abdomen of wind-heat type

13. add Manchurian Wildginger Herb(细辛, Xixin)——sciatica

14. add White Peony Root (白芍药, Baishaoyao)——release cold obstruction of cold evils and relieve pain, treat all kinds of pain belonging to cold type, such as precordial pain, stomachache, hypochondriac pain, dysmenorrhea, and arthralgia

Prescriptions: 1. Jin Gui's Bolus for Tonifying the Kidney Yin(金匮肾气丸, Jinguishenqi Wan)

2. Decoction for Strengthening the Spleen yang and Kidney yang (真武汤, Zhenwu Tang)

3. Pills for Kidney Yang(右归丸, Yougui Wan)

4. Decoction of Ephedra, Aconite and Asarum(麻黄附子细辛汤, Mahuang Fuzi Xixin Tang)

Notes: Being pungent and hot, Prepared Daughter Root of Common Monkshood(附

子,Fuzi)can invigorate heart yang to dredge the vessels and tonify kidney yang, recuperate depleted yang. Therefore, it is one of the most important herbs for recuperating depleted yang and rescuing the patient from collapse. Together with Ginseng (人参, Renshen), Dwarf Lilyturf Root (麦门冬, Maimendong) and Chinese Magnoliavine (五味子, Wuweizi) it is commonly used for coma. It can also be used for cases of deficiency of spleen, kidney and heart yang by tonifying fire and yang. However, Prepared Daughter Root of Common Monkshood (附子, Fuzi) is extremely poisonous. It must be decocted for a long period of time and prescribed in a small dosage. Prepared Daughter Root of Common Monkshood (附子, Fuzi) poisoning will be manifested by symptoms of hypervagotonia, i.e. Salivation, vomiting, numbness of the limbs, slow pulse. Licorice Root (甘草, Gancao) and Dried Ginger (干姜, Ganjiang) may reduce poisoning from Prepared Daughter Root of Common Monkshood (附子, Fuzi). Severe cases should be treated in a hospital.

Daughter Root of Common Monkshood (附子, Fuzi) "tends to act on all meridians", "warms up five-zang organs and recuperates the depleted yang", makes the fire back to its origin and clears heat due to yin deficiency". It is "one of the most important herbs for invigorating Primary yang, and it can act in an upwards, downwards, inwards or outwards direction. Thus it is applied for chronic cases of cold syndrome which originated in zang and fu organs, gradually spreading to tendons and bones and obstructed meridians and blood vessels." Therefore, transactions of Famous Physicians says, "it is the first important herb". It must be emphasized that the key point of manifestations is "thin pulse without vitality and qi deficiency without heat".

2. 肉桂, Rougui

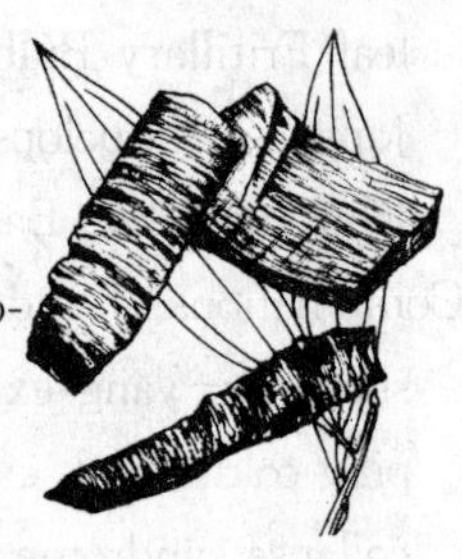
肉 桂

English name: Cassia Bark

Pharmaceutical name: Cortex Cinnamomi Cassiae

Botanical name: Cinnamomum cassia Presl.

Properties and tastes: pungent, hot, sweet

Meridian tropism: kidney, heart, liver, and spleen

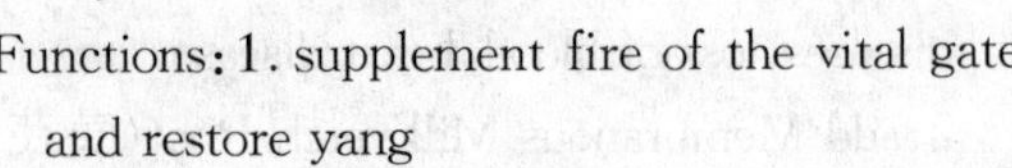

Functions: 1. supplement fire of the vital gate and restore yang

2. expel cold to relieve pain

3. promote the flow of qi-blood by warming the meridians

4. warm yang to promote the functioning of qi

5. stop pain and tranquilize

6. promote circulation of the blood

Indications: 1. insufficiency of the kidney yang, decline of the fire from the vital gate——aversion to cold and cold limbs, soreness of the loin and knee, impotence, frequent urination

2. deficiency of spleen and kidney yang——cold pain in the epigastrium, poor appetite, diarrhea with loose stool

3. blood stasis due to accumulation of cold——dysmenorrhea, amenorrhea and tumor

4. wind-damp arthralgia syndrome——arthralgia and pain in the loins

5. chronic carbuncle of yin type——bone tuberculosis and gangrene

6. un ruptured swelling abscess or slow-healing carbuncles

7. anemia

Dosage: 1.5～4.5g. Make it into powder and take it orally, 1～1.5g each time with water.

Contraindication: Contraindicated in patients with hyperactivity of fire caused by deficiency of yin, interior excessive heat, bleeding due to blood heat and pregnant women.

Combinations: 1. add Prepared Daughter Root of Common Monkshood(附子, Fuzi), Prepared Rhizome of Adhesive Rehmannia (熟地黄, Shoudihuang)——insufficiency of the kidney yang, decline of the fire from the vital gate

2. add Prepared Daughter Root of Common Monkshood (附子, Fuzi), Largehead Atractylodes Rhizome(白术, Baizhu)——deficiency of spleen and kidney yang

3. add Prepared Rhizome of Adhesive Rehmannia(熟地黄, Shoudihuang), Chinese Angelica Root (当归, Danggui)——blood stasis due to accumulation of cold, abdominal pain of amenorrhea

4. add Argy Wormwood Leaf(艾叶, Aiye), Chinese Angelica Root(当归, Danggui)——deficiency cold of qi and blood, dysmenorrhea

5. add Chinese Taxillus Twig (桑寄生, Sangjisheng), Eucommia Bark (杜仲, Duzhong)——pain in the lions due to cold arthralgia

6. add Mulberry Leaf(桑叶, Sangye), Doubleteeth Pulbescent Angelica Root (独活, Duhuo)——arthralgia

7. add Common Anemarrhea Rhizome(知母, Zhimu), Chinese Corktree Bark(黄柏, Huangbai)——diabetes and urine retention, uroschesis due to deficiency of the kidney

8. add Prepared Rhizome of Adhesive Rehmannia(熟地黄, S houdihuang), Ginseng(人参, Renshen)——palpitation, shortness of breath due to deficiency of both qi and blood

9. add Prepared Rhizome of Adhesive Rehmannia(熟地黄, Shoudihuang), Antler Glue(鹿角胶, Lujiaojiao)——chronic carbuncle of yin type, un-ruptured swelling abscess or slow-healing carbuncles

10. add Tuber Fleeceflower Root(何首乌, Heshouwu), Ass-hide Glue (阿胶, Ejiao)——anemia

11. add Yanhusuo (延胡索, Yanhusuo), Chinese Angelica Root(当归, Danggui)——cold pain of the lower abdomen

12. add Coptis Rhizome (黄连, Huanglian)——irritability, insomnia, soreness of loin and knees due to failure of the heart and kidney to integrate, and it is also used to treat chronic diarrhea

13. add White Peony Root (白芍药, Baishaoyao)——suppress the liver yang fry Cassia Bark(肉桂, Rougui) for a short period of time with White Peony Root(白芍药, Baishaoyao)

Prescriptions: 1. Jin Gui's Bolus for Tonifying the Kidney Yin(金匮肾气丸, Jinguishenqi Wan)

2. Decoction of Prepared Rehmannia, cinnamon Bark and Ephedra combination(阳和汤, Yanghe Tang)

Notes: *Herbals for Easy Approaching* (《本草便读》, Bencaobiandu) says, "Cassia Bark(肉桂, Rougui), acting on blood stage of the heart, liver, spleen and kidney meridians, can dispel pathogenic cold in Xuefen and remove blood stasis and lumps. Together with herbs for tonifying the kidney, it can invigorate yang of the gate of life and be used for cases of yang exhaustion. Furthermore, it can let the fire back into its origin. Thus it can invigorate heart yang or spleen yang while combining with assistant or guiding herbs."The function of Cassia Bark(肉桂, Rougui) is similar to that of Prepared Daughter Root of Common Monkshood(附子, Fuzi). Both of them can invigorate the kidney yang. Thus they could be applied to cases of cold syndrome in Lower-jiao due to yang deficiency and mutually reinforce the function of invigorating kidney yang. However, being dry and drastic, Prepared Daughter Root of Common Monkshood(附子, Fuzi) is one of the most important herbs for recuperating yang and rescuing the patient from collapse, while the function of Cassia Bark(肉桂, Rougui) is milder than that of Prepared Daughter Root of Common Monkshood(附子, Fuzi). The main functions of Cassia Bark(肉桂, Rougui) are invigorating the fire of the gate of life, supporting the transformation of qi and letting the fire back into its origin. Furthermore, Cassia Bark(肉桂, Rougui) can act on Blood stage and be applied to cases of amenorrhea and blood arthralgia syndrome due to pathogenic cold in the meridians and blood stasis. Thus small dosage of Cassia Bark(肉桂, Rougui), in combination with herbs for tonifying qi and Blood, may remarkably invigorate the production of Blood and qi, which could be one of its primary functions. Both Cassia Bark(肉桂, Rougui) and Prepared Daughter Root of Common Monkshood(附子, Fuzi) originate from laurel. Cassia Bark(肉桂, Rougui) is bark of laurel while Cassia Twig(桂枝, Guizhi) is the tender branch of it. Both of them have the functions of warming blood, supporting the transformation of qi and dispelling the accumulation of coldness. Cassia Twig(桂枝, Guizhi), being light, tends to go upwards and has the functions of invigorating yang and transforming qi, relieving the exterior syndrome and expelling pathogenic cold. Cassia Twig(桂枝, Guizhi) also acts in the limbs and has the functions of warming and dredging the meridians, and invigorating qi and blood. While Cassia Bark(肉桂, Rougui) is strong and can warm up the interior and alleviate pain. Cassia Bark(肉桂, Rougui) tends to go downwards and has the functions of invigorating Kidney yang and letting the fire back to the gate of life. Thus it is applied to cases due to excessive yin and cold in the interior and Kidney yang deficiency.

3. 吴茱萸, Wuzhuyu

English name: Medicinal Evodia Fruit

Pharmaceutical name: Fructus Evodiae Rutaecarpae

Botanical name: Evodia rutaecarpa Benth.

Properties and tastes: pungent, hot, bitter, poisonous

吴茱萸

Meridian tropism: liver, stomach, and spleen

Functions: 1. smooth stagnated liver qi
2. warm the Middle-jiao to expel cold and arrest vomiting
3. alleviate pain
4. eliminate dampness
5. inhibit bacteria
6. reduce blood pressure
7. diuresis

Indications: 1. cold pain in the epigastrium——abdominal pain, a desire for warmth and pressing, vomiting upon food intake, abdominal distention and less food intake, chronic diarrhea and loose stools, cold limbs due to spleen and stomach cold syndrome

2. headache of Jueyin meridian——vertical headache, retching with salivation

3. pain in cold hernia——distention and cold pain in the lower abdomen and testis due to accamulation of cold in the liver meridian, contraction and cold pain of scrotum, pain exaggerated by catching cold, pain alleviated while getting warmth

4. infertility due to retention of cold in the uterus——accompanied with cold pain in the lower abdomen, cold limbs, and delayed menstruation

5. stomach-cold syndrome——stomachache, vomiting watery fluid and diluted foam-like sputum, acid regurgitation, which can be alleviated by getting warm

6. liver fire invading the stomach——vomiting and acid regurgitation, distending pain in the chest and hypochondrium, irritability, dry throat, stringy and rapid pulse

7. pain in arthralgia of the foot joints due to cold-dampness, disturbance of the lower legs due to pathogenic cold and dampness——fullness and pain, numbness of the legs and, limitation of movement, abdominal distention, restlessness and extremely unbearable irritation

8. deficiency cold of spleen and kidney, morning diarrhea——accompanied with abdominal pain, soreness in the lumbar region, cold limbs, lassitude, loss of appetite, a deep slow and forceless pulse

Dosage: 1.5～6g, proper dosage for external application.

Contraindication: This herb is pungent, hot and intense in properties, has a tendency to impair qi and produce pathogenic fire. It is not suitable to be taken for a long period of time or overtaken, not to be taken for patients with interior heat due to deficiency of yin.

Combinations: 1. add Ginseng (人参, Renshen)——deficiency cold in Middle-jiao, poor appetite, vomiting on food intake

2. add Coptis Rhizome (黄连, Huanglian)——vomiting and acid regurgitation due to stagnation of liver qi producing fire

3. add Common Floweringquince Fruit (木瓜, Mugua)——retention of cold-damp disturbing the spleen, cholera morbus, vomiting, diarrhea and spasm

4. add Chinese Angelica Root (当归, Danggui)——delayed menstruation, scanty and dark-colored blood, cold pain in the lower abdomen due to retention of deficiency cold in the uterus in women

5. add Chinese Magnoliavine (五味子, Wuweizi)——deficiency cold of spleen and kidney, morning diarrhea

6. add Fennel Fruit (小茴香, Xiaohuixiang)——stomachache, abdominal pain, pain hernia due to cold pathogens

7. add Dried Ginger (干姜, Ganjiang)——vomiting and acid regurgitation due to stomach cold

8. add Common Floweringquince Fruit (木瓜, Mugua), Areca Seed (槟榔, Binlang), Fresh Ginger (生姜, Shengjiang)——pain of arthralgia of the foot joints due to cold-damp

9. add Szechwan Chinaberry Fruit (川楝子, Chuanlianzi), Tangerine Seed (橘核, Juhe)——hernia of cold type, swelling, stiffness and regional cold pain of the testis

10. add Argy Wormwood Leaf (艾叶, Aiye)——infertility due to retention of cold in the uterus, metrorrhagia and metrostaxis.

Prescriptions: 1. Fructus Euodia Pill (吴茱

萸汤,Wuzhuyu Tang)

2. Zuojin Bolus(左金丸,Zuojin Wan)

3. Decoction for Warming Channels(温经汤,Wenjing Tang)

Notes: Medicinal Evodia Root (吴茱萸, Wuzhuyu)is pungent for dispersion and bitter for descent. It is one of the most important herbs attributed to the liver meridian. It is also attributed to spleen and stomach meridians. The nature of Medicinal Evodia Root(吴茱萸, Wuzhuyu) is hot, dry and drastic, with functions of dispersing and descending the stagnated liver qi, and warming up Jueyin and expelling pathogenic cold. Therefore it is applied for headache due to ascending of adverse cold qi after flowing downwards extremely. Furthermore, Medicinal Evodia Root(吴茱萸, Wuzhuyu) can warm the Middle-jiao and keep turbid qi downwards, and regulate the liver and stomach to stop vomiting. Its effect of alleviating pain and stopping vomiting is significant. It is successfully applied to diarrhea due to spleen and kidney yang deficiency and gastrointestinal dysfunction. The powder of it can be applied externally to the center of the sole of the foot to cure mouth ulcers and hypertension by letting the fire downwards. It can be mixed with Vaseline and made into 20% or 30% ointment. It also can be mixed with the same amount of zinc oxide and made into ointment. The ointment of Medicinal Evodia Root(吴茱萸, Wuzhuyu)is applied to cases of eczema, neurodermatitis, impetigo and so on. Medicinal Evodia Root(吴茱萸, Wuzhuyu)can kill ascaris of pig in vitro and kill oxyurid by taking the decoction of this herb orally for three to five days. An over dose may cause blurred vision or illusion because of its function of exciting the central nerve.

Both Medicinal Evodia Root(吴茱萸, Wuzhuyu) and Fresh Ginger(生姜, Shengjiang) can stop vomiting. The former can warm the Liver and expel pathogenic cold, and is usually applied to cases of vomiting and acrid regurgitation due to Liver cold invading the stomach. Fresh Ginger(生姜, Shengjiang) can warm the stomach and expel pathogenic cold, and is usually applied in cases of vomiting of watery liquid due to adverse stomach cold.

4. 花椒, Huajiao

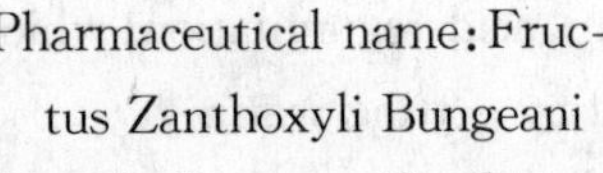

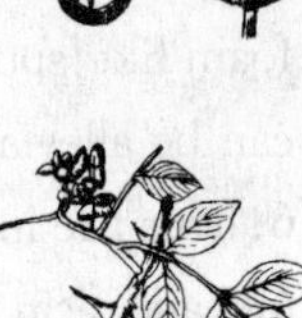

花　椒

English name: Bunge Pricklyash

Pharmaceutical name: Fructus Zanthoxyli Bungeani

Botanical name: Zanthoxylum bungeanum Maxim.

Properties and tastes: pungent, hot and slightly poisonous

Meridian tropism: kidney, stomach, and spleen

Functions: 1. warm the Middle-jiao to relieve pain and control diarrhea

2. destory parasites

3. use it for local anesthesia

Indications: 1. invasion of pathogenic cold in the Middle-jiao——cold pain in the epigastrium, vomiting and diarrhea

2. ascariasis——abdominal pain due to parasitic infestation, ascaris intestinal obstruction, biliary ascariasis(colic caused by ascariasis)

3. scabies, scrotum pruritus due to damp pathogen, female mycotic colpitis, pruritus vulvae(external application)

Dosage: 2～6g, decoct it with water, or grind it into powder. Proper dosage for external application.

Contraindication: Contraindicated in patients with interior heat due to deficiency of yin and pregnant women.

Combinations: 1. add vinegar——fry and boil Bunge Pricklyash(花椒, Huajiao), take the liquid can treat abdominal pain due to ascariasis

2. add Dried Ginger(干姜, Ganjiang)——extreme cold pain in the stomach and abdomen

3. add Tuckahoe(茯苓, Fuling)——cough and asthma due to deficiency cold of the lung and kidney, accompained by cold foot and lumbar path

4. add Lightyellow Sophora Root(苦参, Kushen)——scabies and pruritus decotion being used as a lotion

5. add Smoked Plum(乌梅, Wumei)——incessant chronic diarrhea and dysentery, diarrhea with undigested food, as well as for morbid leukorrhea due to cold-damp

Prescriptions: 1. Dark Pulm Pill (乌梅丸, Wumei Wan)

2. The Middle-jiao-warming and qi-restoring Decoction (大建中汤, Dajianzhong Tang)

Notes: Bunge Pricklyash(花椒, Huajiao), is pungent, hot, fragrant and dry. Li Shizhen (李时珍) said: "It is applied to cases of cough by dispersing Lung cold, Bi syndrome of wind-cold-dampness, edema, diarrhea and dysentery, frequent urination, feet flabbiness, and chronic dysentery due to yang deficiency by invigorating Kidney fire." The regular dosage is 2～6g. It could be decocted or ground into powder, which is put into a capsule.

The seed of Bunge Pricklyash (花椒, Huajiao) is Bunge Tricklyash Seed(椒目, Jiaomu), which is bitter and cold acting on the spleen and urinary bladder meridians. Bunge Tricklyash Seed(椒目, Jiaomu) can promote diuresis to cure edema and alleviate asthma. It is applied in cases of edema, difficulty in urination, adverse qi and asthma. In the light of "Bunge Tricklyash Seed(椒目, Jiaomu) relieving asthma", as stated by Zhu Danxi(朱丹溪), it has been applied successfully to bronchial asthma, asthmatic trachitis, cardiac asthma, pulmonary emphysema and so on in recent years.

Both Bunge Pricklyash (花椒, Huajiao) and Medicinal Evodia Root (吴茱萸, Wuzhuyu) can warm the Middle-jiao to relieve pain and alleviate vomiting. Bumge Prichlyash(花椒, Huajiao) primarily impacts the Stomach Meridian and is good at expelling turbidity and killing parasites, while Medicinal Evodia Root(吴茱萸, Wuzhuyu) acts on the liver meridian and is good at keeping adverse qi downwards.

5. 干姜, Ganjiang

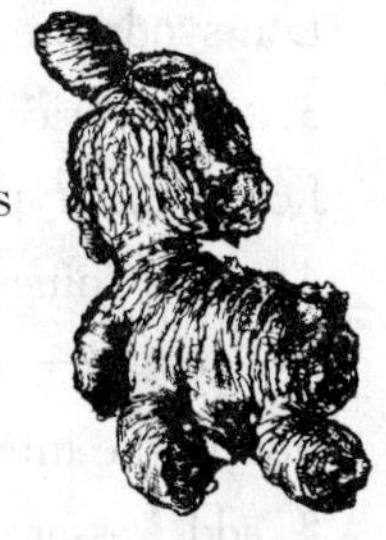
干姜

English name: Dried Ginger

Pharmaceutical name: Rhizoma Zingiberis Officinalis

Botanical name: Zingiber officinale Rose

Properties and tastes: pungent, warm

Meridian tropism: spleen, stomach, heart, and lung

Functions: 1. warm the Middle-jiao and dispel cold

2. recuperating depleted yang

3. warm the lungs to resolve fluid retention

4. warm the meridians for arresting bleeding

Indications: 1. invasion of pathogenic cold in the spleen and stomach-cold-pain in the epigastrium, vomiting, diarrhea and a slow, moderate pulse

2. yang exhaustion syndrome——extreme cold of the extremities, faint pulse which is about to disappear

3. cold-fluid in the lung——cough and asthma, coldness of the body with chills, profuse and thin phlegm

4. hemorrhage of deficient cold syndrome——hematemesis, epistaxis, hematochezia, metrorrhagia and metrostaxis accompanied with cold sensation in the palms and soles, sallow complexion, a pale tongue with thin white coating

Dosage: 3～9g

Contraindication: Contraindicated in patients with interior heat caused by deficiency of yin and pregnant women.

Combinations: 1. add Coptis Rhizome(黄连, Huanglian)——pain in the epigastrium, vomiting, diarrhea and dysentery and intermingling cold and heat

2. add Prepared Daughter Root of Common Monkshood(附子, Fuzi)——yang exhaustion syndrome

3. add Licorice Root(甘草, Gancao)——deficient cold type of consumptive lung disease

4. add Chinese Magnoliavine (五味子, Wuweizi)——cold phlegm and fluid retention in the interior, cough with dyspnea

5. add Lesser Galangal Rhizome(高良姜, Gaoliangjiang)——cold pain in the epigastrium

6. add Pinellia Rhizome(半夏, Banxia)——vomiting without discharging or spitting saliva due to stomach cold

7. add Largehead Atractylodes Rhizome(白术, Baizhu)——diarrhea due to deficiency of the spleen

8. add Longstament Onion Bulb (薤白, Xiebai)——obstruction of qi in the chest

9. add Smoked Plum(乌梅, Wumei)——metrorrhagia due to cold blood

10. add Ass-hide Glue(阿胶, Ejiao)——hematemesis of cold deficiency type, hematochezia

11. add Chinese Angelica Root(当归, Danggui)——postpartum abdominal pain

Prescriptions: 1. Bolus for Regulating the Middle Warmer(理中丸, Lizhong Wan)

2. Decoction for Collapse (四逆汤, Sini Tang)

3. Dark Pulm Pill(乌梅丸, Wumei Wan)

Notes: Baked Ginger (炮姜, Paojiang) is a preparation of Dried Ginger(干姜, Ganjian g), while Fresh Ginger (生姜, Shengjiang) is fresh Dried Ginger(干姜, Ganjiang). Being warm in property, Fresh Ginger(生姜, Shengjiang) is good at dispersing pathogenic wind-cold and warming the Middle-jiao to stop vomiting. Being hot, Dried Ginger(干姜, Ganjiang) is good at recuperating the depleted yang and rescuing the patient from collapse as well as warming the Lung to resolve the phlegm. Baked Ginger(炮姜, Paojiang) is good at warming the Middle-jiao to stop diarrhea and arrest bleeding.

Both Dried Ginger (干姜, Ganjiang) and Prepared Daughter Root of Common Monkshood(附子, Fuzi) can recuperate the depleted yang. Dried Ginger (干姜, Ganjian g) impacts primarily the spleen and stomach, and has the function of warming the Middle-jiao and dispersing pathogenic cold, whereas Prepared Daughter Root of Common Monkshood(附子, Fuzi) primarily invigorates Primary yang in the Lower-jiao. If the patient is suffering from diarrhea due to deficient cold of the stomach and spleen, and has a cold feeling in the limbs, Prepared Daughter Root of Common Monkshood(附子, Fuzi), then can be used to generate earth by invigorating fire. Prepared Daughter Root of Common Monkshood (附子, Fuzi) and Dried Ginger (干姜, Ganjiang) could be used simultaneously in order to recuperate the depleted yang and restore the pulse. They can mutually enhance the function of recuperating the depleted yang and rescuing the patient from collapse. Thus there was a saying in ancient times that "Prepared Daughter Root of Common Monkshood(附子, Fuzi) is not hot unless it is used together with Dried Ginger(干姜, Ganjiang)."

Both Dried Ginger (干姜, Ganjiang) and Medicinal Evodia Root(吴茱萸, Wuzhuyu) can warm the Middle-jiao and disperse pathogenic cold. They can be used in cases of cold feeling and pain in the abdominal area due to pathogenic cold accumulated in the Middle-jiao. Dried Ginger (干姜, Ganjiang) also warms the Upper-jiao to remove water retention and alleviate cough. Medicinal Evodia Root (吴茱萸, Wuzhuyu) can warm the Lower-jiao. It is applied to hernia due to pathogenic cold by warming the liver. It is also used for diarrhea due to pathogenic cold by warming the kidney.

6. 小茴香, Xiaohuixiang

English name: Fennel Fruit

Pharmaceutical name: Fructus Foeniculi Vulgaris

Botanical name: Foeniculum vulgare Mill.

Properties and tastes: pungent, warm

Meridian tropism: liver, kidney, spleen, and stomach

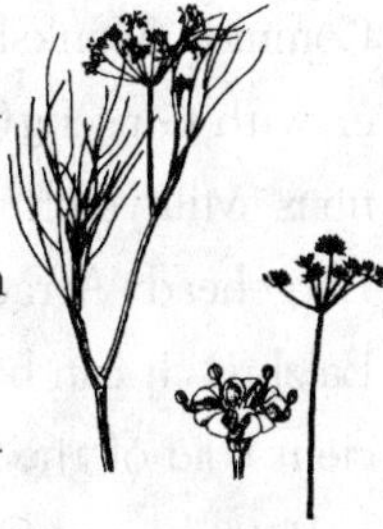
小茴香

Functions: 1. dispel cold and stop pain

2. regulate the flow of qi and the stomach

Indications: 1. pain in cold hernia, due to pathogenic cold (weighing down of the testis)

2. vomiting and poor appetile due to stomach cold, pain and distention in the epigastrium

Dosage: 3～9g. Proper amount for external application.

Contraindication: Not to be taken for patients with interior heat due to deficiency of yin.

Combinations:

1. add Medicinal Evodia Root (吴茱萸, Wuzhuyu), Common Aucklandia Root (木香, Muxiang)——cold hernia, cold pain in the lower abdomen

2. add Cassia Bark(肉桂, Rongui) Combined Spicebush Root (乌药, Wuyiao)——cold hernia, cold pain in the lower abdomen

3. add Chinese Angelica Root(当归, Danggui), Nutgrass Galingale Rhizome (香附, Xiangfu)——Dysmenorrhea

4. add Common Floweringquince Fruit (木瓜, Mugua)——arthralgia of foot joints due to cold-damp, soreness and pain of the feet and knees, weakness in walking

5. add Tangerine Seed (橘核, Juhe), Hawthorn Fruit (山楂, Shanzha)——swelling and pain in the testis, and scrotum with a feeling of falling

6. add Dried Ginger(干姜, Ganjiang), Common Aucklandia Root(木香, Muxiang)——vomiting due to stomach cold, poor appetile, distention and pain in the epigastrium

7. add Fresh Ginger(生姜, Shengjiang), Officinal Magnolia Bark (厚朴, Houpu)——dyspepsia

8. add Fresh Ginger (生姜, Shengjiang),

Pinellia Rhizome(半夏,Banxia)——stomachache due to cold,hiccup,vomiting

Notes: Fennel Fruit(小茴香,Xiaohuixiang) can disperse the stagnated liver qi,warm the kidney and expel pathogenic cold to alleviate pain. When used with herbs for warming the liver and kidney and promoting the circulation of qi to alleviate pain,Fennel Fruit (小茴香,Xiaohuixiang)is usually applied to cases of hernia,manifested as pain and malposition of testis due to pathogenic cold. Furthermore,it can regulate qi and improve appetite. It is also applied to cases of vomiting,poor appetite,distention and pain in the gastric and abdominal area due to Stomach cold.

7.高良姜,Gaoliangjiang

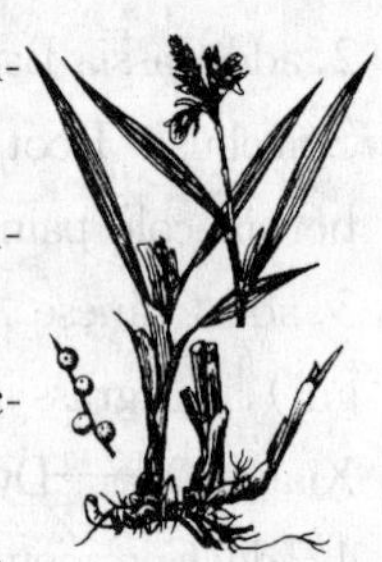

English name: Lesser Galangal Rhizome

Pharmaceutical name: Rhizoma Alpiniae Officinari

Botanical name:Aplinia officinarum Hance.

高良姜

Properties and tastes: pungent,hot

Meridian tropism:spleen,stomach

Function:warm the spleen and stomach

Indication: invasion of cold in the spleen and stomach——cold pain in the epigastrum, vomiting with discharging thin cold saliva, etc.

Dosage:3～9g

Contraindication:Do not use for patients with interior heat due to yin deficiency.

Combinations:1. add Nutgrass Galingale Rhizome(香附,Xiangfu)——cold-evil invading the stomach, cold pain in the stomach and epigastrium

2. add Dried Ginger(干姜,Ganjiang)——cold pain in the epigastrium, nausea and vomiting,or diarrhea with loose stools,etc.

3. add Scorpion(全蝎,Quanxie)——toothache due to pathogenic wind-fire, a new infection or a chronic disease. It can also treat tumefaction of the parotid

4. add Pinellia Rhizome(半夏,Banxia), Lesser Galangal Rhizome(高良姜,Gaoliangjiang)——stomach cold, reversed upward flow of qi,vomiting of watery fluid

5. add Prepared Daughter Root of Common Monkshood(附子,Fuzi),White Peony Root (白芍药,Baishaoyao)——cold pain in the abdomen and diarrhea with undigested food

6. add Officinal Magnolia Bark(厚朴, Houpu), Chinese Angelica Root(当归, Danggui)——sudden onset of angina in the chest and abdomen,fullness sensation in the hypochondrium,intolerable restlessness

7. add Fennel Fruit(小茴香,Xiaohuixiang)——hernia due to pathogenic cold, stabbing pain in the lower abdomen and women's pain in the lower abdomen due to stagnation of cold evil

Prescription: Pill of Galangal and Nutgrass lastedge(良附丸,Liangfu Wan)

Notes:Lesser Galangal Rhizome(高良姜,Gaoliangjiang) is pungent in taste and hot in property, and a kind of pure-yang herb, which can expel chronic cold. The function of it is similar to that of Cassia Bark(肉桂, Rongui) and Prepared Daughter Root of Common Monkshood(附子,Fuzi). Together with Ginseng(人参,Renshen),Membranous Milkvetch Root(黄芪,Huanfqi) and Largehead Atractylodes Rhizome(白术, Baizhu),it can be effectively applied to deficient cold of the Spleen and Stomach.

Both Lesser Galangal Rhizome(高良姜, Gaoliangjiang) and Dried Ginger (干姜,

Ganjiang) are pungent and hot and the most important herbs for warming the Middle-jiao and dispersing pathogenic cold. The main function of Lesser Galangal Rhizome (高良姜, Gaoliangjiang) is dispersing Stomach cold. Thus it is good at curing a cold feeling and pain in the gastric and abdominal area, belching, vomiting. While the main function of Dried Ginger (干姜, Ganjiang) is dispersing Spleen cold, it is also good at curing abdominal pain and diarrhea.

Both Lesser Galangal Rhizome (高良姜, Gaoliangjiang) and Fresh Ginger (生姜, Shengjiang) have the functions of warming the Middle-jiao and dispersing pathogenic cold. Lesser Galangal Rhizome (高良姜, Gaoliangjiang) tends to act on the interior, disperses Stomach cold to relieve pain. While Fresh Ginger (生姜, Shengjiang) tends to act on the exterior, disperses wind-cold to relieve the exterior syndrome and regulates Stomach qi to stop vomiting.

8. 丁香, Dingxiang

English name: Clove Flower-bud

Pharmaceutical name: Flos Caryophylli

Botanical name: Eugenia caryopyllata Thunb. Also known as Syzygium aromaticum (L.) Merr. Et Perry

丁 香

Properties and tastes: pungent, warm

Meridian tropism: spleen, stomach, and kidney

Functions: 1. warm the Middle-jiao and dispel the cold

2. lower the adverse flow of qi to relieve hiccup

3. warm the kidney to strengthen yang

Indications: 1. vomiting, hiccup, accompanied with poor appetite, diarrhea due to stomach cold

2. impotence, soreness and weakness of the legs accompanied with aversion to cold, soreness and weakness of the back and knees due to kidney yang deficiency

Dosage: 3～6g

Contraindication: Do not use with patients with interior heat due to yin deficiency, antagonistic to Tumeric Root-tuber (郁金, Yujin)

Combinations: 1. add Persimmon Calyx and Receptacle (柿蒂, Shidi)——hiccups, vomiting, fullness and oppression in the abdomen and epigastrium due to stomach cold

2. add Pinellia Rhizome (半夏, Banxia), Medicinal Evodia Root (吴茱萸, Wuzhuyu)——vomiting, abdomind pain due to stomach cold

3. add Largehead Atractylodes Rhizome (白术, Baizhu), Villous Amomum Fruit (砂仁, Sharen)——poor appetite, vomiting due to insufficiency and cold of the spleen and stomach

4. add Prepared Daughter Root of Common Monkshood (附子, Fuzi), Cassia Bark (肉桂, Rongui)——impotence due to deficiency of the kidney, pudendal coldness, morbid leukorrhea due to cold-dampness

5. add Tangerine Peel (橘红, Juhong)——vomiting and diarrhea in children

Prescription: Decoction of Flossyzygii Aromatica and calyx Kaki (丁香柿蒂汤, Dingxiang Shidi Tang)

Notes: Clove Flower-bud (丁香, Dingxiang) warms the Middle-jiao and disperses pathogenic cold. It is good at keeping the adverse qi downwards. It is one of the most important herbs applied to vomiting and hiccup due to Stomach cold. It can also invigorate the Kidney yang and be applied to hernia due to deficiency of Kidney yang.

9. 细辛, Xixin

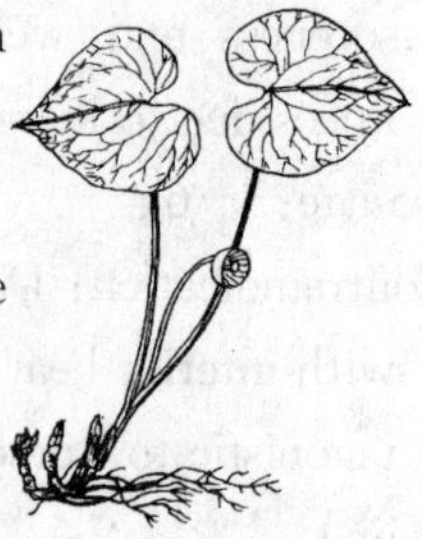

English name: Manchurian Wildginger Herb

Pharmaceutical name: Herba Asari cum Radice

Botanical name: Asarum sieboldii Miq. or A. heteropoides Fr. Schm. Var. mandshuricum (Maxim.) Kitag.

细 辛

Properties and tastes: pungent, warm

Meridian tropism: lung, stomach

Functions: 1. expel cold to relieve pain

2. expel pathogenic wind from the body surface

3. warm the lung to resolve fluid retention

4. reduce resuscitation

5. use it for local anesthesia

Indications: 1. wind-cold headache, severe pain all over the body

2. headache, toothache, lower back pain, pain in the joints, chest blockage and cardiac pain, sciatica etc.

3. cough and asthma due to lung cold, obstruction of cold fluid in the lung, discharging profuse thin white sputum and fluid, and coldness of the body with chills

4. rhinorrhea——stuffy nose, headache, occasional turbid nasal discharge

Dosage: 2～6g.

Contraindication: Contraindicated in make it into patients with profuse sweating due to deficiency of qi, headache caused by hyperactivity of yang due to deficiency of yin, cough due to lung heat and deficiency of yin, incompatible with Black False Bellebore (藜芦, Lilu)

Combinations: 1. add Rhizome or Root of Forbes Notopterygium (羌活, Qianghuo), Divaricate Saposhnikovia Root (防风, Fangfeng)——wind cold, headache, stuffy nose

2. add Dahurian Angelica Root (白芷, Baizhi), Szechwan Lovage Rhizome (川芎, Chuanxiong)——headache

3. add Gypsum (石膏, Shigao)——toothache due to stomach heat

4. add Coptis Rhizome (黄连, Huanglian)——ulceration on the oral musosa and the tongue

5. add Ephedra (麻黄, Mahuang)——arthralgia and shaoyin cold

6. add Tatarian Aster Root (紫苑, Ziyuan), Common Coltsfoot Flower (款冬花, Kuandonghua)——cough with profuse thin sputum due to lung cold

7. add Dahurian Angelica Root (白芷, Baizhi), Divaricate Saposhnikovia Root (防风, Fangfeng)——rhinorrhea

8. add Officinal Magnolia Bark (厚朴, Houpu)——cough, fullness in the chest

9. add Dried Ginger (干姜, Ganjiang), Chinese Magnoliavine (五味子, Wuweizi)——cough and asthma with profuse thin sputum caused by obstruction of cold fluid in the lung

Prescriptions: 1. Decoction of Ephedra, Aconite and Asarum (麻黄附子细辛汤, Mahuang Fuzi Xixin Tang)

2. Small Blue Dragon Decoction (小青龙汤, Xiaoqinglong Tang)

Notes: Manchurian Wildginger Herb (细辛, Xixin) can expel pathogenic cold in the interior as well as the exterior. It also has the functions of relieving pain and arresting cough. Its function of expelling pathogenic cold is much stronger than that of relieving the exterior syndrome and diaphoresis. Therefore it could not be considered as one of the important herbs for relieving the exterior syndrome. It is pungent and can activate yang. Thus it is usually applied to cases of the exterior syndrome due to yang deficiency and cough and asthma due to cold phlegm. It is also applied to headache, arthralgia and rhinorrhea to relieve pain. Using Manchurian Wildginger Herb(细辛, Xixin)with herbs of cold nature may modify the action of those herbs and disperse the stagnated fire.

Collected Decoction of Herbals (《本草汇言》, Bencaohuiyan) says, "with Dried Ginger(干姜,Ganjiang)and Cassia Bark(肉桂, Rongui), Manchurian Wildginger Herb(细辛,Xixin)can expel pathogenic cold in zang and fu organs. If it is used in combination with Prepared Daughter Root of Common Monkshood(附子, Fuzi), it can disperse pathogenic cold of various diseases, with Doubleteeth Pulbescent Angelia Root(独活, Duhuo), it can cure headache of Shaoyin; with Fineleaf Schizomepeta Herb (荆芥,Jingjie)and Divaricate Saposhnikovia Root(防风, Fangfeng), it can disperse pathogenic wind of various meridians; with Baikal Skullcap Root(黄芩, Huangqin), Coptis Rhizome(黄连, Huanglian), and Wild Mint(薄荷, Bohe), it can cure toothache due to pathogenic wind-fire and it has a remarkable effect on dispersing the stagnated heat of various meridians."

Both Manchurian Wildginger Herb(细辛,Xixin) and Ephedra(麻黄, Mahuang) have the functions of relieving the exterior syndrome and dispersing pathogenic cold. Ephedra(麻黄, Mahuang) mainly disperses pathogenic wind-cold of Taiyang meridian and is usually applied to the exterior excessive syndrome without sweating. Ephedra (麻黄,Mahuang)also promotes the dispersing function of the Lung and diuresis. Thus it can be applied to cough and asthma due to exterior pathogenic factors imparring the dispersing function of the Lung, and the exterior syndrome with edema. Manchurian Wildginger Herb(细辛, Xixin) mainly disperses wind-cold of the Shaoyin meridian. It has the functions of dredging the orifices to relieve pain, keeping the adverse qi downwards and removing phlegm. Thus it is applied to cases of fever with deep pulse due to pathogenic cold invading Shaoyin and cases of headache, pain of the body and stuffy nose due to wind-cold, cases of Bi syndrome due to wind-dampness, and cough and asthma due to water retention.

10. 荜茇, Biba

English name: Long Pepper Fruit

Pharmaceutical name: Fructus Piperis Longi

Botanical name: Piper longum L.

Properties and tastes: pungent, hot

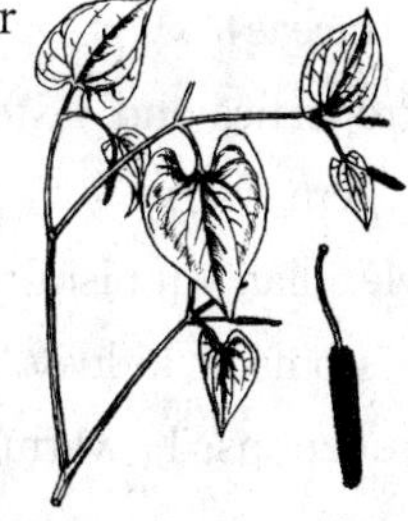

荜 茇

Meridian tropism: stomach, large intestine

Functions: warm the Middle-jiao and alleviate pain.

Indications: 1. cold syndrome of stomach and intestines-vomiting, hiccup, abdominal pain, diarrhea

2. pain of dental caries

Dosage: 3～6g

Combination: add Officinal Magnolia Bark(厚朴, Houpu), Common Aucklandia Root(木

香,Muxiang), Lesser Galangal Rhizome(高良姜, Gaoliangjiang)——cold syndrome of stomach and intestines

Notes: Long Pepper Fruit(荜茇,Biba) is pungent and hot. It tends to act on the gastrointestinal area. It functions to warm the Middle-jiao and disperse cold, especially chronic Stomach cold as well as stagnated cold of the Large Intestine. Thus it is applied to vomiting and abdominal pain due to Stomach cold. This herb can be used single-handed. The powder of it can relieve toothache by nasal feeding or being put into the tooth cavity. Thus Li Shizhen(李时珍) said, "it is one of the most important herbs for headache, rhinorrhea and toothache."

11. 荜澄茄, Bichengqie

English name: Mountain Spicy Tree Fruit

Botanical name: Litsea cubeba(Lour) Pers(Lauraceae)

Properties and tastes: pungent, warm

Meridian tropism: spleen, stomach, kidney, and bladder

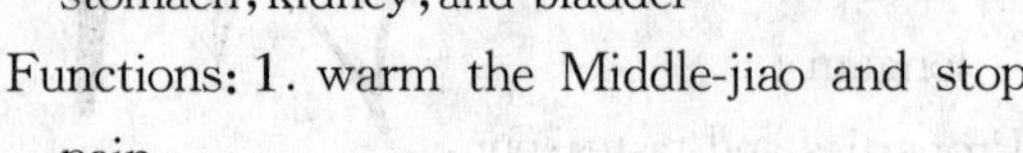

荜澄茄

Functions: 1. warm the Middle-jiao and stop pain

2. warm the bladder

Indications: 1. Stomach cold syndrome: vomiting, hiccups, pain of the epigastrium

2. difficulty in urination due to stagnation of cold

3. turbid urine due to stagnation of cold and dampness

4. colic pain of cold type

Dosage: 3～6g

Contraindication: Contraindicated in patients with interior heat due to yin deficiency.

Combinations: 1. add Lesser Galangal Rhizome (高良姜, Gaoliangjiang), Nutgrass Galingale Rhizome(香附, Xiangfu)——Stomach cold syndrome

2. add Cassia Bark(肉桂, Rongui), Tuckahoe(茯苓, Fuling)——difficult urine due to cold

3. add Sevenlobed Yam Rhizome(萆薢, Bixie), Grassleaf Sweetflag Rhizome(石菖蒲, Shichangpu)——turbid urine due to stagnation of cold and dampness

4. add Medicinal Evodia Root (吴茱萸, Wuzhuyu), Common Aucklandia Root (木香, Muxiang)——colic pain of cold type

Notes: Mountain Spicy Tree Fruit(荜澄茄, Bichengqie) is not only good at warming the Middlejiao and keeping the adverse qi downwards but also has the strong function of warming the kidney and urinary bladder and expelling cold to relieve pain. Thus it is applied to gastric pain, vomiting and hiccup due to Stomach cold and hernia due to cold. This simple herb is enough, however, it is usually applied to patients with herbs for warming the Middle-jiao and that of promoting the circulation of qi in a compound prescription.

Both Mountain Spicy Tree Fruit(荜澄茄, Bichengqie) and Long Pepper Fruit(荜茇, Biba) can warm the Middle-jiao and disperse cold and be applied to deficient cold syndrome in the Middle-jiao. The differences between them are as follows: Long Pepper Fruit(荜茇, Biba) is pungent, hot and strong, having the strong function of warming the Middle-jiao and expelling chronic and stagnated cold. Mountain Spicy Tree Fruit(荜澄茄, Bichengqie) is pungent and warm, having the functions of warming the Middle-jiao and keeping the adverse qi downwards, warming the spleen and Stomach and removing qi stagnation. It also can warm qi of the kidney and urinary bladder. It can be applied to cases of hernia and abdominal pain, difficulty in urination and turbid urine due to pathogenic cold.

Appendix: Other Drugs For Warming Interior

Name	Properties and tastes	Meridian tropism	Functions	Indications	Dosage	Contraindication
Common Monkshood's Mother Root (乌头, Wutou)	pungent, bitter, hot and with great poisonous	heart, liver, spleen	Clear away wind, eliminate cold and stop pain, arrest swelling	Bi syndrome, headache, abdominal pain, carbuncle (external use)	1.5~4.5g Decoct 30 to 60 minutes earlier than other herbs	It is as toxic as Prepared Daughter Root of Common Monkshood (附子, Fuzi) but more stronger, contraindicated during pregnancy. Not to combine with Tendrilleaf Fritillary Bulb (贝母, Beimu), Snakegourd Fruit (瓜蒌, Gualou), Pinellia Rhizome (半夏, Banxia), Japanese Ampelopsis Root (白蔹, Bailian), Bletilla Rhizome (白及, Baiji)
Galanga Galangal Fruit (红豆蔻, Hongdoukou)	pungent, warm	spleen, stomach	warm middle jiao and expel cold, regulate qi stop pain, and excite spleen	Damp heat cold attack middle jiao (warmer), epidemic and abdominal pain, vomit, diarrhea poor appetite	3~6g	It is forbidden for cases with interior heat due to yin deficiency.
Black Pepper Fruit (胡椒, Hujiao)	pungent, hot	stomach, large intestine	Warm middle jiao and arrest pain, antiepilepsy	abdominal, cold pain vomit, diarrhea, epilepsy	2~3g proper dosage for external use	Contraindicated in heat due to deficiency of yin
Star Anise (大茴香, Dahuixiang)	pungent, sweet, warm	liver, kidney, spleen	Eliminate cold, warm liver meridian, warm kidney, stop pain, regulate stomach qi, its function is similar to that of Fennel Fruit (小茴香, Xiaohuixiang) but more stronger	Cold hernia, abdominal pains, hernia in testis (scrotal hernia), vomiting, poor, appetite, epigastric region cold pain	3~9g	Contraindicated in yin deficiency, excessive fire. Overdosage will cause eyes injury and carbuncle.

Part Ⅲ
Drugs for Qi and Blood Diseases

Introduction: It is said in *Classic of Yellow Emperor* (内经, Neijing): The coordination between the qi and blood is vital for body health. Diseases occur because of the qi and blood deficiency, or qi and blood stagnation, or the adverse flow of qi and blood. We discussed deficiency deseases in the chapter on Tonics, so the last two kinds of diseases are the focuses of this chapter. The flow of the qi and blood is under the influence of the deficiency or excess of Zang and Fu organs, changes of the mood and hot or cold pathogens. Generally, qi stagnation proceeds blood stagnation, that is, blood circulation is driven by the flow of the qi, and blood stagnation is caused by qi stagnation. But diseases in the blood stage sometimes procced those in the qi stage. The key to the diagnosis is determining which one is the main pathogen and which one occurs first when qi and blood stagnation combine. Other diseases of qi and blood include the adverse flow of the qi due to qi stagnation and hemorrhage due to blood disorders. Different rules should be followed to lower the adverse flow of qi or to stop bleeding.

Qi, blood and body fluid are the only substances circulating in the human body, so diseases in the qi or blood stage influence the body fluid. Physicians should carefully seek to find the cause of phlegm and fluid retention.

Chapter 6
Drugs for Regulating Qi

Definition: Drugs with the functions of regulating the functional activities of qi and driving the flow of qi are called drugs for regulating qi. They are indicated for qi stagnation and reversed flow of qi due to disorders of the functional activities of qi.

Functions: Most drugs for regulating qi are fragrant in flavor and warm in nature with the functions of regulating the activities of qi to invigorate the spleen, promote the flow of qi to relieve pain, removing liver-qi stagnation, checking the upwardly adverse flow of qi, or dissolving mass due to the obstruction of qi.

Indications: Disorders of the functional activities of qi caused by dysfunction of Zang and Fu organs include a distress feeling in the chest, cough and asthma due to impairment of function of the lung, distending pain in the hypochrondrium and breasts, hernia pain and irregular menstruation due to stagnation of the liver-qi. In addition, there may be distending pain in the stomach and abdomen, belching and acid regurgitation, nausea and vomiting, constipation or diarrhea due to qi stagnation of the spleen and stomach. Qi stagnation generally manifests as an oppressed and distending feeling with pain; while the adverse flow of qi manifests as nausea and vomiting, hiccup or asthma.

Cautions: With different functions of promoting the flow of qi, removing qi stagnation and descending the upwardly adverse flow of qi, proper drugs should be chosen for qi stagnation in varying degrees.

Most drugs of regulating qi with pungent flavor are prone to excessively consume qi and yin, so they should be cautiously used for patients with qi deficiency or yin deficiency.

Liver, a yin organ of storing the blood, acts as a yang organ to regulate the flow of qi and blood, therefore, the treatment of qi stagnation which is generally closely related to the dysfunction of liver should be combined with drugs of nourishing yin and liver blood.

1. 橘皮, Jupi

English name: Tangerine Peel

Pharmaceutical name: Pericarpium Citri Reticulatae

Botanical name: Citrus reticulata Blanco which is a name for one of many orange or tangerine-like plants such as Citrus tangerina Hort. Et Tanaka or C. erythrosa Tanaka.

橘 皮

Properties and tastes: bitter, sour, warm

Meridian tropism: spleen, lung

Functions: 1. regulate the qi and normalize the function of the spleen and stomach, and improve digestion

2. eliminate the dampness and resolve phlegm, arrest asthma

3. inhibit staphylococci

4. increase blood pressure and exciting the heart

5. inhibit gastrospasm and enterospasm

6. prevent capillary hemorrhage by lowering the fragility of the capillary wall

7. anti-inflammatory and antiallergic functions

8. ulcer-preventive effect and cholagogic effect

Indications: 1. stagnation of qi in the stomach and spleen manifested as gastric and abdominal distention, poor appetite, nausea and vomiting, indigestion, abdominal pain and diarrhea

2. retention of damp pathogen in the Middle-jiao manifested as oppressed feeling in the chest, abdominal distension, poor appetite, lassitude, loose stool, and a thick greasy tongue coating

3. accumulation of phlegm-dampness characterized by cough, abundant expectoration, white sticky sputum, oppressed feeling in the chest and shortness of breath

Dosage: 3～9g

Contraindication: For patients with heat in the body, dry cough due to yin deficiency or asthma due to qi deficiency, Tangerine Peel (橘皮, Jupi) is not suggested for use.

Combinations: 1. add Fresh Ginger (生姜, Shengjiang)——vomiting of cold type and discomfort in the stomach

2. add White Mulberry Root-bark (桑白皮, Sangbaipi)——cough, asthma, and abundant expectoration due to lung heat

3. add Bamboo Shavings (竹茹, Zhuru)——gastric and abdominal distention, vomiting,

hiccup or pernicious vomiting

4. add Medicine Terminalia Fruit(诃子, Hezi)——hoarseness, and discomfort in the throat

5. add Immature Bitter Orange(枳实, Zhishi)——gastritis, enteritis and ulcers with distention and pain in the stomach and abdomen.

6. add Largehead Atractylodes Rhizome(白术, Baizhu)——poor appetite due to retention of dampness in the spleen and stomach

7. add Green Tangerine Peel(青皮, Qingpi)——distention and pain in the hypochrondrium, oppressed feeling in the chest and abdominal distention due to incoordination between the liver and spleen

8. add Dang-shen Root(党参, Dangshen) and Largehead Atractylodes Rhizome(白术, Baizhu)——cough and asthma due to reversed flow of qi with profuse and watery sputum

9. add Perilla Leaf(苏叶, Suye) and Tuckahoe(茯苓, Fuling)——cough, profuse sputum, vertigo and palpitation

10. add Licorice Root(甘草, Gancao)——acute mastitis

11. add Christina Loosetrife Herb(金钱草, Jinqiancao)——gallstones

12. add Chinese Eaglewood Wood(沉香, Chenxiang)——distention in the stomach and abdomen

Prescription: Erchen Decoction(二陈汤, Erchen Tang)

Notes: Green Tangerine Peel(青皮, Qingpi) noticed for regulating qi of the spleen and lung can be used to eliminate dampness and phlegm due to its drying flavor. Green Tangerine Peel(青皮, Qingpi) and Pinellia Rhizome(半夏, Banxia) are usually used in combination for damp-phlegm in the lung and phlegm retention in the stomach. They are called "two cheng"(two old ones) since aged drugs are preferred.

To prevent the impairment of qi or the stagnation of qi when regulating-qi drugs or invigorating-qi drugs are used. Dang-shen Root(党参, Dangshen) and Largehead Atractylodes Rhizome(白术, Baizhu) which can reinforce the spleen are combined for patients with qi deficiency.

Tangerine Peel(橘皮, Jupi) is used in a wide range. Li Shizhen(李时珍) said: Tangerine Peel(橘皮, Jupi) is effective for many kinds of diseases due to its regulating the flow of qi and eliminating dampness. To invigorate qi, it is combined with tonifying drugs; to purge qi stagnation, it is combined with purging drugs; to ascend the flow of qi, it is combined with ascending drugs; and to descend the flow of qi, it is combined with depressant drugs. So caution should be taken when Tangerine Peel(橘皮, Jupi) is combined with other drugs in the application.

In addition, Tangerine Seed(橘核, Juhe), with bitter flavor and warm nature, descends the flow of qi, dissolves the mass and relieves pain. It is used for hernia, distention and pain in testis and nodules of breast, Tangerine Peel(橘皮, Jupi) is also named Tangerine Peel(陈皮, Chenpi) and etc. 3～9g are prescribed every time.

2. 青皮, Qingpi

English name: Green Tangerine Peel

Pharmaceutical name: Pericaropium Citri Reticulatae Viride

Botanical name: Citrus reticulata Blanco which is a name for one of many orange or tangerine-like plants such as

Citrus tangerina Hort. Et Tanaka or C. erythrosa Tanaka.

Properties and tastes: bitter, pungent, warm

Meridian tropism: liver, gallbladder, and stomach

青 皮

Functions: 1. soothe the liver, relieve the stagnation of qi

2. relieve the internal stagnation

3. relax the smooth muscle of intestine

Indications: 1. distention feeling and pain in the chest and hypochondrium due to liver-qi stagnation or problems between the liver and stomach

2. distending pain in the breasts, acute mastitis, hyperplasia of mammary glands of hernia pain

3. full feeling and distending pain in the stomach due to dyspepsia

4. mass in the abdomen and hepatosplenomegaly

Dosage: 3～9g

Contraindication: Cautions should be taken for patients with hyperhidrosis or qi deficiency.

Combinations:

1. add Tumeric Root-tuber(郁金, Yujin) is combined for qi stagnation manifested as hypochrondric pain, pain in the liver area, cholecystitis and chronic hepatitis

2. add Chinese Thorowax Root(柴胡, Chaihu) is combined for intercostal neuralgia

3. add Tangerine Peel (陈皮, Chenpi) is combined for food stagnation, abdominal pain and dyspepsia

4. add Pangolin Scales(穿山甲, Chuanshanjia) is combined for swelling pain in the breasts and acute mastitis

5. add Common Burreed Rhizome(三棱, Sanleng) and Zedoray(莪术, Ezhu) are combined for cirrhosis, fatty liver, mass in the abdomen

6. add Fennel Fruit(小茴香, Xiaohuixiang) is combined for hernia pain

Prescription: Powder of Radix Bupleuri for Dispersing the Depressed Liver Qi(柴胡疏肝散, Chaihushugan San)

Notes: *Herbals for Easy Approaching* (《本草便读》, Bencaobiandu) says that: Green Tangerine Peel(青皮, Qingpi), with its warm nature and strong functions can be used for all that are caused by liver and gall bladder disorders such as hernia, phlegm retention, mass in the abdomen etc. It is said that injections made of Green Tangerine Peel(青皮, Qingpi) are effective for shock and supraventcular tachycardia.

Green Tangerine Peel(青皮, Qingpi) is the green skin of the immature fruit of the tangerine, and acts on the liver meridian with intense nature and strong functions of dissolving mass and relieving stagnation; while Tangerine Peel(橘皮, Jupi) is the yellow skin of the mature fruit acts on the spleen meridian with mild nature and drying flavor. It reinforces the spleen to relieve the dampness.

Green Tangerine Peel(青皮, Qingpi) is used for liver-qi stagnation and diseases along the liver meridian such as pain in the chest and hypochondrium, distention in the breasts, and hernia; while Tangerine Peel (橘皮, Jupi) is used for feeling of fullness and distending pain in the stomach and abdomen, oppressed feeling in the chest with abundant expectoration. They are combined in coordination between the liver and stomach.

3. 枳实, Zhishi

English name: Immature Bitter Orange

Pharmaceutical name: Fructus Citri seu Ponciri Immaturus

Botanical name: Citrus aurantium L., Poncirus trifoliata (L.) Raf., or C. wilsonii Tanaka

枳 实

Properties and tastes: bitter, pungent, and slightly cold

Meridian tropism: spleen, stomach, and large intestine

Functions: 1. relieve qi stagnation to remove food stagnation

2. resolve phlegm to relieve the feeling of fullness

3. strengthen the function of heart

4. increase blood pressure

5. promote urination

6. increase gastrointestinal peristalsis

7. increase uterine contraction

Indications: 1. abdominal distention and pain, eructation with fetid odor and constipation due to food stagnation

2. fullness and distending feeling in the abdomen due to dysfunction of the spleen and stomach in transporting and distributing nutrients

3. diarrhea and dysentery with tenesmus

4. obstruction of qi in the chest with the feeling of stiffness and fullness in the chest and upper abdomen, poor appetite and profuse phlegm due to obstruction of the flow of qi

5. gastroptosis, gastric dilatation, prolapse of rectum and hysteroptosis

6. the injection made of Immature Bitter Orange(枳实, Zhishi) can be used in the treatment of shock and heart failure

Dosage: 3～9g, 15g in some cases.

Contraindication: Cautions should be taken when it is prescribed for pregnant women.

Combinations: 1. add Largehead Atractylodes Rhizome(白术, Baizhu) and Baikal Skullcap Root(黄芩, Huangqin)——a fullness feeling in the chest, abdominal pain, diarrhea and dysentery due to the damp-heat of the spleen and stomach

2. add Nutgrass Galingale Rhizome(香附, Xiangfu) and Medicated Leaven(神曲, Shenqu)——dyspepsia, feeling of stiffness and fullness in the chest and upper abdomen

3. add Membranous Milkvetch Root(黄芪, Huangqi) and Shunk Bugbane Rhizome(升麻, Shengma)——gastroptosis, prolapse of rectum, and hysteroptosis

4. add Coptis Rhizome(黄连, Huanglian) and Pinellia Rhizome(半夏, Banxia)——yellow sticky phlegm and feeling of stiffness and fullness in the chest due to the accumulation of phlegm-heat in the chest

5. add Largehead Atractylodes Rhizome(白术, Baizhu)——dyspepsia, dysfunction of the spleen and stomach, hepatosplenomagaly, gastroptosis, prolapse of rectum

6. add Rhubarb(大黄, Dahuang) and Coptis Rhizome(黄连, Huanglian)——abdominal pain and dysentery with tenesmus

7. add Snakegourd Fruit(瓜蒌, Gualou) and Cassia Twig(桂枝, Guizhi)——chest pain, coronary heart diseases, angina cordis

8. add Officinal Magnolia Bark(厚朴, Houpo) and Rhubarb(大黄, Dahuang)——constipation due to heat, distention and pain in the abdomen

9. add Bamboo Shavings(竹茹, Zhuru)——nausea and vomiting due to stomach-heat and phlegm accumulation

Prescriptions: 1. Minor Decoction for Purgation(小承气汤, Xiaochengqi Tang)

2. Fructus Anrranttii Immaturus and Rhi-

zoma Atractylodis Macrocep Halae Pill(枳术丸,Zhizhu Wan)

Notes: Immature Bitter Orange (枳实, Zhishi), with intense functions of dissipating qi stagnation and promoting the flow of qi, is commonly used for dyspepsia, distention in the abdomen, dysentery with tenesmus due to accumulation of the damp-heat, and feeling of stiffness and fullness in the chest due to obstruction of the flow of qi by phlegm. Zhu Zhenheng, an ancient doctor, said: Immature Bitter Orange(枳实, Zhishi) is the herb which can purge the phlegm retention, dredge the orifice obstruction and relieve qi stagnation with the strength of destroying the wall of a building. Modern research indicates that it can increase heart contraction and increase blood pressure. Its injection is used for infectious shock and allergic shock by venous inflow. It is also used for visceroptosis due to its effect of increasing the rate of the smooth muscle contraction.

Bitter Orange(枳壳, Zhiqiao) is almost the same as Immature Bitter Orange(枳实, Zhishi) in flavor, nature and functions except that Immature Bitter Orange(枳实, Zhishi), with vigorous nature and bitter flavor, relieves qi stagnation to dissolve mass, resolves phlegm to relieve the feeling of fullness; while Bitter Orange(枳壳, Zhiqiao), with mild nature, regulates the flow of qi to relieve the distention and is used for mild cases of distending feeling in the chest and abdomen and food stagnation.

4. 佛手, Foshou

English name: Finger Citron Fruit

Pharmaceutical name: Fructus Citri Sarcodactylis

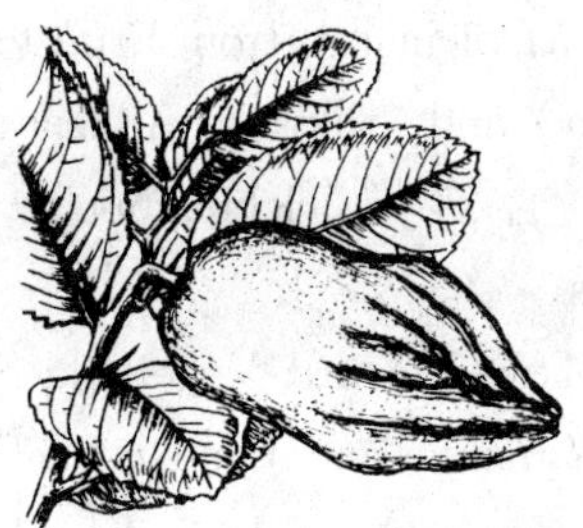

佛 手

Botanical name: citrus medica L. var. sarcodactylis(Noot.)Swingle

Properties and tastes: pungent, bitter, warm

Meridian tropism: liver, spleen, stomach, and lung

Functions: 1. soothe the liver and eliminate qi stagnation

2. promote the flow of qi to relieve pain

3. regulate the function of the stomach to promote digestion

4. relieve cough, reduce sputum and allay asthma

Indications: 1. dyspepsia: feeling of fullness and distention in the abdomen, poor appetite, eructation and stomach pain

2. chronic bronchitis, emphysema of lungs: cough with abundant expectoration

3. liver and gall bladder diseases: distention and pain in hypochondrium and abdomen

4. anxiety neurosis: mental depression, sighing

Dosage: 3~9g

Combinations: 1. add Hawthorn Fruit(山楂, Shanzha), Medicated Leaven(神曲, Shenqu) and Malt(麦芽, Maiya)——dyspepsia

2. add Pinellia Rhizome(半夏, Banxia) and Tuckahoe(茯苓, Fuling)——chronic bronchitis and emphysema of lungs

3. add Tumeric Root-tuber(郁金, Yujin) and Bitter Orange(枳壳, Zhiqiao)——liver and gall bladder diseases

4. add Medicinal Citron Fruit(香橼, Xiangyuan) and Silktree Albizia Immature Flower(合欢花, Hehuanhua)——anxiety neurosis

5. add Towel Gourd Vegetable Sponge(丝瓜络, Sigualuo) and Loquat Leaf(枇杷叶, Pipaye)——prolonged cough and chest pain

Notes: Finger Citron Fruit(佛手, Foshou), with fragrant flavor and mild nature, can relieve the qi stagnation of the spleen and stomach, soothe the liver to eliminate the qi stagnation, and promote the flow of qi to relieve pain. It is used especially for prolonged cough with profuse phlegm and chest pain due to its mild effect of eliminating dampness to reduce phlegm.

Finger Citron Fruit(佛手, Foshou) and Medicinal Citron Fruit(香橼, Xiangyuan), with similar fragrant flavor and functions for soothing the liver and regulating the flow of qi, and regulating the function of the stomach to eliminate phlegm, are often combined for mutual reinforcement in the treatment of liver-qi stagnation, or lack of cooperation between the liver and stomach, or cough due to damp-phlegm. The difference between them lies in that Finger Citron Fruit(佛手, Foshou) is more effective in regulating the flow of qi of the liver and stomach to reinforce the stomach and relieve pain; while Medicinal Citron Fruit(香橼, Xiangyuan) is more effective in regulating the flow of qi of the spleen and lung to eliminate the phlegm and stop cough.

5. 木香, Muxiang

English name: Common Aucklandia Root

Pharmaceutical name: Radix Saussureae seu Vladimiriae

Botanical name: There are two major types of plant used for this herb. One is Saussurea lappa Clark which is usually from Guangdong Province and the other is either Vladimiria souliei (Franch.) Ling or V. denticulata Ling which are from Sichuan Province. S. Lappa is also known as Aucklandiae lappa Decne.

木 香

Properties and tastes: pungent, bitter, warm

Meridian tropism: spleen, stomach, large intestine, gallbladder

Functions: 1. promote the flow of qi to relieve pain

2. regulate the function of the stomach to relieve qi stagnation

3. promote the gastrointestinal peristalsis

4. anti-inflammatory effect(Colibacillus and Bacillus dysenteriae)

Indications: 1. distending pain in the abdomen, qi stagnation in the spleen and stomach, indigestion

2. dyspepsia, poor appetite, vomiting, diarrhea, abdominal distention

3. dysentery with tenesmus

4. cholecystitis, cholelithiasis

5. gastroduodenal ulcer

6. It is added into the tonics to prevent the qi stagnation.

Dosage: 3～9g. The crude drug is used for relieving the qi stagnation, roasted one for tonifying the intestine to relieve diarrhea.

Contraindication: Caution should be taken for patients with hyperactivity of fire due to yin deficiency or body fluid deficiency.

Combinations: 1. add Green Tangerine Peel(青皮, Qingpi)——distending pain in the abdomen due to qi stagnation in the spleen and stomach

2. add Coptis Rhizome (黄连, Huanglian)——abdominal pain, dysentery with tenesmus
3. add Radish Seed(莱服子, Laifuzi)——abdominal distention, borborymus, dyspepsia, frequent intestinal flactus from anus
4. add Fennel Fruit (小茴香, Xiaohuixiang)——hernia pain
5. add Combined Spicebush Root (乌药, Wuyao)——abdominal pain due to adverse flow of qi
6. add Largehead Atractylodes Rhizome(白术, Baizhu)——poor appetite, distending pain in abdomen
7. add Dang-shen Root (党参, Dangshen) and Villous Amomum Fruit (砂仁, Sharen)——chronic diarrhea.
8. add Rhubarb(大黄, Dahuang) and Capillary Wormwood Herb (茵陈蒿, Yinchenhao)——cholecystitis and cholelithiasis.
9. add Areca Seed(槟榔, Binlang)——food stagnation, dysentery, and difficult defecation
10. add tonics to prevent the stagnation of qi

Prescription: Pill of Aucklandia and Areca (木香槟榔丸, Muxiang Pinglang Wan)

Notes: Common Aucklandia Root(木香, Muxiang) is a major herb with the function of promoting the flow of qi to relieve pain, and is mainly used for distending pain in the abdomen. The *Pearl Bag* (《珍珠囊》, Zhenzhunang) said: Common Aucklandia Root (木香, Muxiang) can disperse qi-stagnation, regulate the flow of qi of the whole body, normalize the function of the stomach and spleen, and purge the lung-qi. Modern research has shown that Common Aucklandia Root(木香, Muxiang) can promote gastriointestinal peristalsis and has an inhibitory effect on Colibacillus and Bacillus dysenteriae. To prevent qi stagnation, Common Aucklandia Root(木香, Muxiang) is added into the tonifying prescription to promote the flow of qi.

6. 香附, Xiangfu

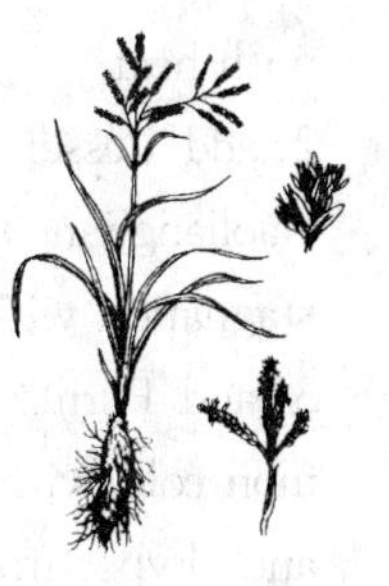
香附

English name: Nutgrass Galingale Rhizome

Pharmaceutical name: Rhizoma Cyperi Rotundi

Botanical name: Cyperus rotundus L.

Properties and tastes: pungent, slightly bitter, slightly sweet, medium

Meridian tropism: liver, San-jiao

Functions: 1. soothe the liver and regulate the flow of qi
2. regulate the flow of qi to disperse the stagnation
3. regulate menstruation and relieve pain
4. anti-inflammation effect and antipyretic effect
5. tranquilize the central nerve
6. cordial effect and reduce blood pressure

Indications: 1. liver-depressed syndromes: depression, restlessness, stress, distending pain in the hypochrondrium
2. incoordination between the liver and stomach: acid regurgitation, vomiting, eructation, hiccup, poor appetite, and distending pain in the stomach
3. pain due to qi stagnation: dysmenorrhea, distending pain in the breasts, stomach pain, hypochrondric pain, and hernia
4. irregular menstruation due to qi stagnation
5. common cold with qi stagnation

Dosage: 6 ~ 12g. Vinegar processed herb has better effect in relieving pain.

Contraindication: Cautions should be taken for patients without qi stagnation or with heat due to yin deficiency, or with proceeded menstrual cycle.

Combinations: 1. add Cape Jasmine Fruit (栀子, Zhizi)——stomache due to qi stagnation with heat

2. add Lesser Galangal Rhizome (高良姜, Gaoliangjiang)——stomach pain due to qi stagnation with cold or stomach spasm

3. add Perilla Leaf (苏叶, Suye)——common cold with distending pain in the chest and hypochrondrium, eructation, hiccup, poor appetite

4. add Chinese Angelica Root (当归, Danggui) and Argy Wormwood Leaf (艾叶, Aiye)——dysmenorrhea, irregular menstruation

5. add Chinese Thorowax Root (柴胡, Chaihu)——distending pain in the hypochondrium

6. add Fennel Fruit (小茴香, Xiaohuixiang)——hernia pain of cold type

7. add Snakegourd Fruit (瓜蒌, Gualou)——distending pain in the breasts

Prescription: Pill of Galangal and Nutgrass lastedge (良附丸, Liangfu Wan)

Notes: In Chinese medicine, Nutgrass Galingale Rhizome (香附, Xiangfu) is regarded as the first choice for woman diseases and diseases due to qi disorders. Nutgrass Galingale Rhizome (香附, Xiangfu) with the most mild nature of qi regulation can be used in the treatment of exterior or interior syndromes, excess or deficient syndromes, internal diseases or woman diseases which always become worsened under the influence of mental irritation. Studies have proved the anti-inflammation effect, analgetic effect and estrogen-like effect of Nutgrass Galingale Rhizome (香附, Xiangfu).

Nutgrass Galingale Rhizome (香附, Xiangfu) and Common Aucklandia Root (木香, Muxiang), with similar bitter and sour flavors, all can promote the flow of qi to relieve pain. Common Aucklandia Root (木香, Muxiang) can regulate the flow of qi in the Middle-jiao to disperse the qi stagnation and to promote digestion, and it is used for distending pain in the abdomen and dysentery with tenesmus; while Nutgrass Galingale Rhizome (香附, Xiangfu) can soothe the depressed liver, regulate menstruation to relieve pain, and is used for hypochondriac pain, irregular menstruation and dysmenorrhea.

7. 乌药, Wuyao

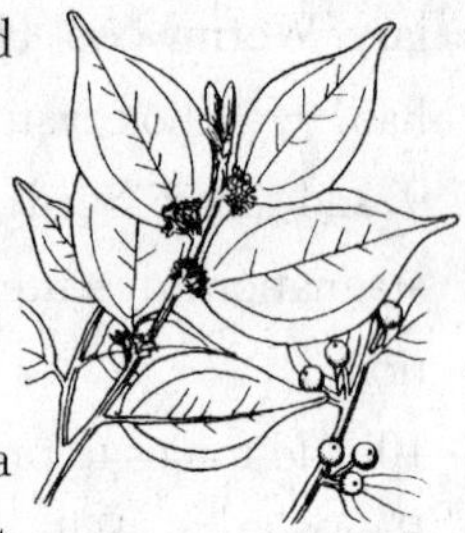

English name: Combined Spicebush Root

Pharmaceutical name: Radix Linderae Strychnifoliae

Botanical name: Lindera strychnifolia (Sieb. et Zucc.) Villar; in southeastern China L. chunii Merr. Is used instead.

乌 药

Properties and tastes: pungent, warm

Meridian tropism: lung, spleen, kidney, urinary bladder

Functions: 1. promote the flow of qi to relieve pain

2. disperse the cold evil to warm the kidney

3. dual regulation on gastrointestinal smooth muscle

Indications: 1. pain in the chest and abdomen: qi stagnation due to cold manifested as oppressed feeling in the chest, hypochondriac pain, distending pain in the abdomen, and hernia due to cold evil, dysmenorrhea, and etc.

2. frequency of micturition, enuresis with lassitude in loin and legs, cold extremities and aversion to cold due to kidney yang deficiency

Dosage: 3～12g

Contraindication: Cautions should be taken in condition of qi deficiency with heat.

Combinations: 1. add Sharpleaf Galangal Fruit (益智仁, Yizhiren)——kidney yang deficiency of cold type manifested as frequency of micturition, urinary incontinence and children enuresis

2. add Chinese Angelica Root(当归, Danggui)——cold pain in the abdomen due to derangement of qi and blood caused by cold pathogen, dysmenorrhea, and postpartum abdominal pain

3. add Common Aucklandia Root (木香, Muxiang)——lower abdominal pain due to adverse flow of qi

4. add Cassia Bark(肉桂, Rougui)——abdominal pain due to spleen and kidney yang deficiency, and lower abdominal pain of cold type

5. add Nutgrass Galingale Rhizome(香附, Xiangfu)——pain due to qi disorders

6. add Chinese Eaglewood Wood (沉香, Chenxiang)——an oppressed feeling in the chest, and cold pain in the abdomen

7. add Fennel Fruit(小茴香, Xiaohuixiang) and Tangerine Seed(橘核, Juhe)——hernia of cold type, abdominal pain, and a swelling pain of the scrotum

8. add Longstament Onion Bulb (薤白, Xiebai)——oppressed pain in the chest and hypochrondrium

Prescription: Linderae Powder(天台乌药散, Tiantaiwuyao San)

Notes: Though they have the same effect of promoting the flow of qi to relieve pain, Combined Spicebush Root(乌药, Wuyao) and Nutgrass Galingale Rhizome(香附, Xiangfu) act on different meridians. Nutgrass Galingale Rhizome(香附, Xiangfu) is effective for soothing the depressed liver, regulating menstruation to relieve pain; while Combined Spicebush Root(乌药, Wuyao) is known for warming and promoting the qi in the Lower-jiao, and relieving the qi stagnation of liver and kidney. So Nutgrass Galingale Rhizome (香附, Xiangfu) is used for stagnation of liver-qi, and Combined Spicebush Root(乌药, Wuyao) for qi stagnation with cold-dampness in the Lower-jiao, and Common Aucklandia Root(木香, Muxiang) for qi stagnation in the stomach.

8. 沉香, Chenxiang

English name: Chinese Eaglewood Wood

Pharmaceutical name: Lignum Aquilariae

Botanical name: Aquilaria agallocha Roxb. or A. sinensis(Lour.)Gilg

沉 香

Properties and tastes: pungent, bitter, warm

Meridian tropism: spleen, stomach, and kidney

Functions: 1. promote the flow of qi to relieve pain

2. descend the adverse flow of qi and regulating the qi in the Middle-jiao

3. warm the kidney yang to help inspiration to relieve asthma

Indications: 1. qi stagnation due to cold accumulation manifested as distending pain in the chest and abdomen, irregular menstruation, and lower abdominal pain

2. vomiting due to the cold in the stomach, hiccup

3. asthma due to failure of the kidney in receiving air

4. bronchial asthma

Dosage: 1 ~ 1.5g. It should be decocted later in a decoction, or to be taken after the fine powder is infused in boiling water and mixed with juice.

Contraindication: Chinese Eaglewood Wood (沉香, Chenxiang), with its sour flavor and warm nature, reinforces the heart in the body. So cautions should be taken for patients with hyperactivity of fire due to yin deficiency, or prolapse syndromes due to qi deficiency.

Combinations: 1. add Prepared Daughter Root of Common Monkshood (附子, Fuzi) and Cassia Bark (肉桂, Rougui)——dyspnea due to cold of deficiency type

2. add Villous Amomum Fruit (砂仁, Sharen) and Szechwan Chinaberry Fruit (川楝子, Chuanlainzi)——gastric and abdominal pain due to qi stagnation

3. add Combined Spicebush Root (乌药, Wuyao) and Ginseng (人参, Renshen)——an oppressed feeling in the chest, abdominal distention, frequent eructation, lassitude etc

4. add Clove Flower-bud (丁香, Dingxiang) and Cassia Bark (肉桂, Rougui)——acute gastritis, vomiting due to cold

5. add Desertliving Gistanche (肉苁蓉, Roucongrong)——constipation due to qi deficiency accompanied by shortness of breath, spontaneous perspiration, and lassitude

6. add Nutgrass Galingale Rhizome (香附, Xiangfu) and Villous Amomum Fruit (砂仁, Sharen)——stuffiness, distending pain in the chest, hypochondrium, and irregular menstruation

7. add Chinese Arborvitae Leafy Twig (侧柏叶, Cebaiye)——bronchial asthma

8. add Prepared Daughter Root of Common Monkshood (附子, Fuzi) and Actinolite (阳起石, Yangqishi)——impotence due to cold

9. add Horse Bezoar (马宝, Mabao)——hiccup, inatentative treatment of carcinoma of the esophagus (take powders of these two kinds of herbs in same quantity, 0.9 ~ 1.5g every time, tid.)

Prescription: Decoction of Calyx Kaki (柿蒂汤, Shidi Tang)

Notes: Chinese Eaglewood Wood (沉香, Chenxiang), with sour and fragrant flavor and warm nature, can descend the upwardly adverse flow of qi, relieve asthma and stop vomiting, and is used for pain in the chest and abdomen due to cold, vomiting, hiccup and asthma due to cold of deficiency type.

Chinese Eaglewood Wood (沉香, Chenxiang) and Combined Spicebush Root (乌药, Wuyao) both can warm the spleen and stomach, promote the flow of qi to relieve pain for symptoms such as distending pain in the chest and abdomen, asthma due to upwardly adverse flow of qi. Chinese Eaglewood Wood (沉香, Chenxiang) is noted for descending adverse flow of qi and warming the kidney yang to help inspiration to relieve asthma without excessive consumption of qi; while Combined Spicebush Root (乌药, Wuyao), with its extremely intense nature to travel through the whole body, is used for all diseases due to cold accumulation in San-jiao, qi obstruction or blood stagnation.

9. 川楝子, Chuanlianzi

English name: Szechwan Chinaberry Fruit

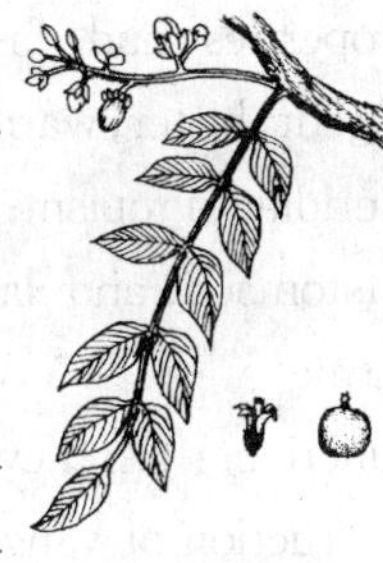
川楝子

Pharmaceutical name: Fructus Meliae Toosendan

Botanical name: Meliz toosendan Sieb. et Zucc.

Properties and tastes: bitter, cold, and slightly poisonous

Meridian tropism: liver, stomach, small intestine, urinary bladder

Functions: 1. promote the flow of qi to relieve pain

2. clear away the heat and purging the fire

3. functions on tinea and parasitosis

Indications: 1. pain syndromes: the liver fire or incoordination between the liver and spleen manifested as hypochondriac pain, gastric and abdominal pain and hernial pain

2. parasitosis

3. tinea capitis

4. acute mastitis

Dosage: 3 ~ 9g. Proper amount for external use.

Contraindication: With bitter flavor and cold nature, it is unsuitable for patients with spleen-yang deficiency. Long term use or taking in large quantity is not suggested due to its slight toxic effect.

Combinations:

1. add Yanhusuo(延胡索, Yanhusuo)——pain syndromes due to liver fire such as hypochondriac pain, epigastric pain or abdominal pain

2. add Nutgrass Galingale Rhizome(香附, Xiangfu)——liver-qi stagnation manifested as an oppressed feeling in the chest, frequent sighing, hypochondriac pain, distention feeling in the breasts, dysmenorrhea, hernia pain

3. add Medicinal Evodia Root(吴茱萸, Wuzhuyu) and Fennel Fruit(小茴香, Xiaohuxiang)——pain due to hydrocele testis, epididymitis, hernia

4. add Areca Seed(槟榔, Binlang)——abdominal pain due to parasitosis

5. add Szechwan Chinaberry Bark(苦楝皮, Kulianpi)——acute mastitis

Prescriptions: 1. Sichuan Chinaberry Powder (金铃子散, Jinlingzi San)

2. Decoction for Nourishing Liver and Kidney(一贯煎, Yiguan Jian)

Notes: Li Shizhen(李时珍) named it as one of the most effective herbs for pain in the chest and abdomen, and hernial pain, because it can clear away the heat in the small intestine and bladder and conduct the fire in the pericardium downwardly. The ointment made of the powder of the drug should be applied to the head where it has been cleared with saline for tinea in the head.

10. 荔枝核, Lizhihe

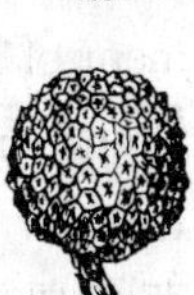
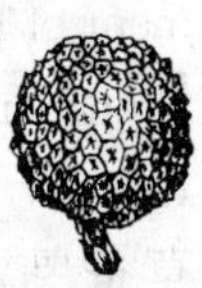
荔枝核

English name: Lychee Seed

Pharmaceutical name: Semen litchi Chinensis

Botanical name: Litchi chinensis Sonn.

Properties and tastes: sweet, astringent, warm

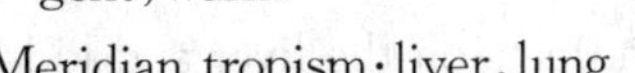

Meridian tropism: liver, lung

Functions: 1. dispel cold and disperse stagnation

2. regulate the flow of qi to disperse qi stagnation

3. relieve pain

Indications: Pain syndromes: hernia pain, distending pain in the testicle prolonged stomach pain, dysmenorrhea, and postpartum abdominal pain.

Dosage: 9 ~ 15g.

Contraindication: Cautions should be taken for patients without qi stagnation due to cold-dampness.

Combinations: 1. add Fennel Fruit (小茴香, Xiaohuixiang) and Medicinal Evodia Root (吴茱萸, Wuzhuyu)——hernia pain, and distending pain in the testicles due to cold accumulation in the Liver Meridian

2. add Chinese Gentian Root (龙胆草, Longdancao) and Cape Jasmine Fruit (栀子, Zhizi)——fire of excess in the liver meridian, downward flow of damp-heat manifested as distending pain in the testicles, and swelling of the scrotum

3. add Nutgrass Galingale Rhizome (香附, Xiangfu)——prolonged stomach pain due to liver-qi stagnation

4. add Nutgrass Galingale Rhizome (香附, Xiangfu)——premenstrual abdominal pain due to qi and blood stagnation or postpartum abdominal pain

Notes: Lychee Seed (荔枝核, Lizhihe), sweet in flavour and warm in nature, acts on the liver meridian and disperses qi stagnation in the liver meridian, and is used in the treatment of hernia due to cold accumulation the liver meridian and of distending pain in the testicle. *Essentials of Materia Medica* (《本草备要》, Bencaobeiyao) said: Lychee Seed (荔枝核, Lizhihe) acts on the liver and kidney meridians, and scatters the qi stagnation and dispels the cold evil. It is used for stomach pain, pain syndromes in the qi and blood stage of woman diseases.

11. 薤白, Xiebai

English: Longstament Onion Bulb

Pharmaceutical name: Bulbus Allii

Botanical name: Allium macrostemon Bge. or A. chinensis G. Don

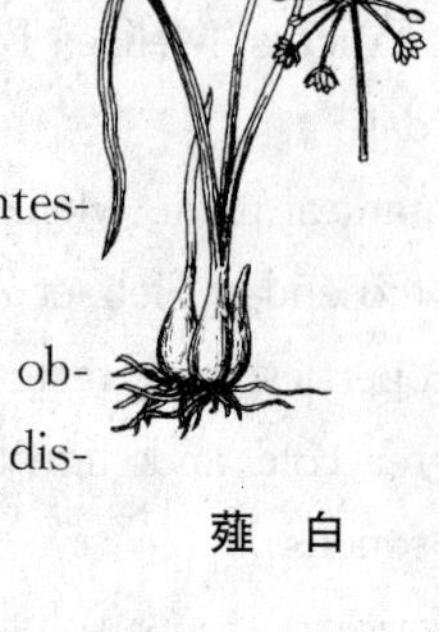

薤 白

Properties and tastes: pungent, bitter, warm

Meridian Tropism: lung, stomach, and large intestine

Functions: 1. relieve the obstruction of yang-qi to disperse accumulation of pathogen

2. promote the circulation of qi to remove stagnation

3. relieve asthma

4. anti-inflammatory effect

5. inhibitory effect on bacillus dysenteriac and staphlococcus

6. lower the blood lipid and have inhibitory action on platelet aggregation

Indications: 1. obstruction of qi in the chest: oppressed feeling in the chest, chest pain accompanied by cough and asthma due to accumulation of cold phlegm and distruction of yang in the chest. It is used in the clinic for coronary diseases and angina pectoris

2. prevent arteriosclerosis

3. bronchial asthma

4. dysentery

Dosage: 5～9g

Contraindication: It is not advisable for patients with qi deficiency and without qi stagnation, poor appetite due to dysfunction of stomach, or for patients who can not endure the odor of garlic.

Combinations: 1. add Snakegourd Fruit (瓜蒌, Gualou)——obstruction of qi in the chest, coronary disease and angina pectoris due to cold accumulation

2. add Coptis Rhizome (黄连, Huanglian) and Chinese Corktree Bark (黄柏, Huangbai)——dysentery, diarrhea with pus and blood stool

3. add Common Aucklandia Root(木香, Muxiang) and Immature Bitter Orange(枳实, Zhishi)——dysentery with tenesmus

4. add Trogopterus Dung(五灵脂, Wulingzhi) and Dan-shen Root(丹参, Danshen)——chest pain due to blood stagnation, and arterio scleorsis

5. add Sandalwood(檀香, Tanxiang)——obstruction of qi in the chest

Prescription: Decoction of Trichosanthis Allii Macrostemi and Rhizoma(瓜蒌薤白半夏汤, Guolou Xiebai Banxia Tang)

Notes: Longstament Onion Bulb(薤白, Xiebai), sour in flavor and warm in nature, is noted for scattering the stagnation, dispersing the obstruction of qi in the chest, dispelling the qi stagnation downwardly, and is regarded as the principal herb for the obstruction of qi in the chest. It is also used for cough with profuse phlegm, dysentery with tenesmus, qi stagnation in the Lower-jiao, and leukorrhea with reddish discharge. Presently, coronary disease, angina pectoris and intercostal neuralgia are the main indications in clinic.

12. 檀香, Tanxiang

English name: Sandalwood

Pharmaceutical name: Lignum Santali Albi

Botanical name: Santalum album L.

Properties and tastes: pungent, warm

檀 香

Meridian tropism: spleen, stomach, and lung

Functions: 1. regulate the flow of qi and coordinate the functions of the spleen and stomach

2. disperse the cold and relieve pain

Indication: pain syndromes——chest pain, abdominal pain, stomach pain, and angina pectoris due to qi stagnation

Dosage: 1～3g. Decocting for a longer time is not recommended. Proper amount for external use.

Combinations:

1. add Balloonflower Root(桔梗, Jiegeng) and Tumeric Root-tuber(郁金, Yujin)——chest pain

2. add Villous Amomum Fruit(砂仁, Sharen) and Combined Spicebush Root(乌药, Wuyao)——gastric and abdominal pain

3. add Long Pepper Fruit(荜茇, Biba) and Manchurian Wildginger Herb(细辛, Xixin)——angina pectoris

4. add Common Aucklandia Root(木香, Muxiang)——stomach pain due to qi stagnation

5. add Dan-shen Root(丹参, Danshen)——chest pain, stomach pain, angina pectoris

Notes: Sandalwood(檀香, Tanxiang), with sour flavor to dispel, and warm nature to disperse cold, can regulate qi of the diaphragm and scatter the qi obstruction in the chest, and promote the flow of qi to relieve pain. It also can excite the spleen and regulate the function of the Middle-jiao due to its fragant flavor, and is used for chest and diaphragm pain and stomach pain due to cold accumulation. For external use, it can stop bleeding.

Longstament Onion Buib(薤白, Xiebai) is noted for warming yang in the chest and scattering the blockage; while Sandalwood (檀香, Tanxiang) is noted for relieving the stagnation such as qi stagnation in the chest and diaphragm with cold pathogen. The functions of warming yang and relieving stagnation, reducing mass and relieving the obstruction of yang-qi are promoted when they are combined for the treatment of obstruction of qi in the chest.

13. 柿蒂, Shidi

English name: Persimmon Calyx and Receptacle
Pharmaceutical name: Calyx Diospyros Kaki
Botanical name: Diospyros kaki L.
Properties and tastes: bitter, astringent, medium

柿 蒂

Meridian tropism: stomach
Function: lower the upwardly adverse flow of qi and relieve hiccup
Indication: hiccup due to failure of descending the stomach-qi
Dosage: 6～12g
Combinations: 1. add Clove Flower-bud(丁香, Dingxiang)——cold in the stomach manifested as hiccups
2. add Reed Rhizome (芦根, Lugen) and Bamboo Shavings(竹茹, Zhuru)——heat in the stomach manifested as hiccups
Prescription: Decoction of Calyx Kaki(柿蒂汤, Shidi Tang)
Notes: Persimmon Calyx and Receptacle (柿蒂, Shidi), bitter in flavor and mild in nature, can lower the upwardly adverse flow of qi and is especially useful for relieving hiccups. *Seeking Truth of Herbals* (《本草求真》, Bencaoqiuzhen) said: Persimmon Calyx and Receptacle (柿蒂, Shidi) and Clove Flower-bud(丁香, Dingxiang) both can relieve hiccups. One is bitter and mild, while the other is sour and hot. When they are used in combination, it will be more effective for diseases with heat and cold at the same time. But Persimmon Calyx and Receptacle(柿蒂, Shidi) also acts as an adjuvant herb of Clove Flower-bud (丁香, Dingxiang) for cold diseases, and Clove Flower-bud(丁香, Dingxiang) acts as an adjuvant herb of Persimmon Calyx and Receptacle(柿蒂, Shidi) for heat diseases. Sometimes, it is effective when many herbs are in combination, and sometimes it is effective when only one kind of herb is used. So, the prescription should be given according to the nature of the diseases.

Appendix: Other Drugs For Regulating Qi

Name	Properties and tastes	Meridian tropism	Functions	Indications	Dosage	Contraindications
Medicinal Citron Fruit (香橼, Xiangyuan)	acid, slightly bitter sour, warm	Liver, spleen, lung	Smooth liver qi, regulate the functions of the middle-jiao, and remove phlegm	Indigestion, cough with profuse phlegm, distending pain in the abdomen and hypochoindriac, depression and making a deep sigh	3～9g	Be cautious for yin deficiency and blood-dryness case and pregnant women

Name	Properties and tastes	Meridian tropism	Functions	Indications	Dosage	Contraindications
Thickleaf Vladimiria Root (青木香, Qingmuxiang)	acid, bitter slightly cold	Liver, stomach	Promote the flow of qi to relieve pain, remove toxic substances and promote subsidence of swelling and descend the blood pressure	Distending pain in the chest, abdomen and hypochondriac area, food poisoning, snake-biting, hypertension	3～9g	Overdosage may cause gastrio-intestinal side effects. Don't overtake
Sword Jackbean Seed (刀豆子, Daodouzi)	sweet, warm	Stomach, kidney	Lower the upwardly adverse flow of qi and relieve hiccup	Hiccup due to cold of deficiency type, vomiting	9～15g	
Chinese Nardostachys Root and Rhizome or Spoonleaf Nardostachys Root and Rhizome (甘松, Gansong)	acrid, sweet, warm	Spleen, stomach	Promote the flow of qi to relieve pain, relieve stagnation and activate the spleen, tranquilize to relieve muscle spasm	Oppressed feeling in the chest due to qi stagnation distending pain in the stomach and abdomen, poor appetite. premature pulsation	3～6g	
Rugose Rose Flower (玫瑰花, Meiguihua)	sweet, slightly bitter, warm	Liver, spleen	Promote the flow of qi to scatter qi stagnation, regulate the flow of qi to relieve stagnation	Distending pain in the chest, stomach and hypochondriac, irregular menstruation, breast pain proceeding the menstruation period and relieving alcoholism	3～6g	
Plum Flower Bud (绿萼梅, Lüemei)	sour, astringent, medium	Stomach	Soothe the liver qi and regulate the functions of the stomach, regulate the flow of qi to scatter stagnation	Distending pain in the chest and hypochondriac, restlessness and globus hystericus	3～9g	
Aspongopus (九香虫, Jiuxiangchong)	salty, warm	Spleen, liver, kidney	Promote the flow of qi to relieve pain, warm the kidney yang	Oppressed feeling in the stomach, abdominal distention, chest and hypochondrac pain, stomach pain, aching pain in the lumbar region and knee joints, impotence	3～9g	

Chapter 7
Drugs for Treating Blood Disorders

Definition: Drugs which can adjust diseases in Blood System are divided into drugs for activating blood, removing blood stasis and hemostats. The former has the principal function of dredging blood vessels and dispersing stagnant blood. And the latter has the principal function of stopping internal and external bleedings.

Function: Drugs for activating blood and removing blood stasis play the effects of circulating blood, removing blood stasis with drastic drugs, dispersing stasis, clearing the meridians, removing obstruction of qi and blood, reducing swelling and relieving pain. Hemostatics have the effects of not only stopping bleeding, but also cooling blood, astrigenging, removing blood stasis and warming meridians.

Indications: Diseases in Blood System can be divided into four types: blood deficiency, blood heat, blood stasis and hemorrhage. It is advisable to tonify blood for blood deficiency, cool blood for blood heat, activate blood for blood stasis and stop bleeding for hemorrhage. Blood tonics and cooling-blood drugs are respectively listed into chapter 3 (drugs for Invigorating deficiency) and chapter 4 (drugs for clearing away heat). This chapter only introduces drugs for activating blood and removing blood stasis and hemostatics. Drugs for activating blood and removing blood stasis are indicated for stagnant blood syndrome. The main manifestations of it are pain (with fixed place) or numbness; mass found in the exterior or interior of the body, or hematoma caused by traumatic injury; hemorrhage with purplish dark clots; ecchymosis appeared in the skin and mucosa or purple tongue with spots.

Hemostatics are indicated for bleedings in both internal and external part of the body, such as hemoptysis, epistaxis, hematemesis, hematuria, hemafecia, metrorrhagia and metrostaxis, purpura and traumatic bleeding.

Cautions: 1. Qi and blood of the human body have a close relationship. Qi is the commander of blood. Circulation of qi leads to circulation of blood and stagnation of qi leads to stagnation of blood. Therefore, at the time of applying drugs for activating blood, drugs for circulating qi should be added in order to strengthen the function of circulating blood and removing stasis.

2. It is improper to prescribe drugs for activating blood and removing stasis to women with profuse menstruation. And these drugs should be avoided to pregnant women.

3. When drugs for activating blood and removing stasis are prescribed, stagnation of heat and cold should be distinguished. And select hemostatics by warming meridians or hemostatics by cooling blood.

4. When hemostatics are used, according to bleeding of blood-heat type of deficient cold type, of stagnant blood type or with continuous blood prostration, hemostatics should be properly selected by cooling blood, by warming meridians, by removing stagnation and by astringency.

5. When hemostatics by cooling blood drugs

and by astringent drugs are used, pay attention to the stagnation to avoid the side effect of hemostasis. If there is any sign of blood stasis, drugs for activating blood and removing stasis should be given as well.

Section 1
Drugs for Activating Blood and Removing Stasis

1. 川芎, Chuanxiong

English name: Szechwan Lovage Rhizome

Pharmaceutical name: Radix Ligustici Wallichii

Botanical name: Ligusticum wallichii Franch.

Properties and tastes: pungent, warm

川 芎

Meridian tropism: liver, gall bladder, and pericardium

Functions: 1. activate blood and circulate qi

2. expel wind and relieve pain

3. tranquilize and allay excitement

4. expand coronary artery and strengthen coronary blood flow

5. increase cerebral blood flow and relieve encephaledema

6. control platelet agglutination and inhibit thrombosis

7. expand peripheral blood vessels and reduce blood pressure

8. antiradiation function and bacteriostasis

Indications: 1. headache caused by wind-cold, wind-dampness, wind-heat and stagnant blood. If this drug is combined with other compatible drugs, it can also treat headache due to blood deficiency.

2. gynecological diseases——menoxenia, amenorrhoea, dysmenorrhea, dystocia and postpartum abdominal pain which belong to stagnation of qi and blood syndrome

3. coronary heart disease and angina pectoris

4. pricking pain in hypochondriac region caused by stagnation of qi and blood

5. cerebral thrombosis, cerebral embolism, ischemic cerebrovascular disease and transient cerebral ischemia

6. sequela of cerebrovascular accident numbness of limbs hemiplegia

7. arthralgia due to wind-cold and dampness, athrodynia of the body and limbs, and traumatic injury

8. carbuncle, cellulitis, skin diseases and swelling

Dosage: 3～9g

Contraindication: Contraindicated in cases of menorrhagia, bleeding diseases, and patients with vigorous fire due to yin deficiency as well as pregnant women.

Combinations: 1. add Nutgrass Galingale Rhizome (香附, Xiangfu)——abdominal pain due to postpartum stagnation of blood, menoxemia and dysmenorrhea

2. add Chinese Angelica Root (当归, Danggui)——impairment of fetus during pregnancy, dystocia and retention of placenta.

3. add Glabrous Greenbrier Rhizome (土茯苓, Tufuling)——headache due to liver depression and damp-heat

4. add Gypsum (石膏, Shigao)——headache and distention of head caused by wind-fire

5. add Tall Gastrodia Rhizome (天麻, Tian-

ma)——dizziness and headache caused by liver wind

6. add Manchurian Wildginger Herb(细辛, Xixin)——headache due to exogenous wind-cold

7. add Dahurian Angelica Root(白芷, Baizhi)——lingering migraine which has its onset with pricking pain when there is wind, and belongs to cold type

8. add Cassia Twig(桂枝, Guizhi)——arthralgia of the limbs and joints due to wind cold

9. add Spine Date Seed(酸枣仁, Suanzaoren) and Tuckahoe(茯苓, Fuling)——insomnia due to deficiency and restlessness

10. add Dandelion(蒲公英, Pugongying) and Snakegourd Fruit(瓜蒌, Gualou)——carbuncle, swelling, cellulitis

11. add Dan-shen Root(丹参, Danshen)——angina pectoris, coronary heart disease

12. add Chinese Thorowax Root(柴胡, Chaihu)——pain in the chest and hypochondriac region

13. add Peach Seed(桃仁, Taoren), Frankincense(乳香, Ruxiang) and Myrrh(没药, Moyao)——pain and swelling due to traumatic injury

14. add Medicated Leaven(神曲, Shenqu)——diarrhea due to dampness

15. add Twotooth Achyranthes Root(牛膝, Niuxi)——retrograde menstruation

16. add Safflower(红花, Honghua)——amenorrhoea

17. add Chinese Angelica Root(当归, Danggui) and Membranous Milkvetch Root(黄芪, Huangqi)——numbness of the limbs, hemiplegia

18. add Chrysanthemum Flower(菊花, Juhua)——headache due to wind heat

19. add Peach Seed(桃仁, Taoren) and Safflower(红花, Honghua)——headache due to blood stagnation

20. add Scorpion(全蝎, Quanxie)——trigeminal neuralgia

Prescriptions: 1. Powder of Radix Bupleuri for Dispersing the Depressed Liver Qi(柴胡疏肝散, Chaihushugan San)

2. Chuanxiong Mixture(川芎茶调散, Chuanxiongchatiao San)

3. Decoction Containing Four Drugs(四物汤, Siwu Tang)

Notes: Szechwan Lovage Rhizome(川芎, Chuanxiong) has the action of activating blood, regulating qi and expels wind. Dr. Li Shizhen(李时珍) called it as "qi drug within blood". Dr. Zhang Yuansu(张元素) summarized its function as "ascending upward to the head and eyes, descending downward to the Sea of Blood. As it is pungent, dispersing and ascending in property, it is said that "Szechwan Lovage Rhizome(川芎, Chuanxiong) must be used for headache." It is the first drug to be selected for headache caused by wind-cold, wind-damp and stagnation of qi and blood. *The Complete Works of Jingyue*(《景岳全书》, Jingyuequanshu) says "both Szechwan Lovage Rhizome(川芎, Chuanxiong) and Chinese Angelica Root(当归, Danggui) are drugs for blood. But the dispersing function of Szechwan Lovage Rhizome(川芎, Chuanxiong) is stronger than that of Chinese Angelica Root(当归, Danggui). Thus it can expel wind-cold, treat headache, scatter blood stasis, smooth blood vessels, remove accumulated qi, relieve pain, evacuate pus, reduce swelling, eliminate blood stagnation and dredge meridians. Decoct it with Manchurian Wildginger Herb(细辛, Xixin), it can be used to treat pain caused by trauma".

2. 乳香, Ruxiang

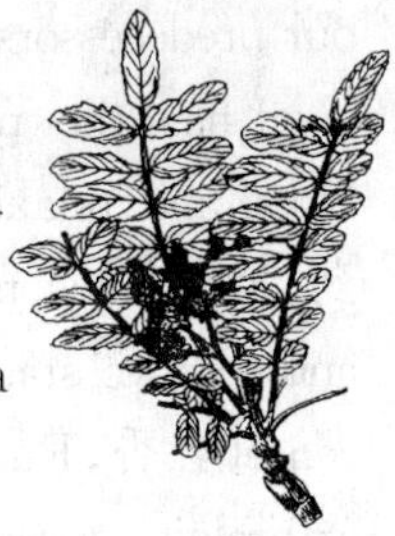

English name: Olibanum, Frankincense

Pharmaceutical name: Gummi Olibanum

Botanical name: Boswellia carterii Birdw.

Properties and tastes: pungent, bitter, warm

乳 香

Meridian tropism: heart, liver, and spleen

Functions: 1. activate blood and relieve pain

2. reduce swelling and promote tissue regeneration

Indications: 1. pain syndrome——epigastric pain, arthralgia due to wind-dampness, traumatic pain, swelling pain due to carbuncle and cellulitis, pain caused by acute appendicitis and hepatalgia after hepatitis

2. gynecological syndrome due to stagnation of blood——dysmenorrhea, amenorrhoea and postpartum abdominal pain, etc.

3. unhealed cellulitis (external application to the affected area)

Dosage: 3～9g. Proper amount should be given for external use.

Contraindication: This drug has a bitter taste and the liquid becomes turbid when it is decocted in water. It may cause vomit for those with sensitive stomach. So a large dosage is not advisable. It should be cautiously used for patients with sensitive stomach. It should not be used for pregnant women and those without blood stagnation.

Combinations: 1. add Chinese Angelica Root (当归, Danggui), Szechwan Lovage Rhizome (川芎, Chuanxiong), Nutgrass Galingale Rhizome (香附, Xiangfu)——dysmenorrhea and amenorrhoea

2. add Szechwan Chinaberry Fruit (川楝子, Chuanlianzi), Yanhusuo (延胡索, Yanhusuo)——epigastric pain

3. add Rhizome or Root of Forbes Notopterygium (羌活, Qianghuo), Chinese Angelica Root (当归, Danggui)——arthralgia due to wind-cold and dampness, pain in the limbs and joints

4. add Myrrh (没药, Moyao), Safflower (红花, Honghua)——traumatic pain

5. add Myrrh (没药, Moyao), Mush (麝香, Shexiang)——carbuncle, cellulitis with swelling and pain

6. add Honeysuckle Flower (金银花, Jinyinhua), Weeping Forsythia Capsule (连翘, Lianqiao)——acute appendicitis

7. add Myrrh (没药, Moyao)——promote the function of Zang and fu organs, smooth meridians. It is used for all kinds of pain in the heart, stomach, hypochondrium, abdomen, limbs and joints. The powder is applied externally to the affected area to treat unhealed skin diseases.

Notes: In addition to its action to activate blood and remove blood stagnation, Frankincense (乳香, Ruxiang) has the action of not only activating blood removing blood stasis, but also circulating qi and dispersing stagnation of qi. It is good for the treatment of pain syndrome caused by stagnation. It is used in internal medicine gynecology, surgery and traumatology. Dr. Li Shizhen (李时珍) said: "The fragrant smell of Frankincense (乳香, Ruxiang) goes into the heart meridian to activate blood and relieve pain. That is why it is a principal drug to treat pain caused by carbuncles, cellulitis and cardiac and abdominal pain."

3. 没药, Moyao

English name: Myrrh

Pharmaceutical name: Myrrha

Botanical name: Commiphora myrrha Engl. or Balsamodendron ehrenbergianum Berg.

Properties and tastes: bitter, medium

Meridian tropism: heart, liver, and spleen

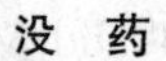

没 药

Functions: 1. activate blood and relieve pain

2. subdue swelling and promote the regeneration of tissues

3. reduce blood-lipid

Indications: 1. pain syndrome——dysmenorrhea, amenorrhoea, gastric and abdominal pain, arthralgia due to wind-damp, pain caused by traumatic injury, swelling pain caused by carbuncle and cellulitis, abdominal pain caused by acute appendicitis.

2. resistant cellulitis

3. hyperlipemia

Dosage: 3～9g. Proper dosage for external use.

Contraindication: The contraindications are the same as that of Frankincense (乳香, Ruxiang). When Myrrh (没药, Moyao) is used in combination together with Frankincense (乳香, Ruxiang), the dosage of the two drugs should be decreased accordingly because they have almost the similar functions.

Combinations: 1. add Safflower (红花, Honghua)——cardiac and abdominal pain caused by blood stasis, amenorrhoea and dysmenorrhea.

2. add Nutgrass Galingale Rhizome (香附, Xiangfu), Yanhusuo (延胡索, Yanhusuo)——gastric pain due to stagnation of blood and qi.

Notes: The function of this drug is similar to that of Frankincense (乳香, Ruxiang). Thus the two are used together to treat various kinds of pain caused by blood stagnation. According to the experience (summed up) by our predecessors, Frankincense (乳香, Ruxiang) has the main function of activating blood and relaxing tendons and Myrrh (没药, Moyao) is mainly used to dispel blood and remove stagnation. Therefore, Frankincense (乳香, Ruxiang) is often used to treat arthralgia caused by wind-dampness and Myrrh (没药, Moyao) is used to treat gastric pain caused by blood stagnation.

4. 延胡索, Yanhusuo

English name: Yanhusuo

Pharmaceutical name: Rhizoma Corydalis Yanhusuo

Botanical name: Corydalis yanhusuo W. T. Wang; in northeastern China C. bulbosa Dc. Or C. Ambigua Cham. et Schlecht. Var. amurensis Maxim are used locally.

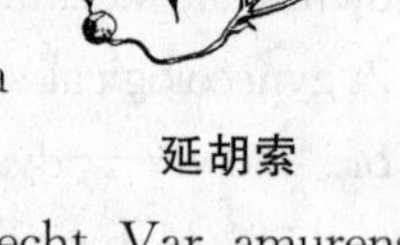

延胡索

Properties and tastes: pungent, bitter, warm

Meridian tropism: heart, liver, and spleen

Functions: 1. activate blood and promote the circulation (flow) of qi

2. relieve pain

3. induce sleep and tranquilize the mind

4. relax muscles

5. expand coronary artery, increase blood flow and decrease coronary resistance.

6. anti-gastric ulcer function has effect on gastric ulcer

Indications: 1. pain syndrome——dysmenorrhea, pain in the chest and hypochondriac region, hernia pain, swelling pain caused by traumatic injury, arthralgia due to wind-dampness, abdominal pain due to acute appendicitis and pain in the limbs or whole body pain caused by stagnation of qi and blood.

2. hypertention in earlier stage

3. angina pectoris, coronary heart disease

4. atrial early beating and paroxysmal auricular fibrillation

Dosage: 6 ~ 9g. Each time take 1.5 ~ 3g of powder with warm water. Its effect of relieving pain is strengthened if it is stir-baked with vinegar.

Contraindication: This drug is contraindicted in pregnant women.

Combinations: 1. add Frankincense (乳香, Ruxiang), Myrrh (没药, Moyao), Sappan Wood (苏木, Sumu)——traumatic injury and pain caused by stagnation and swelling.

2. add Nutgrass Galingale Rhizome (香附, Xiangfu), Chinese Angelica Root (当归, Danggui), White Peony Root (白芍药, Baishaoyao)——abdominal pain during menstruation.

3. add Cassia Bark (肉桂, Rougui), Common Aucklandia Root (木香, Muxiang), Chinese Angelica Root (当归, Danggui)——stagnation of qi and blood, cardiac and abdominal pain, hernia pain, sore and pain of the four limbs.

4. add Snakegourd Fruit (瓜蒌, Gualou), Longstament Onion Bulb (薤白, Xiebai), Dan-shen Root (丹参, Danshen)——disention feeling and pain in the chest, angina pectoris.

5. add Lesser Galangal Rhizome (高良姜, Gaoliangjiang), Dried Ginger (干姜, Ganjiang)——cold pain in the abdomen.

6. add Chinese Taxillus Twig (桑寄生, Sangjisheng), Twotooth Achyranthes Root (牛膝, Niuxi)——pain in the lower limbs.

7. add Szechwan Chinaberry Fruit (川楝子, Chuanlianzi), Nutgrass Galingale Rhizome (香附, Xiangfu)——epigastric pain

8. add Immature Bitter Orange (枳实, Zhishi), Tumeric Root-tuber (郁金, Yujin)——hypochondriac pain and hepatalgia

9. add Cassia Twig (桂枝, Guizhi), Rhizome or Root of Forbes Notopterygium (羌活, Qianghuo)——pain in the upper limbs.

10. add Fennel Fruit (小茴香, Xiaohuixiang), Combined Spicebush Root (乌药, Wuyao)——swelling pain of scrotum caused by cold hernia

11. add Szechwan Lovage Rhizome (川芎, Chuanxiong)——headache

12. add Bletilla Rhizome (白及, Baiji)——gastro-duodenal ulcer

13. add Common Selfheal Fruit-spike (夏枯草, Xiakucao)——early hypertension

14. add Dan-shen Root (丹参, Danshen), Safflower (红花, Honghua), Szechwan Lovage Rhizome (川芎, Chuanxiong)——angina pectoris coronary heart disease

15. add Dan-shen Root (丹参, Danshen), Hawthorn Fruit (山楂, Shanzha)——arrhythmia

Prescription: Sichuan Chinaberry Powder (金铃子散, Jinlingzi San)

Notes: This drug has the action of both to promote the circulation of qi and to activate the blood and effect of relieving pain. Dr. Li Shizhen (李时珍) said: " Yanhusuo (延胡索, Yanhusuo) can activate blood and qi, which belongs to the first class of drugs", and "It is wonderful to use it to treat all kinds of pain no matter whether it is in interior or exterior of the body". In the recent years, clinically it is often used with drugs for activating blood and qi to treat coronary heart diseases and relieve angina pectoris. Modern pharmacological research shows that this drug also has the function of inducing sleep, to tranguilethe mind and to relax muscles.

Yanhusuo(延胡索, Yanhusuo), Frankincense (乳香, Ruxiang), Myrrh (没药, Moyao) and Trogopterus Dung (五灵脂, Wulingzhi) all have the effect of activiting blood and relieving pain, but with different degrees. Yanhusuo(延胡索, Yanhusuo) has the strongest effect of relieving pain. Trogopterus Dung(五灵脂, Wulingzhi) has less effect, Frankincense (乳香, Ruxiang), Myrrh(没药, Moyao) have the least effect.

5. 郁金, Yujin

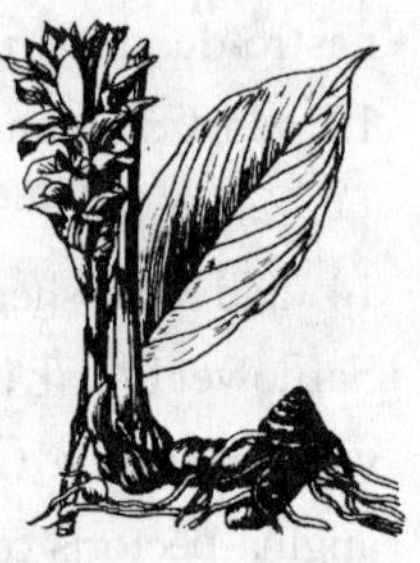
郁 金

English name: Turmeric Root-tuber

Pharmaceutical name: Tuber Curcumae

Botanical name: Curcuma longa L., C. aromatica Salisb., or less frequently C. zedoaris (berg) Rosc.

Properties and tastes: pungent, bitter, cold

Meridian tropism: heart, liver, and gallbladder

Functions: 1. activate blood and relieve pain

2. circulate qi and relieve depression

3. cool blood and clear away the heart-fire

4. cholagogue function and treat jaundice

Indications: 1. stagnation of qi and blood syndrome——distentional pain in the chest, abdomen and hypochondriac region, irregular menstruation and dysmenorrhea

2. coronary heart disease and angina pectoris

3. hepatosplenomegaly, jaundice and cholelithiasis

4. damp-warm disease——lethargy and unconciousness caused by invasion of damp-heat to the pericardium

5. epilepsy and madness

6. hemorrhage syndrome——hematemesis, epistaxis, hematuria and vicarious menstruation caused by depression of liver qi, which transforms into heat and leads to bleedings.

Dosage: 6～12g.

Contraindication: It is incompatible with Clove Flower-bud(丁香, Dingxiang)

Combinations: 1. add Capillary Wormwood Herb(茵陈蒿, Yinchenhao), Wrinkled Gianthyssop Herb (藿香, Huoxiang)——to treat jaundice, hypochondriac pain, as well as fullness in the chest, oliguria and poor appetite which are caused by damp-warm disease

2. add Tree Peony Bark (牡丹皮, Mudanpi), Cape Jasmine Fruit (栀子, Zhizi)——macular eruption caused by febrile disease, hematemesis and epistaxis

3. add Christina Loosetrife Herb (金钱草, Jinqiancao), Common Aucklandia Root (木香, Muxiang)——cholelithiasis

4. add Rehmannia Dried Root (生地黄, Shengdihuang), Twotooth Achyranthes Root (牛膝, Niuxi)——hematemesis, epistaxis, hematuria and retrograde menstruation caused by blood-heat and stasis

5. add Dan-shen Root (丹参, Danshen), Turtle Carapace (鳖甲, Biejia)——hepatosplenomegaly

6. add Green Tangerine Peel (青皮, Qingpi), Tangerine Peel (橘皮, Jupi)——invasion of liver qi to the stomach, distentional pain in the epigastrium and hypochondriac region

7. add Chinese Angelica Root (当归, Danggui), Nutgrass Galingale Rhizome (香附, Xiangfu)——oligmenstruation and abdominal pain for women

8. add Balloonflower Root (桔梗, Jiegeng), Snakegourd Fruit (瓜蒌, Gualou)——

hypochondriac pain after hepatitis

9. add Safflower (红花, Honghua), Snakegourd Fruit(瓜蒌, Gualou)——coronary heart disease, angina pectoris

10. add Centipede (蜈蚣, Wugong)——spasm due to epilepsy

11. add Grassleaf Sweetflag Rhizome(石菖蒲, Shichangpu)——unconsciousness of epidemic encephalitis and encephalitis B

Prescription: Rhizoma Acori Graminei and Radix Curcumae Decoction(菖蒲郁金汤, Changpu Yujin Tang)

Notes: The function of Tumeric Root-tuber(郁金, Yujin) is similar to those of Zedoray(莪术, Ezhu) and Turmeric Rhizome(姜黄, Jianghuang). They have the actions of activating blood, removing blood stasis, promoting circulation of qi and relieving pain. They are indicated for stagnation of qi and blood syndrome. But Tumeric Root-tuber(郁金, Yujin) is cold in property, used for dispersing qi of liver, relieving depression, cooling blood, clearing away heart-fire, cholagogic function and treating jaundice. Thus, it is used for unconsciousness during febrile disease and jaundice caused by stagnation of qi and blood together with heat syndromes. Zedoray(莪术, Ezhu) and Turmeric Rhizome(姜黄, Jianghuang) have the property of warmth and are mainly used for all kinds of pain syndromes caused by stagnation of qi and blood together with cold syndromes. Zedoray(莪术, Ezhu) has a strong effect which can scatter blood stasis and ablate stagnations.

6. 姜黄, Jianghuang

English name: Turmeric Rhizome

Pharmaceutical name: Rhizoma Curcumae

Botanical name: Currcuma longa L. or C. aromatica Salisb.

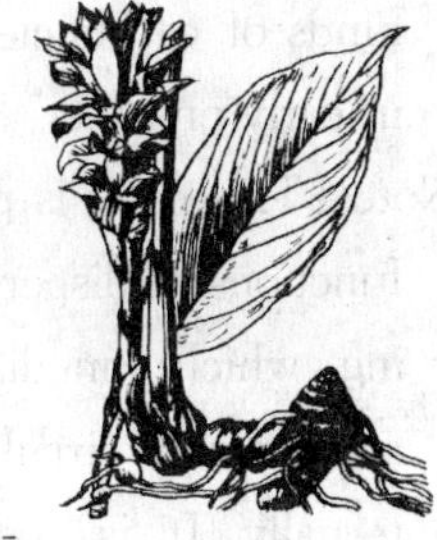

姜黄

Properties and tastes: pungent, bitter, warm

Meridian tropism: liver, spleen

Functions: 1. disperse bloods stasis and promote circulation of qi

2. dredge meridians and relieve pain

3. reduce blood-lipid

4. anti-angina pectoris

5. anti-inflammation

6. excite the uterus

Indications: 1. pain due to blood stagnation——pain in the chest and hypochondriac region, amenorrhea, abdominal pain and traumatic injury

2. arm pain due to wind-dampness——rheumarthritis, periomethritis

3. early onset of carbuncles, cellulitis and furuncle——reduce swelling and relieve pain if applied externally

4. angina pectoris and coronary heart disease

Dosage: 6 ~ 9g. Proper dosage for external use.

Contraindication: Do not use for women with menorrhagia and during pregnancy.

Combinations: 1. add Chinese Angelica Root (当归, Danggui), Safflower (红花, Honghua), Yanhusuo (延胡索, Yanhusuo)——pain due to blood stagnation

2. add Rhizome or Root of Forbes Notopterygium(羌活, Qianghuo), Chinese Angelica Root(当归, Danggui), White Peony Root(白芍药, Baishaoyao)——arm pain due to wind-dampness

3. add Rhubarb(大黄, Dahuang), Dahurian Angelica Root(白芷, Baizhi), Snakegourd Root(天花粉, Tianhuafen)——Grind into powder for external application to treat all

kinds of carbuncles, cellulitis and furuncles in early onset

Notes: This drug is pungent in taste, with the functions of dispersing, warming and dredging, which can dispel wind-cold externally and activate circulation of qi and blood internally. It is good to treat pain on the shoulder and in the arm.

7. 莪术, Ezhu

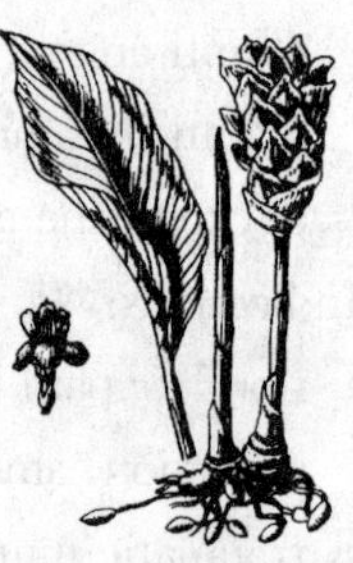
莪 术

English name: Zedoary

Pharmaceutical name: Rhizoma Curcumae Zedoariae

Botanical name: Curcuma zedoaria (Berg.) Rosc.

Properties and tastes: pungent, bitter, warm

Meridian tropism: liver, spleen

Function: 1. scatter and remove blood stasis
2. circulate qi and relieve pain
3. ablate stagnation and invigorate stomach
4. antitumor function
5. antithrombosis
6. antibacteria
7. increase the number of white blod cells (WBC)

Indications: 1. abdominal pain of amenorrhoea caused by stagnation of qi and blood
2. distention, fullness and pain in epigastrium and abdominal region caused by inability of the spleen to transport and transform the retained food
3. cervix cancer, ovarian cancer, leukemia, lymphadenoma and liver cancer, etc.
4. hepatosplenomegaly, abdominal mass
5. coronary heart diseases

Dosage: 3～9g. To bath this drug in vinegar may strengthen its function of relieving pain.

Contraindication: Do not use for women with menorhagia and during pregnancy.

Combinations: 1. add Green Tangerine Peel (青皮, Qingpi)——fullness, suffocation and pain in the chest and abdomen caused by stagnation of qi
2. add Coptis Rhizome (黄连, Huanglian), Medicinal Evodia Root (吴茱萸, Wuzhuyu)——acid regurgitation
3. add Common Aucklandia Root (木香, Muxiang), Officinal Magnolia Bark (厚朴, Houpo)——retention of food, borborygmus, distention pain in the epigastrium
4. add Common Burreed Rhizome (三棱, Sanleng)——hepatosplenomegaly, abdominal pain due to retention of food, amenorrhoea resulting from blood stasis, cancer or tumor
5. add Common Burreed Rhizome (三棱, Sanleng), Turtle Carapace (鳖甲, Biejia)——tumor and masses
6. add Common Burreed Rhizome (三棱, Sanleng), Szechwan Lovage Rhizome (川芎, Chuanxiong)——amenorrhoea and abdominal pain caused by stagnation of qi and blood
7. add Chinese Angelica Root (当归, Danggui), Red Peony Root (赤芍药, Chishaoyao), Szechwan Lovage Rhizome (川芎, Chuanxiong)——oligomenorrhoea, amenorrhoea complicated by pain in the lower abdomen, mental depression, wiry pulse or mass in the lower abdomen

Notes: Zedoray (莪术, Ezhu) has the actions both of dispersing, removing blood stasis, activating the circulation of qi and relieving pain. Hence it is used for pain caused by stagnation of qi and blood and mass syndrome. Modern research indicates that it has the effect of preventing tumour and thrombosis and increasing white blood cells (WBC).

8. 三棱, Sanleng

English name: Common Burreed Rhizome

Pharmaceutical name: Rhizoma Sparganii

Botanical name: Sparganium simplex Huds., S. Stoloniferum Buch.-Ham., or S stenophyllum Maxim. In some regions Scirpus flabiatilis (Torr.) is used locally in place of this herb.

三 棱

Properties and tastes: bitter, medium

Meridian tropism: liver, spleen

Functions: 1. dissipate and remove blood stasis

2. activate the flow qi and relieve pain

3. inhibit growth of cancer cells

Indications: 1. stagnant blood syndrome——amenorrhoea, abdominal pain and abdominal mass

2. syndrome of food retention——distentional pain in the epigastrium and abdomen

3. primary liver cancer, stomach cancer and carcinoma of the esophagus

Dosage: 3～9g

Contraindication: Do not use for women with menorrhagia or who are pregnant.

Combinations: 1. add Zedoray (莪术, Ezhu)——hepatosplenomegaly, abdominal pain due to retention of food, amenorrhea resulting from blood stasis, swelling due to cancer

2. add Green Tangerine Peel (青皮, Qingpi), Malt (麦芽, Maiya)——retention of food due to stagnation of qi, distentional pain in epigastrium and abdomen

3. add Dang-shen Root (党参, Dangshen), Largehead Atractylodes Rhizome (白术, Baizhu)——weakness of spleen and stomach, retention of food due to stagnation of qi

Notes: The effect of this drug is same as that of Zedoray (莪术, Ezhu) and the two are often used together. In the detailed comparison, Common Burreed Rhizome (三棱, Sanleng) has stronger effect in scattering blood stasis and Zedoray (莪术, Ezhu) is stronger in activating qi and relieving pain. It is said in *Annotation on Shennong's Herbal Classic* (《本草经疏》, Bencaojingshu): "Common Burreed Rhizome (三棱, Sanleng) can be used to treat blood disease with blood drugs and treat qi disease with qi drugs. Blood stasis, qi obstruction or food retention cause all kinds of the masses. Drugs with bitter flavor have the function of expelling, drugs with pungent flavor have the function of dispersing, drugs with sweat flavor have the function of regulating and benifitting the spleen, therefore, it can treat all kinds of hard masses caused by obstruction or retention."

9. 丹参, Danshen

English name: Dan-shen Root

Pharmaceutical name: Radix Salviae Miltiorrhizae

Botanical name: Salvia miltiorrhiza Bge.

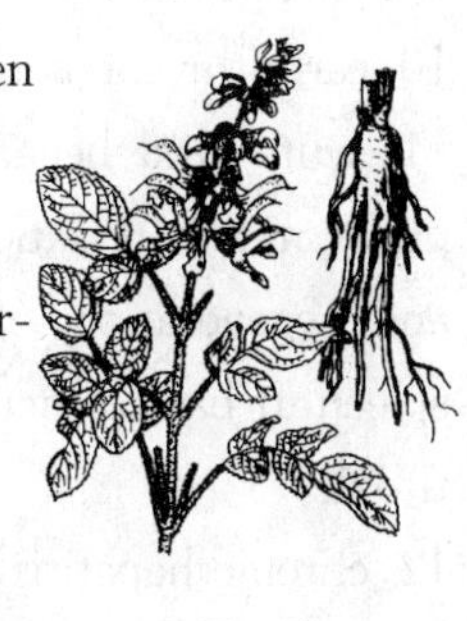

丹 参

Properties and tastes: bitter, slightly cold

Meridian tropism: heart, liver

Functions: 1. activate blood and dredge meridians

2. cool blood and subdue swelling

3. clear away heart fire and calm the mind

4. expand blood vessels, increase coronary

blood flow and lower blood pressure

5. tranquilize and ease pain

Indications: 1. angina pectoris, coronary heart disease——caused by obstruction of collaterals due to blood stagnation

2. obstruction of qi in the chest, cardialgia and epigastric pain——caused by stagnation of qi and blood

3. gynecological disease——menoxemia, amenorrhoea due to blood stasis, hysteromyoma and postpartum abdominal pain due to stagnation and hysteromyoma

4. abdominal mass

5. ischemic apoplexy, cerebral thrombosis

6. viral myocarditis, chronic pulmonary heart disease

7. neurasthenia——palpitation, insomnia, restlessness which belong to insufficiency of heart blood

8. epidemic febrile disease——high fever, restlessness, insomnia and even unconsciousness, delirium, dull macular eruption, deep red tongue, all caused by invasion of the Ying and Blood System by pathogenic heat

9. hypertention, atheroscleorsis

10. early thrombosed obliterative angiitis

11. acute viral hepatitis (this drug can improve microcirculation, promote renovation and regeneration of tissues, retract liver spleen. It has a function of antivirus and antitoxic)

12. chronic hepatitis, early cirrhosis (can relieve hepatic pain, retract liver and spleen)

13. arthralgia due to wind-damp-heat, red swelling and hot pain in joints

14. swelling and pain due to sores, carbuncles as well as due to traumatic injury and stagnation

Dosage: 6～15g.

Contraindication: This drug should be used cautiously for patients with hemorrhage disease and it is antagonistic to Black Falsehellebore (藜芦, Lilu).

Combinations: 1. add Tree Peony Bark (牡丹皮, Mudanpi)——yin deficiency and blood heat, low fever which fails to be reduced, or invasion of the Ying and Blood System by pathogenic heat, macular eruption, hematemesis, epistaxis or red, swelling and pain of joints due to heat arthralgia

2. add Rosewood (降香, Jiangxiang), Sanchi Root (三七, Sanqi)——angina pectoris, coronary heart disease

3. add Chinese Angelica Root (当归, Danggui)——postpartum lochiorrhea

4. add Nutgrass Galingale Rhizome (香附, Xiangfu)——dysmenorrhea

5. add Chinese Magnoliavine (五味子, Wuweizi), Spine Date Seed (酸枣仁, Suanzaoren)——neurasthenia

6. add Lobed Kudzuvine Root (葛根, Gegen)——diabetis manifested by dark tongue or with spots, ecchymosis

7. add Snakegourd Fruit (瓜蒌, Gualou), Pangolin Scales (穿山甲, Chuanshanjia)——acute mastitis, sores

8. add Common Burreed Rhizome (三棱, Sanleng), Zedoray (莪术, Ezhu)——abdominal mass

9. add Capillary Wormwood Herb (茵陈蒿, Yinchenhao), Tumeric Root-tuber (郁金, Yujin), Indigowoad Root (板蓝根, Banlangen)——acute and chronic hepatitis, pain in the two sides of hypochondriac region

10. add Frankincense (乳香, Ruxiang), Myrrh (没药, Moyao), Peach Seed (桃仁, Taoren)——ectopic pregnancy, abdominal pain and amenorrhoea due to blood stasis

11. add Weeping Forsythia Capsule (连翘, Lianqiao), Honeysuckle Flower (金银花,

Jinyinhua)——carbuncle, swelling, sore and toxin

12. add Suberect Spatholobus Stem(鸡血藤, Jixueteng), Chinese Angelica Root(当归, Danggui), Figwort Root(玄参, Xuanshen)——early thrombosing obliterative angitis

13. add Suberect Spatholobus Stem(鸡血藤, Jixueteng), Magnetite(磁石, Cishi)——hypertension

14. add Sandalwood(檀香, Tanxiang)——gastralgia due to stagnant blood, angina pectoris

15. add Szechwan Lovage Rhizome(川芎, Chuanxiong)——ischemic apoplexy, cerebral thrombosis

Prescriptions: 1. Drink of Red Sage Root(丹参饮, Danshen Yin)

2. Tonic Pill for Mental Discomfort(补心丹, Buxin Dan)

Notes: Dan-shen Root(丹参, Danshen) acts on blood stages of the heart and liver, and has the action of cooling blood, activating blood, removing blood stasis, promoting blood production. Its property is neutral and it is a principle drug in harmonizing the blood system. The forefathers said that one Dan-shen Root(丹参, Danshen) plays the effect of Decoction Containing Four Drugs(四物汤, Siwu Tang). It is said in *Herbals for Easy Approaching* (《本草便读》, Bencaobiandu): "Although Dan-shen Root(丹参, Danshen) has the mild function of tonifying blood and strong function of activating blood, which is a main drug to adjust blood system. The main reason why it is used to treat arthralgia and stagnations is that it has the functon of promoting blood circulation"

Dan-shen Root (丹参, Danshen) and Szechwan Lovage Rhizome(川芎, Chuanxiong) are both drugs for activating blood and are used to treat all kinds of pain due to blood stagnation. But Szechwan Lovage Rhizome(川芎, Chuanxiong) is warm in property and good for treating stagnation of qi and blood due to congealing. Dan-shen Root(丹参, Danshen) is cold in property and good for treating stagnation due to blood heat. Szechwan Lovage Rhizome (川芎, Chuanxiong) can be used to expel wind and relieve pain, so that it is indicated for headache. Dan-shen Root(丹参, Danshen) can be used to clear away the heart-fire, calm the mind and treat unconsciousness due to blood heat in combination with Szechwan Lovage Rhizome(川芎, Chuanxiong). Dan-shen Root(丹参, Danshen) and Tumeric Root-tuber(郁金, Yujin) are used together to treat pain in the chest and hypochondriac region and mental disorder. But Dan-shen Root(丹参, Danshen) is mainly used to activate blood, relieve pain, and calm the mind. Tumeric Root-tuber(郁金, Yujin) is mainly used to regulate qi, relieve pain, and induce resuscitation with fragrant flavor.

10. 虎杖, Huzhang

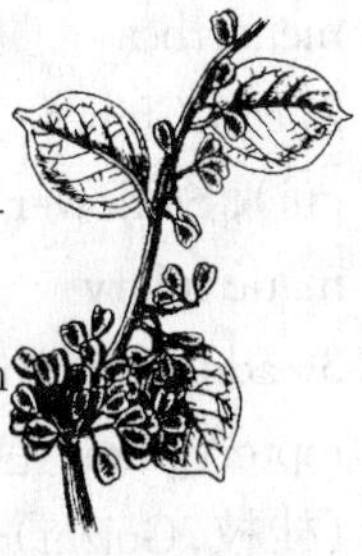

English name: Giant Knotweed Rhizome

Pharmaceutical name: Rhizoma Polygoni Cuspidati

Botanical name: Polygonum cuspidatum Sieb. et Zucc.

Properties and tastes: bitter, cold

虎 杖

Meridian tropism: liver, gallbladder, and lung

Functions: 1. activate blood and ease pain

2. clear away heat and remove dampness

3. detoxificate and reduce swelling

4. remove phlegm and relieve cough
5. relieve constipation by purgation
6. benefit gallbladder to treat jaundice
7. promote urine and remove gallbladder stone
8. broad spectrum bacteriostasis

Indications: 1. amenorrhoea and dysmenorrhea due to blood stasis
2. jaundice due to damp-heat and cholelithiasis
3. difficulty and pain in micturition, stranguria with turbid urine and morbid leukorrhea, urolith caused by accumulation of damp-heat in urinary bladder
4. scald by water and fire, sore, carbuncle, swelling, toxins and bite by venomous snake
5. cough due to lung heat
6. constipation due to accumulation of heat
7. arthralgia caused by wind-dampness and swelling pain due to traumatic injury
8. infection in biliary tract, chronic hepatitis, epidemic jaundice hepatitis

Dosage: 9～30g

Contraindication: Do not use for pregnant women.

Combinations: 1. add Motherwort Herb(益母草, Yimucao), Nutgrass Galingale Rhizome(香附, Xiangfu)——amenorrhoea and dysmenorrhea
2. add Chinese Angelica Root(当归, Danggui), Safflower(红花, Honghua)——traumatic injury
3. add Rhizome or Root of Forbes Notopterygium(羌活, Qianghuo), Cassia Twig(桂枝, Guizhi)——arthralgia due to wind-damp
4. add Capillary Wormwood Herb(茵陈蒿, Yinchenhao), Christina Loosetrife Herb(金钱草, Jinqiancao)——jaundice due to damp-heat, cholelithiasis, urinary calculus
5. add Sevenlobed Yam Rhizome(萆薢, Bixie), Coix Seed(薏苡仁, Yiyiren)——thin and white morbid leukorrhea
6. add Baikal Skullcap Root(黄芩, Huangqin), Honeysuckle Flower(金银花, Jinyinhua)——cough with yellow sputum due to lung heat
7. add Rhubarb(大黄, Dahuang)——constipation due to accumulation of heat
8. add Capillary Wormwood Herb(茵陈蒿, Yinchenhao), Rhubarb(大黄, Dahuang)——biliary infection
9. add Chinese date(大枣, Dazao)——chronic hepatitis

Notes: For treating scald, select proper amount of the fresh and cleaned Giant Knotweed Rhizome(虎杖, Huzhang) to grind into paste with strong tea water and put it on the affected area, or grind the fresh or dry drug into powder and spread it on the affected area. For sore, toxic and snakebite, it can be taken orally or pound the fresh drug into pieces for external application. According to modern pharmacological research, this drug has the effect of antibacteria, antivirus, easing cough, relieving asthma, tranquilizing and decreasing cholesterol as well as stopping bleeding. Giant Knotweed Rhizome(虎杖, Huzhang) is similar to Rhubarb(大黄, Dahuang) in property, effect and also in their chemical components. But it is weaker than Rhubarb(大黄, Dahuang) in purgation. Function of Giant Knotweed Rhizome(虎杖, Huzhang) is between clearing away heat to detoxificate and purging by bitter flavor and cold property.

11. 益母草, Yimucao

English name: Motherwort Herb

Pharmaceutical name: Herba Leonuri Heterophylli

Botanical name: Leonurus heterophyllus Sweet

Properties and tastes: pungent, bitter, and slightly cold

Meridian tropism: heart, liver, and urinary bladder

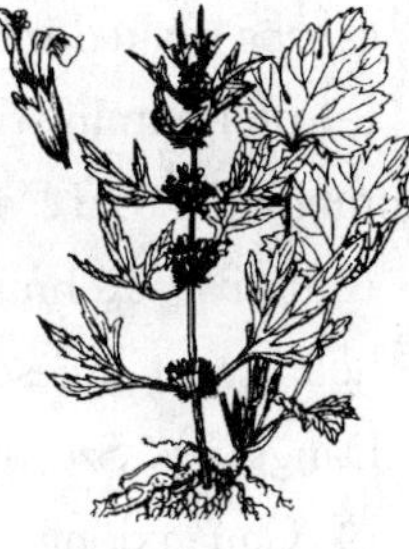
益母草

Functions: 1. activate blood and regulate menstruation

2. promote urine and reduce swelling

3. clear away heat and detoxificate

4. expel wind and relieve itching

5. stimulate an uterus

6. antimyocardial ischemia and antiangina pectoris

7. antithrombosis

Indications: 1. gynecological stagnant blood syndrome——menoxemia, irregular menstruation, distentional pain in lower abdomen, amenorrhoea, abdominal pain due to postpartum stagnation and lochiostasis

2. acute nephritis edema, difficulty in urination

3. swelling and toxin of sores, carbuncles, itching skin

4. angina pectoris, coronary heart disease

5. traumatic injury

Dosage: 9～15g. Decoct it into paste or use it to make a pill. Pound the proper amount of this herb for external application or decoct it in water for external washing.

Contriandication: Do not use for pregnant women.

Combinations: 1. add Rehmannia Dried Root (生地黄, Shengdihuang), White Peony Root(白芍药, Baishaoyao), Chinese Angelica Root (当归, Danggui)——menoxenia, diseases before and after childbirth

2. add Szechwan Lovage Rhizome (川芎, Chuanxiong), Chinese Angelica Root(当归, Danggui), Charred Hawthorn Fruit (山楂炭, Shanzhatan)——postpartum abdominal pain, subinvolution of uterus

3. add Charred Hawthorn Fruit (山楂炭, Shanzhatan), Argy Wormwood Leaf(艾叶, Aiye), Chinese Angelica Root(当归, Danggui)——postpartum hemorrhage or lochiorrhea, distentional pain in the abdomen caused by inertia of uterus

4. add Lalang Grass Rhizome (白茅根, Baimaogen), Baikal Skullcap Root (黄芩, Huangqin)——acute nephritis, edema.

5. add Christina Loosetrife Herb(金钱草, Jinqiancao)——haematuria due to nephrolithiasis

6. add Nutgrass Galingale Rhizome(香附, Xiangfu), Chinese Angelica Root (当归, Danggui)——stagnation of qi and blood manifested as menoxenia, distentional pain in the abdomen before menstruation, postpartum abdominal pain and traumatic injury

Notes: This drug disperses by its pungent flavor and descends by its bitter flavor. With slippery nature, it is good for gynecological diseases. So it is named "benefiting mother", or "female herb". It has the action of activating blood and removing liquid to promote menstruation, which make it an important drug for menstruation and delivery. In the recent years, it has been clinically used to treat coronary heart disease, hypertension and edema in cases of nephropathy. In addition, its seed is called Leonurus Furit (茺蔚子 Chongweizi) with a sweet flavor and slightly cold property. *Shennong's Herbal Classic* (《神农本草经》, Shennongbencaojing) says: "It has the function of brightening eyes, benefiting essence and removing water-qi", which is almost the same indication of Motherwort Herb (益母草,

Yimucao) but with a little bit more of tonifying function. But *Essentials of Materia Medica* (《本草备要》, Bencaobeiyao) says "*Shennong's Herbal Classic* (《神农本草经》, Shennongbencaojing) indicates it has the function of brightening eyes and tonification within circulation, and is used for stagnation of liver blood and for irrigation of blood to the pupil. If there is no stagnation, the tonification function doesnot play its effect".

12. 鸡血藤, Jixueteng

English name: Suberect Spatholobus Stem

Pharmaceutical name: Radix et Caulis Jixuetent

Botanical name: Millettia dielsiana Harms, Millettia reticulata Benth., Mucuna birdwoodiana Tutcher, or Spatholobus suberectus Dunn.

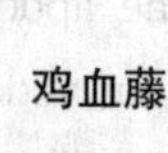

鸡血藤

Properties and tastes: bitter, medium

Meridian tropism: heart, liver, lung, large intestine

Functions: 1. circulate and tonify blood

2. relax the muscles and smooth collaterals

3. remove stasis and regulate menstruation

4. induce white blood cells (WBC)

Indications: 1. gynecological diseases——menoxenia, irregular menstruation, dysmenorrhea, amenorrhoea, which are caused either by blood stasis, blood deficiency or by blood deficiency complicated by stagnation

2. arthralgia due to wind-damp

3. numbness of hands and feet, paralysis of limbs and body

4. leukopenia after radiotherapy

5. coronary heart disease

Dosage: 9～15g. The largest dosage is 30g. It can be soaked into wine or decocted in paste for oral administration.

Combinations: 1. add Prepared Rhizome of Adhesive Rehmannia (熟地黄, Shoudihuang). Chinese Angelica Root (当归, Danggui), Szechwan Lovage Rhizome (川芎, Chuanxiong)——amenorrhoea, menoxenia and dysmenorrhea caused by blood deficiency or blood stagnation

2. add Rhizome or Root of Forbes Notopterygium (羌活, Qianghuo), Doubleteeth Pulbescent Angelica Root (独活, Duhuo)——arthralgia due to wind-dampness

3. add Cassia Twig (桂枝, Guizhi), Mulberry Twig (桑枝, Sangzhi)——numbness of hands and feet due to blood deficiency or blood stasis

4. add Tuber Fleeceflower Root (何首乌, Heshouwu), Earth Worm (地龙, Dilong)——paralysis

5. add Glossy Privet Fruit (女贞子, Nuzhenzi), Largehead Atractylodes Rhizome (白术, Baizhu)——leukopenia after radiotherapy

6. add Szechwan Lovage Rhizome (川芎, Chuanxiong)——coronary heart disease

Notes: This drug is bitter and sweet in flavor and warm in property. It has the function not only of activating and tonifying blood, but also of relaxing muscles and smoothing collaterals and is especially good at activating blood. It is indicated for amenorrhoea, dysmenorrhea and delayed menstruation caused by blood deficiency complicated by stagnation, as well as numbness of the limbs and body, arthralgia of wind-dampness type and hemiplegia which are due to unnourishment of tendons by blood in old people or a weak person. Modern pharmacological research shows that it has the functions of exciting uterus, triqulizing the mind, hypnosis and reducing blood pressure.

13. 桃仁, Taoren

English name: Peach Seed

Pharmaceutical name: Semen Persicae

桃 仁

Properties and tastes: bitter, medium

Meridian tropism: heart, liver, lung, and large intestine

Functions: 1. activate blood and remove blood stasis

2. loosen the bowel to relieve constipation

3. stop cough and relieve asthma

4. expand blood vessels and increase blood flow volume

Indications: 1. gynecological stagnant blood syndrome——dysmenorrhea, amenorrhoea due to blood stagnation, postpartum abdominal pain due to blood stasis, hysteromyoma, pelvic mass, ovarian cyst

2. internal carbuncle——pulmonary abscess, acute appendicitis

3. traumatic injury

4. constipation due to intestinal dryness

5. cough and asthma

Dosage: 6～9g. Pound into pieces and decoct it with water

Contraindication: Contraindicated in pregnant women

Combinations: 1. add Rhubarb (大黄, Dahuang), Tree Peony Bark (牡丹皮, Mudanpi)——acute appendicitis

2. add Rhubarb (大黄, Dahuang), Ground Beetle (䗪虫, Zhechong)——abdominal fullness and pain due to blood stagnation

3. add Safflower (红花, Honghua)——swelling pain with blood stagnation caused by traumatic injury, amenorrhoea and dysmenorrhea due to blood stagnation, angina pectoris and stomach-ache cause by stagnation of heart blood

4. add Cassia Twig (桂枝, Guizhi), Tuckahoe (茯苓, Fuling), Tree Peony Bark (牡丹皮, Mudanpi)——hysteromyoma and cophocytic cyst

5. add Hemp Seed (火麻仁, Huomaren), Chinese Angelica Root (当归, Danggui), Immature Bitter Orange (枳实, Zhishi)——constipation due to intestinal dryness after delivery, after illness or in aged people, especially constipation caused by internal accumulation of stagnant heat after traumatic injurry

6. add Safflower (红花, Honghua), Szechwan Lovage Rhizome (川芎, Chuanxiong), Chinese Angelica Root (当归, Danggui)——amenorrhoea, dysmenorrhea due to blood stagnation, abdominal pain due to stagnation after delivery

7. add Ephedra (麻黄, Mahuang), White Mulberry Root-bark (桑白皮, Sangbaipi)——cough, respiratory asthma

8. add Reed Rhizome (芦根, Lugen), 冬瓜, Coix Seed (薏苡仁, Yiyiren)——pulmonary abscess

9. add Ginseng (人参, Renshen)——cough and asthma due to lung deficiency

10. add Dan-shen Root (丹参, Danshen), Peach Seed (桃仁, Taoren)——vasculitis

11. add Apricot Seed (杏仁, Xingren)——all kinds of pain caused by stagnation of qi and blood, chronic tracheitis, constipation due to consumption of body fluid, and esophagus cancer

Prescriptions: 1. Peech Seed and Safflower Decoction of Four Ingredients (桃红四物汤, Taohongsiwu Tang)

2. Semen Pericae Decoction for Purgation

(桃仁承气汤,Taohechengqi Tang)

Notes:Peach Seed(桃仁,Taoren)has a strong effect in removing stasis. It is often used to treat diseases caused by obstruction due to blood stagnation. Pulmonary abscess and acute appendicitis are often caused by existance of both heat and blood stasis,and ulcered flesh into abscess. Therefore, if the drugs for clearing away heat are used,Peach Seed(桃仁,Taoren)is often selected as an adjuvant drug to remove stasis and help purge heat and remove carbuncle.

14.红花,Honghua

English name:Safflower

Pharmaceutical name:Flos Calthami

Botanical name:Carthamus tinctorius L.

Properties and tastes:pungent,warm

红 花

Meridian tropism:heart,liver

Functions:1. activate blood and remove blood stasis

2. dredge meridians and relieve pain

3. decrease oxygen consumption in myocardium

4. inhibit thrombosis

5. lower blood pressure

6. protect against ischemic anaerobic encephalopathy

7. contract uterus

Indications:1. stagnant blood syndrome in gynecology——dysmenorrhea, amenorrhoea due to blood stasis, postpartum abdominal pain due to stagnation, hysteromyoma, pelvic inflammatory mass and dystocia, retention of placenta

2. coronary heart disease,angina pectoris

3. vascular embolic disease——cerebral thrombosis, cerebral embolism and thromboangitis obliterans

4. traumatic injury and bedsores

5. dark colored exanthema maculosum——exanthema maculosum caused by febrile disease measles with dark colour caused by stagnation and heat

Dosage:3~9g

Contraindication:Not to be used by pregnant women.

Combinations:1. add Szechwan Lovage Rhizome(川芎,Chuanxiong),Peach Seed(桃仁,Taoren),Dan-shen Root(丹参,Danshe n)——angina pectoris and coronary heart disease

2. add Chinese Angelica Root(当归,Danggui),Nutgrass Galingale Rhizome(香附,Xiangfu),Yanhusuo(延胡索,Yanhusuo)——menoxenia and dysmenorrhea

3. add Root of Sinkiang Arnebia(紫草,Zicao),Indigowoad Leaf(大青叶,Daqingye),Great Burdock Achene(牛蒡子,Niubangzi)——exanthema maculosum caused by febrile disease or measles with dark colored eruption

4. add Weeping Forsythia Capsule(连翘,Lianqiao),Dandelion(蒲公英,Pugongying)——swelling and toxic sores and carbuncles

5. add Common Burreed Rhizome(三棱,Sanleng),Zedoray(莪术,Ezhu),Peach Seed(桃仁,Taoren)——tumor and mass caused by obstruction of stagnant blood

6. add Chinese Thorowax Root(柴胡,Chaihu),Chinese Angelica Root(当归,Danggui),Rhubarb(大黄,Dahuang)——traumatic injury,local hematoma and pain

7. add Frankincense(乳香,Ruxiang),Myrrh(没药,Moyao),Red Peony Root(赤芍药,Chishaoyao)——thromboangitis obliterans

8. add Chinese Angelica Root(当归, Danggui), Dan-shen Root (丹参, Danshen), Peach Seed(桃仁, Taoren)——oligmenorrhoea, amenorrhoea and abdominal pain due to stagnation of blood

9. add Szechwan Lovage Rhizome(川芎, Chuanxiong)——cerebral thrombosis and cerebral embolism

10. add Chinese Angelica Root(当归, Danggui), Twotooth Achyranthes Root(牛膝, Niuxi), Cassia Bark(肉桂, Rougui)——lochiorrhea and distentional pain in the abdomen after birth

11. add Chinese Date(大枣, Dazao)——duodenal bulbar ulcer

Prescription: Peech Seed and Safflower Decoction of Four Ingredients(桃红四物汤, Taohongsiwu Tang)

Notes: This drug has a good effect for activating blood and removing stagnation. Safflower(红花, Honghua) is a principal drug to scatter blood stasis, activate blood circulation, harmonize and regulate blood. It is indicated for many kinds of women diseases caused by blood disorder. In recent years it has been widely applied to syndromes caused by obstruction of stagnant blood or unsmooth circulation of blood, such as cardiocerebral vascular diseases, thromboangitis obliterans and phlebitis, etc. It is reported that it can be used to treat cerebral thrombosis and cerebral embolism and one can get good results by vein injection. In addition, it can also be used to treat duodenal bulbarulcer, neurodermatitis and plane warts, etc. As for the dosage and effect, Li Shizhen(李时珍) said that a large dosages may promote blood circulation and a small dosage may nourish blood. It is explained in *Developed Interpretation of the Herbs* (《药品化义》, Yaopinhuayi) that: "If it is overdosed 3 or 4 Qian(9~12g), its pungent flavor and warm property become stronger and may cause the dispersion of blood. When used with Sappan Wood(苏木, Sumu), it may expel stagnant blood, with Cassia Bark(肉桂, Rougui), it may smooth amenorrhoea. With adjuvant drugs like Chinese Angelica Root(当归, Danggui), and White Peony Root(白芍药, Baishaoyao), the effect is conducting and activating blood, so it may treat pucking pain all over the body. If it is underdosed 7 or 8 Fen(2~2.5g), it has the effect of regulating and harmonizing blood, so it promotes the circulation of qi and then helps the blood sea to tonify the blood. If the dosage is only 2 or 3 Fen(0.6~0.9g), it plays the effect of nourishing and producing blood, removes pathogenic fire in the heart meridian and adjusts qi and blood." The dosage of drugs is important in both cases of reinforcement and reduction.

15. 五灵脂, Wulingzhi

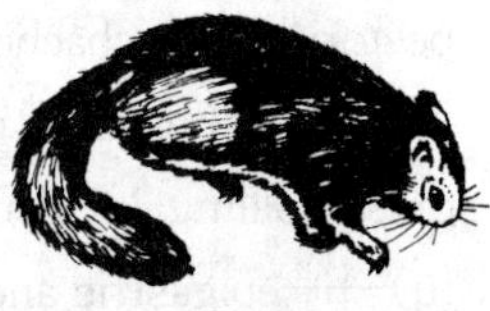

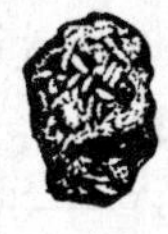

五灵脂

English name: Trogopterus Dung

Pharmaceutical name: Faeces Trogopterori

Botanical name: Trogopterus xanthipes Milne-Edwards

Properties and tastes: bitter, warm

Meridian tropism: liver

Functions: 1. circulate qi and activate blood

2. remove blood stasis and relieve pain

3. detoxicate and reduce swelling

Indications: 1. pain due to stagnant blood——dysmenorrhea, amenorrhoea, postpartum abdominal pain due to stagnation as well as chest pain, epigastric pain and pain from swelling due to fracture

2. haemorrhage syndrome due to stagnant blood——such as uterine bleeding, metrorrhagia, purplish color with clots and pricking pain in the lower abdomen

3. angina pectoris of coronary heart disease

4. haemorrhage and pain caused by gastric and duodenal ulcer

5. endometrial hyperplasia syndrome

6. bitten by snake, Scorpion(全蝎,Quanxie) bite and centipede bite-oral administration and external application.

Dosage: 3～9g. Decoct the packed drug. Proper dosage for external application. Parching it into charcoal can remove stasis and stop bleeding

Contraindication: The drug should be given cautiously. It is antagonistic to Ginseng(人参,Renshen).

Combinations: 1. add Cattail Pollen (蒲黄, Puhuang)——gynecological pain due to stagnation, infertility due to endometrial hyperplasia syndrome, and chest pain, angina pectoris, stomachache, hernia pain

2. add Yanhusuo(延胡索,Yanhusuo), Nutgrass Galingale Rhizome (香附, Xiangfu)——epigastric and abdominal pain

3. add Sanchi Root(三七,Sanqi), Rehmannia Dried Root (生地黄, Shengdihuang)——haemorrhage with internal stagnation

4. add Capillary Wormwood Herb(茵陈蒿, Yinchenhao), Cattail Pollen (蒲黄, Puhuang)——viral hepatitis

5. add Figwortflower Picrorhiza Rhizome (胡黄连, Huhuanglian)——infantile malnutrition

6. add Szechwan Lovage Rhizome(川芎, Chuanxiong)——coronary heart disease, angina pectoris

Prescription: Powder for Stopping Pain by Dissipating Blood Stasis(失笑散, Shixiao San)

Notes: Trogopterus Dung(五灵脂,Wulingzhi) can purge by its bitter flavor and dredge by its warm property, acting on the blood stage of liver and with the effect of circulating qi, activating blood, removing stasis and relieving pain, which is a principal drug to treat all kinds of diseases caused by stagnation of qi and blood. Used together with Cattail Pollen(蒲黄,Puhuang), it is called Powder for Stopping Pain by Dissipating Blood Stasis (失笑散, Shixiao San), the formula which was highly appraised by Li Shizhen (李时珍). "Powder for Stopping Pain by Dissipating Blood Stasis (失笑散, Shixiao San) can not only treat cardialgia or pain caused by blood stagnation in women, but also treat all kinds of pain in the heart, abdomen, hypochondrium, lower abdomen and hernia of men, women, the old and children, as well as pain caused by stagnation of qi and blood and uterine bleeding before and after delivery. It plays an effect on diseases which can not be treated by many other drugs and it is always effective, it is considered a magical formula at the time." According to modern research, Trogopterus Dung(五灵脂, Wulingzhi) has the function of restraining the growth of mycobacterium tuberculosis and relieving spasm of smooth muscles.

16. 牛膝, Niuxi

English name: Twotooth Achyranthes Root

Pharmaceutical name: Radix Achyranthis Bidentatae

Botanical name: Achyranthes bidentata BI.

Properties and tastes: bitter, sour, medium

Meridian tropism: liver, kidney

Functions: 1. activate blood and restore menstruation

2. conduct blood (fire) to descend

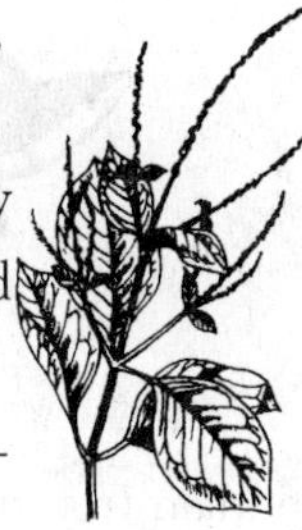

3. reinforce the liver and kidney and strengthen bones and tendons

牛 膝

4. promote urination and treat stranguria

5. relieve cough

6. reduce blood sugar

7. reduce plasma cholesterol

8. stimulate uterus and expand cervical canal

Indications: 1. menstrual diseases in women——menoxenia, dysmenorrhea, amenorrhoea, postpartum obstruction and abdominal pain which are all caused by stagnant blood

2. soreness and pain in waist and knee——caused by deficiency of the liver and kidney or prolonged arthralgia

3. stranguria——urethral pain and lumbago caused by blood stranguria, heat stranguria, chyluria stranguria or urinary stones

4. headache and dizziness——caused by hypertension or cerebrovascular spasm

5. upward perversion of fire syndrome——toothache, aphtha, hematemesis and epitasis

6. dysfunctional uterine bleeding

7. dystocia

8. edema and difficult urination

Dosage: 6～15g.

Contraindication: It is not advisable to prescribe for women in pregnancy or with menorrhagia

Combinations: 1. add Plantain Seed (车前子, Cheqianzi)——edema due to yang deficiency

2. add Cluster Mallow Seed (冬葵子, Dongkuizi)——retention of placenta

3. add Gambirplant Hooked stem and Branch (钩藤, Gouteng)——dizziness, vertigo, distented feeling of head, headache, hemiplegia and hypertension due to hyperactivity of liver yang

4. add Honeysuckle Flower (金银花, Jinyinhua), Red Peony Root (赤芍药, Chichaoyao)——thromboangitis obliterans

5. add Chinese Corktree Bark (黄柏, Huangbai), Swordlike Atractylodes Rhizome (苍术, Cangzhu)——artharalgia due to damp-heat, flaccidity and weakness in the lower limbs and erysipelas or eczema in the lower part of the body

6. add Chinese Angelica Root (当归, Danggui), Safflower (红花, Honghua)——amenorrhoea

7. add Eucommia Bark (杜仲, Duzhong), Chinese Taxillus Twig (桑寄生, Sangjisheng)——pain in the waist and knees

8. add Chinese Angelica Root (当归, Danggui), Baikal skullcap Root (黄芩, Huangqin)——blood stranguria, difficult urination and dysuria

9. add Rehmannia Dried Root (生地黄, Shengdihuang), Hematite (代赭石, Daizheshi)——swelling pain in tooth and gum caused by upward perversion of deficient fire

10. add Szechwan Lovage Rhizome (川芎, Chuanxiong), Safflower (红花, Honghua)——dystocia

11. add Chinese Angelica Root (当归, Danggui), Peach Seed (桃仁, Taoren), Safflower (红花, Honghua)——diseases caused by stagnant blood in gynecology and traumotology

Prescription: Decoction of Pubesent Angelica

and Loranthus(独活寄生汤,Duhuo Jisheng Tang)

Notes: Twotooth Achyranthes Root(牛膝,Niuxi) is good for the"going downward"function, indicated for various kinds of diseases in the waist, abdomen, knees and feet caused by stagnant blood in internal, external. When we prescribe drugs for headache, dizziness and vertigo due to the flaming upwards of fire and hyperactivity of liver yang, this drug can be used to conduct blood or fire going downward, the effect of drugs downward.

Twotooth Achyranthes Root(牛膝,Niuxi) has the effect of tonifying the liver and kidney and strengthen tendons and bones, but only mildly. Together with the related drugs for tonifying the liver and kidney, strengthening tendons and bone, removing wind and damp and eliminating damp-heat, it has the function of smoothing joints to treat arthralgia and flaccidity.

These are two types of Twotooth Achyranthes Root(牛膝, Niuxi). One is made in Sichuan province and called Medicininal Cyathula Root(川牛膝,Chuanniuxi) which is good for activating blood, removing stasis, conducting blood downward, inducing diuresis and treating stranguria. The other is made in Henan province and called Achyranthis Root(怀牛膝, Huainiuxi) which is good for tonifying liver and kidney and strengthening tendons and bones.

17. 穿山甲, Chuanshanjia

English name: Pangolin Scales

Pharmaceutical name: Squama Manitis

Botanical name: Manis pentadactyla Linnaeus

Properties and tastes: salty, slightly, cold

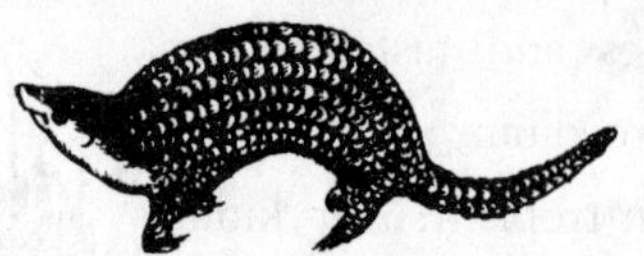

穿山甲

Meridian tropism: liver, stomach

Functions: 1. activate blood and remove mass
2. reduce swelling and evacuate pus
3. dredge meridians and promote lactation
4. raise white blood cells(WBC)

Indications: 1. amenorrhoea due to blood stagnation
2. lumps, in the chest and abdomen
3. galactostasis
4. early onset of carbuncle or undiabrotic of formed pus
5. scrofula(lymph tuberculosis, chronic lymphadenitis)
6. artharalgia due to wind-dampness
7. ovarian tumor

Dosage: 3～9g

Contraindication: It is not advisable for pregnant women and patients with diabrotic carbuncles snd boils. Patients with a weak constitution should cautiously use it.

Combinations: 1. add Chinese Angelica Root (当归, Danggui), Szechwan Lovage Rhizome(川芎, Chuanxiong), Safflower(红花, Honghua)——amenorrhoea
2. add Common Burreed Rhizome(三棱, Sanleng), Zedoray(莪术, Ezhu)——lumps in the abdomen and ovarian tumor
3. add Membranous Milkvetch Root(黄芪, Huangqi), Chinese Angelica Root(当归, Danggui)——galactostasis due to insufficiency of qi and blood
4. add Honeysuckle Flower(金银花, Jinyinhua), Snakegourd Root(天花粉, Tianhuafe n), Red Peony Root(赤芍药,

Chichaoyao)——carbuncle

5. add Chinese Angelica Root(当归, Danggui), Membranous Milkvetch Root(黄芪, Huangqi), Chinese Honeylocust Spine(皂角刺, Zaojiaoci)——carbuncle, undiabrotic of formed pus

6. add Common Selfheal Fruit-spike(夏枯草, Xiakucao), Oyster Shell(牡蛎, Muli), Tendrilleaf Fritillary Bulb(贝母, Beimu)——scrofula and subcutaneous nodule

7. add Chinese Angelica Root(当归, Danggui), Szechwan Lovage Rhizome(川芎, Chuanxiong), Rhizome or Root of Forbes Notopterygium(羌活, Qianghuo)——artharalgia of wind-dampness

8. add Cowherb Seed(王不留行, Wangbuliuxing)——galactostasis

Prescription: Fairy Decoction for Treating Cutancous Infections(仙方活命饮, Xianfanghuoming Yin)

Notes: Pangolin Scales(穿山甲, Chuanshanjia) has good function of dispersion, which can dredge meridians and it is beneficial to the affected area. The main functions are to activate blood, promote meastruation, and reduce carbuncle and diabrotic pus. Li Shizhen (李时珍) said: "This drug was not used in ancient times. Nowadays it is a principal drug for treatment of malaria, carbuncles, promoting menstruation and lactation." For syndrome of blood stagnation, it can be ground into powder for oral use. 1～1.5g per dose.

18. 䗪虫, Zhechong

English name: Ground Beetle

Properties and tastes: salty, cold

Meridian tropism: liver

Functions: 1. disperse blood stasis and remove

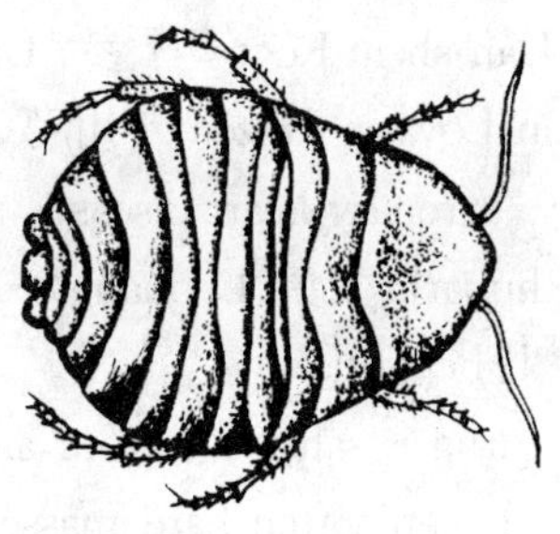

䗪 虫

stagnation

2. promote joining of fractured bones

Indications: 1. obstruction of stagnation in gynecology——amenorrhoea, postpartum pain due to stagnation

2. lumps in the chest and abdomen and hepatosplenomegaly, placental remnants, incomplete abortion

3. fracture, injury pain, stagnant pain due to traumatic injury

4. coronary heart disease

Dosage: 3～9g. Grind into powder for oral use. 1～1.5g per dose, when it is orally taken, it is better with millet wine.

Contraindication: It is contraindicated in pregnant women.

Combinations: 1. add Rhubarb(大黄, Dahuang)——stagnant blood syndrome in gynecology, such as amenorrhoea, abdominal mass, lump, squamous and dry skin, dark complexion around the eyes as well as traumatic swelling and pain

2. add Turtle Carapace(鳖甲, Biejia), Tree Peony Bark(牡丹皮, Mudanpi)——hepotosplenomegaly and liver sclerosis

3. add Frankincense(乳香, Ruxiang), Myrrh(没药, Moyao)——fracture, swelling and pain in injuries

4. add Turtle Carapace(鳖甲, Biejia)——resolve blood stasis, remove distention and lumps in the abdomen

5. add Dan-shen Root(丹参, Danshen), Szechwan Lovage Rhizome(川芎, Chuanxiong)——coronary heart disease

6. add Rhubarb(大黄, Dahuang)——chronic active B hepatitis

Notes: The drug is salty in flavour and cold in property. It can soften hard masses, remove stagnant blood. It is a principal drug for treating traumatic injury. The function of dispersing blood and removing stagnation is almost the same as that of Leech(水蛭, Shuizhi), but it is mild in nature. In addition, when treating lumbar sprain, the drug can be used alone by drying it over a fire and grinding it into powder for oral use.

19. 水蛭, Shuizhi

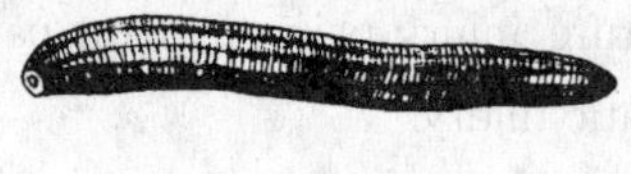

水 蛭

English name: Leech
Pharmaceutical name: Hirudo
Botanical name: Hirudo nipponica Whitman
Properties and tastes: salty, bitter, medium
Meridian tropism; liver
Functions: 1. scatter blood stasis and remove stagnation

2. remove abdominal mass

3. anticoagulant and reduce blood-lipid function

Indications: 1. amenorrhoea due to blood stagnation, abdominal mass and lump

2. pain due to traumatic injury

3. hyperlipemia

4. angina pectoris, coronary heart disease

5. acute onset of pulmonary heart disease

6. thrombocythemia after splenectomy

7. intracranial hematoma due to cerebral haemorrhage

8. thrombophlebitis

Dosage: 3～6g. Dry it over a fire and grind it into powder for oral administration. 0.3～0.6g each time.

Contraindication: It is contraindicated in pregnant women.

Combinations: 1. add Peach Seed(桃仁, Taoren), Common Burreed Rhizome(三棱, Sanleng), Sappan Wood(苏木, Sumu)——amenorrhoea due to blood stasis, tumor, mass and traumatic injury

2. add Gadfly(虻虫, Mengchong), Ground Bettle(地鳖虫, Dibiechong)——thrombocythemia

3. add Rhubarb(大黄, Dahuang), Pharbitis Seed(牵牛子, Qianniuzi)——abdominal pain with difficult bowel movement.

4. add Ginseng(人参, Renshen), Membranous Milkvetch Root(黄芪, Huangqi), Chinese Angelica Root(当归, Danggui)——weak constitution with amenorrhoea, abdominal mass due to stagnant blood.

5. add Chinese Angelica Root(当归, Danggui), Szechwan Lovage Rhizome(川芎, Chuanxiong), Safflower (红花, Honghua)——thrembophlebitis.

Notes: Leech(水蛭, Shuizhi) is good at dissipating blood stasis. In recent years, this drug has been used with drugs for activating blood and removing stagnation to treat thrombocythemia and is quite effective. It shows the drug does have the effect of dissipating blood stasis.

20. 虻虫, Mengchong

English name: Gadfly
Pharmaceutical name: Tabanus
Botanical name: Tabanus budda Portshinsky
Properties and tastes: bitter, slightly cold, slightly toxic

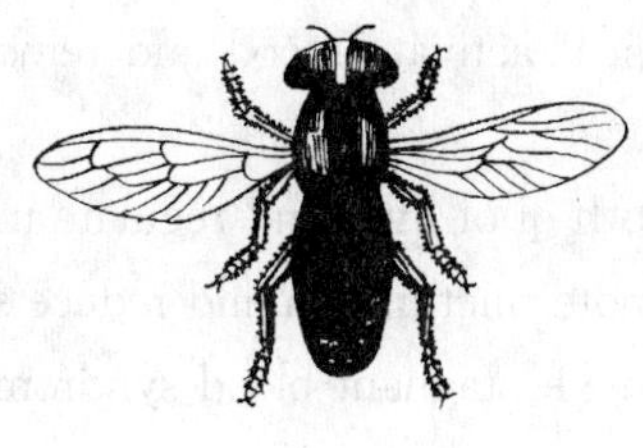

虻 虫

Meridian tropism: liver

Functions: 1. dissipate blood stasis and remove stagnation

2. remove abdominal mass

Indications: 1. amenorrhoea, abdominal mass due to blood stagnation

2. pain caused by traumatic injury

3. angina pectoris, coronary heart disease

Dosage: 1～1.5g. Dry it over a fire and grind it into powder for oral administration. 0.3g per dose.

Contraindication: It is contraindicated in pregnant women.

Combinations: 1. add Leech (水蛭, Shuizhi), Ground Beetle (䗪虫, Zhechong), Peach Seed (桃仁, Taoren)——amenorrhoea, abdominal mass

2. add Rhubarb (大黄, Dahuang), Frankincense (乳香, Ruxiang), Myrrh (没药, Moyao)——traumatic injury, pain due to blood stasis

3. add Tangerine Peel (橘皮, Jupi)——angina pectoris, coronary heart disease

Notes: Gadfly (虻虫, Mengchong) has the function of dissipating blood stasis, the same as that of Leech (水蛭, Shuizhi), but with drastic effect. It may cause abdominal diarrhea after taking it.

Leech (水蛭, Shuizhi), Gadfly (虻虫, Mengchong) and Ground Beetle (䗪虫, Zhechong) are all worm drugs with toxicity. They are drastic drugs for dissipating blood stasis and removing mass. Amomg them, Gadfly (虻虫, Mengchong) has the strongest effect on dissipating blood stasis. Leech (水蛭, Shuizhi) has less effect and Zhechong is milder. Therefore, select the proper drug according to the degree of stagnation and the condition of antipathogenic qi.

21. 降香, Jiangxiang

English name: Rosewood

Pharmaceutical name: Lignum Dalbergiae Odoriferae

Botanical name: Dalbergia odorifera T. Chen

Properties and tastes: pungent, warm

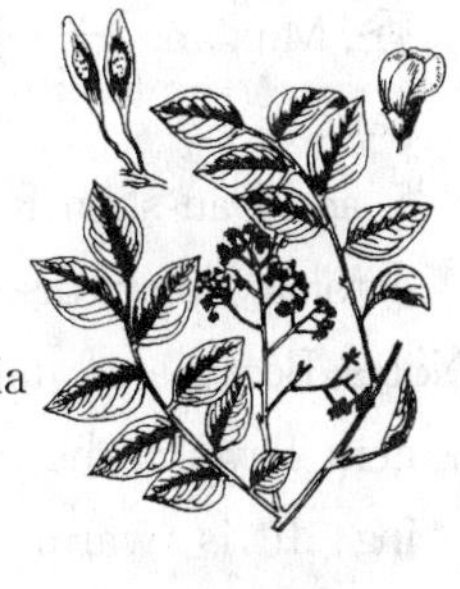

降 香

Meridian tropism: heart, liver, spleen

Functions: 1. activate blood and remove stagnation

2. stop bleeding and relieve pain

3. eliminate filth and remove turbidity

4. harmonize the Middle-jiao and relieve vomiting

Indications: 1. pain in the chest and hypochondrium which is caused by stagnation of qi and blood

2. traumatic injury and wounds hemorrhage

3. vomiting and abdominal pain due to internal obstruction of filth and turbidity

4. angina pectoris, coronary heart disease

Dosage: 3 ～ 6g. Proper amount for external use.

Contraindication: It is not advisable to use for people with deficiency of yin and excess of fire and bleeding due to blood-heat but without stagnation.

Combinations: 1. add Tumeric Root-tuber (郁金, Yujin), Peach Seed (桃仁, Taoren), Towel Gourd Vegetable Sponge (丝瓜络,

Sigualuo)——pain in the chest and hypochondrium

2. add Frankincense (乳香, Ruxiang), Myrrh(没药, Moyao)——pain caused by the swelling of traumatic injury

3. add Sanchi Root(三七, Sanqi)——bleeding due to trauma for external use

4. add Wrinkled Gianthyssop Herb(藿香, Huoxiang), Common Aucklandia Root(木香, Muxiang)——vomiting and abdominal pain

5. add Dan-shen Root(丹参, Danshen)——coronary heart disease, angina pectoris

Notes: Because of its fragrant smell and pungent flavour, the drug is good for dispersing. It is warm in property, it dredges meridians and has the effects of removing stagnation, stopping bleeding and relieving pain. Clinically, it is mainly used to treat pain in the chest and hypochondrium, as well as traumatic injury. Pharmacological research shows that due to its component of Dalbergia hupeana contained in this drug, it has an anticoagulation function and can obviously increase the flow of coronary blood volume and cardiac amplitude. That is why it is mostly used for treating coronary heart disease in recent years.

22. 泽兰, Zelan

English name: Hirsute Shiny Bugleweed Herb

Pharmaceutical name: Herba Lycopi

Botanical name: Lycopus lucidus Turcz. Var. Hirtus Reg.

泽兰

Properties and tastes: bitter, pungent, slightly warm

Meridian tropism: liver, spleen

Functions: 1. activate blood and remove stagnation

2. smooth qi of liver and regulate meridians

3. promote micturation and reduce swelling

Indications: 1. stagnant blood syndrome in gynecology——amenorrhoea, dysmenorrahea, menoxenia, abdominal mass and postpartum abdominal pain caused by blood stagnation

2. pain caused by traumatic injury

3. pain in the chest and hypochondrium

4. swelling of carbuncle

5. edema, difficulty in micturation

Dosage: 9 ~ 15g. Proper amount for external use.

Contraindication: It should be used cautiously for those without stagnation.

Combinations: 1. add Chinese Angelica Root (当归, Danggui), Nutgrass Galingale Rhizome(香附, Xiangfu)——stagnant blood syndrome in gynecology

2. add Peach Seed(桃仁, Taoren), Safflower (红花, Honghua)——amenorrhoea due to blood stasis

3. add Common Burreed Rhizome(三棱, Sanleng), Zedoray(莪术, Ezhu)——abdominal mass

4. add Immature Bitter Orange(枳实, Zhishi), White Peony Root(白芍药, Baishaoyao)——postpartum abdominal pain caused by blood stagnation

5. add Chinese Angelica Root(当归, Danggui), Szechwan Lovage Rhizome(川芎, Chuanxiong)——swelling pain due to stagnant blood an injury at the sitw of an injury

6. add Dan-shen Root(丹参, Danshen), Tumeric Root-tuber(郁金, Yujin)——pain in the chest and hypochondrium

7. add Chinese Angelica Root(当归, Danggui), Honeysuckly Flower(金银花, Jinyinhua), Licorice Root(甘草, Gancao)——

swelling of carbuncle

8. add Fourstamen Stephania Root(防己, Fangji)——difficult urination and puffiness in the body and face after delivery

Notes: Hirsute Shiny Bugleweed Herb(泽兰, Zelan) disperses blood by its pungent flavour and dredges mendians by its warm property. It strengthens the spleen by fragrancy and benefits liver by discharging. It is mild so it can circulate qi of liver so as to smooth the meridians. Removing stagnation and promoting urination without damaging the anti-pathogenic qi, characterize it. Thus, it is a commonly used drug for stagnation of blood, irregular menstruation, edema and fullness in women. It is said in *Compendium of Materia Medica* (《本草纲目》, Bencaogangmu): "Hirsute Shiny Bugleweed Herb (泽兰, Zelan) goes into the Blood System to treat edema, remove carbuncle, scatter stagnant blood, and eliminate abdominal mass. It is a prinicipal drug for women."

Hirsute Shiny Bugleweed Herb(泽兰, Zelan) and Motherwort Herb(益母草, Yimucao) are both drugs for activating blood and removing stagnation and are often used together to treat syndromes of blood stasis., Hirsute Shiny Bugleweed Herb (泽兰, Zelan) has less effect than Motherwort Herb (益母草, Yimucao). In addition, these two drugs can both treat swelling of a carbuncle, but Motherwort Herb(益母草, Yimucao) is cold in property and treats swelling of a carbuncle by dispersing stagnation and detoxication. Hirsute Shiny Bugleweed Herb (泽兰, Zelan) is slightly warm in property and disperses by its pungent flavour. It only has the effect of removing stagnation and reducing swelling, without the detoxicating function to treat the primary cause, while its function of promoting urination and reducing swelling is better than that of Motherwort Herb(益母草, Yimucao).

23. 王不留行, Wangbuliuxing

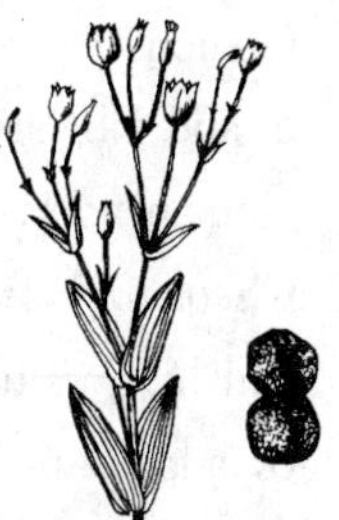
王不留行

English name: Cowherb Seed

Pharmaceutical name: Semen Vaccariae

Botanical name: Vaccaria segetalis(Neck.) Garcke

Properties and tastes: bitter, medium

Meridian tropism: liver, stomach

Functions: 1. activate blood and promote menstruation

2. stimulate milk secretion

3. reduce carbuncle

4. promote urination and treat stranguria

5. stimulate uterine contraction

6. restrain lung cancer and ascite tumor

Indications: 1. amenorrhoea due to blood stasis

2. postpartum retention of breast milk

3. swelling pain of acute mastitis

4. heat stranguria, blood stranguria and urinary stone

5. prostatitis

Dosage: 6～9g

Contraindication: It should be cautiously used for pregnant women.

Combinations: 1. add Immature Bitter Orange (枳实, Zhishi), White Peony Root(白芍药, Baishaoyao)——unsmooth menstruation and abdominal pain

2. add Chinese Angelica Root(当归, Danggui), Szechwan Lovage Rhizome (川芎, Chuanxiong), Safflower(红花, Honghua)——amenorrhoea due to blood stagnation

3. add Membranous Milkvetch Root(黄芪,

Huangqi), Chinese Angelica Root (当归, Danggui)——lack of lactation caused by deficiency of both qi and blood after delivery

4. add Dandelion (蒲公英, Pugongying), Common Selfheal Fruit-spike (夏枯草, Xiakucao), Snakegourd Fruit (瓜蒌, Gualou)——swelling pain of acute mastitis

5. add Christina Loosetrife Herb (金钱草, Jinqiancao), Plantain Seed (车前子, Cheqianzi), Immature Bitter Orange (枳实, Zhishi)——urinary stone

6. add Dan-shen Root (丹参, Danshen), Whiteflower Patrinia Herb (败酱草, Baijiangcao), Peach Seed (桃仁, Taoren)——chronic prostatitis

Notes: In recent years, Cowherb Seed (王不留行, Wangbuliuxing) has been used to treat urinary stone and prostatitis due to its function of promoting urination and activate blood with drugs for promoting urination, activating blood and reducing swelling, . In addition, it is a principal drug for promoting lactation and often used with Pangolin Scales (穿山甲, Chuanshanjia). The common saying is that women will have a smoothing flow of breast milk after taking Pangolin Scales (穿山甲, Chuanshanjia) and Cowherb Seed (王不留行, Wangbuliuxing).

24. 刘寄奴, Liujinu

English name: Diverse Wormwood Herb

Pharmaceutical name: Heaba Artemisiae Anomalae

Botanical name: Artemisia anomala S. Moore

Properties and tastes: bitter, warm

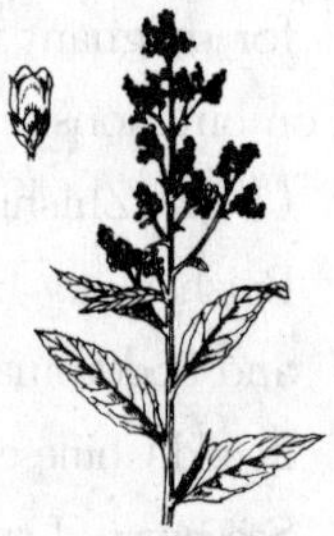

刘寄奴

Meridian tropism: heart, liver, spleen

Functions: 1. disperse blood stasis and dredge meridians

2. remove stagnation and relieve pain

3. remove food retention

4. stop bleeding and reduce swelling

Indications: 1. amenorrhoea and postpartum abdominal pain due to blood stagnation

2. abdominal mass

3. bleeding and pain caused by trauma

4. indigestion, retention of food, distentional pain in the epigastrium and abdomen

5. acute bacteric dysentery

6. heat stroke

Dosage: 3～9g. Proper dosage for external use.

Contraindication: It is not advisable for pregnant women.

Combinations: 1. add Chinese Angelica Root (当归, Danggui), Safflower (红花, Honghua)——amenorrhoea

2. add Motherwort Herb (益母草. Yimucao), Suberect Spatholobus Stem (鸡血藤, Jixueteng)——blood stasis of postpartum.

3. add Safflower (红花, Honghua), Yanhusuo (延胡索, Yanhusuo)——swelling pain caused by trauma

4. add Charred Hawthorn Fruit (焦山楂, Jiaoshanzha), Medicated Leaven (神曲, Shenqu)——indigestion

5. add Common Burreed Rhizome (三棱, Sanleng), Pangolin Scales (穿山甲, Chuanshanjia)——abdominal mass

Notes: The drug can descend because of its bitter flavor and circulate due to its warm property and is good at scattering blood stasis and removing distention. It is the most suitable drug for postpartum blood stagnation and pain caused by traumatic iujury. In addition, the powder can be externally used for bleeding and pain due to trauma.

Diverse Wormwood Herb (刘寄奴, Liujinu) is divided into a south and north kind.

There is no clear difference between the two. But one is cool and the other is warm in property and with a different flavor. The south one is stronger in scattering blood stasis. Pay attention to their use in the clinical treatment.

25. 苏木, Sumu

English name: Sappan Wood

Pharmaceutical name: Lignum Sappan

Botanical name: Caesalpinia sappan L.

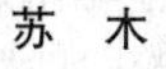

苏 木

Properties and tastes: sweet, salty, slightly pungent, medium

Meridian tropism: heart, liver and spleen

Functions: 1. activate blood and dredge meridians

2. remove stagnation and relieve pain

3. broad-spectrum bacteriostasis

4. tranquilization and hypnosis

Indications: 1. blood stagnation syndrome in gynecology——amenorrhoea and postpartum abdominal pain due to blood stasis

2. traumatic injury and pain due to blood stagnation

Dosage: 3～9g

Contraindication: It is not advisable for pregnant women.

Combinations: 1. add Dang-shen Root (党参, Dangshen), Dwarf Lilyturf Root (麦门冬, Maimendong)——dizziness, vertigo and shortness of breath caused by great loss of blood after delivery.

2. add Chinese Angelica Root (当归, Danggui), Red Peony Root (赤芍药, Chichaoyao), Safflower (红花, Honghua)——traumatic injury.

3. add Frankincense (乳香, Ruxiang), Myrrh (没药, Moyao)——traumatic injury.

4. add Nutgrass Galingale Rhizome (香附, Xiangfu), Lesser Galangal Rhizome (高良姜, Gaoliangjiang)——epigastric pain caused by stagnant blood.

5. add Peach Seed (桃仁, Taoren), Safflower (红花, Honghua), Szechwan Lovage Rhizome (川芎, Chuanxiong)——amenorrhoea due to blood stasis, dysmenorrhea, postpartum abdominal pain due to blood stagnation

Notes: Li Shizhen (李时珍) said: "Little dosage of the drug may activate blood and a large dosage may scatter blood stasis." Zhao Xuemin (赵学敏) said that Sappan Wood (苏木, Sumu) has a better effect for scattering blood if it is decocted in wine.

Sappan Wood (苏木, Sumu) is an important drug for activating blood, smoothing collaterals and removing stagnation, which is effective on treating postpartum, dysmenorrhea, mass and traumatic injury. Recently, it is mostly used for treating cardiovascular disease. The function of Sappan Wood (苏木, Sumu) is similar with that of Safflower (红花, Honghua). But Safflower (红花, Honghua) is slightly warm and Sappan Wood (苏木, Sumu) is slightly cold in property.

Appendix: Other Drugs For Activating Blood And Removing Stasis

Name	Properties and tastes	Meridian tropism	Functions	Indications	Dosage	Contraindication
Saffron Crocus Stigma(藏红花, Zanghonghua)	sweet, cold	Heart, Liver	Activate blood, remove stagnation, and dredge meridians, the effects of which are similar with that of Safflower (红花, Honghua) but with stronger force. It can also cool blood and detoxicate.	High fever caused by macular eruption. The color is not fresh red. Pathogenic heat invades the blood stage in mild febrile disease. Long-term use may nourish the lower Yuan, pleasure the complexion and make happy sensation.	1.5～3g	
Chinese Rose Flower (月季花, Yuejihua)	sweet, warm	Liver	Activate blood, regulate menses, reduce swelling, disperse accumulation	Amenorrhoea, menoxenia, scrofula.	3～6g	It is cautiously used for those with weakness of the spleen and stomach
Chinese Trumpetcreeper Flower (凌霄花, Lingxiaohua)	pungent, slightly cold	Liver, pericadium	Activate blood, scatter blood stasis, cool blood, expel wind	Amenorrhoea due to blood stasis, abdominal mass, itching sensation of the skin	3～9g	It is not advisable for pregnant women.
Pyrite (自然铜, Zirantong)	pungent, neutral	Liver	Remove blood relieve pain, setting of fracture, treat injury	Traumatic injury, fracture, swelling pain due to stagnation	9～15g, 0.3g for powder each time	It is not advisable for pregnant women
Ture Lacquertree Dried Lacquer (干漆, Ganqi)	pungent, bitter, warm, slightly poisonous	Liver, Stomach	Scatter blood stasis, dredge meridians, treat parasites.	Amenorrhoea, abdominal mass, abdominal pain caused by parasite, schistosomiasis.	0.06～0.1g. It is only used in bolus and powder, can't be decocted in water	It is not advisable for pregnant women and those with kidney deficiency
Pubescent Holly Root(毛冬青, Maodongqing)	bitter, astringent, medium	Heart, Lung	Activate blood, smooth blood vessels, clear away heat and detoxicate	Hemiplegia, coronary heart disease, cough due to lung heat, swelling pain in the throat	30～60g	It is not proper for syndrome of deficient coldness.
European Verbena Herb(马鞭草, Mabiancao)	bitter, slightly, cold	Liver, Spleen	Activate blood, remove stagnation, clear away heat, detoxicate, treat malaria, promote urination, reduce swelling	Amenorrhoea due to stagnant blood, dysmenorrhea, abdominal mass, soreness and pain of the joints, pain due to traumatic injury, pain of heat-toxin, swelling pain of gums, inflammation of throat, dysentary, malasia, heat stranguria, edema, ascites	15～30g	It is cautiously used for pregnant women.

Name	Properties and tastes	Meridian tropism	Functions	Indications	Dosage	Contraindication
Princesplume Ladysthumb Fruit (水红花子, Shuihonghuazi)	salty, slightly warm	Liver, Stomach	Expel blood stasis, reduce abdominal mass, eliminate accumulation, relieve pain	Abdominal pain, goiter, indigestion of food, epigastric pain, primary liver cancer, and various kinds of tumor	15～30g	
Chinese Sage Herb(石见穿, Shijianchuan)	bitter, pungent, medium		Activate blood, relieve pain	Pain of the bone, swelling of carbuncle and of cancer	9～15g	
But Dung (夜明砂, Yemingsha)	pungent, cold	Liver	Remove stagnation, reduce accumulation, clear away liver fire and brighten eyes	Traumatic injury, infantile malnutrition, red eyes, suffusion of white eyes	3～9g (decoction of a wrapped drug)	It is not proper for eye diseases due to obstruction of blood stagnation.
Dung Beetle (蜣螂, Qianglang)	salty, cold, slightly, poisonous	Liver	Scatter blood stasis, relieve convulsion, eliminate toxin by purgation	Abdominal mass, epilepsy, insane, constipation, swelling and toxin of sores and carbuncles	1.5～3g	It is not used for pregnant women.

Section 2
Hemostatic Drugs

1. 大蓟, Daji

English name: Japanese Thistle Herb or Root

Pharmaceutical name: Herba Cirsii Japonici

Botanical name: Cirstium japonicum DC

大 蓟

Properties and tastes: sweet, bitter, slightly cold

Meridian tropism: heart, liver

Functions: 1. remove heat from the blood, arrest bleeding

2. dissipate blood stasis and remove carbuncle

3. clear away heat and toxic materials

4. hepataprotective and cholagogic function

5. lower blood pressure

Indications: 1. hemorrage——hematemesis, hemoptysis, epistaxis, metrorrhagia, and hematuria due to blood-heat

2. carbuncle——both exterior and interior carbuncles, such as mastadenitis, intestinal abscess and pulmonary abscess

3. hypertension

4. hepatitis, jaundice——especially for the syndrome of retention of damp-heat in the interior

Dosage: 9～15g. 30～60g for the fresh herb. The fresh herb is better than the dried one. The slightly carbonized herb is especially effective for astringing to arrest bleeding.

Contraindication: It should not be used for cold syndrome of the spleen and deficient stomach.

Combinations: 1. add Rehmannia Dried Root (生地黄, Shengdihuang) and Common Cephalanoplos Herb (小蓟, Xiaoji)——hemorrhage due to blood-heat

2. add Garden Burnet Root(地榆, Diyu) and Twotooth Achyranthes Root(牛膝, Niuxi)——various, carbuncles due to noxious heat

3. add Cattail Pollen (蒲黄, Puhuang), Rehmannia Dried Root (生地黄, Shengdihuang)——functional metrorrhagia and profuse metrorrhagia

4. add Common Selfheal Fruit-spike(夏枯草, Xiakucao)——hypertension

5. add Capillary Wormwood Herb(茵陈蒿, Yinchenhao)——hepatitis and jaundice

Notes: Japanese Thistle Herb or Root(大蓟, Daji) removes heat from the blood to arrest bleeding. It is used to treat various hemorrhages due to blood-heat. It can be taken orally or used externally to treat carbuncle.

2. 小蓟, Xiaoji

English name: Common Cephalanoplos Herb

Pharmaceutical name: Herba Cirsii

Botanical name: Cirsium setosum(Willd.)MB.

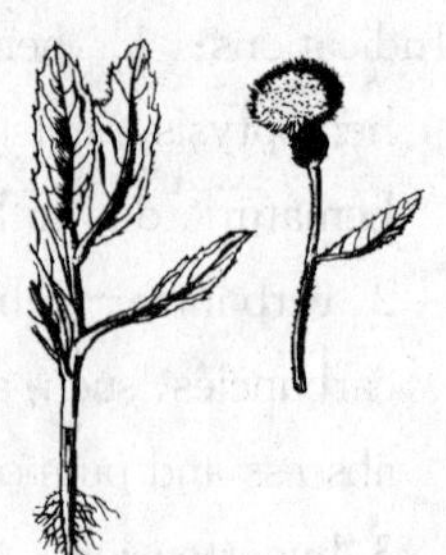

小 蓟

Properties and tastes: sweet, bitter, slightly cold

Meridian tropism: heart, liver

Functions: 1. remove heat from the blood to arrest bleeding

2. clear away toxic materials and remove carbuncle

3. quench evil heat in the liver and cholagogic

4. lower blood pressure

5. promote urination

Indications: 1. hemorrhage——hemoptysis, epistaxis, metrorrhagia and hematuria due to blood-heat

2. carbuncle due to noxious heat

3. jaundice by damp-heat, hepatitis

4. nephritis

5. hypertension

Dosage: 9～15g. 30～60g if it is fresh. Pound the proper amount to paste for external application or decoct it for external washing. Slightly carbonized Field Thistle is used to arrest bleeding. The raw herb is used for other purposes.

Contraindication: It should not be used for deficiency cold syndrome of the spleen and stomach.

Combinations:

1. add Lalang Grass Rhizome (白茅根, Baimaogen)——hematuria, stranguria and nephritis

2. add Gambirplant Hooked Stem and Branch(钩藤, Gouteng) and Common Selfheal Fruit-spike(夏枯草, Xiakucao)——hypertension

3. add Janpanese Thistle Herb or Root(大蓟, Daji)——for various hemorrhages due to blood-heat

4. add Rehmannia Dried Root (生地黄, Shengdihuang) and Cattail Pollen (蒲黄, Puhuang)——menorrhagia

5. add Honeysuckle Flower(金银花, Jinyinhua) and Weeping Forsythia Capsule(连翘, Lianqiao)——noxious heat, carbuncle

6. add Motherwort Herb (益母草, Yimucao)——threatened abortion and hemor-

rhage

Prescription: Herba Cephalanoploris Decoction (小蓟饮子, Xiaoji Yinzi)

Notes: It removes heat from the blood to arrest bleeding. It also induces diuresis. Therefore, except for various hemorrhages due to blood-heat, it is especially effective for hematuria. The fresh herb is better than the dried one for arresting bleeding. The effect decreases after carbonization for arresting bleeding.

Common Cephalanoplos Herb (小蓟, Xiaoji) and Janpanese Thistle Herb or Root (大蓟, Daji) have similar functions. Both of them can remove heat from the blood to arrest bleeding and dissipate blood stasis. However, Janpanese Thistle Herb or Root (大蓟, Daji) has higher effect to dissipate blood stasis and to diminish swelling, Common Cephalanoplos Herb (小蓟, Xiaoji) is more effective in treating bloody gonorrhea and hematuria.

3. 地榆, Diyu

English name: Garden Burnet Root

Pharmaceutical name: Radix Sanguisorbae Officinalis

Botanical name: Sanguisorba officinalis L.

Properties and tastes: bitter, sour, and slightly cold

地 榆

Meridian tropism: liver, stomach, and large intestine

Functions: 1. remove heat from the blood to arrest bleeding

2. clear away toxic materials and remove carbuncle

Indications: 1. hemorrhage——hemoptysis, epistaxis, hematemesis, hematuria, hematochezia, hemorrhoidal bleeding, bloody flux, metrorrhagia

2. scald, eczema, derma ulcer, carbuncle etc.

Dosage: 9 ~ 15g. Proper amount for external application.

Contraindication: External application of the Garden Burnet Root (地榆, Diyu) preparation for the large area scald is prohibited, as a large amount of the hydrolyzed tannic acid contained in it may be absorbed by the body to cause toxic hepatitis. It is not used for hemorrhages due to asthenia cold and the early stage of heat dysentery.

Combinations: 1. add Japanese Pagodatree Flower-bud (槐米, Huaimi) and Japanese Pagodatree Flower (槐花, Huaihua)——hematochezia, hemorrhoidal bleeding

2. add Chinese Corktree Bark (黄柏, Huangbai)——scald and dermal eczema for external application

3. add Spreading Hedyotis Herb (白花蛇舌草, Baihuasheshecao)——typhoid

4. add Dandelion (蒲公英, Pugongying) and Honeysuckle Flower (金银花, Jinyinhua)——carbuncle due to noxious heat

5. add Coptis Rhizome (黄连, Huanglian) and Smoked Plum (乌梅, Wumei)——chronic dysentery

6. add Rehmannia Dried Root (生地黄, Shengdihuang) and Baikal Skullcap Root (黄芩, Huangqin)——metrorrhagia due to blood-heat

Notes: It removes heat from the blood and astringes to arrest bleeding. It may be used for various hemorrhages, especially for hematochezia, hemorrhoidal bleeding, bloody dysentery and metrorrhagia due to pathogenic heat in the blood of the Lower-jiao. It is also a major herb to treat scald. Garden Burnet Root (地榆, Diyu) powder mixed with sesame oil can decrease the extravasation, thus decreasing the pain and speeding up the healing.

4. 白茅根, Baimaogen

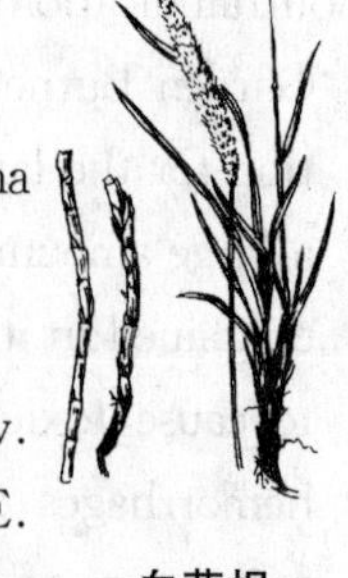
白茅根

English name: Lalang Grass Rhizome
Pharmaceutical name: Rhizoma Imperatae Cylindricae
Botanical name: Imperata cylindrica (L.) P. Beauv. Var. major (Nees) C. E. Hubb.
Properties and tastes: sweet, cold
Meridian tropism: lung, stomach, and bladder
Functions: 1. remove heat from the blood to arrest bleeding
2. clear away heat and induce diuresis
3. nourish the liver and benefit the gallbladder
4. kill bacteria
Indications: 1. hemorrhage——epistaxis, hematemesis, hemoptysis, and hematuria due to blood-heat
2. acute and chronic nephritis
3. stranguria with blood due to damp-heat of bladder, stranguria due to heat, difficult urination
4. acute hepatitis and jaundice due to damp-heat
5. cough due to lung heat
6. vomiting due to stomach heat
7. excessive thirst with fever
Dosage: 9 ~ 15g. 30 ~ 60g if it is fresh. The fresh herb is better than the dried one.
Contraindication: It can not be used for deficiency cold syndrome of the spleen and stomach.
Combinations:
1. add Rehmannia Dried Root (生地黄, Shengdihuang) and Common Cephalanoplos Herb (小蓟, Xiaoji)——hematemesis, epistaxis, and hematuria due to blood-heat
2. add Plantian Seed (车前子, Cheqianzi) and Akebia Stem (木通, Mutong)——stranguria due to heat, and edema
3. add Capillary Wormwood Herb (茵陈蒿, Yinchenhao) and Baikal Skullcap Root (黄芩, Huangqin)——jaundice due to damp-heat
4. add Rice Bean (赤小豆, Chixiaodou)——acute nephritis
5. add Ephedra (麻黄, Mahuang) and Weeping Forsythia Capsule (连翘, Lianqiao)——the early stage of nephritis
6. add Reed Rhizome (芦根, Lugen)——excessive thirst with fever, vomiting due to stomach heat, cough due to lung heat and sore throat
7. add Membranous Milkvetch Root (黄芪, Huangqi)——chronic nephritis
8. add Herb of Christina Loosetrife Herb (金钱草, Jinqiancao) and Capillary Wormwood Herb (茵陈蒿, Yinchenhao)——acute hepatitis
9. add Chinese Arborvitae Leafy Twig (侧柏叶, Cebaiye) and Janpanese Thistle Herb or Root (大蓟, Daji)——hematemesis, epistaxis and hematuria due to blood-heat

Notes: Lalang Grass Rhizome (白茅根, Baimaogen) removes heat from the blood to arrest bleeding, induces diuresis and expels wind-dampness evil. It is especially effective to treat syndromes of bloody gonorrhea and hematuria, such as acute nephritis. Its flavor is sweet but not greasy. Its property is cold, but not harmful for qi of Middle-jiao. It replenishes vital essence when the stomach meridian is entered, and thus promotes the production of the body fluid and quenches the thirst.

Lalang Grass Rhizome(白茅根,Baimaogen) and Reed Rhizome(芦根,Lugen) have similar function of clearing away intrinsic heat from the lung and stomach, and clearing away heat to induce diuresis. However, the function of Reed Rhizome(芦根, Lugen) lean to the qi phase. It mainly clears away the heat of qi stage. It also removes pus. The function of Lalang Grass Rhizome (白茅根, Baimaogen) lean to the blood phase. It removes heat from the blood stage to arrest bleeding. Both of them are used for vomiting due to stomach heat and cough due to lung heat.

5. 槐花, Huaihua

English name: Japanese Pagodatree Flower

Pharmaceutical name: Flos Sophorae Japonicae Immaturus

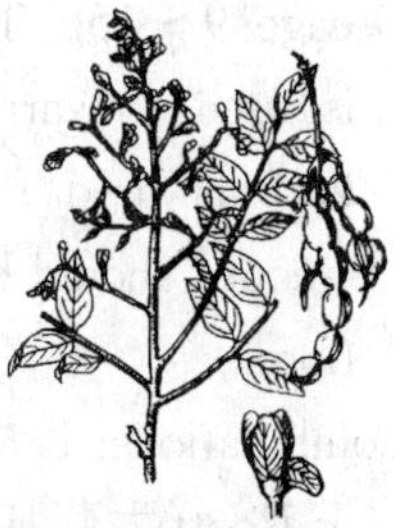

Botanical name: Sophora japonica L.

槐 花

Properties and tastes: bitter, slightly cold

Meridian tropism: liver, large intestine

Functions:

1. remove heat from the blood to arrest bleeding
2. remove the liver fire
3. reduce blood pressure
4. decrease the permeability and friability of the capillary vessel
5. decrease the blood-lipid
6. spasmolysis, treat ulcer
7. anti-inflammation

Indications: 1. hemorrhages due to blood-heat——hematochezia, hemorrhoidal bleeding, hematuria, metrorrhagia, hemoptysis, and epistaxis etc.

2. syndrome of flaring liver-fire——conjunctival congestion, headache with heaviness, and dizziness

3. hypertension

Dosage: 9～15g. The slightly carbonized herb is used for arresting bleeding. The fresh herb is used for the clearing away heat.

Contraindication: It can not be used for the cold syndrome of the spleen and the stomach of deficiency type.

Combinations:

1. add Garden Burnet Root(地榆, Diyu) and Chinese Arborvitae Leafy Twig(侧柏叶, Cebaiye)——hematochezia, hemorrhoidal bleeding.
2. add Baikal Skullcap Root (黄芩, Huangqin) and Common Selfheal Fruit-spike (夏枯草, Xiakucao)——hypertension.
3. add Chinese Arborvitae Leafy Twig(侧柏叶, Cebaiye) and Chniese Date(大枣, Dazao)——bleeding pelioma.
4. add Lalang Grass Rhizome (白茅根, Baimaogen) and India Madder Root(茜草, Qiancao)——hemoptysis, epistaxis, hematuria.
5. add Chrysanthemum Flower (菊花, Juhua)——liver heat and conjunctival congestion.
6. add slightly carbonized Garden Burnet Root(地榆, Diyu) and slightly carbonized Fineleaf Schizomepeta Herb (荆芥, Jingjie)——metrorrhagia and hematochezia.

Notes: The herb removes heat from the blood phase. Thus it is applied for hemorrhages due to blood-heat, especially for hemorrhages in the lower part of the body. The study of the modern pharmacology has shown that the Japanese Pagodatree Flower (槐花, Huaihua) has clear efficacy of decreasing blood-lipid. It arrests bleeding through decreasing the permeability and friability of the capillary vessel.

Japanese Pagodatree Flower-bud(槐米, Huaimi)and Japanese Pagodatree Flower(槐花,Huaihua)are the same and have similar functions. The functions of them are similar. Therefore these two herbs are not distinguished from each other in the Meteria Madica. The efficacy of Japanese Pagodatree Flower-bud(槐米,Huaimi)is slighly better. The function of Japanese Pagodatree Flower (槐花, Huaihua) and Japanese Pagodatree fruit (槐角, Huaijiao) are similar, too. Japanese Pagodatree Flower (槐花, Huaihua) is better for the arresting bleeding, while Japanese Pagodatree(槐角,Huaijiao) has higher efficacy of clearing away heat and purging fire. Japanese Pagodatree (槐角,Huaijiao) moisturizes the intestine. It is effective for hemorrhoidal bleeding and hematochezia. Thus it is usually used for hemorrhage due to hemorrhoid.

6. 侧柏叶, Cebaiye

English name: Chinese Arborvitae Leafy Twig

Pharmaceutical name: Cacumen Biotae Orientalis

Botanical name: Biota orientalis(L.)Endl.

侧柏叶

Properties and tastes: bitter, astringent, and slightly cold

Meridian tropism: lung, liver, and large intestine

Functions: 1. remove heat from the blood to arrest bleeding

2. dissolve phlegm, relieve cough and asthma

3. inhibit bacteria and prevent tuberculosis

4. tranquilize the mind and decrease blood pressure

Indications: 1. various hemorrhages in the interior or exterior of the body——hemoptysis, hematemesis, epistaxis, hematuria, metrorrhagia, hemorrhoidal bleeding and bleeding wounds. Especially for hemorrhages due to bloo-heat.

2. hemorrhage of gastroduodenal ulcer

3. cough due to lung heat, viscid sputum difficult to be expectorated and large amount of yellow sputum

4. chronic bronchitis and chincough

5. tuberculosis

6. seborrheic alopecia

7. empyrosis

Dosage: 9～15g. The slightly carbonized herb is used for arresting bleeding. The fresh herb is used for other cases. The proper amount should be used for external application.

Combinations: 1. add Janpanese Thistle Herb or Root(大蓟, Daji), Common Cephalanoplos Herb (小蓟, Xiaoji) and Lalang Grass Rhizome (白茅根, Baimaogen)——hematemesis, hemoptysis, epistaxis, metrorrhagia, hematuria, etc, due to blood-heat

2. add Arge Wormwood Leaf(艾叶, Aiye) and Baked Ginger (炮姜, Paojiang)——hemorrhage due to asthenia cold

3. add Common Yam Rhizome (山药, Shanyao)and Shorthorned Epimedium Herb (淫羊藿, Yinyanghuo)——chronic bronchitis.

4. add Rehmannia Dried Root (生地黄, Shengdihuang), Argy Wormwood Leaf (艾叶, Aiye) and Hindu Lotus Leaf (荷叶, Heye)——hematemesis and epistaxis due to blood-heat

5. add Honey(蜂蜜, Fengmi)——chincough

6. add Rhubarb(大黄,Dahuang)——hemorrhoidal bleeding

7. add Coptis Rhizome (黄连, Huanglian)——diseases of cutaneous infection

Notes: The property is slightly cold and the flavor is astringent. It is mainly used to treat the syndromes of blood-heat, as it can remove heat from the blood and astringe to arrest bleeding. It is also used to treat hemorrhage due to asthenia cold when combined with Argy Wormwood Leaf(艾叶, Aiye), etc. It is used to treat seborrheic dermatitis as follows: 60g of Chinese Arborvitae Leafy Twig (侧柏叶, Cebaiye) are soaked in proper amount of 60% alcohol for 7 days. The liquid is embrocated on the scalp. It can stop itching and decrease losing hair. The ointment made from the powder of carbonized Chinese Arborvitae Leafy Twig(侧柏叶, Cebaiye) and boiled sesame oil are effective for small and medium sized empyrosis.

7. 仙鹤草, Xianhecao

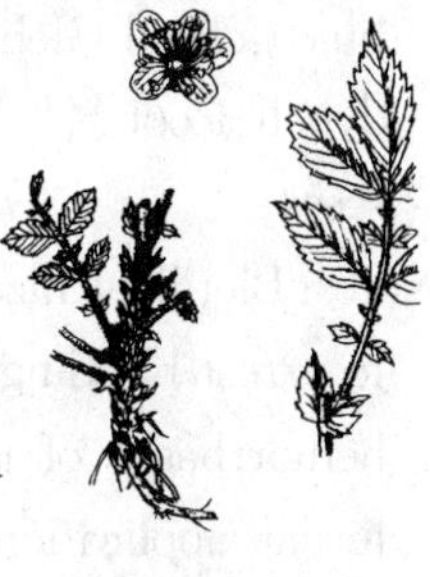

English name: Hairyvein Agrimonia Herb

Pharmaceutical name: Herba Agrimoniae Pilosae

Botanical name: Agrimonia pilosa Ledeb. var. japonica(Miq.) Nakai

仙鹤草

Properties and tastes: bitter, astringent, medium

Meridian tropism: lung, liver, and spleen

Functions: 1. astringe to arrest bleeding

2. remove food stagnancy and arrest dysentery

3. destroy parasites and relieve itching

4. tonify the human body and strengthen the spleen

5. remove toxic substances and promote subsidence of swelling

6. prevent attack of malaria

7. inhibit bacteria and anti inflammation

8. inhibit cancer

9. reduce blood sugar

10. regulate heart rate

Indications: 1. various hemorrhages——hematemesis, hemoptysis, epistaxis, hematochezia, etc.

2. chronic dysentery and bloody dysentery

3. exhaustion and injury caused by strain and sprain

4. trichomonal vaginitis

5. malnutrition of children

6. ulcer, hemorrhoid and breast carbuncle

7. malaria

Dosage: 6～15g. 30～60g, a large amount may be used. Proper amount should be used for external use.

Combinations: 1. add Rehmannia Dried Root (生地黄, Shengdihuang) and Tree Peony Bark(牡丹皮, Mudanpi)——hemorrhage due to blood-heat

2. add Dan-shen Root(丹参, Danshen) and Membranous Milkvetch Root (黄芪, Huangqi)——metrorrhagia due to asthenia cold syndrome

3. add Smoked Plum(乌梅, Wumei) and Common Aucklandia Root(木香, Muxiang)——prolonged diarrhea and dysentery

4. add Longan Aril(龙眼肉, Longyanrou)——exhaustion, injury caused by strain and sprain, fatigue and weakness

Notes: Hairyvein Agrimonia Herb(仙鹤草, Xianhecao) is a drug of astringing to arrest bleeding with the effect of strengthening the physique. It is used for the treatment of various hemorrhages. It is used to treat pruritus of pudendum caused by trichomonal vaginitis as follows: The pudendum is washed with concentrated decoction prepared from 120g of Hairyvein Agrimonia Herb(仙鹤草, Xianhecao). Then a cotton ball with thread dipped in the decoction is put into the vagina for 3～4h. One such treatment is carried out each day for a week. Modern study shows that Hairyvein Agrimonia Herb(仙鹤草, Xianhecao) inhibits cancer cells and eliminates tiredness.

8. 白及, Baiji

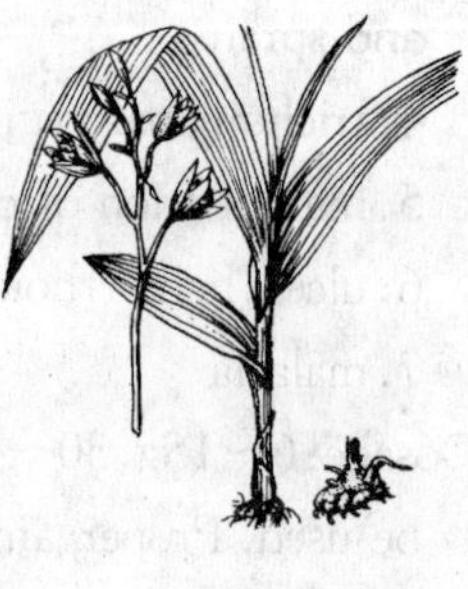
白 及

English name: Bletilla Rhizome

Pharmaceutical name: Rhizoma Bletillae Striatae

Botanical name: Bletilla striata (Thunb.) Reichb. f.

Properties and tastes: bitter, sweet, astringent, slightly cold

Meridian tropism: lung, liver, stomach

Functions: 1. astringe to arrest bleeding

2. diminish swelling and promote tissue regeneration

Indications: 1. hemoptysis, hematemesis and bleeding wounds, especially for hemorrhages due to blood-heat

2. tuberculosis, pulmonary abscess, hemoptysis due to bronchodilatation, as well as pneumoconiosis

3. hemorrhage of alimentary tract ulcer and gastroduodenal perforation, etc.

Dosage: 3～9g. The powder is taken orally for one time each day. Proper amount should be used for external application.

Contraindication: It is incompatible with Common Monkshood(附子, Fuzi).

Combinations: 1. add Parched Baikal Skullcap Root(黄芩, Huangqin) and Common Anemarrhea Rhizome (知母, Zhimu)——hematemesis

2. add Ass-hide Glue (阿胶, Ejiao) and White Peony Root (白芍药, Baishaoyao)——hemorrhage of gastric ulcer

3. add Honeysuckle Flower(金银花, Jinyinhua) and Snakegourd Root(天花粉, Tianhuafen)——carbuncle and ulcer

4. add Lily Bulb(百合, Baihe) and Ass-hide Glue(阿胶, Ejiao)——expectoration with blood due to bronchodilatation

5. add Loquat Leaf(枇杷叶, Pipaye) and Rehmannia Dried Root(生地黄, Shengdihuang)——hemoptysis

6. add Balloonflower Root (桔梗, Jiegeng)——to prepare decoction, which, after sugar is added in, is taken orally for cough due to silicosis and chest pain

7. add Sanchi Root(三七, Sanqi) and Cuttle Bone(乌贼骨, Wuzeigu)——hemorrhage of ulcers

8. add Honeysuckle Flower(金银花, Jinyinhua) Coastal Glehnia Root, and Fourleaf Ladybell Root(沙参, Shashen)——lung abscess

Notes: Bletilla Rhizome(白及, Baiji) astringes to arrest bleeding. It is mainly used to treat hemorrhages of the lung and stomach. External application may be singly used to treat bleeding due to wound. The ointment of the powder of Bletilla Rhizome(白及, Baiji) with sesame oil is externally applied for chapping of the hands and feet. The function of Bletilla Rhizome(白及, Baiji) are reinforcing as well as clearing, and astringing but not leaving pathogenic factors. Therefore, it is often used to treat lung abscess, cough, split purulent sputum, and syndrome that the pathogenic factors are declining. It is reported that Bletilla Rhizome (白及, Baiji) can be used to treat tuberculosis remained unhealed over a long period.

9. 棕榈炭, Zonglutan

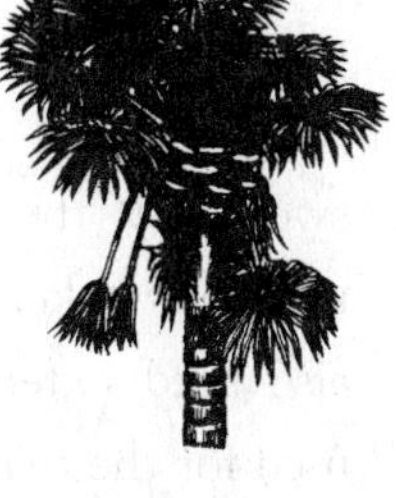
棕榈炭

English name: Fortune Windmillpalm

Pharmaceutical name: Trachycarpus

Botanical name: Palmaceae

Properties and tastes: bitter, astringent, medium

Meridian tropism: lung, liver, and large intestine

Function: astringe to arrest bleeding

Indication: hemorrhage without stagnation of blood stasis——hematemesis, hemoptysis, epistaxis, hematochezia, hemorrhoidal bleeding, hematuria, and metrorrhagia

Dosage: 3～9g.

Contraindication: It cannot be used for hemorrhage due to blood stasis.

Combinations: 1. add Largehead Atractylodes Rhizome (白术, Baizhu), Membranous Milkvetch Root (黄芪, Huangqi) and India Madder Root (茜草, Qiancao)——metrorrhagia due to asthenia cold syndrome and debility of Chong and Ren meridians

2. add Janpanese Thistle Herb or Root (大蓟, Daji), Common Cephalanoplos Herb (小蓟, Xiaoji) and Cape Jasmine Fruit (栀子, Zhizi)——hemorrhage due to blood-heat

3. add Red Peony Root (赤芍药, Chishaoyao) and Chinese Pulsatiall Root (白头翁, Baitouweng)——pus and blood in stool due to dysentery

Prescription: Powder of Ten Drugs Ashes (十灰散, Shihui San)

Notes: It is bitter and asringent in taste and medium in property. The potency is strong for arresting bleeding. It is a drug of astringing to arrest bleeding in common use. It is believed in traditional point that old fortune Windmillpalm (棕榈炭, Zonglutan) is better. It is said in *Compendium of Materia Medica* (《本草纲目》, Bencaogangmu) "Old spoild fortune Windmillpalm (棕榈炭, Zonglutan) used as medicine is excellent." The experimental investigations also showed that the arresting blood of old bark of Cabbage Palm and carbonized old Cabbage Palm is more effective than that of new ones.

10. 三七, Sanqi

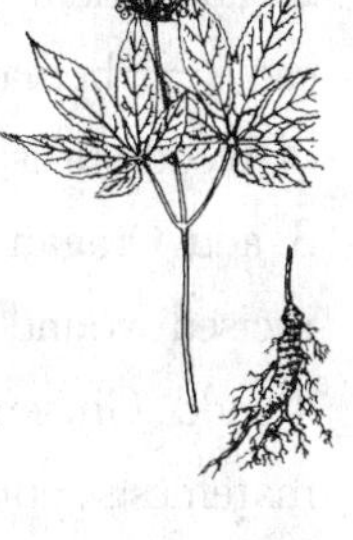
三 七

English name: Sanchi Root

Pharmaceutical name: Radix Pseudoginseng

Botanical name: Panax pesudoginseng Wall. Var. notoginseng (Burkill) Hoo et Tseng

Properties and tastes: sweet, slightly bitter, warm

Meridian tropism: liver, stomach

Functions: 1. dissolve blood stasis to arrest bleeding

2. relieve pain

3. eliminate tiredness, tranquilize the mind and treat insomnia

4. tonify the heart

5. lower the cholesterol level in the blood

Indications: 1. various interior and exterior hemorrhages, especially for hemorrhage with blood stasis

2. traumatic injury, swelling and pain due to blood stagnation, carbuncle and ulcer, and poisonous snake bites

3. coronary heart disease and cardiac neuralgia

4. ischemic cerebrovascular diseases, sequela of cerebral hemorrhage and brain trauma
5. chronic liver disease
6. high blood-lipid

Dosage: 3～9g。1～1.5g of powder is taken orally. Proper amount should be used for external application.

Contraindication: It should be applied with great care for pregnant women and patients with deficiency of yin.

Combinations: 1. add powder of Bletilla Rhizome (白及, Baiji)——hemoptysis due to tuberculosis and bronchodilatation, hematemesis, hematuria, hematochezia and epistaxis
2. add India Madder Root (茜草, Qiancao)——hematemesis, epistaxis and macule of blood stasis
3. add Dragan's Blood (血竭, Xuejie)——incised wound, trauma, carbuncle and ulcer
4. add Ginseng (人参, Renshen)——hematemesis, epistaxis, hematochezia, metrorrhagia, cough due to asthenic disease, coronary heart disease and cardiac neuralgia
5. add Lotus Rhizome Note (藕节, Oujie) and Lalang Grass Rhizome (白茅根, Baimaogen)——hematemesis, epistaxis and macule of blood stasis
6. add Divaricate Saposhnikovia Root (防风, Fangfeng) and Red Halloysite (赤石脂, Chishizhi)——hematochezia
7. add Dan-shen (丹参, Danshen)——coronary heart disease and cardiac neuralgia due to blood stasis

Notes: Sanchi Root (三七, Sanqi) has the function of arresting bleeding, activating blood circulation and nourishing the blood. It arrests bleeding without blood stasis and nourishes the blood without exhausting blood. Thus it is widely used for various blood diseases, and it has excellent efficacy in both internal and external applications. Li Shizhen (李时珍) said: "It can be used as a principal drug for incised wound in Southern Army and has amazing effect". Sanchi Root (三七, Sanqi) eliminates swellings and relieves pains. Thus it is also widely used for the treatment of intractable pain, painful swelling of the body surface and oncosis. It is usually taken orally as powder. But it is also used externaly. Recently, it has been used for the treatment of coronary heart disease, cardiac neuralgia and angina pectoris. It has also been used for the treatment of liver diseases, high blood-lipid, and brain trauma and stomach ulcer. It is a strengthening drug. The function is similar to that of Ginseng (人参, Renshen).

Sanchi Root (三七, Sanqi) activates blood circulation, dissipates blood stasis, arrests bleeding, eliminates swelling and relieves pains. Bletilla Rhizome (白及, Baiji) nourishes the lung, promotes tissue regeneration and astringes to arrest bleeding, while that of Sanchi Root (三七, Sanqi) is mainly dispersion. The function of Bletilla Rhizome (白及, Baiji) is mainly astringency. The former is dispersion and the latter is astringency. When they are combined, they restrict each other. The combination is very effective for various hemorrhages. According to the custom of the Traditional Chinese Medicine, the powder of the equal amount of the two herbs is taken orally. 1.5～3g each time, 2～3 times each day.

11. 血余炭, Xueyutan

English name: Charred Human Hair
Pharmaceutical name: Crinis Carbonisatus
Properties and tastes: bitter, medium

Meridian tropism: liver, stomach

Functions: 1. astringe to arrest bleeding

2. induce diuresis

3. promote tissue regeneration and wound healing (external application)

4. restrain bacteria

Indications: 1. various hemorrhages

2. difficult urination

3. ulceration of carbuncle and empyrosis (external application)

4. pus and blood in stool due to dysentery

Dosage: 6～9g. 1～1.5g of powder is taken for oral use.

Contraindication: It has unpleasant odor to cause vomiting. Thus it is not advisable for patients with digestive trouble.

Combinations: 1. add Juice of Lotus rhizome (鲜藕汁, Xianouzhi)——hemorrhage of the upper part of the body. The powder of Charred Human Hair (血余炭, Xueyutan) is added to half of a glass of Juice of Lotus rhizome (鲜藕汁, Xianouzhi). The mixture is taken orally

2. add Charred Fortune Windmillpalm (陈棕炭, Chenzongtan) and Garden Burnet Root (地榆, Diyu)——hemorrhage of the lower part of the body

3. add Talc (滑石, Huashi)——difficult urination

4. add Coptis Rhizome (黄连, Huanglian)——pus and blood in stool due to dysentery

Notes: It astringes to arrest bleeding and activate blood circulation. It is characterized by aressting bleeding without blood stasis. Therefore, it is used for various hemorrhages. Modern research shows that it can shorten the time of bleeding and blood coagulation as well as recalcification plasma. The effect of arresting bleeding is better than that of Hairyvein Agrimonia Herb (仙鹤草, Xianhecao) and vitamin K.

12. 茜草, Qiancao

茜草

English name: India Madder Root

Pharmaceutical name: Radix Rubiae Cordifoliae

Botanical name: Rubia cordifolia L. In various parts of China R. Cordifolia L. var longifolia Hand.-Mazz., R. Chinensis Reg. Et Maach, R. Truppeliana Loes., or R. Cordifolia L. var pratensis Maxim. are used instead.

Properties and tastes: bitter, cold

Meridian tropism: liver

Functions: 1. remove heat from blood and stop bleeding

2. activate blood flow and absorb clots

3. dredge the meridians

4. relieve cough and reduce sputum

5. inhibit the formation of the calculus and remove the calculus

6. inhibit cancer

7. increase white cells

Indications:

1. various hemorrhages due to blood heat with blood stasis

2. amenorrhea due to blood stasis

3. traumatic injury, swelling and pain due to blood stagnation, toothache caused by dental caries

4. arthralgia syndrome

Dosage: 6～15g. The slightly carbonized herb is used for astringing to arrest bleeding. The crude herb or the herb parched with wine is used for activating blood flow and clearing the channels.

Contraindication: It should be applied with great care for the asthenia of the spleen and the stomach deficiency, the pregnant women, and the bleeding patients without blood stasis.

Combinations: 1. add Janpanese Thistle Herb or Root(大蓟, Daji), Common Cephalanoplos Herb(小蓟, Xiaoji) and Chinese Arborvitae Leafy Twig(侧柏叶, Cebaiye)——hemorrhage due to blood-heat

2. add Chinese Angelica Root(当归, Danggui), Nutgrass Galingale Rhizome(香附, Xiangfu) and Red Peony Root(赤芍药, Chichaoyao)——amenorrhea due to blood stagnation

3. add Safflower(红花, Honghua), Chinese Angelica Root(当归, Danggui) and Szechwan Lovage Rhizome(川芎, Chuanxion g)——traumatic injury, swelling and pain

4. add Suberect Spatholobus Stem(鸡血藤, Jixueteng) and Yanhusuo(延胡索, Yanhusuo)——arthralgia

5. add Chinese Caterpillar Fungus(冬虫夏草, Dongchongxiacao) and Giant Gecko(蛤蚧, Gejie)——chronic bronchitis

6. add Japanese Climbing Fern Spores(海金沙, Haijinsha) and Chinese Honeylocust Spine(皂角刺, Zaojiaoci)——urinary calculus

7. add Rehmannia Dried Root(生地黄, Shengdihuang), Sanchi Root(三七, Sanqi) and Lalang Grass Rhizome(白茅根, Baimaogen)——allergic purpura

8. add Membranous Milkvetch Root(黄芪, Huangqi) and Cuttle Bone(乌贼骨, Wuzeigu)——metrorrhagia due to debility of Chong and Ren Meridians

9. add Coptis Rhizome(黄连, Huanglian) and Garden Burnet Root(地榆, Diyu)——dysentery

Notes: The India Madder Root(茜草, Qiancao) cools and arrests blood, and absorbs clots. It is suitable for hemorrhages due to blood-heat and blood stasis, and bleeding wounds, especially for the metrorrhagia due to blood-heat. It is also used for amenorrhea due to blood stasis, traumatic injury and articular reddish swelling due to arthritis of heat type. It was said in *Seeking Truth of Herbals* (《本草求真》, Bencaoqiuzhen): "The function of India Madder Root(茜草, Qiancao) is similar to that of Groomwell Root of Sinkiang Arnebia(紫草, Zicao). However, Groomwell Root of Sinkiang Arnebia(紫草, Zicao) only enters the liver and removes heat from the blood, leading the blood to circulate smoothly. Thus it can enter the liver and pericardium, activate the blood flow. Therefore, if patients with amenorrhea, wind arthralgia and jaundice due to blood stasis in the interior, take India Madder Root(茜草, Qiancao) orally, the blood stasis would flow downward. It is more effective to remove blood stasis and to arrest bleeding for syndrome of hematemesis, metrorrhagia and hematuria due to blood stasis and difficulty of blood flow. In a word, it is a drug to remove blood stasis. The function of India Madder Root(茜草, Qiancao) should not be confused with that of Groomwell Root of Sinkiang Arnebia(紫草, Zicao) which removes all heat from the blood. India Madder Root(茜草, Qiancao) can not be used for syndrome of fever due to blood deficiency."

13. 蒲黄, Puhuang

English name: Cattail Pollen

Pharmaceutical name: Pollen Typhae

Botanical name: Typha latifolia L., T. Angustifolia L., T. Angustata Bory et Chaub., T. Orientalis. Or numerous other plants of the same genus.

Properties and tastes: sweet, medium

蒲 黄

Meridian tropism: liver, pericardium

Functions: 1. astringe to arrest bleeding

2. activate the blood and absorb clots

3. expand coronary artery and decrease blood pressure

4. decrease cholesterol and triglyceride in blood serum

5. inhibit atherosclerosis

6. contract womb

7. inhibit inflammation

8. anti-tuberculosis

9. induce diuresis, Promote the function of the gallbladder, relieve asthma

Indications: 1. various hemorrhages—hemoptysis, hematemesis, hematuria, epistaxis, metrorrhagia and persistent lochia after delivery

2. pain in the chest and abdomen, dysmenorrhea and abdominal pain after delivery due to blood stasis

3. coronary heart disease and cardiac neuralgia

4. syndrome of high blood——lipid

5. chronic and non——specific colonitis

Dosage: 3～9g. The crude herb is used to activate blood and remove blood stasis. The slightly carbonized herb is used for astringing to arrest bleeding. The proper amount should be used for external application.

Combinations:

1. add Ass-hide Glue(阿胶, Ejiao) and Argy Wormwood Leaf(艾叶, Aiye)——metrorrhagia

2. add Trogopterus Dung(五灵脂, Wulingzhi) and Smoked Plum(乌梅, Wumei)——chronic colonitis

3. add Chinese Angelica Root(当归, Danggui) and Nutgrass Galingale Rhizome(香附, Xiangfu)——dysmenorrhea and abdominal pain after delivery

4. add Lalang Grass Rhizome(白茅根, Baimaogen) and Rehmannia Dried Root(生地黄, Shengdihuang)——hematuria

5. add Bletilla Rhizome(白及, Baiji)——hematemesis and hemoptysis

6. add Dan-shen(丹参, Danshen) and Sanchi Root(三七, Sanqi)——coronary heart disease and cardiac neuralgia

7. add Oriental Waterplantain Rhizome(泽泻, Zexie) and Hawthorn Fruit(山楂, Shanzha)——high blood-lipid

Prescription: Powder for Stopping Pain by Dissipating Blood Stasis(失笑散, Shixiao San)

Notes: Cattail Pollen(蒲黄, Puhuang) has a fairly good effect for arresting bleeding. It is used for the treatment of various hemorrhages. It has multifunction: arresting bleeding as well as activating blood and dissipating blood stasis. It arrests bleeding but does not leave blood stasis. It is reported that the function of removing blood stasis from woman lies in contracting the uterus; and it has the function of arresting bleeding. In addition, it was reported by Li Shizhen(李时珍) that Cattail Pollen(蒲黄, Puhuang) combined withTrogopterus Dung(五灵脂, Wulingzhi) is effective in treating pains in the chest and abdomen.

14. 卷柏, Juanbai

English name: Tamariskoid Spikemoss Herb

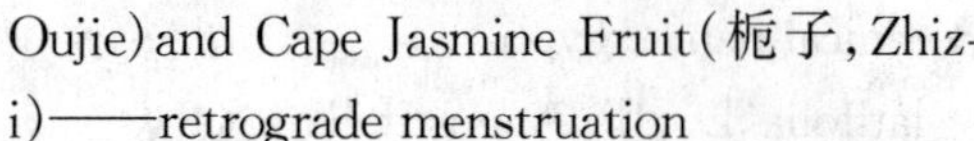

Pharmaceutical name: Herba Selaginellae

Botanical name: Selaginella tamariscina(Beauv.) Spring

Properties and tastes: pungent, medium

Meridian tropism: liver, heart

卷柏

Functions: 1. arrest bleeding

2. activate blood flow and dredge and meridians

3. absorb clots and stop pain

4. astringe leukorrhea

5. treat prolapse of the anus

Indications: 1. various hemorrhages, especially for hematochezia, hemorrhoidal bleeding

2. amenorrhea due to blood stasis and dysmenorrhea

3. abdominal masses

4. traumatic injury, swelling and pain due to blood stagnation

5. increasing leukorrhea

6. lung cancer, throat cancer

Dosage: 3~9g.

Contraindication: It should not be used for pregnant women.

Combinations: 1. add Szechwan Lovage Rhizome(川芎, Chuanxiong), Peach Seed(桃仁, Taoren) and Safflower(红花, Honghua)——amenorrhea and dysmenorrhea

2. add Chinese Arborvitae Leafy Twig(侧柏叶, Cebaiye) and Garden Burnet Root(地榆, Diyu)——hematochezia

3. add Hairyvein Agrimonia Herb(仙鹤草, Xianhecao), charred India Madder Root(茜草炭, Qiancaotan) and Cattail Pollen(蒲黄, Puhuang)——metrorrhagia

4. add Hindu Lotus Rhizome-node(藕节, Oujie) and Cape Jasmine Fruit(栀子, Zhizi)——retrograde menstruation

5. add Asiatic Plantian Seed(车前子, Cheqianzi) and Fineleaf Schizomepeta Herb(荆芥, Jingjie)——leukorrhea

6. add Parched Baikal Skullcap Root(黄芩, Huangqin) and Shunk Bugbane Rhizome(升麻, Shengma)——rectocele

Notes: Tamariskoid Spikemoss Herb(卷柏, Juanbai) activates blood flow, absorbs clots and clears the meridians. It is singly used for the treatment of amenorrhea and dysmenorrhea. The slightly carbonized Tamariskoid Spikemoss Herb(卷柏, Juanbai) has the function of arresting bleeding and is used for hematochezia, and metrorrhagia.

15. 艾叶, Aiye

English name: Argy Wormwood Leaf

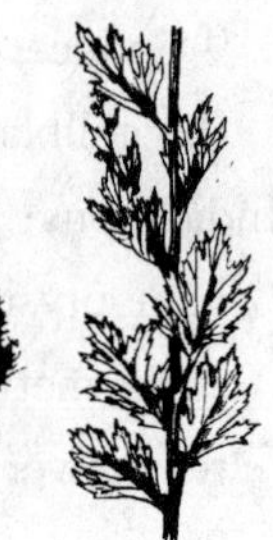

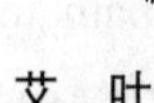

Pharmaceutical name: Folium Artemisiae

Botanical name: Artemisia argyi Levl. et Vant., A. vulgaris L. or A. vulgaris L. var. indica Maxim.

艾叶

Properties and tastes: bitter, pungent, warm

Meridian tropism: liver, spleen, and kidney

Functions: 1. warm the meridian and arrest bleeding

2. dispel cold and stop pain

3. regulate menstruation and prevent miscarriage

4. expel dampness and relieve itching

5. relieve cough and asthma, and dissolve phlegm

6. inhibit bacteria

Indications: 1. hemorrhages due to deficiency cold

2. dysmenorrhea, irregular menstruation and leukorrhea

3. threatened abortion or vaginal bleeding during pregnancy

4. cold syndrome of spleen and stomach of deficiency type, abdominal cold-pain and the feeling of cold and abdominal pain after delivery

5. chronic bronchitis and asthma

6. bacillary dysentery

7. allergic dermatitis, allergic rhinitis, drug alergy and asthma

8. used to prepare moxa rolls and moxa cones for moxibustion

Dosage: 3～9g. Proper amount should be used for the external applications. The slightly carbonized Argy Wormwood Leaf (艾叶, Aiye) is used for warming the meridians and arresting bleeding. The crude herb is used for the other applications.

Contraindication: It should be carefully used for the syndrome of yin deficiency and blood heat. Oral intake of large amount of Argy Wormwood Leaf (艾叶, Aiye) may cause acute gastroenteritis, toxic hepatitis and jaundice.

Combinations: 1. add Nutgrass Galingale Rhizome (香附, Xiangfu)——irregular menstruation, inability of pregnancy caused by cold womb, leukorrhea, threatened abortion, and cold pains of the lower abdomen and spermary of man

2. add Chinese Angelica Root (当归, Danggui) and Prepared Rhizome of Adhesive Rehmannia (熟地黄, Shoudihuang)——irregular menstruation or metrorrhagia due to cold womb

3. add Rehmannia Dried Root (生地黄, Shengdihuang) and Chinese Arborvitae Leafy Twig (侧柏叶, Cebaiye)——hemorrhage due to blood-heat

4. add Cicada Slough (蝉蜕, Chantui) and Divaricate Saposhnikovia Root (防风, Fangfeng)——itching due to eczema

5. add Ass-hide Glue (阿胶, Ejiao)——dysmenorrhea, menorrhagia, metrorrhagia or hemorrhage after delivery

6. add Tangerine Peel (橘皮, Jupi)——diarrhea due to qi and abdominal pain

Prescription: Decoction of Colla Corii Asini and Artemisiae Argyi (胶艾汤, Jiaoai Tang)

Notes: Argy Wormwood Leaf (艾叶, Aiye) is mainly used for hemorrhages due to deficiency cold. It is especially effective for metrorrhagia. The external application of its decoction is used to treat itching due to eczema. The moxibustion with moxa rolls and moxa cones made of dry moxa makes warm qi influx into the body. It warms qi and blood and reaches the meridians. Recently it has been found that oil of Argy Wormwood Leaf (艾叶, Aiye) has the function of relieving cough and asthma, and dissolving phlegm. The long-time administration of Argy Wormwood Leaf (艾叶, Aiye) has better effect. The amount to be taken orally should not be too large, as the large amount may cause acute inflammation of digestive track, even disturbance of metabolism of liver cells, or even poisoning.

Both Argy Wormwood Leaf (艾叶, Aiye) and Cassia Bark (肉桂, Rougui) have the function of warming qi and blood of the Lower-jiao. However, the flavors of Cassia Bark (肉桂, Rougui) are pungent and sweet and the property is extremely heat. It can activate blood but can not arrest bleeding. It can abort but can not prevent miscarriage. The flavors of Argy Wormwood Leaf (艾叶, Aiye) are bitter and pungent and the property is warm. It can warm qi and blood to regulate menstruation, and arrest bleeding to prevent miscarriage.

16. 灶心土, Zaoxintu

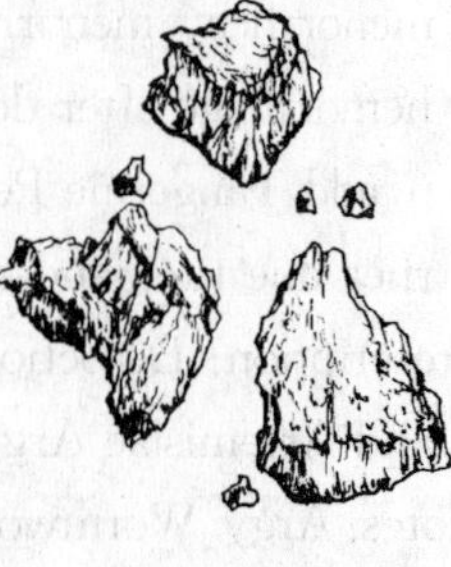

English name: Burnt Clay-lining of Kitchen Range

Properties and tastes: pungent, slightly warm

Meridian tropism: spleen, stomach

Functions:

1. warm the Middle-jiao to stop bleeding
2. lower the adverse flow of qi to stop vomiting
3. astringe intestine to relieve dysentery

Indications: 1. dysfunction of the spleen in keeping the blood flowing within the vessels——hematemesis, epistaxis, hematochezia, metrorrhagia, etc. with deficiency of qi

2. vomiting due to deficiency cold of the Middle-jiao and disorder of the stomach qi, pregnant reactions
3. prolonged diarrhea due to deficiency of spleen
4. infantile bacillary dysentery

Dosage: 15～30g. It should be wrapped with chandar and decoct first. In addition, the decoction of 60～120g of the herb is used as drinking water.

Contraindication: It is not suitable for patients with vomiting caused by bleeding due to deficiency of yin or stomach-heat.

Combinations: 1. add Rehmannia Dried Root (生地黄, Shengdihuang), Prepared Daughter Root of Common Monkshood (附子, Fuzi) and Ass-hide Glue (阿胶, Ejiao)——hemorrhages due to dysfunction of the spleen in keeping the blood flowing within the vessels

2. add Pinellia Rhizome (半夏, Banxia) and Dried Ginger (干姜, Ganjiang)——vomiting due to cold syndrome of spleen and stomach
3. add Perilla Stem (苏梗, Sugeng), Villous Amomum Fruit (砂仁, Sharen) and Bamboo Shavings (竹茹, Zhuru)——vomiting during pregnancy and vomiting without appetite
4. add Prepared Daughter Root of Common Monkshood (附子, Fuzi), Dried Ginger (干姜, Ganjiang) and Largehead Atractylodes Rhizome (白术, Baizhu)——chronic diarrhea due to deficiency of spleen

Notes: Burnt Clay-lining of Kitchen Range (灶心土, Zaoxintu) is the scorched earth in the bottom center of the chamber of a stove in which bavin is burnt. It is mainly composed of silicates, alumina and ferric oxide. It also contains sodium oxide, potassium oxide, magnesium oxide and calcium oxide etc.

Appendix: Other Hemostatic Drugs

Name	Properties and tastes	Meridian tropism	Function	Indications	Dosage	Contraindications
Ramie Root (苎麻根, Zhumagen)	sweet, cold	Heart, liver	Remove heat from blood, arrest bleeding, prevent miscarriage, remove toxic materials	Various hemorrhages due to heat, threatened abortion due to blood heat, vaginal bleeding during pregnancy, damp-heat and dripping urination, carbuncle and ulcer due to toxic heat	9～30g	Can not be used by patients with deficiency cold of the spleen and the stomach, and less heat in the blood system.
Japanese Dock Root (羊蹄, Yangti)	bitter, astringent, cold	Heart, liver, large intestine	Remove heat from blood, arrest bleeding, slow purging, relieve constipation, kill intestinal worms, treat tinea	Various hemorrhages due to heat, constipation, glae, tinea, pelioma due to blood platelet decreasing	9～15g	Can not be used by patients with loose stool due to asthenia of the spleen.
Taiwan Beautybetter Leaf(紫珠, Zizhu)	bitter, astringent, slightly cold	Liver, lung, stomach	Astringe to arrest bleeding, remove toxic materials, treat carbuncle	Various hemorrhages due to heat, bleeding wounds, burn, carbuncle and ulcer	9～15g	Carefully used for bleeding due to deficiency cold
Soot (百草霜, Baicaoshuang)	pungent, warm	Lung, stomach, large intestine	Arrest bleeding, eliminate stagnated food, relieve diarrhea	hematemesis, epistaxis, hematochezia, metrorrhagia, stagnated food, diarrhea	1.5～6g Wrapped with chandar when decoction is made. Proper amount for external applications	Can not be used for patients with deficient yin inducing vigorous fire. External application may leave black marking on the skin.
Hindu Lotus Rhizome-node(藕节, Oujie)	sweet, astringent, medium	Liver, lung, stomach	Astringe to arrest bleeding	hematemesis, hemoptysis, hematuria, hematochezia,	9～30g	
Copperleaf Herb(铁苋菜, Tiexiancai)	slightly bitter, astringent, slightly cold	Heart, liver, lung, large intestine	Astringe to arrest bleeding, relieve diarrhea, remove heat and toxic materials	Various hemorrhages, diarrhea, dermatitis, tetter	9～30g	Can not be used for pregnant women
Ophicalcite (花蕊石, Huaruishi)	sour, astringent, medium	Liver	Remove blood stasis, arrest bleeding	hemoptysis, hematemesis, bleeding wounds	9～15g. 1～1.5g of powder is taken by oral.	Carefully used for pregnant women.

PARTⅣ
Drugs For Expelling Water-dampness

Drugs which can regulate water metabolism of body, eliminate water-damp evil ofthe exterior and the interior, upper and lower part of body are named Drugs For Water-dampness. The drugs are divided into antirheumatics, aromatics and drugs for promoting diuresis to eliminate damp pathogen.

Nature produces water and water produces everything. The normal metabolism is the essential condition to maintain normal life. All of the normal water of the body is called essential substance from body fluid by traditional Chinese medicine. The fluid is produced by functioning of qi after entering into stomach and is transported to every part of body with the circulation of qi and blood. If functions of an organ fail or qi and blood stagnate or turbid evil invades, the circulation of fluid will be abnormal, store up in body and change into water, dampness, phlegm, fluid evil. In general, the evil which has no-shape and spreads all over the place is named dampness; the evil which has shape and stores up in body is named water evil. Phlegm and fluid belong to water evil. The evil can be expelled from skin by the treatment of lung when it stays in skin, muscle, meridian, and joints. The evil which in Middle-jiao can be removed from Middle-jiao by the treatment of spleen; the evil which in Lower-jiao can be expelled through promoting urination by the treatment of kidney. As to the sputum spitted out from the lung, there is a chapter for it. As to the stubbon water-fluid which should be eliminated by purgation, it is classified into purgatives.

Chapter 8
Drugs for Expelling Wind-dampness

Definition: The herbs which expel wind-dampness evil and relieve pain of arthritis are named antirheumatics.

Functions: This kind of herbs can expel wind-dampness evil from the exterior and meridians. Some of them have the effect of relaxing muscles, removing obstruction of meridians, relieving pain, expelling the exterior evil, tonifying liver and kidney and strengthening tendons and bones. Recent research shows that this kind of herbs functions as a sedative, analgestic and antiphlogistic. Some also have the effect of reducing fever and function as an analgesic

Indications: Used for arthralgia, spasm of muscles, numbness, hemiparalysis, aching pains of the waist and kness, flaccidity in the lower part of body. In the clinic this kind of herb is usually used to treat rheumatic arthritis, rheumatoid arthritis, sciatica, migratory arthralgia, hyperosteogeny and sequela of cerebral vascular accident.

Cautions: This kind of herbs are pungent, warm, fragrant and dry, they easily weaken yin and blood, so should be cautiously used for patients with yin and blood-deficiency.

1. 独活, Duhuo

English name: Doubleteeth Pulbescent Angelica Root

Pharmaceutical name: Radix Duhuo

Botanical name: Angelica pubescens Maixm. or A. pubescens Maxim.

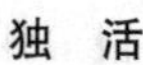

独 活

F. biserrata Shan et Yuan are the plants most commonly used. Other plants used include A. porphyrocaulis Nankai et Kitag. A. dahurica (see Dahurian Angelica Root (白芷, Baizhi) in chapter1), Heraclelum hemsleyanum Diels, Heracleum lanatum Michx., Aralia atropurpurea Franch., and Aralia cordata Thunb.

Properties and tastes: sour, bitter, warm

Meridian tropism: liver, kidney, and urinary bladder

Functions: 1. expel wind-dampness evil, relieve arthralgia

2. induce diaphoresis and expel exterior evil

3. analgesic and antiphlogistic

Indications: 1. arthralgia of wind-dampness——rheumatic arthritis, rheumatoid arthritis etc. especially in the lower part of the body

2. exterior syndrome due to wind-cold with dampness——aversion to cold, fever, headache, heavy sensation of the body and arthralgia

3. toothache and headache caused by wind-fire

4. skin eczema

Dosage: 3～9g

Contraindication: Use cautiously for patients with yin-deficiency and dry-blood. Do not use in cases of exogenous wind syndrome.

Combinations: 1. add Divaricate Saposhnikovia Root (防风, Fangfeng), Eucommia Bark (杜仲, Duzhong)——arthralgia of wind-cold-dampness, aching pains of the waist and kness

2. add Rhizome or Root of Forbes Notopterygium (羌活, Qianghuo)——exterior syndrome due to wind-cold with dampness; wind-arthralgia, moving pain of the whole body, severe and migratory arthralgia

3. add Dahurian Angelica Root (白芷, Baizhi), Szechwan Lovage Rhizome (川芎, Chuanxiong)——parietal headache caused by wind-cold-dampness

4. add Gypsum (石膏, Shigao), Shunk Bugbane Rhizome (升麻, Shengma)——toothache caused by wind-fire

5. add Rhizome or Root of Forbes Notopterygium (羌活, Qianghuo), Chinese Pine Node (松节, Songjie)——rheumatoid arthritis

6. add Bunge Pricklyash (花椒, Huajiao)——vitiligo (Exteral use, shine upon)

Prescription: Decoction of Pubesent Angelica and Loranthus (独活寄生汤, Duhuo Jisheng Tang)

Notes: Doubleteeth Pulbescent Angelica Root (独活, Duhuo) is sour, bitter, and dry. It is good at expelling wind dampness evil, relieving arthralgia, indicated for invasion of arthralgia of wind-cold-dampness to the muscles and joints, no matter it is a newly or lingering disease, it is usually in the lower part of the body. So Doubleteeth Pulbescent Angelica Root(独活, Duhuo) is a major herb for treating pain of the waist and legs caused by cold-dampness. *Orthodox Interpretation of Materia Medica* (《本草正义》, Bencaozhengyi) said: Doubleteeth Pulbescent Angelica Root(独活, Duhuo) is usually used for the lower part of the body and for wind in the waist and lower abdome. It can not only cure wind-cold-dampness, flaccidity and arthralgia but also cure sore syndrome of Yin Fen. It is good at reducing the sore if it is not diabrotic, or easily astringe the sore if it is diabrotic. Doubleteeth Pulbescent Angelica Root(独活, Duhuo) is similar to Rhizome or Root of Forbes Notopterygium(羌活, Qianghuo) in property, taste and function. Both can expel wind and dampness evil, disperse cold, relieve arthralgia and treat arthralgia of wind-cold-dampness with combination. Rhizome or Root of Forbes Notopterygium (羌活, Qianghuo) acts on Taiyang meridian, it is good at dispersing wind-cold-dampness evil in meridian of Taiyang, inducing diaphoresis and expelling exterior evil, especially for evil in upper and exterior; Doubleteeth Pulbescent Angelica Root(独活, Duhuo) acts on Shaoyin meridian, it is good at expelling wind-dampness in lower part of the body and it has a good effect to relieve pain of waist and legs caused by wind-dampness. In treating headache, Rhizome or Root of Forbes Notopterygium (羌活, Qianghuo) treats headache of Taiyang meridian from vertex to occiput, Doubleteeth Pulbescent Angelica Root (独活, Duhuo) treats the headache of Shaoyin meridian affecting teeth and face. Moreover, Rhizome or Root of Forbes Notopterygium(羌活, Qianghuo) is usually used as conducting herb of Taiyang meridian. Doubleteeth Pulbescent Angelica Root (独活, Duhuo) is mostly used as conducting herb of Shaoyin meridian.

2. 威灵仙, Weilingxian

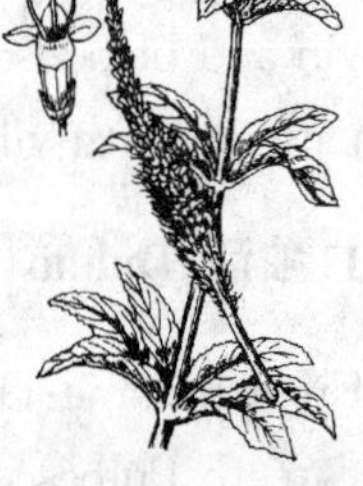
威灵仙

English name: Chinese Clematis Root

Pharmaceutical name: Radix Clemetidis Chinensis

Botanical name: Clematis chinensis Osbeck

Properties and tastes: sour, salty, warm

Meridian tropism: urinary bladder

Functions: 1. expel wind-dampness and remove obstruction of meridians
2. relieve arthralgia
3. treat a fishbone stuck in the throat
4. eliminate retained fluid and ablate stagnation
5. regulate functions of the gallbladder

Indications: 1. arthralgia muscular constricture and traumatic injury
2. any small bone stuck in the throat (decoct this herb with water and swallow it gradually)
3. dysphagia, phlegm fluid, abdominal mass
4. hiccups
5. cholelithiasis
6. hypertrophic rachitis (made into injecting liquid for point injection)

Dosage: 6～9g, 30 grams for a bone stuck in the throat.

Contraindication: The herb is spreading in property, and impairs vital qi in case of long term administration. Use cautiously for weak persons.

Combinations: 1. add Chinese Taxillus Twig

(桑寄生, Sangjisheng)——arthralgia of wind-dampness caused by blood deficiency, unsmooth movement of limbs and body, pain of body

2. add Rhizome or Root of Forbes Notopterygium (羌活, Qianghuo)——rheumatic arthritis, especially for pain of the upper body

3. add Twotooth Achyranthes Root(牛膝, Niuxi)——stagnation of wind-dampness in the meridian, pain of joints, especially the lower body

4. add Largeleaf Gentian Root(秦艽, Qinjiao), Mulberry Twig(桑枝, Sangzhi)——chronic rheumatic arthralgia, pain and unsmooth movement of joint, numbness of hands and feet etc.

5. add Peach Seed(桃仁, Taoren), Safflower (红花, Honghua)——pain of traumatic injury

6. add Arisaema With Bile(胆南星, Dannanxing), Indigwoad Root(板蓝根, Banlangen)——esophageal cancer

Notes: Chinese Clematis Root(威灵仙, Weilingxian) has the effects of removing obstruction of meridians, expelling wind-dampness and relieving arthralgia. *Orthodox Interpretation of Materia Medica* (《本草正义》, Bencaozhengyi) said: "Chinese Clematis Root(威灵仙, Weilingxian) is good at moving and anti-inflammation. And it is proper to treat excess syndrome such as the stagnation of dampness and phlegm, blood stasis and qi stagnation." So it is used for the syndrome of stasis, stagnation of qi, arthritis of wind-dampness, numbness of the body, spasm of muscles and unsmooth movement of joints. So Zhu Zhenheng(朱震亨) called it as "a major herb for treating wind evil". In modern clinics, it is used to treat esophageal cancer since it can remove food stagnation and phlegm. Moreover, according to *Revised Materia Medica in Kaibao Period* (《开宝本草》, Kaibaobencao), Chinese Clematis Root(威灵仙, Weilingxian) has the effect of preventing pestilence and malaria.

Both Chinese Clematis Root(威灵仙, Weilingxian) and Largeleaf Gentian Root (秦艽, Qinjiao) have the effect of expelling wind and dampness evil, so both of them can treat arthritis, unsmooth movement of the limbs, especially for the lower body. But Chinese Clematis Root(威灵仙, Weilingxian) is warm and moving. It is properly used for pain due to wind-dampness with cold nature or unsmooth movement of the limbs, even numbness paralysis. Largeleaf Gentian Root(秦艽, Qinjiao) is a little bit cold, good at expelling dampness, indicating for wind-dampness with excessive dampness. Moreover, Chinese Clematis Root(威灵仙, Weilingxian) is salty in property and can resolve hard lumps. So it can treat stagnation and bone stuck in the throat, Largeleaf Gentian Root(秦艽, Qinjiao) reduces asthenia heat, so it treats bone-heating and consumptive disease and jaundice due to dampness-heat.

3. 防己, Fangji

English name: Fourstamen Stephania Root

Pharmaceutical name: Radix Stephaniae Tetrandrae

Botanical name: Stephania tetrandra S. Moore

Properties and tastes: bitter, sour, cold.

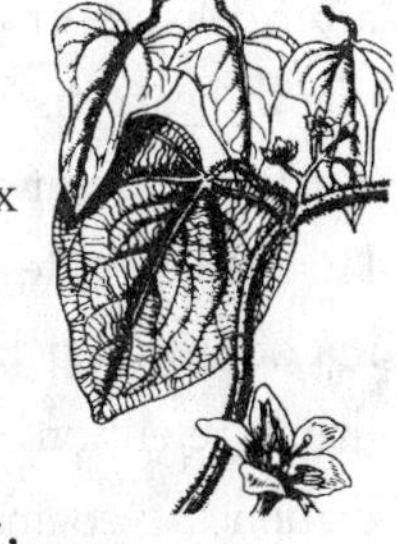

防　己

Meridian tropism: urinary bladder, kidney, spleen.

Functions: 1. expel wind-dampness evil and relieve arthritis
2. promote urination to alleviate edema
3. relax the functions of striated muscle
4. reduce blood pressure
5. dilate coronary arteries
6. anti-carcinoghic
7. anti-inflammatory effect, anti-allergic, reduce fever

Indications: 1. arthritis of wind-dampness, especially to dampness-heat type.
2. edema, ascites, puffiness caused by beriberi
3. hypertention, coronary heart disease
4. carcinoma of the lung and silicosis
5. all types of nervous pain. Pain in the chest caused by tuberculosis disease, intercostal neuralgia

Dosage: 6～9 g

Contraindication: The herb is too bitter and cold to be used much for protecting vital qi. Do not use in cases of spleen and stomach-deficiency and yin-deficiency without dampness-heat.

Combinations: 1. add Chinese Clematis Root (威灵仙, Weilingxian)——pain of shoulder, back and joints caused by wind-dampness in meridians
2. add Hirsute Shiny Bugleweed Herb (泽兰, Zelan)——edema of women in period or after delivery or at the early stage of ascites due to heart disease
3. add Membranous Milkvetch Root (黄芪, Huangqi)——fever, aversion to wind, edema of face and limbs, bone and joint pain, urine retention, treating arthritis due to dampness, edema caused by wind evil, chronic nephritis, edema due to heart disease
4. add Dang-shen Root (党参, Dangshen), Cassia Twig (桂枝, Guizhi)——edema, floating pulse, heavy body, shortness of breath, asthma also treating hydrops of thoracic cavity
5. add Common Anemarrhea Rhizome (知母, Zhimu), Chinese Cotktree Bark (黄柏, Huangbai)——obvious red swelling and hot pain of joints, fever, more thirsty, which belong to heat arthritis
6. add Ephedra (麻黄, Mahuang), Gypsum (石膏, Shigao)——acute nephritis
7. add Membranous Milkvetch Root (黄芪, Huangqi), Cassia Twig (桂枝, Guizhi)——chronic nephritis
8. add Dan-shen Root (丹参, Danshen)——coronary heart disease, hypertension
9. add Spreading Hedyotis Herb (白花蛇舌草, Baihuasheshecao)——lung cancer
10. add Coix Seed (薏苡仁, Yiyiren), Silkworm Feculae (蚕砂, Cansha)——arthritis of dampness-heat type

Prescription: Decoction of Radix Stephaniae Tetrandrae and Radix Astragali seu Hedysari in Combination (防己黄芪汤, Fangji Huangqin Tang)

Notes: Fourstamen Stephania Root (防己, Fangji) is good at expelling wind-dampness and relieving arthritis. It is used to treat arthritis caused by dampness-heat evil for it is cold in property. Root of Dutchman-Spipe is named Root of Dutchman-Spipe (木防己, Mufangji) which has a good effect for expelling wind and relieving arthritis. So Chen Zangqi (陈藏器), an ancient physician, said: Root of Dutchman-Spipe (木防己, Mufangj i) is used for treating wind evil, Fourstamen Stephania Root (防己, Hanfangji) is used for treating water evil.

Animal experiment shows that large dosage are obviously toxic to the liver, kidney and adrenal. Attention must be paid in the clinic.

4. 秦艽, Qinjiao

English name: Largeleaf Gentian Root

Pharmaceutical name: Radix Gentianae Macrophyllae

Botanical name: Gentiana macrophylla Pall. In parts of southwest China and Tibet G. Crassicaulis Duthie ex Burkill or G. Tibetica King are used instead.

秦 艽

Properties and tastes: bitter, sour, slightly, cold

Meridian tropism: stomach, liver, and gallbladder

Functions: 1. expel wind-dampness, relieve arthritis

2. relax muscles

3. reduce fever

4. remove dampness and treat jaundice

5. anti-carcinogenic, tranquilize the mind, reduce fever, antianaphylaxis shock and antihistamine functions

6. lower blood sugar

7. reduce blood pressure

8. promote urination

9. bacteriostasis

Indications: 1. arthritis——rheumatic arthritis, rheumatoid arthritis

2. hemiplagia after apoplexy——especially for muscular constricture of upper limbs

3. hectic fever, tidal fever and infantile malnutrition fever

4. jaundice due to dampness-heat

Dosage: 6～9 g

Contraindication: It can lower blood sugar, do not use for diabetes patients.

Combinations: 1. add Chinese Clematis Root (威灵仙, Weilingxian), Divaricate Saposhnikovia Root (防风, Fangfeng)——rheumatic arthritis, rheumatoid arthritis

2. add Chinese Angelica Root (当归, Danggui), White Peony Root (白芍药, Baishaoyao)——hemiplagia after apoplexy

3. add Capillary Wormwood Herb (茵陈蒿, Yinchengao), Cape Jasmine Fruit (栀子, Zhizi)——jaundice due to damp-heat

4. add Baikal skullcap Root (黄芩, Huangqin), Swordlike Atractylodes Rhizome (苍术, Cangzhu)——infantile acute epidemic hepatitis of jaundice.

5. add Common Anemarrhea Rhizome (知母, Zhimu), Chinese Wolfberry Root-bark (地骨皮, Digubi)——yin-deficiency and vigorous fire, low fever.

6. add Turtle Carapace (鳖甲, Biejia)——hectic fever and tidal fever

7. add Oriental Variegated Coralbean Bark (海桐皮, Haitongpi)—muscular constricture of limbs, sequela of infantile paralysis.

Prescription: Large Leaf Gentian and Turtle Powder (秦艽鳖甲散, Qinjiao Biejia San)

Notes: Largeleaf Gentian Root (秦艽, Qinjiao) can expel wind and dampness evil, relax muscles and remove the obstruction of meridians. It can be used in combination no matter whether the rheumatic arthritis is of long or short duration; cold or heat type. It is slightly cold in property and can clear away heat, especially for arthritis with heat symptoms, ie fever, redness and swelling in the joints. It also has an effect on paralysis of limbs after apoplexy. Largeleaf Gentian Root (秦艽, Qinjiao) is bitter, medium, not dry, so there has been the saying: All herbs of expelling wind are drying except Largeleaf Gentian Root (秦艽, Qinjiao) which is humidifying, and it is demulcent of expelling wind drugs and tonic of dispersing drugs.

Both Largeleaf Gentian Root(秦艽,Qinjiao) and Chinese Gentian Root (龙胆草, Longdancao) can expel dampness, and reduce fever, so it can treat jaundice due to dampness-heat. Largeleaf Gentian Root(秦艽,Qinjiao)expels wind and dampness evil, and it is medium and not drying. So it is usually used for treating arthritis of wind-dampness, hectic fever. Chinese Gentian Root(龙胆草,Longdancao)is extremely bitter and cold and purges excessive fire of the lower meridian, dampness-heat in Lower-jiao, conjunctival congestion, dizziness, deafness, chronic convulsion due to liver heat and swelling of valvae, pruritus valvae and profuse leukorrhea due to dampness-heat.

5. 豨莶草, Xixiancao

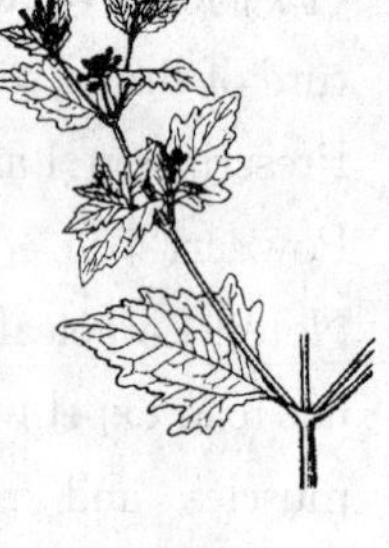

豨莶草

English name: Common St. Paulswort Herb

Pharmaceutical name: Herba Siegesbeckiae Orientalis

Botanical name: Siegesbeckia orientalis L. var. pubescens Mak., or S. Orientalis L., or S. Orientalis L. var. glabrescens Mak.

Properties and tastes: bitter, sour, cold

Meridian tropism: liver, kidney

Functions: 1. expel wind-dampness

2. remove obstruction of meridian

3. clear away heat and detoxicate

4. reduce blood pressure

5. diastolizate blood vessels

6. anti-inflammation

7. restrain malarial parasite

Indications: 1. arthritis of wind-dampness, pain of joint, muscular contracture, preferable for heat type

2. flaccidity-numbness of limbs, feeble feet, paralysis of limbs

3. swelling of carbuncle, toxic of sores, eczema itching

4. jaundice hepatitis

5. hypertension

Dosage: 9 ～ 15 g. The processed drug is for arthritis, the unprepared drug is for clearing away heat and detoxicating.

Combinations: 1. add Rhizome or Root of Forbes Notopterygium (羌活, Qianghuo), Doubleteeth Pulbescent Angelica Root (独活, Duhuo)——arthritis of wind-dampness

2. add Swordlike Atractylodes Rhizome(苍术, Cangzhu), Medicininal Cyathula Root (川牛膝, Chuanniuxi)——flaccidity

3. add Chinese Taxillus Twig (桑寄生, Sangjisheng), Peach Seed (桃仁, Taoren)——paralysis of limbs due to apoplexy

4. add Honeysuckle Flower(金银花, Jinyinhua), Licorice Root (甘草, Gancao)——swelling of carbuncle and toxic of sore

5. add Mulberry Twig (桑枝, Sangzhi), Densefruit Pittany Root-bark (白鲜皮, Baixianpi)——eczema and itching

6. add Chinese Wolfberry Root-bark(地骨皮, Digubi), Abalone Shell (石决明, Shijueming)——for hypertension

7. add Harlequin Glorybower Leaf(臭梧桐, Chouwutong)——arthritis of wind-dampness and hypertension

8. add Oriental Variegated Coralbean Bark (海桐皮, Haitongpi)——arthritis of wind-dampness, hemipalegia and sequela of infantile paralysis

Notes: Common St. Paulswort Herb(豨莶草, Xixiancao) is pungent, bitter and cold, it is good at resolving dampness-heat, expelling wind and relieving itching, so Siegesbeckia is useful for pyogenic infection and ulceration of skin due to dampness-heat and rubella, itching due to monious dampness; After steaming of wine, the property of bitter and cold changes into sweet and warmth. It has the effect to replenish liver and kidney except expelling wind-dampness. So it treats numbness of limbs, pain of muscles, sore and softness in waist and legs, dizziness, tinntus, insomnia, worry etc. Especially for numbness of limbs. *Annotation on Shennong's Herbal Classic* (《本草经疏》, Bencaojingshu) said: "Common St. Paulswort Herb(豨莶草, Xixiancao) is a serious herb for expelling wind, resolving dampness and removing blood stasis." It is proved true in the clinic.

6. 木瓜, Mugua

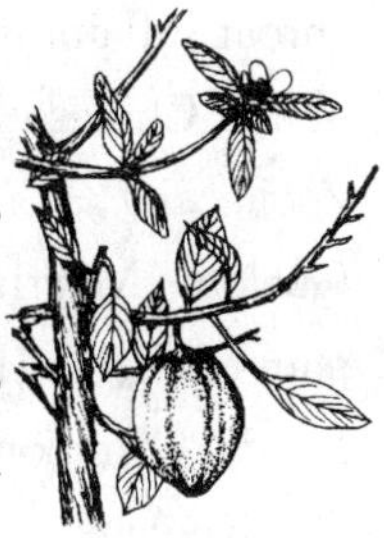

English name: Common Floweringquince Fruit

Pharmaceutical name: Fructus Chaenomelis Lagenariae

Botanical name: Chaenomeles lagenaria(Loisel.) Koidz. In some parts of China C. sinensis(Thouin) Koehne or C. speciosa(Sweet) Nankai are used instead.

木 瓜

Properties and tastes: sour, warm

Meridian tropism: liver, spleen

Functions: 1. relax muscles and promote collateral circulation

2. resolve dampness and regulate the stomach

3. remove food stagnation

4. protect liver and lower enzyme functions

Indications: 1. arthritis of wind-dampness——prolonged arthritis, muscular contracuture, unable to turn

2. flaccidity of lower limbs——cold-dampness, swelling and pain of feet, restlessness due to heart attack

3. spasm due to vomiting diarrhea, obstruction of excessive vomiting, chronic convulsion muscular contracture

4. dyspepsia

5. acute jaundice hepatitis

6. acute bacteric dysentery

Dosage: 6～15 g.

Contraindication: Use cautiously for patients with hyperacidity.

Combinations: 1. add Twotooth Achyranthes Root(牛膝, Niuxi)——arthritis of dampness, unsmooth movement of joints

2. add Coix Seed(薏苡仁, Yiyiren)——suffering from summer-heat, vomiting and diarrhea, and abdominal pain, spasm or foot pain and softness caused by dampness in meridian, heaviness and numbness, flaccidity of lower limbs and edema

3. add Smoked Plum(乌梅, Wumei)——chronic gastritis

4. add Medicinal Evodia Root(吴茱萸, Wuzhuyu)——systremma, flaccidity of lower limbs, abdominal pain, abdominal pain of hernia and flaccidity of the lower body

5. add Chinese Angelica Root(当归, Danggui), White Peony Root(白芍药, Baishaoyao)——muscular spasm caused by blood deficiency

6. add Hawthorn Fruit(山楂, Shanzha), Medicated Leaven(神曲, Shenqu)——dyspepsia

7. add Fourstamen Stephania Root(防己, Fangji), Chinese Clematis Root(威灵仙, Weilingxian)——pain and numbness of joints

8. add Doubleteeth Pulbescent Angelica Root(独活, Duhuo)——flaccidity of waist and knees caused by wind-dampness, pain of

joint

Notes: Common Floweringquince Fruit(木瓜, Mugua) has a good effect for relaxing muscles, promoting collateral circulation and resolving dampness. So it is usually used for arthritis of wind-dampness, especially for muscular contracture. So Zhang Jing yue said: "Common Floweringquince Fruit (木瓜, Mugua) is necessary to conduct meridions in treating feeble of waist and knees, flaccidity of lower limbs. And it can harmonize the stagnation of qi and check the prolapse of qi." Common Floweringquince Fruit (木瓜, Mugua) can treat spasm due to vomitting and diarrhea, because it can resolve dampness and regulate Middle-jiao. Also it can relax muscles, promote collateral circulation, and relieve systremma. It is sour and astringent, so take cautions when it is used at the beginning of pain for the vigorousness of pathogenic qi to avoid damaging anti-pathogenic qi.

7. 络石藤, Luoshiteng

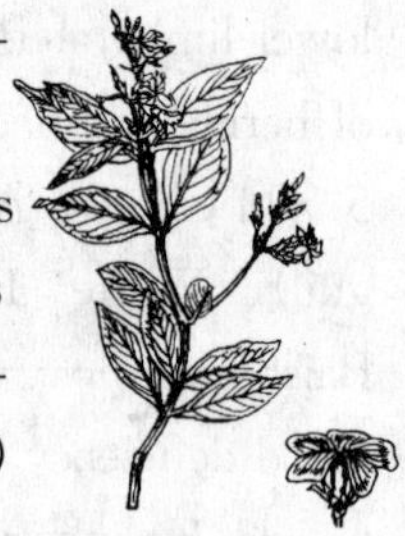

English name: Chinese Starjasmine Stem

Pharmaceutical name: Caulis Trachelospermi Jasminoidis

Botanical name: Trachelospermum jasminoides (Lindl.) Lem.

络石藤

Properties and tastes: bitter, slightly cold

Meridian tropism: heart, liver

Functions: 1. expel wind and remove obstruction of meridians

2. remove heat from the blood and detumescentify

3. expand blood vessels

4. reduce blood pressure

Indications:

1. arthritis of wind-dampness - especially for heat-arthritis of wind-dampness, red swelling of joints

2. throat inflammation, swelling of throat

3. swelling pain of carbuncle

4. hypertension

Dosage: 6～15 g.

Combinations: 1. addCommon Floweringquince Fruit (木瓜, Mugua), Chinese Taxillus Twig(桑寄生, Sangjisheng), Coix Seed(薏苡仁, Yiyiren)——arthritis of wind-dampness

2. add Barbary Wolfberry Fruit (枸杞子, Gouqizi), Chinese Angelica Root (当归, Danggui)——pain of muscle and bone, feeble waist and knees

3. add Blackberrylily Rhizome (射干, Shegan), Figwort Root (玄参, Xuanshen)——throat inflammation

4. add Chinese Honeylocust Spine(皂角刺, Zaojiaoci), Snakegourd Fruit (瓜蒌, Gualou), Myrrh(没药, Moyao)——swelling pain of carbuncle

5. add Common St. Paulswort Herb (豨莶草, Xixiancao)——hypertension or feeble lower limbs

6. add Kadsura Pepper Stem (海风藤, Haifengteng)——arthritis of wind-dampness and hemiparalgia

Notes: Chinese Starjasmine Stem(络石藤, Luoshiteng) expels the wind and removes obstruction of meridians, and clears away heat, especially for arthritis of heat. It can be used individually in tonic wine. It can be boiled alone with water to treat sorethroat.

8. 桑枝, Sangzhi

English name: Mulberry Twig

Pharmaceutical name: Ramulus Mori Albae

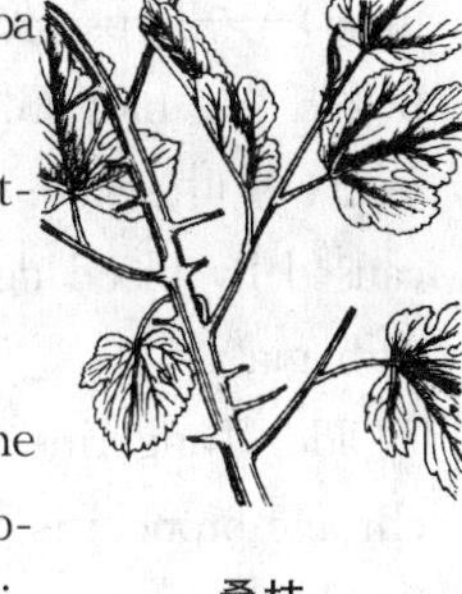
桑枝

Botanical name: Morus alba L.

Properties and tastes: bitter, medium

Meridian tropism: liver

Functions: 1. expel the wind and remove obstruction of the meridians

2. regulate functions of joints

3. promote urination and detumescentify

4. reduce blood pressure

Indications: 1. arthritis of wind-dampness——unsmooth movement of joints, muscular constricture, especially for heat-arthritis of wind-dampness in the upper extremities

2. numbness of limbs after apoplexy or hemiparalgia

3. edema, urine retention, pain of limbs

Dosage: 9～30 g.

Combinaitons: 1. add Fourstamen Stephania Root (防已, Fangji), Chinese Clematis Root (威灵仙, Weilingxian), Rhizome or Root of Forbes Notopterygium (羌活, Qianghuo)——arthritis of wind-dampness

2. add Tumeric Rhizome (姜黄, Jianghuang), Dahurian Angelica Root (白芷, Baizhi), Szechwan Lovage Rhizome (川芎, Chuanxiong)——pain of arms

3. add Tuckahoe (茯苓, Fuling), White Mulberry Root-bark (桑白皮, Sangbaipi)——edema

4. add Cassia Twig (桂枝, Guizhi)——arthritis of arms

5. add Mulberry Leaf (桑叶, Sangye)——arthritis of wind-dampness, eruption due to wind-heat, exterior syndrome of wind-heat

Notes: Mulberry Twig (桑枝, Sangzhi) is good at expelling the wind, dampness, removing obstruction of meridians, and clear away heat. It is proper to treat numbness, muscular contracture and skin itching caused by wind and dampness. It is especially used for arthritis of wind-dampness-heat.

Both Mulberry Twig (桑枝, Sangzhi) and Cassia Twig (桂枝, Guizhi) can remove obstruction of meridians. Mulberry Twig (桑枝, Sangzhi) is good at expelling the wind, dampness and removing obstruction of meridians; Cassia Twig (桂枝, Guizhi) is good at warming yang and removing obstruction of meridians. It can be used to treat the arthritis of wind-dampness. But Mulberry Twig (桑枝, Sangzhi) is bitter and purgative, therefore it can be used to treat syndrome of wind-dampness-heat. Cassia Twig (桂枝, Guizhi) is sour and warm, therefore it can be used to treat the arthritis caused by wind-cold-dampness. Since Mulberry Twig (桑枝, Sangzhi) is good at dispersing wind and clearing away dampness, it treats itching of skin. Cassia Twig (桂枝, Guizhi) has an effect of warming meridians.

9. 桑寄生, Sangjisheng

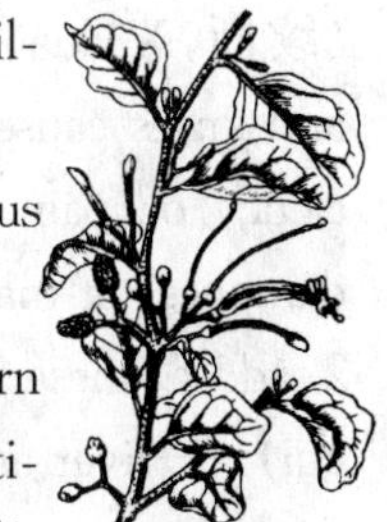
桑寄生

English name: Chinese Taxillus Twig

Pharmaceutical name: Ramus Loranthi seu Visci

Botanical name: In southern China Loranthus parasiticus (L.) Merr.. L. gracilifolius Schult., or L. yadoriki Sieb is used as the source of this herb. In northern China Viscum coloratum (Kom.) Nankai or V. album L. are used.

Properties and tastes: bitter, medium

Meridian tropism: liver, stomach

Functions: 1. expel wind-dampness

2. tonify liver and kidney, strengthen the

muscles, bones and tendons

3. nourish the blood and prevent miscarriage

4. reduce blood pressure and promote urination

5. reduce blood lipid

6. dilate coronary artery and strengthen coronary flow

7. inhibit platelet aggregation, antithrombosis

Indications: 1. arthritis of wind-dampness, especially for sourness of waist and knees, prolonged arthritis impairment of the liver and kidney

2. vaginal bleeding during pregnancy, threatened abortion accompanied by lumbago

3. primary hypertension, hypertension of arteriosclerosis

4. chronic nephritis

5. coronary heart disease, angina pectoris and arrhythmia

6. chronic bronchitis

7. poliomyelitis

Dosage: 9～20 g

Combinations: 1. add Himalayan Teasel Root(续断, Xuduan)——soreness of the waist and knees caused by liver and kidney deficiency or pain of limbs caused by wind-dampness or massive metrorrhagia

2. add Chinese Angelica Root(当归, Danggui)——liver and kidney-deficiency, threatened abortion

3. add Gambirplant Hooked stem and Branch(钩藤, Gouteng)——hypertension

4. add Twotooth Achyranthes Root(牛膝, Niuxi)——pain of waist and legs caused by wind-dampness, flaccidity of waist and knees

5. add Common Selfheal Fruit-spike(夏枯草, Xiakucao), Cassia Seed(决明子, Juemingzi)——hypertension, arteriosclerosis

6. add Ass-hide Glue(阿胶, Ejiao), Perilla Leaf(苏叶, Suye)——threatened abortion caused by blood deficiency, incessant metrorrhagia

7. add Tangerine Peel(橘皮, Jupi)——chronic bronchitis

8. add Shorthorned Epimedium Herb(淫羊藿, Yinyanghuo)——poliomyelitis

9. add Mulberry Twig(桑枝, Sangzhi)——pain and unsmooth movement of joint, and hypertension, dizziness, tinnitus, numbness of limbs

Prescriptions: 1. Decoction of Pubesent Angelica and Loranthus(独活寄生汤, Duhuo Jisheng Tang)

2. Pills for Preventing Habitual Abortion(寿胎丸, Shoutai Wan)

Notes: Chinese Taxillus Twig(桑寄生, Sangjisheng) expels wind, dispels dampness, relaxes muscles and promotes collateral circulation and treats arthritis of wind-dampness. It is especially good at replenishing liver and kidney, strengthening the muscles and bones. So it is proper to be used for liver-kidney deficiency, pain of waist and knees. Modern research shows that this herb can dilate coronary, reduce blood pressure. In the clinic, it treats hypertension and coronary artery heart disease.

10. 五加皮, Wujiapi

English name: Slenderstyle Acanthopanax Root-bark

Pharmaceutical name: Cortex Acanthopanacis Radicis

Botanical name: Acanthopanax gracilistylus W. W. Smith, A. sessiliflours (Rupr. et

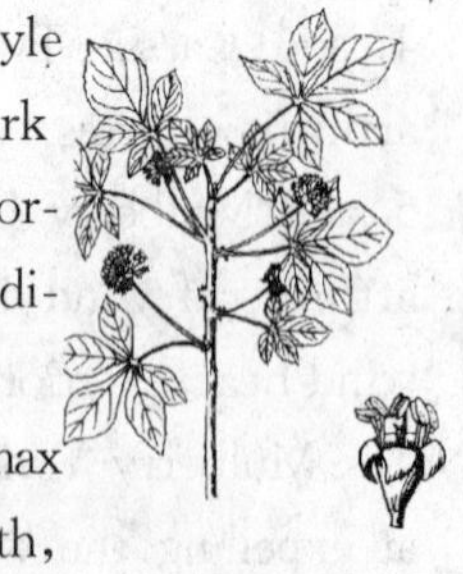
五加皮

Maxim.)seem., A. senticosus (Rupr. et Maxim.) Harms, or A. henryi (Oliv.) Harms.

Properties and tastes: sour, bitter, warm

Meridian tropism: liver, kidney

Functions: 1. expel wind-dampness

2. strengthen the tendons and bones

3. promote urination and detumessentify

4. strengthen immunity

5. anti-inflammation

6. antitumor

7. expel phlegm, relieve cough and asthma

8. tranquilize, relieve pain

9. expand blood vessels, promote coronary flow

10. regulate blood pressure

Indications: 1. arthritis of wind-dampness—swelling and pain of joints, spasm of four limbs whether deficiency or excess is present

2. pain of waist and knees caused by liver and kidney deficiency, feeble walking, retarded development in children

3. edema, urine retention, especially for subscutaneous edema

4. angina pectoria

5. hyperlipemia

6. leukopenia

7. cerebral thrombosis

8. hypotension

9. chronic bronchitis

Dosage: 3～9 g

Contraindication: Not to be taken by patients with yin deficiency and vigorous fire. North Slenderstyle Acanthopanax Root-bark(北五加皮, Beiwujiapi) is poisonous, which can't be overtaken or taken for a period of time.

Combinations: 1. add Rhizome or Root of Forbes Notopterygium (羌活, Qianghuo), Largeleaf Gentian Root (秦艽, Qinjiao), Chinese Clematis Root(威灵仙, Weilingxian)——arthritis of wind-dampness

2. add Twotooth Achyranthes Root(牛膝, Niuxi), Common Floweringquince Fruit(木瓜, Mugua), Himalayan Teasel Root(续断, Xuduan)——liver and kidney-deficiency, pain of waist and knees, flalccidity of lower body

3. add Indian Bread Exodermis (茯苓皮, Fulingpi), Areca Peel(大腹皮, Dafupi)——edema, urine retention

4. add Prepared Rhizome of Adhesive Rehmannia (熟地黄, Shudihuang), Danshen Root(丹参, Danshen), Eucommia Bark (杜仲, Duzhong), Chinese Wolfberry Rootbark(地骨皮, Digubi)——dripping urine, pudendal coldness of women, pain of waist and knees

5. add Chinese Taxillus Twig (桑寄生, Sangjisheng), Hairy Antler (鹿茸, Lurong)——retarded development of infants in walking.

Notes: Li Shizhen(李时珍) said: Slenderstyle Acanthopanax Root-bark(五加皮, Wujiapi) is an effective herb to treat flaccidity and arthritis of wind-dampness and strengthen the tendons and bones "It not only supports healthy energy but also expels evil." So, it is the best herb for wind-dampness syndrome with pain of the waist and legs caused by liver-kidney deficiency and feeble tendons and bones. It should be incompatible with herbs for expelling dampness or clearing away heat for pruritus valve, it can also treat infantile retardation in walking caused by yang-deficiency with herbs for nourishing liver and kidney.

Slenderstyle Acanthopanax Root-bark(五加皮, Wujiapi) grow in different parts, south and north. South Slenderstyle Acanthopanax Root-bark(南五加皮, Nanwujiapi)is not poisonous and good at replenishing liver and kidney, strengthening tendons and bones, especially for arthritis of deficiency syndrome, while North Slenderstyle Acanthopanax Root-bark(北五加皮, Beiwujiapi) can strengthen the heart, induce duresis and has poison and can not be used in large dosages.

11. 白花蛇, Baihuashe

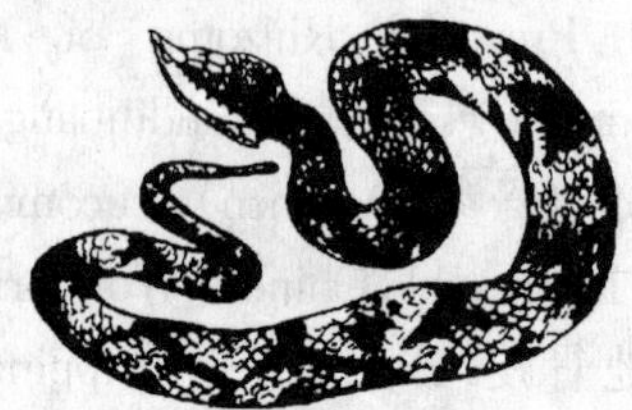

白花蛇

English name: Agkistrodon Acutus

Pharmaceutical name: Agkistrodon seu Bungarus

Properties and tastes: sweet, salty, warm, poisonous

Meridian tropism: liver

Functions: 1. expel wind and promote collateral circulation

2. calm the frightened mind and relieve spasm

3. anticoagulation, antithrombosis

4. relieve pain and tranquilize

5. antitumor

6. expand blood vessels, reduce plood pressure

Indications: 1. arthritis of wind-dampness——stubbon arthritis lasting for a long time, numbness and pain of limbs

2. sequela of windstroke

3. leprosy, meurodermatitis, itching, scrofula, malignant boil etc.

4. tetanus, infantile convulsion

5. obliterative vascular disease——angiitis, phlebitis etc.

6. coronary heart disease

7. vascular nerve headache

8. peripheral neuralgia

Dosage: 3～9 g. Powder: 1～1.5 grams.

Contraindication: Use cautiously in cases of yin-deficiency and blood-dryness and deficiency.

Combinations: 1. add Tall Gastrodia Rhizome (天麻, Tianma), Scorpion(全蝎, Quanxie)——neurodermatitis, apoplexy, distortion of face, itching, scrofula

2. add Garter Snake(乌梢蛇, Wushaoshe), Centipede(蜈蚣, Wugong)——tetanus, infantile convulsion

Notes: Agkistrodon Acutus (白花蛇, Baihuashe) apts to arrest wind, dredge meridians, remove toxin and relieve pain, indicating for excessive internal wind-toxic syndromes. It is effective in treating leprosy, tetanus and infantile convulsion syndromes because it acts on the liver meridian and arrests convulsions, Li Shizhen(李时珍) said: "It can penetrate bones to arrest wind, treat convulsion. It is a major herb for wind arthritis, convulsion, tinea and malignant boil. This is because it goes into five Zang organs internally and comes to skins externally and nowhere it can not reach." Agkistrodon Acutus(白花蛇, Baihuashe) is similar to Garter Snake(乌梢蛇, Wushaoshe) in action, but Agkistrodon Acutus (白花蛇, Baihuashe) is poisonous and has a stronger effect when compared with Garter Snake (乌梢蛇, Wushaoshe) which has no toxicity and has slight effect.

Snake Slough(蛇蜕, Shetui) is sweet and salty in taste and medium in nature. The action is arresting wind, arresting convulsion, arresting itching and treating eye disease. Snake Slough(蛇蜕,Shetui)can treat infantile convulsion, itching of skin, and eye disease. Dosage: 2～3 g. Powder: 0.3～0.6 g.

12. 伸筋草, Shenjincao

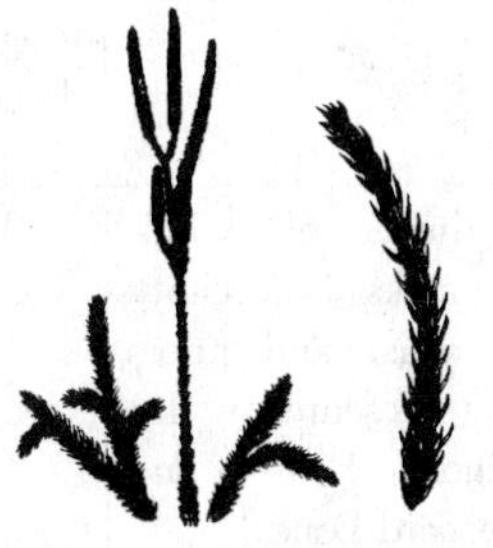

伸筋草

English name: Common Clubmoss Herb

Pharmaceutical name: Herba Lycopodii

Botanical name: Lycopodium japonicum Thunb.

Properties and tastes: bitter, sour, warm

Meridian tropism: liver

Functions: 1. expel wind and dampness

2. relax muscular contracture and promote collateral circulation

3. relieve pain

Indications: arthritis due to wind-dampness——muscular spasm, unsmooth movement of joints due to lingering disease

Dosage: 9～15 g

Combinations: 1. add Common St. Paulswort Herb(豨莶草, Xixiancao)——arthritis due to wind-dampness, unsmooth movement of joints

2. add White Peony Root(白芍药), Chinese Angelica Root (当归, Danggui)——unsmooth circulation of collaterals due to systremma and traumatic injury

Notes: Common Clubmoss Herb (伸筋草, Shenjincao) has the action of expelling wind, eliminating dampness, relaxing muscles and removing obstruction of the meridian. Especially good at relaxing muscles and arresting spasm, so the herb is named Common Clubmoss Herb(伸筋草, Shenjincao). It is mostly used to treat arthritis due to wind-dampness, muscular contracture and unsmooth movement syndromes, also for unsmooth circulation of collaterals due to systremma and traumatic injury, because it can relax muscles and tendons and activate the circulation of meridians.

Both Common Clubmoss Herb(伸筋草, Shenjincao) and Common St. Paulswort Herb(豨莶草, Xixiancao) can expel wind dampness and treat pain and numbness of the body caused by wind-cold-dampness evil, but Common Clubmoss Herb(伸筋草, Shenjincao) is moving not fixing, it is good at relaxing muscles, promoting blood stasis, removing obstruction of the meridian So spasm and unsmooth movement of limbs can be better treated by it; Common St. Paulswort Herb(豨莶草, Xixiancao) expels wind-dampness and replenishes liver and kidney, so it is used to treat pain and numbness of waist and legs caused by wind-dampness evil or liver and kidney-deficiency, dizziness, and tinnitus.

Appendix: Other Drugs For Expelling Wind-dampness

Name	Properties and tastes	Meridian tropism	Functions	Indications	Dosage	Contraindication
Harleguin Glorybower Leaf (臭梧桐, Chouwutong)	acid, bitter, sweet, cold	liver	Expel wind-dampness, reduce blood pressure	Arthritis of wind-dampness hemiplegia hypertension	6～15 grams	

Name	Properties and tastes	Meridian tropism	Functions	Indications	Dosage	Contraindication
Paniculate Swallowwort Root (徐长卿, Xuchangqing)	acid, warm	Liver, stomach	Expel wind, relieve pain and itching, detoxify, relieve pain, tranquilize, reduce blood pressure, reduce blood grease antibiosis	Arthritis, traumatic injury, itching, snake bite	3～9 grams 1 to 3 grams for powder, external use: Appropriate dosage. Don't decoct for a long time	
Dog Bone (狗骨, Gougu)	sweet, warm	Spleen, liver, kidney	Expel wind, relieve pain, strengthen the tendons and bones	Arthritis of wind-dampness, flaccidity of waist and knees (represented for Tiger Bone and Leopard Bone)	3～6 grams	
Oriental Variegated Coralbean Bark (海桐皮, Haitongpi)	bitter, acid, medium	liver	Expel wind-dampness, remove obstruction of meridians	Arthritis of wind-dampness, scabies, eczema	6～12 grams external use: Appropriate dosage	
Silkworm Feculae (蚕砂, Cansha)	sweet, acid, warm	liver spleen stomach	Expel wind and dampness, regulate the stomach and remove dampness	Arthritis of wind-dampness, eczema, itching conoulsion due to vomiting and diarrhoea, massive, metrorrhagia and incessant metrorrhagia	6～9 grams external use: Appropriate dosage	
Kadsura Pepper Stem (海风藤, Haifengteng)	acid, bitter, slightly warm	liver	Expel wind-dampness, remove obstruction of meridian	Arthritis of wind-dampness traumatic injury coronary heart disease and cerebral thrombosis	6～9 grams	
Obscured Homalamena Rhizome (千年健, Qiannianjian)	bitter, acid, warm	Liver, kidney	Expel wind-dampness, strengthen the tendons and bones	Arthritis of wind-dampness spasm and numbness	6～9 grams	can cause nausea, vomiting, dizziness and spasm. Detoct Licorice Root(甘草, Gancao) for detoxication
Chinese Pine Node(松节, Songjie)	bitter, warm	liver	Expel wind, dampness, relieve pain,	Arthritis of wind-dampness, traumatic injury	9～15 grams	
Orientvine Stem or Hair Orientvine Stem (青风藤, Qingfengteng)	bitter, medium	liver	Expel wind, relieve pain, anti inflammation, relieve pain, relieve cough	Arthritis of wind-dampness, flaccidity of lower limbs	6～12 grams	

Name	Properties and tastes	Meridian tropism	Functions	Indications	Dosage	Contraindication
Common Threewingnut Root Leaf or Flower (雷公藤, Leigongteng)	bitter, acid, cold, poisonous	liver	Expel wind and dampness, destroy tuberculomyces and detoxicate, the functions of immunity suppression and antibiotic immunosuppressant	Arthritis of wind-dampness Kill maggot and mouse, snake bite, rheumatoid arthritis, Behcet's syndrome, multiple aphtha and lupus erythematosus etc.	6～12 grams, decoct without peel. The patient with heart, liver, kidney spleen and stomach disease and young women should use cautiously.	This herb may cause digestive tract reaction, CNS damagement, hemorrhage of internal organs and necrosis. Treat with general acute poisoning measures
Nippon Yam Rhizome (穿山龙, Chuanshanlong)	bitter, slightly cold	liver, lung	Expels wind and dampness, promotes circulation and remove obstruction of meridians, relieves cough and expels phlegm	Arthritis of wind-dampness, obstruction in the chest, heart-pain, asthma caused by lung heat, skin infection	9～15 grams	
Decumbent Corydalis Rhizome (夏天无, Xiatianwu)	acid, bitter, warm	liver	Expel wind and dampness promote circulation, relieve pain	Arthritis of wind-dampness, traumatic injury, abdominal pain and near sighted	6～15 grams	
Common Heron's Bill Herb or Wilford Cranesbill Herb (老鹳草, Laoguancao)	acid, bitter, medium	liver, large intestine	Expel wind and dampness, relieve diarrhoea	Arthritis of wind-dampness, diarrhoea caused by dampness-heat	15～30 grams	
Chinese Pyrola Herb (鹿衔草, Luxiancao)	sweet, bitter, warm	liver, kidney	Expel wind-dampness, strengthen the tendons, and bones, tonify lung and kidney arrest bleeding	Arthritis of wind-dampness, flaccidity of tendons and bones, waist-pain caused by kidney deficiency, cough caused by lung deficiency, asthma caused by kidney deficiency, vomiting and epistaxis, massive metrorrhagia and incessant metrorrhagia	9～30 grams	

Chapter 9
Drugs for Resolving Dampness with Fragrant Taste

Definition: The herbs, which are fragrant and have effect of resolving dampness and activating spleen are called herbs for resolving dampness with fragrant drugs.

Functions: The herb is sour, fragrant, warm and dry. It has the effect of smoothing qi, dispersing and eliminating the turbid dampness, invigorating the spleen and activating stomach, etc.

Indications: Dampness stranding the spleen, syndrome epigastric distension and oppression, vomiting with acid regurgitation, anorexia and tiredness, sweet taste in the mouth and salivation, white and grease tongue coating due to dysfunctions of the spleen in transportation and transformation. In addition, it is also applicable for damp-warm syndrome and summer-heat damp syndrome.

Cautions: 1. There are two kinds of dampness. One is cold-dampness, the other is heat-dampness, so we should combine other herbs according to different character of dampness when using herbs for eliminating dampness. Cold-dampness syndrome should be combined with drugs for warming internal cold; heat-dampness syndrome should be combined with drugs for clearing away heat and drying dampness. For damp pathogen being sticky and stagnant in nature, obstruction of dampness may lead to stagnation of qi, promoting the circulation of qi benefits to eliminate dampness, so the drugs for eliminating dampness should be combined with drugs for promoting circulation of qi. So, insufficiency of the spleen resulting in production of dampness syndrome should be combined with drugs for invigorating the spleen and benefiting original qi.

2. Take cautions for yin-deficiency in use because the drugs tend to be warm and dry and easy to damage yin.

3. These drugs are fragrant, containing volatile oil, so they are not advisable to be decocted for a long time so as to prevent low effect.

1. 苍术, Cangzhu

English name: Swordlike Atractylodes Rhizome

Pharmaceutical name: Rhizoma Atractylodis

Botanical name: Atractylodes lancea Thunb., A. chinensis Koida., or A. japonica Koidz. Ex Kitam.

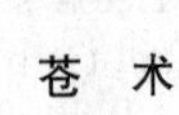

苍 术

Properties and tastes: sour, bitter, warm

Meridian tropism: spleen, stomach

Functions: 1. dry dampness and strengthen the spleen

2. eliminate the wind-dampness

3. diaphoretic and relieve the exterior

4. eliminate the diffuse opacity and improve eyesight

5. reduce the level of blood sugar

6. prevent virus and germs

Indications: 1. stagnation of dampness in Middle-jiao syndrome——abdominal distention, loose stools, anorexia, nausea, vomiting, greasy tongue coating. It can also treat damp pathogens, loose stools and diarrhea in infants

2. arthritis of dampness——feeling of heaviness, numbness of the limbs, swelling and pain of the joints

3. flaccidity of dampness-warm, eczema and leukorrhea

4. the exterior syndrome with pathogenic wind-cold and damp in the exterior——chilly sensation, fever, headache, heavy feeling, toothache, nasal obstruction

5. prevent respiratory infections, chickenpox, mumps, and scarlet fever

6. infantile rickets

7. night blindness and dryness of eyes

8. diabetes

Dosage: 6～9 g

Contraindication: Do not use in conditions of yin deficiency with heat signs and excessive sweating due to exterior deficiency.

Combinations: 1. add Chinese Corktree Bark (黄柏, Huangbai), Twotooth Achyranthes Root(牛膝, Niuxi)——swelling and pain of feet and knees, paralysis and flaccidity due to the downward flow of damp-heat

2. add Ningpo Figwort Root(玄参, Xuanshen)——diabetes

3. add Largehead Atractylodes Rhizome(白术, Baizhu), Officinal Magnolia Bark(厚朴, Houpo)——stagnation of dampness in the Middle-jiao

4. add Doubleteeth Pulbescent Angelica Root(独活, Duhuo), Largeleaf Gentian Root(秦艽, Qinjiao)——arthritis due to wind, cold and dampness

5. add boiled pig liver(猪肝, Zhugan)——night blindness, keratomalocia

6. add Dahurian Angelica Root(白芷, Baizhi)——female leukorrhea due to damp evil

7. add Tangerine Peel(橘皮, Jupi)——dropsy due to deficiency

8. add Nutgrass Galingale Rhizome(香附, Xiangfu), Medicated Leaven(神曲, Shenqu), Cape Jasmine Fruit(栀子, Zhizi)——stagnation of food and heat

9. add Medicated Leaven(神曲, Shenqu)——summer diarrhea

10. add Sichuan Pepper(川椒, Chuanjiao)——diarrhea

Prescription: Peptic Powder(平胃散, Pingwei San)

Notes: Swordlike Atractylodes Rhizome(苍术, Cangzhu) promotes aromatic dryness and has a strong effect to dry dampness. It is used to treat the syndrome of dampness retention involving spleen yang, sputum, edema, eczema, etc. This herb is sour, dispersing, warm and dry. It can expel wind-dampness evil, especially for arthritis due to cold damp.

This drug eliminates filth with aromatics and defends anti-pathogenic qi of the four seasons. Burned in room, Swordlike Atractylodes Rhizome(苍术, Cangzhu) and Largehead Atractylodes Rhizome(白术, Baizhu) have the function of eliminating germs.

To understand their combined use, please refer to Largehead Atractylodes Rhizome (白术, Baizhu).

2. 厚朴, Houpo

English name: Officinal Magnolia Bark

Pharmaceutical name: Cortex Magnoliae Officinalis

Botanical name: Magnolia officinalis Rehd. et Wils or M. officinalis Rehd. et Wils var. hiloba Rehd. et Wils.

Properties and tastes: bitter, sour, warm

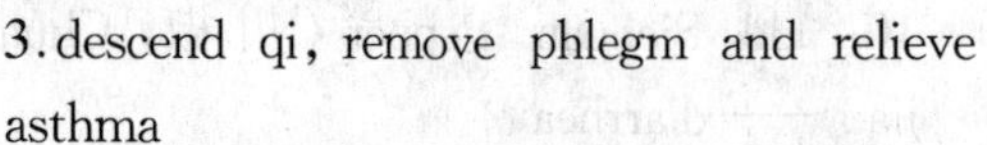

厚 朴

Meridian tropism: spleen, stomach, lung, large intestine

Functions: 1. promote circulation of qi, dry dampness

2. remove stagnation and relieve fullness

3. descend qi, remove phlegm and relieve asthma

4. inhibiti bacteria

5. inhibit secretion of acidity

6. relax striated muscles

7. reduce blood pressure

Indications: 1. abdominal distention and fullness: due to stagnation of dampness, food and qi paralyoic ileus. It also can prevent introperation and intestinal tympanites

2. cough, asthma, profuse sputum

3. acute enteritis, baçillary or amebic dysentery

4. abdominal postoperative distension

Dosage: 3～9 g

Contraindication: use cautiously for women during pregnancy

Combinations: 1. add Pinellia Rhizome(半夏, Banxia), Tuckahoe(茯苓, Fuling)——enteritis, hepatitis, abdominal distention due to gastrointestinal neurosis

2. add Immature Bitter Orange(枳实, Zhishi), Rhubarb(大黄, Dahuang)——stagnation of food, distentional pain in the abdomen, constipation, neurosis

3. add Cassia Twig(桂枝, Guizhi), Apricot Seed(杏仁, Xingren)——cough due to wind-cold from the exterior

4. add Tangerine Peel(橘皮, Jupi), Round Cardamom Seed(白豆蔻, Baidoukou)——a white and greasy tongue coating, loss of appetite

5. add Green Tangerine Peel(青皮, Qingpi), Tumeric Root-tuber(郁金, Yujin)——stagnation of liver-qi, reversal upward flow of qi, abdominal distention, fullness and pain

6. add Swordlike Atractylodes Rhizome(苍术, Cangzhu)——fullness and pain in the abdomen, indigested food stagnated in the stomach, acid regurgitation and eructating foul odor, vomitng

7. add Coptis Rhizome(黄连, Huanglain), Cape Jasmine Fruit(栀子, Zhizi)——vomiting, diarrhea, chest congestion, loss of appetite, yellowish and greasy tongue coating

8. add Ginseng(人参, Renshen), Largehead Atractylodes Rhizome(白术, Baizhu), Malt(麦芽, Maiya)——deficiency-fullness

9. add Immature Bitter Orange(枳实, Zhishi), Radish Seed(莱菔子, Laifuzi)——lowering of qi, relaxing the bowels

10. add Immature Bitter Orange(枳实, Zhishi), Hawthorn Fruit(山楂, Shanzha)——regulating circulation of qi, promoting digestion

Prescriptions: 1. Peptic Powder(平胃散, Pingwei San)

2. Minor Decoction for Purgation(小承气汤, Xiaochengqi Tang)

Notes: Officinal Magnolia Bark(厚朴, Houpo) is bitter, dry, and sour in taste, dispersing and warm in property and can expel cold. Officinal Magnolia Bark(厚朴, Houpo) is good at promoting circulation of qi, drying dampness and ablating stagnation. It is an important drug for relieving distention and fullness. It is often used for abdominal distention and fullness due to stagnation of dampness, indigestion and stagnation of qi, especially for excessive distention. Ye Tianshi(叶天士) said: "Normal dosage of Officinal Magnolia Bark(厚朴, Houpo) can dispel qi, while a small dosage for activating yang." Officinal Magnolia Bark (厚朴, Houpo) has different effects with different dosage.

Both Officinal Magnolia Bark (厚朴, Houpo) and Immature Bitter Orange (枳实, Zhishi) can treat the symptoms of indigestion and stagnation of sputum, distension and fullness in the abdomen and chest and constipation. Officinal Magnolia Bark (厚朴, Houpo) strengthens the spleen with warm, relieves sputum and indigestion, disperses lumps and expels distension; however, Immature Bitter Orange (枳实, Zhishi) has the effect of removing mass and activating circulation of qi.

3. 藿香, Huoxiang

English name: Wrinkled Gianthyssop Herb

Pharmaceutical name: Herba Agastaches seu Pogostemi

Botanical name: Agastache rugosa (Fisch et Mey.) O. Ktze. or Pogostemon cablin (Blanco) Benth.

藿 香

Properties and tastes: sour, slightly warm

Meridian tropism: spleen, stomach and lung

Functions: 1. resolve dampness in the Middle-jiao.

2. eliminate summer-heat and relieve exterior syndrome

3. regulate the stomach and prevent vomiting

4. treat tinea

5. inhibiti bacteria

Indications: 1. stagnation of dampness in the Middle-jiao——abdominal distention and fullness, loss of appetite, nausea, vomiting and diarrhea

2. summer heat damp, cold and influenza——aversion to cold and fever, retention of dampness in the interior, manifested as chilliness, fever, heaviness, headache and pain of body, fullness of the chest, nausea, vomiting and diarrhea due to affection of exogenous wind-cold in summer

3. the initial stage of febrile disease caused by damp-warm evil in summer, dampness is more serious than heat. Both dampness and heat are equally serious.

4. tinea manuum, athlete's foot, tinea pedis

5. rhinorrhea with turbid discharge, nasal obstruction

6. vomiting due to stagnation of dampness in the Middle-jiao, stomach and spleen deficiency, morning sickness.

Dosage: 6～9 g. Fresh herbs should be doubled.

Contraindication: Not to be taken for hyperactivity of fire due to yin deficiency and dry tongue without coating.

Combinations: 1. add Foutune Eupatorium Herb (佩兰, Peilan)——being attacked by pathogenic heat in summer, feeling of fullness in the head, chest congestion, dizziness, nausea, vomiting or pain in the abdomen and diarrhea

2. add Clove Flower-bud (丁香, Dingxiang), Fresh Ginger (生姜, Shengjiang)——vomiting due to a cold in stomach, and distending pain of the abdomen

3. add Perilla Leaf (紫苏, Zisu), Dahurian Angelica Root (白芷, Baizhi)——affection of exogenous wind-cold in summer

4. add Villous Amomum Fruit (砂仁, Sharen), Nutgrass Galingale Rhizome (香附, Xiangfu)——vomiting during pregnancy, poor appetite

5. add Tangerine Peel (橘皮, Jupi), Sword-

like Atractylodes Rhizome (苍术, Cangzhu)——acute gastritis

6. add Coptis Rhizome(黄连, Huanglain), Bamboo Shavings(竹茹, Zhuru)——vomiting due to dampness-heat

7. add Weeping Forsythia Capsule(连翘, Lianqiao), Pinellia Rhizome(半夏, Banxia) - sunstroke with fever, thirst, nausea, and vomiting

8. add Pig Gall(猪胆, Zhudan)——rhinorrhea with turbid discharge

Prescription: Herbal Agastachis Powder for Restoring Healthy Energy(藿香正气散, Huoxiangzhengqi San)

Notes: Wrinkled Gianthyssop Herb (藿香, Huoxiang) is warm in nature but not very dry. It is most applicable for fever, chillness, heaviness and pain of the head and the body, fullness of the chest, nausea, vomiting, and diarrhea due to the affection of exterior wind-cold in summer with retention of dampness in the interior. Officinal Magnolia Bark(厚朴, Houpo) can not only eliminate dampness but also expel the affection of exogenous. Dr. Su Song(苏颂) named Officinal Magnolia Bark (厚朴, Houpo) as the most applicable herb for treating the spleen and stomach with vomiting. *Principles of Materia Medica* (《本草正要》, Bencaozhengyao) also said: Officinal Magnolia Bark(厚朴, Houpo) is the quickest treatment for dampness syndrome involving the spleen, weariness, and poor appetite, thickened greasy tongue coating.

Both Wrinkled Gianthyssop Herb(藿香, Huoxiang) and Perilla Leaf(紫苏, Zisu) have the effect of eliminating exterior evil, activating the circulation of qi, regulating Middle-jiao, but Wrinkled Gianthyssop Herb(藿香, Huoxiang) is aromatic in odor, and good at eliminating dampness and stopping vomiting. Perilla Leaf(紫苏, Zisu) is pungent, dispersing and good at inducing sweet to disperse cold evil.

4. 佩兰, Peilan

English name: Fortune Eupatorium Herb

Pharmaceutical name: Herba Eupatorii Fortunei

Botanical name: Eupatorium fortunei Turcz.

佩兰

Properties and tastes: sour, medium

Meridian tropism: spleen, stomach, lung

Functions: 1. resolve dampness and regulate the Middle-jiao

2. eliminate summer-heat and expel the effect of exogenous summer-heat and dampness

3. stop the influenza virus

Indications: 1. stagnation of dampness in Middle-jiao——abdominal distention and fullness, poor appetite, nausea, vomiting, diarrhea, white and greasy tongue coating, etc.

2. spleen heat syndrome, dampness-heat retention involving the spleen, the feeling of sweetness and greasiness in mouth, vomiting, sticky and turbid saliva, foul smell in the mouth

3. summer-heat dampness syndrome, the beginning of summer-heat febrile disease

Dosage: 6～9 g. The fresh herb should be doubled.

Combinations: 1. add Swordlike Atractylodes Rhizome(苍术, Cangzhu), Officinal Magnolia Bark(厚朴, Houpo), Round Cardamom Seed(白豆蔻, Baidoukou)——the stagnation of dampness in Middle-jiao

2. add Wrinkled Gianthyssop Herb(藿香, Huoxiang), Hindu Lotus Leaf (荷叶, Heye), Sweet Wormwood (青蒿, Qinghao)——summer-heat dampness

3. add Talc(滑石, Huashi), Coix Seed(薏苡仁, Yiyiren)——the beginning of summer-heat febrile disease

Notes: Fortune Eupatorium Herb (佩兰, Peilan) is sour in taste, medium in nature, aromatic in odour and good at eliminating dampness. It not only regulates stomach by eliminating dampness in Middle-jiao but also eliminate the exterior summer-heat dampness pathogens. So it is usually used to treat summer-heat dampness in summer, and it is an effective drug to treat stagnation of dampness involving the spleen, and the feeling of sweetness and greasiness in the mouth, including the foul smell in the mouth.

Both Wrinkled Gianthyssop Herb(藿香, Huoxiang) and Foutune Eupatorium Herb (佩兰, Peilan) have the effect of eliminating dampness and relieving the exterior, treating abdominal distention, vomiting and diarrhea due to dampness involving the spleen or the effect of exterior wind-cold in summer with retention of dampness in the interior. The two herbs are usually used in combination. However, Wrinkled Gianthyssop Herb (藿香, Huoxiang) is the most effective herb for treating vomiting due to dampness. Foutune Eupatorium Herb(佩兰, Peilan) is aromatic in odor, and better than Wrinkled Gianthyssop Herb (藿香, Huoxiang) in eliminating prolonged dampness, So Foutune Eupatorium Herb (佩兰, Peilan) is a major useful herb to treat the feeling of sweetness and a foul smell in the mouth due to dampness.

5. 砂仁, Sharen

English name: Villous Amomum Fruit

Pharmaceutical name: Fructus seu Semen Amomi

Botanical name: Ammomum villsum Lour. or A. xanthioides Wall.

砂 仁

Properties and tastes: sour, warm

Meridian tropism: spleen, stomach

Functions: 1. eliminate dampness and stop vomiting

2. warm Middle-jiao and stop diarrhea

3. promote the circulation of qi and prevent miscarriage

Indications: 1. stagnation of dampness in Middle-jiao——fullness and distending pain in the chest, loss of appetite, vomiting, and diarrhea

2. diarrhea due to deficiency-cold of the spleen——chilliness, cold of limbs, or-agueousgraing diarrhea chiefly marked by watery stools with undigested food

3. hiccup due to cold of the stomach, vomiting, diarrhea with undigested food

4. morning sickness and threatened abortion

Dosage: 3～6 g. Decoct it later than other drugs.

Combinations: 1. add Himalayan Teasel Root (续断, Xuduan)——deficiency of the kidney yang, failure of pregnancy due to uterus-cold

2. add Baikal skullcap Root (黄芩, Huangqin)——threatened abortion or heat due to spleen deficiency

3. add Swordlike Atractylodes Rhizome(苍术, Cangzhu)——acute enteritis

4. add Cassia Bark(肉桂,Rougui)——hyperactivity of the spleen Yang, cold pain in the abdomen, poor appetite, loose stool
5. add Perilla Stem(苏梗,Sugeng), Largehead Atractylodes Rhizome(白术, Baizhu)——threatened abortion, morning sickness
6. add Chinese Taxillus Twig(桑寄生, Sangjisheng)——threatened abortion pain of dropping in the waist
7. add Common Aucklandia Root(木香, Muxiang)——indigestion
8. add Java Amomum Fruit(豆蔻, Doukou)——deficiency-cold of spleen and stomach, stagnation of dampness, loss of appetite, fullness in Middle-jiao, regurgitation, vomiting, and nausea due to blocked circulation of qi

Prescription: Decoction of Six Mild Druges Adding Radix Aucklandiae and Fructus Amomi(香砂六君子汤, Xiangshaliujunzi Tang)

Notes: Villous Amomum Fruit(砂仁,Sharen) is sour in taste, dispersing and warm in nature. It is an effective herb to eliminate dampness and activate the circulation of qi. It can be used to treat symptoms for stagnation of dampness and qi with abdominal distention, poor appetite, and vomiting. Moreover, Villous Amomum Fruit(砂仁,Sharen) is usually used to treat morning sickness, threatened abortion for it has the effect of activating qi and regulating Middle-jiao. *Compendium of Materia Medica* (《本草纲目》, Bencaogangmu) said: Villous Amomum Fruit(砂仁, Sharen) is the herb which warms Middle-jiao and regulates qi. If the qi of Upper-jiao doesn't descend; the qi of Lower-jiao doesn't ascend or the qi of Middle-jiao condenses, Villous Amomum Fruit (砂仁,Sharen) should be used for the quickest effect.

Villous Amomum Fruit(砂仁,Sharen) is same as Round Cardamom Seed(白豆蔻, Baidoukou) in taste and nature. Both have the effect of eliminating dampness, activating qi and regulating Middle-jiao. But Villous Amomum Fruit(砂仁, Sharen) is fragrant and extremely dry, especially useful to the spleen and stomach. It is usually used to treat serious stagnation of cold-dampness in Middle-jiao and morning sickness, threatened abortion. Round Cardamom Seed(白豆蔻,Baidoukou) is slightly fragrant in odor, slightly warm, and mobilizes the pulmonary qi. It is usually used to treat dampness-sputum involving the lung, oppression in the chest and slight symptom of cold-dampness in Middle-jiao.

Moreover, the core of Villous Amomum Fruit(砂仁, Sharen) is named as Villous Amomum Pericarp(砂壳, Shaqiao) whose nature and taste are similar to those of Villous Amomum Fruit(砂仁,Sharen). The effect of Villous Amomum Fruit(砂仁, Sharen) is more greater than that of Villous Amomum Pericarp(砂壳,Shaqiao). Villous Amomum Pericarp(砂壳,Shaqiao) is used to treat stagnation of qi of the spleen and stomach with 3～6 g.

6. 白豆蔻, Baidoukou

English name: Round Cardamom Seed

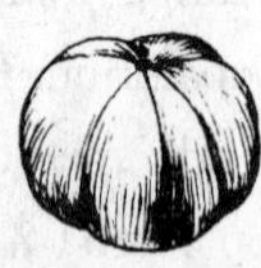

Pharmaceutical name: Fructus Amomi Cardamomi

Botanical name: Amomum cardamomum L. Sometimes Elettaria cardamomum White et Maton is

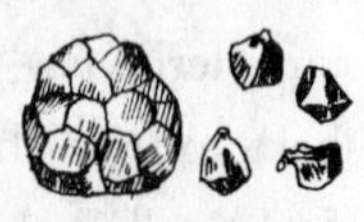

白豆蔻

used but it is of a poorer quality.

Properties and tastes: sour, warm

Meridian tropism: lung spleen, stomach

Functions: 1. promote the circulation of qi and resolve dampness

2. warm the Middle-jiao and arrest vomiting

Indications: 1. stagnation of dampness in Middle-jiao and qi stagnation of the spleen and stomach-fullness in the chest and upper abdomen, loss of appetite, loose stool, turbid greasy tongue coating

2. vomiting——stomach cold syndrome with vomiting, vomiting of milk in infants, morning sickness and regurgitation, hiccups

Dosage: 3～6 g. The herb is fragrant and easy to volatilize. Grind it into pieces and decoct it later.

Contraindication: Not to be taken for patients with yin deficiency and blood dryness.

Combinations: 1. add Coix Seed (薏苡仁, Yiyiren), Apricot Seed (杏仁, Xingren)——early stage of febrile disease caused by damp-warm evil, heaviness of the head, feeling of oppression in the chest, weariness, dark urination, loose stool, and a white and greasy tongue coating

2. add Wrinkled Gianthyssop Herb (藿香, Huoxiang), Tangerine Peel (橘皮, Jupi)——aucte gastritis

3. add Officinal Magnolia Bark (厚朴, Houpo), Swordlike Atractylodes Rhizome (苍术, Cangzhu)——abdominal mass, chest congestion and loss of appetite, anorexia, and turbid and greasy tongue coating caused by the stagnation of dampness in Middle-jiao

4. add Tangerine Peel (橘皮, Jupi), Pinellia Rhizome (半夏, Banxia)——cold-dampness with nausea and vomiting

5. add Apricot Seed (杏仁, Xingren)——distention, fullness and discomfort in the chest and costal regions, excessive damp-sputum

Prescription: Decoction of Three kinds of Kernels (三仁汤, Sanren Tang)

Notes: Round Cardamom Seed (白豆蔻, Baidoukou) is sour, warm and aromatic, so it can eliminate dampness and activate the circulation of qi. It is combined with herbs for eliminating dampness and activating circulation of qi, such as Officinal Magnolia Bark (厚朴, Houpo), Swordlike Atractylodes Rhizome (苍术, Cangzhu), Tangerine Peel (橘皮, Jupi) to treat the stagnation of dampness and qi, distention, fullness in the abdomen, and poor appetite. It activates the circulation of qi, warms the Middle-jiao and stops vomiting, so it is appropriate to treat vomiting duo to cold stomach. It can be used to mobilize the Upper-jiao and eliminate dampness. Moreover, Round Cardamom Seed (白豆蔻, Baidoukou) can treat a drunk person for it removes poison of wine.

Katsumada Galangal Seed (草豆蔻, Caodoukou) has the same effect as that of Round Cardamom Seed (白豆蔻, Baidoukou), but the former is warmer and drier.

7. 草果, Caoguo

English name: Caoguo

Pharmaceutical name: Fructus seu Semen Amomi

Botanical name: Ammomum villosum Lour. or A. xanthioides Wall..

Properties and tastes: sour, warm

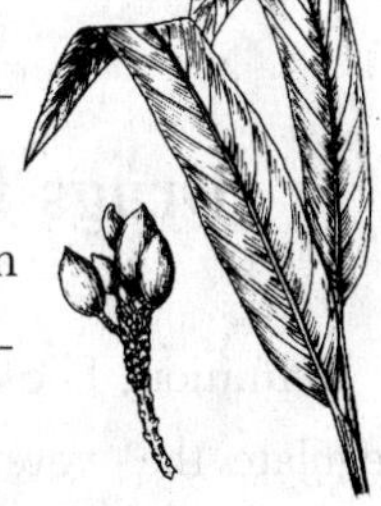

草 果

Meridian tropism: spleen, stomach

Functions: 1. dry dampness

2. warm the Middle-jiao

3. prevent recurrence of malaria

Indications: 1. stagnation of cold-dampness in the spleen and stomach——feeling of fullness, distention, cold pain in the abdomen, vomiting, diarrhea, white, turbid and greasy mass

2. malaria

Dosage: 3 ~ 6 g. The kernel should be used without shell after being pounded.

Combinations: 1. add Officinal Magnolia Bark (厚朴, Houpo), Swordlike Atractylodes Rhizome(苍术, Cangzhu), Pinellia Rhizome (半夏, Banxia)——stagnation of cold-dampness in the spleen and stomach, turbid and greasy masses

2. add Antifebrile Dichroa Root (常山, Changshan), Common Anemarrhea Rhizome(知母, Zhimu)——malaria

3. add Areca Seed(槟榔, Binlang), Officinal Magnolia Bark (厚朴, Houpo), Common Anemarrhea Rhizome (知母, Zhimu), and Baikal skullcap Root(黄芩, Huangqin)——pestilence, panthogens in the space between the exterior and interior, aversion to cold, sthenic heat, oppression in the chest, nausea, vomiting, headache, agitated, string, rapid pulse, and turbid, greasy mass

Notes: It is sour with a heavy aromatic odor and has a strong effect in drying dampness and dispersing cold. It is an important herb not only to treat cold-dampness in the spleen and stomach, but also for episode malaria, especially with cold-dampness.

Herb / Comparision	Villous Amomum Fruit (砂仁, Sharen)	Round Cardamom Seed (白豆蔻, Baidoukou)	Caoguo (草果, Caogou)
The effect of circulating qi	strongest	stronger	ineffective
The characteristic of warming and drying	slight	stronger	strongest
Indications	Stagnation of qi and cold-dampness of spleen and stomach; pain in the abdomen due to cold in the middle-jiao, diarrhea, threatened abortion	Qi stagnation of the stomach and spleen, stagnation of cold-dampness in the middle-jiao	Cold-dampness of the spleen and stomach; malaria

Chapter 10
Drugs for Inducing Diuresis and Excreting Dampness

Definition: The drugs which can dredge and regulate the water passage, promote diuresis are named drugs for inducing diuresis and excreting dampness.

Functions: These herbs have the effect of promoting urination, causing large quantity of urine or increasing diuresis, making dampness in body discharge from urine. Some of these drugs also have the effect of eliminating damp-heat, treating stranguria and discharge of urinary calculus.

Indications: dysuria, edema, stranguria,

phlegm fluid, damp-warm disease, jaundice, eczema syndromes due to water-dampness

Cautions: Uncorrect usage can damage yin, so the drugs should be cautiously used in cases of yin deficiency and consumption of fluid.

1. 茯苓, Fuling

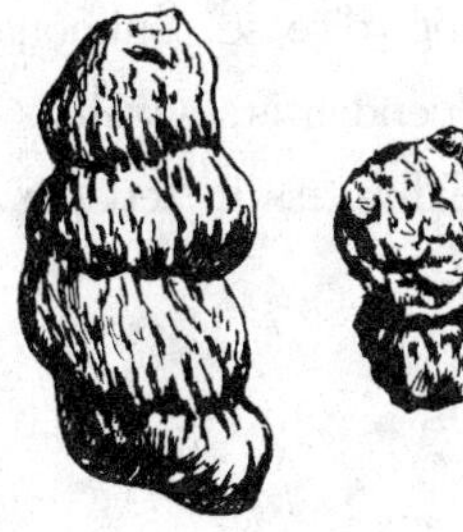

茯 苓

English name: Tuckahoe

Pharmaceutical name: Sclerotium Poriae Cocos

Botanical name: Poria cocos(Schw.) Wolf

Properties and tastes: sweet, medium

Meridian tropism: spleen, heart, stomach

Functions: 1. promote urination

2. invigorate the spleen

3. tranquilize the mind

4. improve immunity function, inhibit tumor

Indications: 1. edema——urine retention and diarrhea due to dampness retention with spleen deficiency

2. urinary infection——frequent of urine, urgent micturition, pain of urination

3. spleen deficiency syndrome——fatigue, poor appetite, diarrhea

4. restlessness of mind——palpitation, insomnia, hypomnesis due to spleen and heart deficiency

5. infant diarrhea

6. after operation of malignant tumor——improve immunity function of body, relieve symptoms, prevent toxin and side effects caused by chemical treatment

Dosage: 6～15 g

Contraindication: Cautions should be taken when it is prescribed for yin-deficiency and fluid impairment.

Combinations: 1. add Akebia Stem(木通, Mutong)——downward flow of damp-heat, dark urination

2. add Largehead Atractylodes Rhizome(白术, Baizhu)——retention of dampness with fluid due to spleen deficiency, abdominal mass and fullness, loss of appetite, dizziness, vertigo, nausea, vomiting, urine retention and Meniere's syndrome

3. add Membranous Milkvetch Root(黄芪, Huangqi)——improve immunity function after operation of tumor

4. add Common Aucklandia Root(木香, Muxiang)——dysentery

5. add Dang-Shen Root(党参, Dangshen)——loss of appetite due to spleen deficiency

6. add Licorice Root(甘草, Gancao), Cassia Twig(桂枝, Guizhi)——palpitation, shortness of breath, edema of face and limbs due to insufficiency of heart and spleen

7. add Thinleaf Milkwort Root(远志, Yuanzhi), Spine Date Seed(酸枣仁, Suanzaoren)——restlessness of the mind, amnesia, palpitation, insomnia

8. add Tangerine Peel(橘皮, Jupi) Tendrilleaf Fritillary Bulb(川贝, Chuanbei)——phlegm in the lung, cough and phlegm, due to asthma

9. add Areca Peel(大腹皮, Dafupi), White Mulberry Root-bark(桑白皮, Sangbaipi)——facial edema, limb edema, urine retention

10. add Umbellate Pore Fungus(猪苓, Zhuling)——edema due to spleen deficiency

11. add Sharpleaf Galangal Fruit(益智仁,

Yizhiren)——stranguria caused by kidney deficiency, and diarrhea

12. add Rice Bean (赤小豆, Chixiaodo u)—— heat stranguria diarrhea and mastadenitis

13. add Red Peony Root (赤芍药, Chishaoyao)——urine retention, such as acute nephritis, cystitis

14. add Indian Bread with Hostwood(茯神, Fushen)——sleeplessness, palpitation, hypomnesis

Prescriptions: 1. Decoction of Four Mild Drugs (四君子汤, Sijunzi Tang)

2. Powder of Radix Ginseng, Poria and Rhizoma Atracthlodis Macrocephalae(参苓白术散, Shenlingbaizhu San)

Notes: Tuckahoe(茯苓, Fuling) is medium in property. It is the most commonly used drug for invigorating the spleen, inducing diuresis, tranquilizing the mind and eliminating phlegm. Clinically it can be divided into Indian Bread Exodermis(茯苓皮, Fulingpi), Indian Bread Pink Epidermis(赤茯苓, Chifuling), Tuckahoe(茯苓, Fuling) and Indian Bread with Hostwood(茯神, Fushen). Indian Bread Exodermis(茯苓皮, Fulingpi) is good at eliminating dampness, used for treating edema. Indian Bread Pink Epidermis(赤茯苓, Chifuling) is good at clearing away heat and eliminating dampness, for treating strangury due to heat and urinary infection. Tuckahoe(白茯苓, Baifuling) is good at invigorating the spleen. Indian Bread with Hostwood(茯神, Fushen) is good at tranquilizing the mind, used for palpitation and insomnia.

Both Tuckahoe(茯苓, Fuling) and Coix Seed(薏苡仁, Yiyiren) can invigorate the spleen and eliminate dampness, used for the syndrome of deficiency of the spleen and excess of dampness. While Tuckahoe(茯苓, Fuling) is sweet and tasteless in flavor and medium in property, it has good effect on tonifying the heart and spleen, calming the heart and tranquilizing the mind. Coix Seed (薏苡仁, Yiyiren) can clear away heat by its cold property and is good at treating consumptive lung disease, pulmonary abscess and acute appendicitis, as well as eliminating pathogenic dampness in tendons, bones and muscles.

2. 猪苓, Zhuling

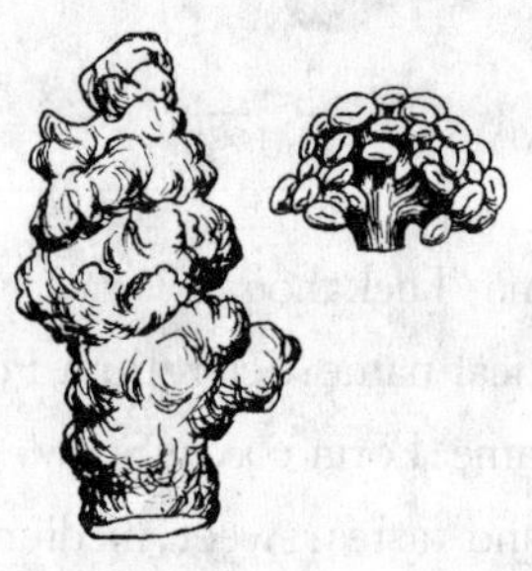

猪　苓

English name: Umbellate Pore Fungus

Pharmaceutical name: Sclerotium Polypori Umbellati

Botanical name: Polyporus umbellatus (Pers.) Fr.

Properties and tastes: sweet, medium, tasteless

Meridian tropism: kidney and urinary bladder

Functions: 1. promote diuresis to eliminate dampness

2. antitumorigenesis

3. protective the liver

4. reduce blood pressure

Indications: 1. edema, urine retention

2. urinary infection——frequent urine, urgent micturition, urodynia

3. diarrhea due to water-damp and cold-damp in the stomach and intestine, prolonged watery diarrhea, white and greasy

tongue coating

4. chronic viral hepatitis

5. malignant tumor——advanced primary pulmonary carcinoma, cancer of liver, acute leukemia, nasopharyngeal

6. psoriasis

Dosage: 6～12g

Contraindication: Use cautiously for patients with consumption of body fluid. Do not use in cases of water-damp.

Combinations: 1. add Pinellia Rhizome(半夏, Banxia)——emission in dream

2. add Oriental Waterplantain Rhizome(泽泻, Zexie), Tuckahoe(茯苓, Fuling)——urine retention, edema, diarrhea, stranguria

3. add Akebia Stem(木通, Mutong), Talc(滑石, Huashi)——urine retention, urodynia, hematuria

4. add Areca Peel(大腹皮, Dafupi), Villous Amomum Fruit(砂仁, Sharen)——edema and fullness, urine retention

5. add Common Yam Rhizome(山药, Shanyao), Largehead Atractylodes Rhizome(白术, Baizhu)——leucorrhagia of cold-dampness

6. add Tree of Heaven Ailanthus Bark(椿根皮, Chungenpi), Cape Jasmine Fruit(栀子, Zhizi)——leucorrhagia of warm-dampness

7. add Capillary Wormwood Herb(茵陈蒿, Yinchenhao), Plantain Seed(车前子, Cheqianzi)——yang jaundice

Prescriptions: 1. Powder of Five Drugs with Poria(五苓散, Wuling San)

2. Decoction of Umberllate Pore(猪苓汤, Zhuling Tang)

Notes: Both Umbellate Pore Fungus(猪苓, Zhuling) and Tuckahoe(茯苓, Fuling) are drugs for promoting diuresis to eliminate damp. The two are used as mutual reinforcement for treating difficult urination, painful stranguric and edema. But Umbellate Pore Fungus(猪苓, Zhuling) is much tasteless and bit sweet, mainly acts on kidney and urinary bladder and good at promoting diuresis to eliminate damp and is without the functions of tonifying the Middle-jiao to benefit the spleen. Tuckahoe(茯苓, Fuling) has less effect in inducing diuresis than Umbellate Pore Fungus(猪苓, Zhuling), but it has a tonifying function when inducing diuresis, which can reinforce the heart and spleen, and tranquilize the mind. Therefore, Li Shizhen(李时珍) said: "Umbellate Pore Fungus(猪苓, Zhuling) excites dampness by its tasteless flavor and qi can be increased or decreased. In this way, it can open striae of skin and muscles and benefit urination, whose function is the same as that of Tuckahoe(茯苓, Fuling). It is not as good as Tuckahoe(茯苓, Fuling) when used as a tonic."

3. 泽泻, Zexie

English name: Oriental Waterplantain Rhizome

Pharmaceutical name: Rhizoma Alismatis Plantago-aquaticae

Botanical name: Alisma plantago-aquatica L. var. orientale Samuels

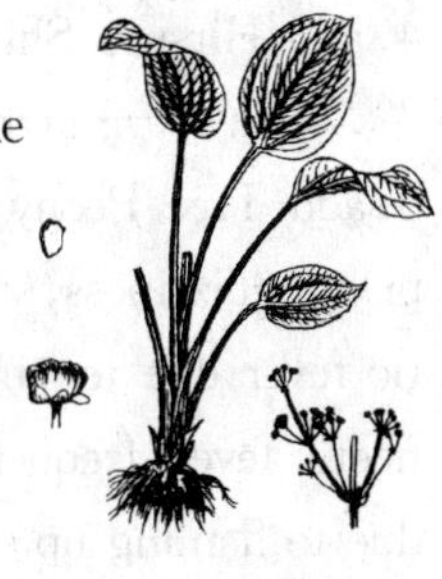

泽 泻

Properties and tastes: sweet, tasteless, cold

Meridian tropism: kidney and urinary bladder

Functions: 1. promote urination to eliminate dampness

2. purge kidney - heat

3. lower limpemia and prevent fatty liver

4. reduce blood pressure, increase coronary artery and anticoagulation

Indications: 1. water-damp and fluid retention

syndrome——urine retention, edema, diarrhea, stranguria, profuse leukorrhea, dizziness due to the retention of phlegm, especially used for otogenic dizziness

2. frequent seminal emission——belongs to hyperactivity of the ministerial fire. Symptom: tidal fever, night sweating, increased dreams during sleep, vexation, dark urine, red tongue, and thready and rapid pulse

3. hyperlipemia and coronary atherosclerotic cardiopathy

Dosage: 6～12 g

Combinations: 1. add Pinellia Rhizome(半夏, Banxia)——abdominal fullness and distention due to dampness retention in Middle-jiao, scanty urine

2. add Largehead Atractylodes Rhizome(白术, Baizhu)——phlegm, dizziness, urine retention, edema, diarrhea, stranguria, profuse leukorrhea etc. It is also used for Meniere's disease

3. add Bitter Orange(枳壳, Zhiqiao)——agitated urine retention and constipation

4. add Hirsute Shiny Bugleweed Herb(泽兰, Zelan)——cirrhotic ascites

5. add Tree Peony Bark(牡丹皮, Mudanpi)——dizziness, soreness of the loins, hectic fever due to yin deficiency, tidal fever, hectic fever, frequent seminal emission etc. due to flaming up of deficiency fire

6. add Tuckahoe(茯苓, Fuling), Umbellate Pore Fungus(猪苓, Zhuling), Largehead Atractylodes Rhizome(白术, Baizhu)——urine retention, edema and acute and chronic nephritis

7. add Talc(滑石, Huashi), Sevenlobed Yam Rhizome(萆薢, Bixie)——turbid urine like grease

8. add Rehmannia Dried Root(生地黄, Shengdihauang), Akebia Stem(木通, Mutong)——stranguria caused by heat, pain of urination, urine retention

9. add Plantain Seed(车前子, Cheqianzi), White Mulberry Root-bark(桑白皮, Sangbaipi)——edema, fullness, and urine retention

10. add Chinese Taxillus Twig(桑寄生, Sangjisheng), Tuckahoe(茯苓, Fuling)——edema during pregnancy

11. add Hawthorn Fruit(山楂, Shanzha), Kelp(海带, Haidai)——hyperlipemia

Prescriptions: 1. Powder of Five Drugs with Poria(五苓散, Wuling San)

2. Bolus of Six Drugs Containing Rhizome Rehmanniae Peaeparatea(六味地黄丸, Liuweidihuang Wan)

Notes: Oriental Waterplantain Rhizome(泽泻, Zexie) is similar to Tuckahoe(茯苓, Fuling), with its sweet and tasteless flavor and the effect of exciting dampness, which are often used for the water damp syndrome. Its cold property can also purge heat of the kidney and urinary bladder, which is fit for treating damp-heat in the Lower-jiao. Modern research shows that Oriental Waterplantain Rhizome(泽泻, Zexie) is also effective on reducing blood lipid. Thus, this drug can be used for treating hyperlipemia and faty liver. *Compendium of Materia Medica* (《本草纲目》, Bencaogangmu) says: "Oriental Waterplantain Rhizome(泽泻, Zexie) has the functions of nourishing five Zang organs, benefiting body strength, treating dizziness and improving ear ability and improving eyesight." But it also says: "Overtaking Oriental Waterplantain Rhizome(泽泻, Zexie) may cause blindness of eyes and violent overtaking may lead to brightness of eyes." Further research is needed.

Both Oriental Waterplantain Rhizome(泽

泻,Zexie)and Akebia Stem(木通,Mutong) can dredge the water passage and treat the syndrome of interior retention of water-dampness or obstruction of the water passage. Akebia Stem(木通,Mutong) is used mainly to clear away heat of the heart and small intestines and smooth qi and blood, while Oriental Waterplantain Rhizome(泽泻,Zexie) is good at clearing away deficient fire of the kidney meridian.

4. 薏苡仁, Yiyiren

English: Coix Seed

Pharmaceutican name: Semen Coicis Lachryma-jobi

Botanical name: Coix lachryma-jobi L.

Properties and tastes: sweet, tasteless, and slightly cold

薏苡仁

Meridian tropism: spleen, lung and large intestine

Functions: 1. promote urination and eliminate dampness
2. invigorate the spleen and stop diarrhea
3. dispel urine and promote urination
4. dispel dampness and expel arthritis
5. clear away heat and promote pus discharge
6. reduce growth of cancer
7. reduce blood sugar
8. sedative analgesic and antipyretic effect

Indications: 1. water-dampness syndrome——urine retention, edema, flaccidity of lower limbs and diarrhea due to spleen-deficiency
2. arthralgia due to wind-dampness type——arthritis due to wind-dampness, rheumatoid arthritis and spasm of muscles and vessels etc., especially for arthralgia due to warm-dampness type
3. stranguria caused by warm-dampness and stranguria caused by the urinary stone
4. pulmonary abscess, appendicitis
5. cancer of alimentary canal
6. plane warts

Dosage: 9～13 g. The theapreutic effect can be seen after it is used for a long time. Fried drug is used for invigorating the spleen, raw herb for the others. It is a good drug for diet therapy.

Combinations:
1. add Dang-Shen(党参,Dangshen), Large-head Atractylodes Rhizome(白术,Baizhu)——insufficiency of the spleen leading to over abundance of dampness, and diarrhea
2. add Chinese Angelica Root(当归,Danggui), Doubleteeth Pulbescent Angelica Root(独活,Duhuo)——arthralgia due to wind-dampness for a long time with blood-deficiency
3. add Whiteflower Patrinia Herb(败酱草,Baijiangcao), Chinese Waxgourd Fruit(冬瓜子,Dongguazi)——acute appendicitis
4. add Talc(滑石,Huashi), Bamboo Leaf(竹叶,Zhuye)——dampness in meridians, fever with pain, dark and scanty urine
5. add Reed Rhizome(芦根,Lugen), Balloonflower Root(桔梗,Jiegeng)——lung abscess
6. add Swordlike Atractylodes Rhizome(苍术,Cangzhu), Tuckahoe(茯苓,Fuling)——chronic enteritis
7. add Apricot Seed(杏仁,Xingren), White Amomum Fruit(白蔻仁,Baikouren)——the beginning of febrile disease caused by damp－warm evil
8. add Snakegourd Root(天花粉,Tianhuafen), Green Gram Spermoderm(绿豆衣,Ludouyi)——diabetes
9. add Fourstamen Stephania Root(防己,

Fangji)——arthralgia of wind-dampness, spasms of muscles and vessels of heat type

10. add Ephedra(麻黄, Mahuang), Chinese Clematis Root(威灵仙, Weilingxian)——arthralgia of wind-dampness, spasm of muscles and vessels of cold type

11. add Swordlike Atractylodes Rhizome(苍术, Cangzhu), Chinese Corktree Bark(黄柏, Huangbai)——arthralgia of wind-dampness, spasm of muscles of damp-heat type.

12. add Spreading Hedyotis Herb(白花蛇舌草, Baihuasheshecao)——cancer of alimentary canal

13. add Chinese Waxgourd Fruit(冬瓜子, Dongguazi), Peach Seed(桃仁, Taoren)——lung abscess

14. add Whiteflower Patrinia Herb(败酱草, Baijiangcao), Peach Seed(桃仁, Taoren)——appendicitis

15. add Six to One Powder(六一散, Liuyi San), Charred Human Hair(血余炭, Xueyutan)—preventing recurrence of lithangiuria

Prescription: Decoction of Ephedra, Apricot, Coix and Licorice(麻杏薏甘汤, Maxingyigan Tang)

Notes: Coix Seed(薏苡仁, Yiyiren) is a bland drug which can induce diuresis and invigorate the spleen, the functions of which are similar with those of Tuckahoe(茯苓, Fuling), indicating retention of water and dampness and excess of dampness due to spleen deficiency. Since it can relieve spasm, smooth and dredge tendons and meridians, clear away heat and evacuate pus, it is a principal drug for treating spasm and pain of tendons and meridians caused by rheumatism as well as for pulmonary abscess and acute appendicitis. Modern research shows that it functions as an anticancer drug and reduces blood sugar, diabetes and plain warts, etc. *Expounding of Herbals* (《本草述》, Bencaoshu) says: "For eliminating dampness, Coix Seed(薏苡仁, Yiyiren) is the same as Swordlike Atractylodes Rhizome(苍术, Cangzhu) and Largehead Atractylodes Rhizome(白术, Baizhu), but it doesn't cause dryness like them. For clearing away heat, Coix Seed(薏苡仁, Yiyiren) is the same as(黄芩, Huangqin) and Coptis Rhizome(黄连, Huanglian), but it doesn't damage yin like them. For benefiting qi, Coix Seed(薏苡仁, Yiyiren) is the same as Ginseng(人参, Renshen) and Largehead Atractylodes Rhizome(白术, Baizhu), but it doesn't produce damp-heat like them. It is actually an important drug for tonifying the middle qi."

5. 车前子, Cheqianzi

English name: Plantain Seed

Pharmaceutical name: Semen Plantaginis

Botainical name: Plantago asiatica L. or P. Depressa Wild.

车前子

Properties and tastes: sweet, cold

Meridian tropism: kidney, liver, lung

Functions: 1. promote urination and relieves stranguria

2. clear away liver heat and improve eyesight

3. quench lung heat and remove phlegm

4. promote urination to control diarrhea

5. antibacteria

Indications: 1. urine retention, edema, stranguria, profuse leukorrhea, frequent seminal emission during dreams

2. diarrhea of summer-heat and dampness type
3. conjunctival congestion, cataract, blurred vision
4. acute and chronic bronchitis of lung-heat type with cough, much yellowish phlegm
5. acute and chronic bacillary dysentery
6. acute viral hephtitis of jaundice type

Dosage: 6 ~ 9 g, wrapped with cloth for boiling.

Combinations: 1. add Twotooth Achyranthes Root(牛膝, Niuxi), Prepared Rhizome of Adhesive Rehmannia (熟地黄, Shoudihuang)——edema of nephritis with kidney deficiency
2. add Chinese Angelica Root(当归, Danggui), Barbary Wolfberry Fruit (枸杞子, Gouqizi)——senile cataract
3. add Chinese Corktree Bark(黄柏, Huangbai), Swordlike Atractylodes Rhizome (苍术, Cangzhu)——profuse leukorrhea of women
4. add Common Selfheal Fruit-spike(夏枯草, Xiakucao), Abalone Shell(石决明, Shijueming)——dizziness and vertigo, hypertension
5. add Apricot Seed(杏仁, Xingren), Balloonflower Root(桔梗, Jiegeng)——cough due to lung heat
6. add Chrysanthemum Flower (菊花, Juhua), Cape Jasmine Fruit(栀子, Zhizi)—acute conjunctivitis
7. add Chinese Corktree Bark(黄柏, Huangbai), Japanese climbing Fern Spores(海金沙, Haijinsha)——heat stranguria, and stranguria caused by urinary stone
8. add Tuckahoe(茯苓, Fuling), Largehead Atractylodes Rhizome(白术, Baizhu)——diarrhea of heat-dampness, urine retention
9. add Yerbadetajo Herb(墨旱莲, Mohanlian)——all kinds of stranguria due to heat, nephritis, urinary infection
10. add Charred human hair (血余炭, Xueyutan)——hematuria, acute nephritis, diarrhea, dysentery

Prescriptions: 1. Eight Health Restoring Powder(八正散, Bazheng San)
2. Bolus of Radix Gentianae for Purging Liver heat (龙胆泻肝汤, Longdanxiegan Tang)

Notes: Plantain Seed (车前子, Cheqianzi) is sweet in taste and cold in property. It can clear away heat while inducing diuresis. It is often used for treating edema and stranguria. Because promoting urination may dry bowel movement, this drug is used for diarrhea due to summer-heat and dampness. It is mostly fit for diarrhea caused by an excess of dampness. *Essentials of Materia Medica* (《本草备要》, Bencaobeiyao) says: "It was said by the ancients that Plantain Seed(车前子, Cheqianzi) could descend but not cause diarrhea and could circulate but not reinforce. But it should be fit for cases with heat in the kidney. It is forbidden for patients with yin deficiency and cold and descended primary qi."

Plantain Seed (车前子, Cheqianzi) and Oriental Waterplantain Rhizome(泽泻, Zexie) are all principal drugs for inducing diuresis, reducing swelling and clearing away damp-heat. It can strengthen the therapeutic effect of distention and fullness due to edema, difficult urination and diarrhea due to summer-heat and dampness when combined with other drugs. Both drugs act on the kidney meridian. Plantain Seed (车前子, Cheqianzi) can tonify yin, indicating infertility due to deficiency of the kidney when used together with drugs for tonifying the kidney. Oriental Waterplantain Rhizome (泽泻, Zexie) purges deficient fire of the kidney, indicating deficiency of yin and vigorousness of fire. In addition, Plantain Seed (车前子, Cheqianzi) also has the effect of clearing away heat of the liver and lung, as well as brightening eyes and removing phlegm.

6. 滑石, Huashi

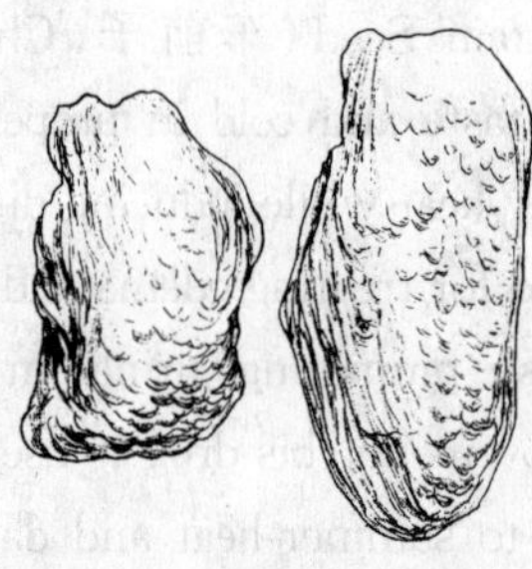

滑　石

English name: Talc

Pharmaceutical name: Talcum

Properties and tastes: sweet, tasteless, cold

Meridian tropism: stomach, urinary bladder

Functions: 1. promote urination and relieve stranguria

2. clear away summer-heat

3. external use for clearing away heat and astringing

Indications: 1. stranguria of heat-dampness——urine retention, dripping and painful urination, acute littritis, cystitis and urinary

2. summer-dampness syndrome with thirst and dysuria, chest congestion due to febrile disease caused by damp heat evil, diarrhea of heat-dampness

3. dermatosis——moist ulcer, eczema, miliaria, etc.

Dosage: 9～15 g. Proper amount for external use

Contraindication: Not to be taken for patients with spleen deficiency, spermatorrhea, consumption of body fluid caused by febrile disease and pregnant women.

Combinations: 1. add Licorice Root (甘草, Gancao)——summer-heat syndrome with thirst and dysuria, dark and scanty urination, diarrhea

2. add Cape Jasmine Fruit(栀子, Zhizi)——acute pyelonephritis, urethritis, urinary stone difficult and dark urine

3. add Chinese Corktree Bark(黄柏, Huangbai)——external use for moist ulcer, eczema, damp and itching of toes, dematitis etc with powder

4. add Wild Mint (薄荷, Bohe), Dahurian Angelica Root (白芷, Baizhi)——external use for miliaria with powder

5. add Plantain Seed(车前子, Cheqianzi), Coix Seed(薏苡仁, Yiyiren)—diarrhea

6. add Baikal Skullcap Root (黄芩, Huangqin), Akebia Stem (木通, Mutong)——febrile disease caused by damp-warm evil, fever disease in summer, etc, perspiration, continuous fever, soreness of the extremities, dark and scanty urination

7. add Hematite (代赭石, Daizheshi)——vomiting and epistaxis

8. add Mole Cricket(蝼蛄, Lougu)——edema of heat-dampness, distention in chest and abdomen, urine retention

9. add Christina Loosetrife Herb (金钱草, Jinqiancao)——stranguria caused by the passage of urinary stone, hypertrophy of prostate

10. add Ark Shell (瓦楞子, Walengzi)——urinary stone

Prescription: Six to One Powder(六一散, Liuyi San)

Notes: Talc(滑石, Huashi) is cold in property

which can clear away heat, and is slippery which is good for the orifice. It can clear away the accumulated heat in the urinary bladder and dredge the water passage, which is a commonly used drug for treating stranguria of damp heat, Zhu Zhenheng(朱震亨), an ancient physician, called it as an important drug for treating stranguria caused by urinary stone. This drug can eliminate dampness, and clear away summer-heat, indicating for summer-heat and damp syndrome. It is often combined with Licorice Root(甘草,Gancao) to form LiuYiSan, which is used for summer-heat syndrome.

Both Talc(滑石,Huashi) and Gypsum(生石膏,Shengshigao) can clear away heat and relieve thirst. But the purpose of Both Talc (滑石,Huashi) is to relieve damp. It is to benefit the orifice, eliminate dampness and harmonize the spleen and stomach. In this way thirst can be relieved. It is indicated for summer-heat with dampness, yellowish urination with difficulty and restless thirst. The purpose of Gypsum(生石膏,Shengshigao) is to relieve restless thirst. This involves in clearing away extreme heat in the Yangming meridian to maintain body fluids. It is indicated for excess heat in Yangming with restless thirst. In addition, for external use, Talc(滑石,Huashi) can treat eczema and the oozing of fluid due to sudamina toxic with an extremely itching sensation. Gypsum(生石膏,Shengshigao) can treat the unhealing of skin and external diseases.

7. 木通, Mutong

English name: Akebia Stem

Pharmaceutical name: Caulis Mutong

Botanical name: Akebia trifoliata(Thunb.) Koidz. Var. australis(Diels) Rehd., Akebia quinata (Thunb.) Decne., Aristolochia Manshuriensis Kom., Clematis armandi Franch., or C. montana Buch.-Ham

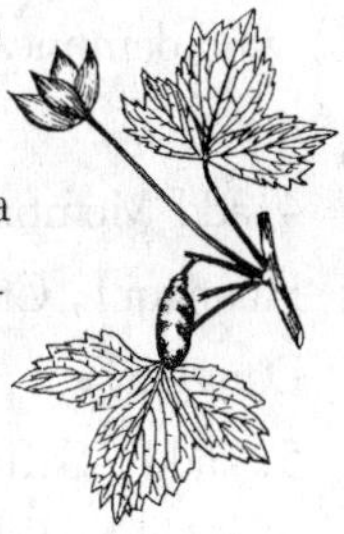

木 通

Properties and tastes: bitter, cold

Meridian tropism: heat, small intestine and urinary bladder

Functions: 1. promote urination and relieve stranguria

2. dispel dampness and clear away heat

3. purge heart heat

4. stimulate and improve lactation

5. promote urination and strengthen the heart

Indications: 1. stranguria of heat-dampness caused by the passage of urinary stone-dark and scanty urination, dripping urine with difficulty and pain

2. flaming up of heart-fire, aphthae with irritability, dark urination

3. galactostasis

4. arthralgia of dampness heat type, immovability of joints

5. amenorrhea due to blood stasis

6. cirrhosis, cardiac and renal edema

Dosage: 3~6 g.

Contraindication: It is reported that large dosage(60g) of this drug once led to acute renal failure. So it can not be overtaken and do not use for pregnant women.

Combinations: 1. add Pig Feet (猪蹄, Zhuti)——lack of lactation after delivery

2. add Plantain Seed (车前子, Cheqianzi)——edema stranguria

3. add Fourstamen Stephania Root(防己, Fangji), Swordlike Atractylodes Rhizome (苍术, Cangzhu)——pain of joints due to

wind-dampness tending to excessive dampness

4. add Membranous Milkvetch Root(黄芪, Huangqi), Chinese Angelica Root(当归, Danggui)——galactostasis

5. add Safflower(红花, Honghua), Twotooth Achyranthes Root(牛膝, Niuxi)——amenorrhea caused by blood stasis

6. add Umbellate Pore Fungus(猪苓, Zhuling), Tuckahoe(茯苓, Fuling)——beriberi, edema of nephritis

7. add Adhesive Rehmannia Root(生地黄, Shengdihuang), Bamboo Leaf(竹叶, Zhuye)——dark and scanty urination, dripping urine with difficulty and pain, aphthae, irritability, insomnia

8. add Bamboo Leaf(竹叶, Zhuye), Baikal Skullcap Root(黄芩, Huangqin), Lalang Grass Rhizome(白茅根, Baimaogen)——urinary infection, hematuria

9. add Oriental Waterplantain Rhizome(泽泻, Zexie), Common Selfheal Fruit-spike(夏枯草, Xiakucao)——ascites due to cirrhosis

Prescriptions: 1. Eight Health Restoring Powder(八正散, Bazheng San)

2. Powder for Dark Urine(导赤散, Daochi San)

Notes: Akebia Stem(木通, Mutong) can induce diuresis, treat stranguria, conduct heat to descend, as well as promote lactation and dredge blood vessels, indicating for stranguria syndrome, difficult urination, edema, lactation and amenorrhea. Modern research shows that it can strengthen the heart and induce diuresis, for ascites due to cirrhosis, cardiac and nephro edema in the clinic, for patients who have no effect in dihydrochlorothiazide, it has the obvious effect of inducing diuresis when together used with this drug.

Both Akebia Stem(木通, Mutong) and Hubo can clear away fire of the small intestine to induce diuresis and also clear away fire of the heart meridian. Akebia Stem(木通, Mutong) is good at treating aphthae, redness of eyes and restlessness of the heart caused by vigorousness of the heart fire. While Amber(琥珀, Hupo) clears away heart fire to relieve convulsions, palpitations, insomnia, dream-disturbed sleep, convulsions and epilepsy due to disturbance of heat to the heart and mind. In the aspect of dredging and smoothing blood vessels, both can treat amenorrhea caused by blood stagnation. But Akebia Stem(木通, Mutong) can be used for galactostasis and arthralgia due to damp-heat. Amber(琥珀, Hupo) can also be used for congestive edema due to injury, sores, carbuncles, swelling and toxin.

8. 通草, Tongcao

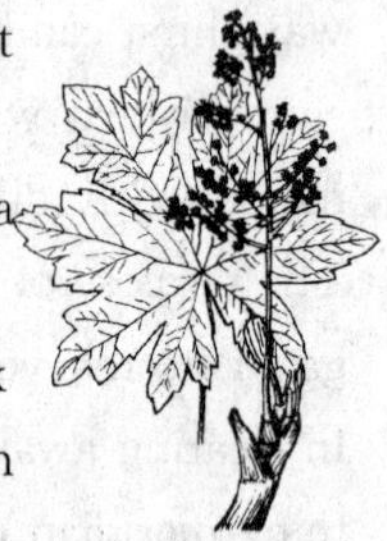

English name: Ricepaperplant Pith

Pharmaceutical name: Medulla Tetrapanacis Papyriferi

Botanical name: Tetrapanax papyriferus(Hook.) K. Koch

Properties and tastes: sweet, tasteless, and slightly cold

通 草

Meridian tropism: lung, stomach

Functions: 1. clear away the heat and promote urination

2. stimulate and improve lactation

Indications: 1. stranguria caused by evil heat——urine retention, dripping urine with difficulty and pain

2. febrile disease caused by damp-warm evil——retention of damp-heat in the interior, dark and short urination

3. galactostasis

Dosage: 3～6g

Contraindication: Not to be taken by pregnant women.

Combinations: 1. add Plantain Seed(车前子, Cheqianzi), Oriental Waterplantain Rhizome (泽泻, Zexie), Cape Jasmine Fruit(栀子, Zhizi)——stranguria caused by evil heat
2. add Coix Seed(薏苡仁, Yiyiren), Talc (滑石, Huashi), Bamboo Leaf (竹叶, Zhuye)——febrile disease caused by damp-warm evil with dark and short urination
3. add Pig Feet(猪蹄, Zhuti), Pangolin Scales(穿山甲, Chuanshanjia), Szechwan Lovage Rhizome(川芎, Chuanxiong)——galactostasis

Notes: Li Shizhen(李时珍) said that "In the upper part, this drug can clear away lung and heart heat, treating headache and remove obstruction of nine orifices. In the lower part, it can reduce damp-heat, induce urination, dredge large intestines and treat pain of the whole body". Ricepaperplant Pith(通草, Tongcao) is sweet, tasteless and cold. When acting on the lung, it purges heat blockage of the lung, conducts heat to descend and dredges water passage to promote urination. When acting on the stomach, it circulates qi to go upward and descends breast milk. But this drug has a soft effect in eliminating dampness, it is fit for cases with less damp-heat.

For the comparison of Ricepaperplant Pith(通草, Tongcao) and Akebia Stem(木通, Mutong), *Orthodox Interpretation of Materia Medica* (《本草正义》, Bencaozhengyi) says: "Ricepaperplant Pith(通草, Tongcao) circulates meridians, clears away heat and induces diuresis, the property of which is similar to that of Akebia Stem (木通, Mutong)." But Ricepaperplant Pith (通草, Tongcao) is sweet and tasteless in flavor and cold in nature, acting on the lungs to purge heat-blockage of the lung in order to dredge water passage and promote urination. It is often used for the damp-warm syndrome. While Akebia Stem(木通, Mutong) is bitter and cold, it can clear and descend fire of the heart and small intestines to promote water passage. Therefore, it is often used for ulceration on the oral mucosa and the tongue, difficult urine and bloody urine caused by excessive fire of the heart and small intestines. Both of them can dredge meridians and are used for lactation, amenorrhoea and painful arthralgia syndrome.

9. 金钱草, Jinqiancao

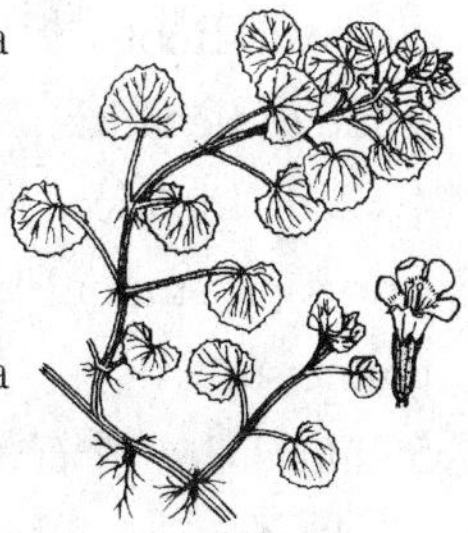

English name: Christina Loosetrife Herb

Pharmaceutical name: Herba Jinqiancao

Botanical name: Glechoma longituba(Nakai) Kupr. [in Jiangsu province], Desmodium styracifolium(Osbeck) Merr. [in Guangdong province], either Lysimachia christinae Hance or Dichondra repens Forst. [in Sichaun province], or Hydrocotyle sibthorpiodes Lam. Bar batrachium (Hance) Hand.-Mazz. [in Jiangxi province].

金钱草

Properties and tastes: sweet, tasteless, medium

Meridian tropism: liver, gallbladder, kidney and urinary bladder

Functions: 1. promote urination and relieve stranguria
2. eliminate dampness and relieve jaundice
3. clear away toxic material and relieve swelling
4. normalize the secretion of gallbladder and

drain the stone away

5. promote urine and drain the stone away

Indications: 1. disease of the liver and gallbladder——cholelithiasis, cholecystitis, jaundice hepatitis

2. urinary stone and stranguria due to damp-heat

3. swelling and toxin of malignent boil snake bite, hemorrhoid, burn and scald

Dosage: 30 ~ 60g. The dosage of fresh herb should be doubled. Proper amount for external use.

Combinations: 1. add Capillary Wormwood Herb(茵陈蒿, Yinchenhao)——cholelithiasis

2. add Bitter Orange (枳壳, Zhiqiao)——dysentery

3. add Dandelion(蒲公英, Pugongying), Indigwoad Root (板蓝根, Banlangen)——jaundice hepatitis

4. add Licorice Root (甘草, Gancao), Chrysanthemum Flower(菊花, Juhua)——plumbism

5. add Talc(滑石, Huashi), Plantain Seed (车前子, Cheqianzi)——stone in the kidney and gallbladder

6. add Tumeric Root-tuber(郁金, Yujin), Common Aucklandia Root (木香, Muxiang)——cholecystitis, obstructive jaundice

Notes: Christina Loosetrife Herb(金钱草, Jinqiancao) is an major drug for treating lithiasis in the urinary system, liver and gallbladder. For urinary system lithiasis, Christina Loosetrife Herb(金钱草, Jinqiancao) can be decocted alone in a large dosage and drunk as tea. Modern research has proved that this drug has the function of benefiting the gallbladder to get rid of stones, inducing diuresis to remove stones and anti-bacteria.

10. 海金沙, Haijinsha

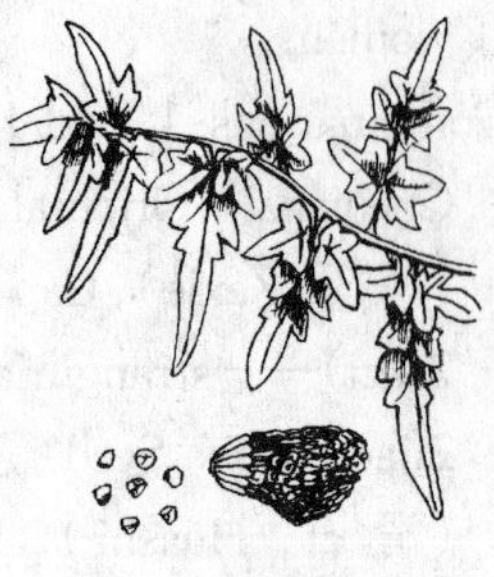
海金沙

English name: Japanese Climbing Fern Spores

Pharmaceutical name: Spora Lygodii

Botanical name: Lygodium haponicum (Thunb.) Sw.

Properties and tastes: sweet, tasteless, cold

Meridian tropism: urinary bladder and small intestine

Functions: 1. promote urination and relieve stranguria

2. normalize the secretion of gallbladder

Indications: 1. stranguria——stranguria caused by evil heat, strangura caused by urinary stones and complicated by hematuria, and stranguria marked by chyluria

2. edema, urine retention

3. jaundice due to dampness-heat

4. acute and chronic tonsillitis, mastitis, erysipelas, etc.

Dosage: 6 ~ 12 g, wrapped with cloth when boiled

Contraindication: Be cautious when prescribed for kidney-yin deficiency.

Combinations: 1. add Talc(滑石, Huashi)——heat stranguria

2. add Japanese Felt Fern Leaf(石韦, Shiwei)——urolitic stranguria

3. add Plantain Seed (车前子, Cheqianzi)——complicated by hematuria stranguria

4. add Sevenlobed Yam Rhizome(萆薢, Bixie)——stranguria marked by chyluria

5. add Pharbitis Seed(牵牛子, Qianniuzi), Kansui Root (甘遂, Gansui)——excessive spleen-deficiency, edema of body, abdominal

distension

6. add Capillary Wormwood Herb(茵陈蒿, Yinchenhao)——jaundice due to dampness-heat

7. add Chicken Gizzard Membrane(鸡内金, Jineijin), Tumeric Root-tuber(郁金, Yujin)——biliary stone

Notes: Japanese climbing Fern Spores(海金沙,Haijinsha)is sweet and tasteless in taste which can induce diuresis, and cold in property which can clear away heat. It has a descending and purging property which can reduce damp-heat of blood stage in the small intestines and urinary bladder meridians to dredge the water passage. It is a principal drug used to treat stranguria and urethra dribbling pain. It can treat all five types of stranguria, especially for urolitic stranguria.

Both Japanese climbing Fern Spores(海金沙, Haijinsha) and Japanese Felt Fern Leaf(石韦, Shiwei) can clear away damp-heat, relieve pain caused by urinary disorders and are often used for treating stranguria due to heat, urolitic stones with blood. Japanese climbing Fern Spores(海金沙, Haijinsha)is mainly used for stranguria due to urinary stones. While Japanese Felt Fern Leaf(石韦, Shiwei)is used mostly for stranguria with blood or due to damp-heat. In addition, Japanese Felt Fern Leaf(石韦, Shiwei) can clear away lung heat to relieve cough and asthma in the upper part, and cool blood to stop metrorrhagia in the lower part.

11. 石韦, Shiwei

English name: Japanese Felt Fern Leaf

Pharmaceutical name: Folium Pyrrosiae

Botanical name: Pyrrosia lingua (Thunb.) Farw., P. Sheareri(Bak.)Ching, P. Drakeana (Franch.) Ching, P. Petiolaos(Christ)Ching, P. Davidii(Gies.)Ching.

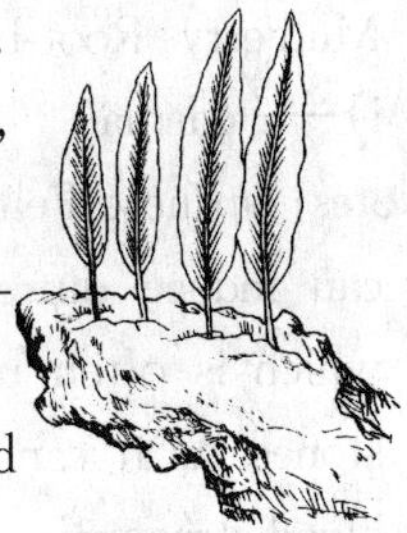

石 韦

Properties and tastes: bitter, sweet, slightly cold

Meridian tropism: lung and urinary bladder

Functions: 1. promote urination and relieve stranguria

2. clear away lung heat and remove phlegm, relieve cough and asthma

3. arrest bleeding

Indications: 1. stranguria——heat stranguria, urolitic stranguria, blood stranguria, stranguria marked by chyluria

2. edema——edema of nephritis

3. cough caused by lung heat——acute and chronic bronchitis and traumatic bleeding

4. bleeding——massive metrorrhagia, hematemesis, epistaxis, hemoptysis and traumatic bleeding

Dosage: 6～9 g, large dosage may be used for 30～60 g.

Combinations: 1. add Umbellate Pore Fungus (猪苓, Zhuling), Talc(滑石, Huashi)——stranguria caused by evil heat

2. add Christina Loosetrife Herb(金钱草, Jinqiancao), Japanese climbing Fern Spores (海金沙, Haijinsha)——urinary stone

3. add Plantain Seed(车前子, Cheqianzi)——blood stranguria, impeded urination during late pregnancy

4. add Areca Seed(槟榔, Binlang), Fresh Ginger(生姜, Shengjiang)——cough and asthma

5. add India Madder Root(茜草, Qiancao), Lalang Grass Rhizome(白茅根, Baimaogen)——massive metrorrhagia, epistaxis, hemoptysis, hematemesis

6. add Areca Peel(大腹皮, Dafupi), White

Mulberry Root-bark (桑白皮, Sangbaipi)——edema

Notes: Japanese Felt Fern Leaf(石韦, Shiwei) can induce diuresis and treat stranguria, which is often used for heat and urinary stones. As it can stop bleeding, it is fit for blood stranguria. Now in the clinic it is effective to use this drug to treat both acute and chronic bronchitis because it can clear lung heat, remove phlegm and relieve cough.

Both Japanese Felt Fern Leaf(石韦, Shiwei) and Talc(滑石, Huashi) are cold in property for treating stranguria, They are effective drugs for dribbling pain in the urethra caused by heat and urinary stones. But Japanese Felt Fern Leaf(石韦, Shiwei) has the functions of cooling blood and stopping bleeding which is mostly used for stranguria with blood. Talc(滑石, Huashi) is slippery in property to eliminate dampness, which is suitable for stranguria caused by damp heat and urinary stones. In addition, Japanese Felt Fern Leaf(石韦, Shiwei) clears away lung heat to relieve cough and cools blood to stop metrorrhagia. Talc (滑石, Huashi) clears away summer-heat to quench thirst.

12. 萹蓄, Bianxu

English name: Common Knotgrass Herb

Pharmaceutical name: Herba Polygoni Avicularis

Botanical name: Polygonum aviculare L.

Properties and tastes: bitter, slightly cold

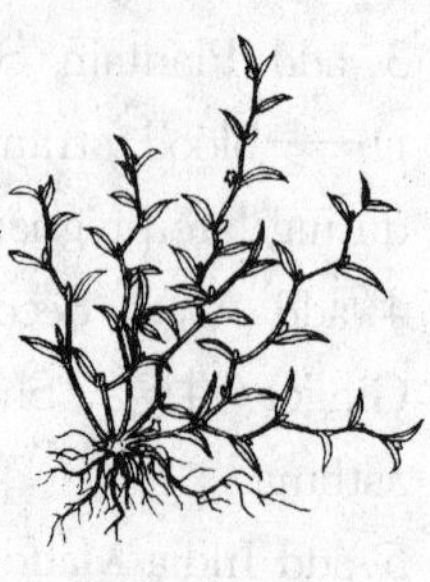

萹 蓄

Meridian tropism: urinary bladder

Functions: 1. promote urination and relieve stranguria

2. kill parasites for relieving itching

3. promote the functions of gallbladder to alleviate jaundice

4. inhibit the growth of Baccilus dysenterly

Indications: 1. stranguria caused by dampness heat, urilotic stranguria, stranguria due to urinary stone-dark and scanty urine, difficulty and pain in micturition, stone in urination

2. eczema, moist ulcer, tinea

3. jaundice due to damp-heat

4. acute bacterial dysentery

5. vaginal trichomoniasis, ascariasis, enterobiasis, hookworm

Dosage: 9 ~ 15g, proper amount for external use

Contraindication: Over taking may cause loss of essence.

Combinations: 1. add Lilac Pink Herb(瞿麦, Qumai), Akebia Stem(木通, Mutong), Talc (滑石, Huashi)——stranguria caused by dampness heat

2. add Japanese Thistle Herb or Root(大蓟, Daji), Common Cephalanoplos Herb(小蓟, Xiaoji), Lalang Grass Rhizome (白茅根, Baimaogen)——blood stranguria

3. add Japanese climbing Fern Spores(海金沙, Haijinsha)——urolitic stranguria

4. add Capillary Wormwood Herb(茵陈蒿, Yinchenhao)——jaundice due to damp heat

5. add Smoked Plum(乌梅, Wumei), Bunge Pricklyash (花椒, Huajiao)——colic cause by ascarid

Notes: Common Knotgrass Herb(萹蓄, Bianxu) is bitter and descending, which can clear away damp heat of the urinary bladder to induce diuresis and treat stranguria, used for dribbling pain of urination caused by heat stranguria. This drug also has the effect of killing parasites and relieving itching sensation, used for skin eczema, ascariasis, enterobiasis as well as pudenda itching sensation caused by vaginal trichomoniasis. This drug can be taken orally.

13. 瞿麦, Qumai

English name: Lilac Pink Herb

Pharmaceutical name: Herba Dianthi

Botanical name: Dianthus superbus L. or D. chinensis L.

瞿 麦

Properties and tastes: bitter, cold

Meridian tropism: heart, small intestine, and urinary bladder

Functions: 1. promote urination and relieve stranguria

2. promote blood circulation to remove obstruction of meridians

3. antisehistosome

Indications: 1. stranguria caused by dampness heat, urolitic stranguria, stranguria due to urinary stone——acute urethritis, cystitis, vesical stone

2. amenorrhea of blood stasis type on irregular menstruation

3. esophageal cancer, cancer of rectum

4. edema, schistosomiasis ascites

Dosage: 9～15 g.

Contraindication: Take cautions when it is prescribed for pregnant women.

Combinations: 1. add Common Knotgrass Herb (萹蓄, Bianxu)——acute urethritis, cystitis, acute nephritis

2. add Dan-shen Root (丹参, Danshen), Common Peony Root (赤芍, Chishao), Motherwort Herb (益母草, Yimucao)——amenorrhea of blood stasis type

3. add Ginseng (人参, Renshen), Tuckahoe (茯苓, Fuling), Largehead Atractylodes Rhizome (白术, Baizhu)——esophageal cancer, cancer of rectum

Prescription: Eight Health Restoring Powder (八正散, Bazheng San)

Notes: Lilac Pink Herb (瞿麦, Qumai) is bitter in taste, cold, descending and slippery in property. It is a major herb for treating heat stranguria. It dredges the heart meridian and goes into the blood stage, scatters blood stasis, and removes masses. It goes into the small intestines to conduct heat and remove obstruction of lower orifices in order to promote urination. It is a commonly used drug for stanuria due to heat. Because it can scatter blood stasis and remove obstruction of orifices, it is also used for gyneacological diseases caused by stagnation of blood.

Both Lilac Pink Herb (瞿麦, Qumai) and Common Knotgrass Herb (萹蓄, Bianxu) are drugs for clearing away heat, inducing diuresis and treating stranguria. For treating dribbling, heat and painful urination, the two herbs are used together for mutual reinforcement. The difference is that Lilac Pink Herb (瞿麦, Qumai) clears small intestines to conduct heat, fitting for hot pain in the urethra or hemaurica with more heat and less dampness, while Common Knotgrass Herb (萹蓄, Bianxu) clears away damp-heat in the urinary bladder, fitting for difficult urination and yellowish oliguria with obstruction of damp-heat. Both of them can be used for sores and swellings caused by toxin heat. But since Common Knotgrass Herb (萹蓄, Bianxu) is good at clearing away damp-heat, it can also be used for diarrhea and jaundice due to damp-heat. Lilac Pink Herb (瞿麦, Qumai) can also scatter blood used for amenorrhea caused by blood stasis.

14. 萆薢, Bixie

English name: Sevenlobed Yam Rhizome

Pharmaceutical name: Rhizoma Dioscoreae

Botanical name: Dioscorea hypolglauca Palib., D. collettii Hook. f., D. tokoro Mak., or D. gracillima Miq.

萆 薢

Properties and tastes: bitter, medium

Meridian tropism: liver, stomach and urinary bladder

Functions: 1. remove dampness

2. expel wind dampness evil

Indications: 1. stranguria marked by chyluria——turbid urine, the color of urine like rice-washing water, such as chronic prostatitis

2. profuse leukorrhea of dampness heat type

3. pain of arthritis caused by wind dampness and lumbago caused by kidney deficiency

Dosage: 9～15g.

Contraindication: Take cautions when it is prescribed for seminal emission and chronic diarrhea due to kidney-deficiency.

Combinations: 1. add Chinese Clematis Root (威灵仙, Weilingxian)——arthritis caused by wind-dampness, immovability of joints, pain in waist and knees

2. add Sharpleaf Galangal Fruit (益智仁, Yizhiren)——turbid urine caused by kidney deficiency with frequency of micturition, dripping urine, chyluria, profuse leukorrhea

3. add Chinese Corktree Bark (黄柏, Huangbai), Coix Seed (薏苡仁, Yiyiren)——eczema, chronic dermatitis or pemphigus belonging to damp-heat syndrome

4. add Plantain Seed (车前子, Cheqianzi), Chinese Corktree Bark (黄柏, Huangbai)--acute urethritis, cystitis

5. add Eucommia Bark (杜仲, Duzhong)——flaccidity of waist and knees with unsteady walking

Prescription: Decoction of Rhizoma Dioscoreae Hypoglaucae for Clearing Turbid Urine (萆薢分清饮, Bixiefenqing Yin)

Notes: Seven lobed Yam Rhizome (萆薢, Bixie) can remove dampness to separate the clear from the turbid, used for damp-turbid disease due to yang deficiency. It is a commonly used drug for treating stranguria. For example, Decoction of Rhizoma Dioscoreae Hypoglaucae for Clearing Turbid Urine (萆薢分清饮, Bixiefenqing Yin) treats stranguria marked by chyluria combined with Sharpleaf Calangal Fruit (益智仁, Yizhiren), Gypsum (石膏, Shigao), and Combined Spicebush Root (乌药, Wuyao). In addition, Li Shizhen (李时珍) said: "The functions of Sevenlobed Yam Rhizome (萆薢, Bixie) is good at eliminating wind-dampness. It can treat chronic and stubborn arthralgia, seminal emission, and malignant boils due to wind-dampness."

15. 茵陈蒿, Yinchenhao

English name: Capillary Wormwood Herb

Pharmaceutical name: Herba Artemesiae Capillaris

Botanical name: Artemisia capillaris Thunb.

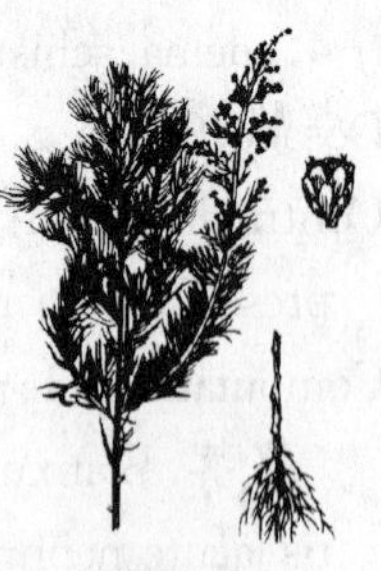

茵陈蒿

Properties and tastes: bitter, slightly cold

Meridian tropism: spleen, stomach, liver, gallbladder channels

Functions: 1. remove dampness-heat evil

2. protect the liver, regulate functions of the gallbladder to alleviate jaundice

3. reduce blood lipids, reduce blood pressure, increase the coronary flow of vitro

4. antibacteria, antiinfluenza virus

5. kill and expel intestinal parasites

6. promote urine, antiinflammation, reduce fever

Indications: 1. jaundice——acute epidemic hepatitis of jaundice type, jaundice of newborn, yang jaundice and yin jaundice

2. billary infection and cholelithiasis

3. ascariasis

4. hypercholesteremia and coronary heart disease

5. febrile disease caused by damp-warm evil, moist ulcer eczema, tinea, corporis, itch etc.

Dosage: 9～30g. Proper dosage for external use

Combinations: 1. add Cape Jasmine Fruit(栀子, Zhizi), Chinese Corktree Bark(黄柏, Huangbai)——jaundice due to dampness heat

2. add Dried Ginger(干姜, Ganjiang), Largehead Atractylodes Rhizome(白术, Baizhu)——jaundice due to cold-dampness

3. add Talc(滑石, Huashi), Weeping Forsythia Capsule(连翘, Lianqiao)——the beginning of febrile disease caused by damp-warm evil, fever of the body, soreness of limbs, chest congestion, abdominal distention, dark urine and constipation

4. add Cape Jasmine Fruit(栀子, Zhizi), Rhubarb(大黄, Dahuang)——jaundice hepatitis

5. add Dandelion(蒲公英, Pugongying), Indigwoad Root(板蓝根, Banlangen)—cellular jaundice of liver

6. add Cape Jasmine Fruit(栀子, Zhizi), Licorice Root(甘草, Gancao), Chinese Date (大枣, Dazao)——acute epidemic hepatitis of infants

7. add Chinese Gentian Root(龙胆草, Longdancao), Indigowoad Leaf(大青叶, Daqingye), Dan-shen Root(丹参, Danshen)——acute epidemic hepatitis

8. add Christina Loosetrife Herb(金钱草, Jinqiancao), Tumeric Root-tuber(郁金, Yujin), Japanese Honeysuckle(银花, Yinhua)——billary infection and cholelithiasis

9. add Smoked Plum(乌梅, Wumei)——ascariasis

10. add Oriental Waterplantain Rhizome(泽泻, Zexie), Lobed Kudzuvine Root(葛根, Gegei)——hyperlipidemia, coronary heart disease

11. add Indigwoad Root(板蓝根, Banlangen)——preventing and treating influenza

Prescription: Decoction of Artemisae Scopariae (茵陈蒿汤, Yinchenhao Tang)

Notes: Traditionally speaking, Capillary Wormwood Herb(茵陈蒿, Yinchenhao) is bitter, purging and descending, it is mainly used to treat jaundice for the functions of clearing away damp-heat. For yin jaundice, it can be used together with drugs for warming yang and invigorating the spleen. Research shows that Capillary Wormwood Herb(茵陈蒿, Yinchenhao) has the functions of not only protecting the liver, promoting the functions of gallbladder, but also reducing blood lipid, expanding coronary artery and lowering blood pressure, and preventing and treating cardiovascular and cerebrovascular diseases. It is reported that it has a good therapeutic effect Capillary Wormwood Herb(茵陈蒿, Yinchenhao), when taken as tea, is used to treat hypercholesterolemia.

Capillary Wormwood Herb(茵陈蒿,

Yinchenhao) and Sweet Wormwood(青蒿, Qinghao) have a fragrant smell which can relieve damp-heat, used for jaundice due to damp-heat, damp-warm syndrome and summer-heat damp syndrome. But Capillary Wormwood Herb(茵陈蒿, Yinchenhao) mainly acts on the spleen and stomach and is a main drug for treating jaundice. Sweet Wormwood(青蒿, Qinghao) acts primarily on the liver and gallbladder, which especially relieves hectic fever and removes summer-heat and purges heat, used for hectic fever due to yin deficiency, cold and heat caused by malaria and high fever due to summer-heat.

16. 赤小豆, Chixiaodou

English name: Rice Bean

Pharmaceutical name: Semen Phaseoli Calcarati

Botanical name: Phaseolus calcaratus Roxb.

Properties and tastes: Sweet, sour, medium

赤小豆

Meridian tropism: heart, small intestine

Functions: 1. promote urination and detumescentify

2. detoxicate and evacuate pus

3. promote urination to alleviate jaundice

Indications: 1. edema——edema and abdominal fullness, flaccidity of lower limbs, edema

2. carbuncle due to toxic heat——mumps, erysipelas, acute mastitis, hematochezia due to toxic heat

3. jaundice due to damp-heat

4. hematoma due to injury, sprain

5. lack of lactation after delivery

Dosage: 9～30 g. Proper dosage for external use.

Combinations: 1. add Lalang Grass Rhizome (白茅根, Baimaogen), White Mulberry Root-bark(桑白皮, Sangbaipi)——edema

2. add Carp(鲤鱼, Liyu)——make soft enough to eat, for edema of nephritis, ascites due to cirrhosis and edema of malnutrition

3. add Ephedra(麻黄, Mahuang), Weeping Forsythia Capsule(连翘, Lianqiao)——aundice with exterior syndrome

4. add Indian Bread Pink Epidermis(赤茯苓, Chifuling)——edema caused by dampness-heat, urine retention, heat stranguria, acute mastitis, diarrhea and dysentery

Notes: Rice Bean(赤小豆, Chixiaodou) is good at descending to dredge the water passage, causing water-dampness to go downward to treat edema. The drug can be decocted alone to treat edema disease. Since it removes toxic substances and promotes pus discharge, it can be used externally for mumps, acute mastitis, erysipelas and carbuncles. Li Shizhen(李时珍) said: "Rice Bean(赤小豆, Chixiaodou) which is smaller and with dark red color can be used as medicine. The one which is bigger and with fresh red or light red color can not treat disease."

Appendix: Others Drugs For Inducing Diuresis And Excreting Dampness

Name	Properties and tastes	Meridian tropism	Functions	Indications	Dosage	Contraindication
Common Rush Stem Pith (灯心草, Dengxincao)	sweet, tasteless, slightly cold	Heart, lung, small intestine	Promote urination and relieve stranguria, clear away heart-heat and conduct heat downward	Stranguria caused by heat evil, edema, insomnia, morbid night crying of infant, insomnia, throat inflammation, also used for moxibustion	1.5～3 grams	
Belvedere Fruit (地肤子, Difuzi)	sweet, bitter, cold	Kidney, urinary bladder	Clear away heat and promote urination and relieve itching	Stranguria caused by dampness-heat, moist ulcer, rubella, itch	9～15 grams, properly for external use	
Toothleaf Goldenray Root and Rhizome (葫芦, Hulu)	sweet, tasteless, cold	Lung, small intestine	Promote urination, detumescentify	Edema, ascites	15～30 grams	It is cautious for deficiency cold of spleen
Chinese Waxgourd Exocarp (冬瓜皮, Dongguapi)	sweet, tasteless, slight cold	Lung, small intestine	Promote urination, detamescentify	Edema	15～30 grams	
Sun Euphorbai Herb (泽漆, Zeqi)	sour, bitter, slightly cold, poisonous	Large intestine, small intestine, lung	Promote urination, detumescentify, remove phlegm	Edema, ascites, cough with dyspnea, scrofula	6～9 grams	Proper amount for external use.
Mazie Style (玉米须, Yumixu)	sweet, tasteless, medium	Kidney, urinary bladder	Promote urination, detumescentify, relieve strangria, clear away liver and gallbladder dampness-heat, regulate functions of the gallbladder, reduce blood sugar, reduce blood pressure, arrest bleeding	Edema, stranguria, hepatitis, cholecystitis, cholelithiasis	1.5～3 grams	
Cluster Mallow Seed (冬葵子, Dongkuizi)	sweet, cold	Large intestine, small intestine, urinary bladder	Relieve stranguria by diuresis, stimulate milk secretion, use lubricant drugs to relieve constipation	Stranguria, edema, galactostasis, distenting pain of the breast, constipation	9～15 grams	
Mole Cricket (蝼蛄, Lougu)	Salty, cold	Urinary bladder	Promote urination, relieve constipation	Edema, stranguria caused by the passage of urinary stone, uroschesis, constipation	3～6 grams	It is forbidden in cases of weakness, qideficiency and in pregnancy
Chinese Cricket (蟋蟀, Xishuai)	pungent, salty and warm		Induce diuresis	Retention of urine, edema, tympanites	4～6 pieces, 1～4 pieces when taking the ground powder	

PART Ⅴ
Drugs for Treating Phlegm, Cough and Asthma

Phlegm, cough and asthma are related in pathogenis. The symptoms among them are complicated. Asthma is usually complicated by phlegm, while phlegm is the main cause of asthma. So they are discussed together.

Asthma results from adverse upward flow of qi, phlegm results from retention of fluid. Therefore, phlegm, cough and asthma are diseases due to disorder of qi and retention of fluid in body. It was said in ancient times "phlegm disease can not be treated by resolving phlegm, and should be treated by regulating qi first."

If fluid disease lasts a long time, the prolonged disease may enter into the collaterals and blood system must be involved. The principle of promoting blood circulation and removing obstruction of collaterals must be better understood.

Chapter 11
Drugs for Removing Phlegm

Definition: Drugs that are used to expel or eliminate phlegm are called drugs which remove phlegm.

Functions: As asthma is often complicated by phlegm and as profuse phlegm also causes cough, these drugs have the function of relieving cough and asthma; vice vesa drugs which relieve cough and asthma also remove phlegm.

Indications: Drugs which remove phlegm are primarily used to treat symptoms such as profuse phlegm, cough, asthma due to phlegm retention, difficulty in expectoration. Drugs which relieve asthma and cough are mainly used to treat cough and asthma due to internal injury and exopathic disease. The pathogenesis of some diseases is influenced by phlegm, such as epilepsy, infantile convulsions, apoplexy, obstruction in the chest, goiter, multiple abscess, subcutaneous nodule, and chronic cellulitis, etc. This phenomenon referred: "all diseases resulting from phlegm". So drugs which remove phlegm also treat the above mentioned symptoms. Phlegm and dampness are basically the same thing, that is why drugs which remove phlegm have an inherent relationship with drugs which resolve dampness and promote urination.

Classification: According to the medical properties, drugs which remove phlegm are divided into two categories: warm and dry drugs, and cold and cool drugs. These categories are used to treat either cold or heat phlegm symptoms respectively.

Cautions: In case of hemoptysis, do not use phlegm-removing drugs with strong and stimulative features because they aggravate the bleeding.

1. 半夏, Banxia

English name: Pinellia Rhizome

Pharmaceutical name: Rhizoma Pinelliae Ternatae

Botanical name: Pinellia ternata(Thunb.) Breit.

半 夏

Properties and tastes: sour, warm, and poisonous.

Meridian tropism: spleen, stomach, and lung.

Functions: 1. dry dampness and remove phlegm

2. descend qi and relieve cough

3. stop the adverse upward flow of stomach qi to prevent vomiting

4. disintegrate masses and scatter blockage

5. detumescentify and relieve pain (external use)

6. tranquilize the mind

7. antitumor effect

Indications: 1. phlegm-damp syndrome——profuse phlegm, coughing, reversed upward flow of qi, thin phlegm, and dizziness due to wind-phlegm.

2. vomiting due to retention of cold fluids, deficient stomach, stomach heat, indigestion, acute or chronic gastritis; neurogenic vomiting and vomiting during pregnancy

3. accumulation of pathogens in the chest——accumulation of heat with stagnancy of phlegm, chest congestion, tenderness, yellow and thick phlegm, yellow and greasy coating of the tongue, slippery and rapid pulse, gastritis, trachitis, and coronary atherosclerotic cardiopathy

4. globus hystericus

5. goiter and subcutaneous nodule, carbuncles cellulitis and snake-bite (External use)

Dosage: 6～9 g. Proper amount is for external use.

Contraindication: Incompatible with Common Monksood (乌头, Wutou). The crude herb can not be used for oral medication. It should be used cautiously if cough is due to yin deficiency, hemorrhagic diseases or if it is accompanied by heat-phlegm symptoms because it is warm and drying.

Combinations: 1. add Tall Gastrodia Rhizome (天麻, Tianma)——dizziness due to wind-phlegm

2. add Tangerine Peel (橘皮, Jupi)——cough due to dampness and phlegm, nausea and vomiting

3. add Dried Ginger (干姜, Ganjiang), Manchurian Wildginger Herb (细辛, Xixin)——cough due to cold-phlegm

4. add Fresh Ginger (生姜, Shengjiang)——vomiting due to an adverse rising of stomach qi

5. add Coptis Rhizome (黄连, Huanglian), Snakegourd Fruit (瓜蒌, Gualou)——chest and abdominal masses and fullness, heat-phlegm syndrome with yellow and thick phlegm

6. add Ginseng (人参, Renshen)——vomiting due to stomach deficiency

7. add Coptis Rhizome (黄连, Huanglian), Bamboo Shavings (竹茹, Zhuru)——restlessness and insomnia due to heat-phlegm

8. add Perilla Stem (紫苏梗, Zisugeng) Villous Amomum Fruit (砂仁, Sharen)——vomiting during pregnancy

9. add Officinal Magnolia Bark (厚朴,

Houpo), Perilla leaf (苏叶, Suye)——chronic pharyngitis due to stagnation of phlegm with qi

10. add Tendrilleaf Fritillary Bulb(贝母, Beimu),Kelp(昆布,Kunbu)——goiter

11. add Motherwort Herb(益母草, Yimucao)——cervix carcinoma

12. add Snakegourd Fruit(瓜蒌, Gualou), Longstament Onion Bulb (薤白, Xiebai)——obstruction in the chest with cold phlegm, and insufficiency of chest-yang

13. add Sorghum(秫米, Shumi)——insomnia due to restlessness of the deficiency type, disorder of the stomach-qi

14. add Common Yam Rhizome (山药, Shanyao)——serious vomiting during pregnancy

15. add Loquat Leaf(枇杷叶, Pipaye)——lingering cough

16. add Tabasheer (天竹黄, Tianzhuhuang)——infantile interaction of phlegm with heat, indigestion, wind-phlegm premonitory

Prescriptions: 1. Erchen Decoction(二陈汤, Erchen Tang)

2. Decoction for Mild Phlegm-heat Syndrome in the chest(小陷胸汤, Xiaoxianxiong Tang)

3. Decoction of Pinellia Rhizome and Official Magnolia Bark(半夏厚朴汤, Banxiahoupo Tang)

4. Decoction of Trichosanthis Allii Macrostemi and Rhizoma Pinelliae(瓜蒌薤白半夏汤, Gualou Xiebai Banxia Tang)

5. Decoction of Pinellia Rhizome for Purging Stomach-Fire(半夏泻心汤, Banxiaxiexin Tang)

Notes: Pinellia Rhizome(半夏, Banxia)' s property is dry, so it is mainly used for the damp-phlegm syndromes. But it is also used for all kinds of phlegm syndromes according to different combinations. It is said in *Origin of Shennong' s Herbal Classic* (《本经逢源》, Benjingfengyuan) that: "Pinellia Rhizome(半夏, Banxia) treats damp phlegm with Swordlike Atractylodes Rhizome(苍术, Cangzhu) and Tuckahoe(茯苓, Fuling); heat phlegm with Snakegourd Fruit(瓜蒌, Gualou) and Baikal skullcap Root(黄芩, Huangqin); wind phlegm with Jackinthepulpit Tuber(南星, Nanxing) and Whiteflower Hogfenel Root(前胡, Qianhu); and treats cold phlegm with White Mustard Seed(白芥子, Baijiezi) and Ginger juice. Pinellia Rhizome(半夏, Banxia) can' t treat dry phlegm. Dry phlegm can be treated by Snakegourd Fruit(瓜蒌, Gualou) and Tendrilleaf Fritillary Bulb(贝母, Beimu)" This herb is good at regulating the functions of the stomach. All kinds of gastric diseases are treated with it, especially vomiting. It also tranquilizes and treats restlessness and insomnia caused by dysfunction of descending. Modern studies indicate that Pinellia Rhizome(半夏, Banxia) can treat cervix carcinoma and cutaneous carcinoma because of its antitumor effect. A mixture of crude Pinellia Rhizome(半夏, Banxia) powder and egg white is applied to the affected part to treat boils on the back and mastadenitis. Clinically, prepared Pinellia Rhizome(半夏, Banxia) is usually used externally.

Pinellia Rhizome (半夏, Banxia) and Fresh Ginger(生姜, Shengjiang) are both useful for regulating the stomach to relieve vomiting. But Pinellia Rhizome (半夏, Banxia) mainly dries dampness and removes phlegm in order to descend adverse qi to relieve vomiting; Fresh Ginger (生姜, Shengjiang), however, mainly warms the stomach and excites the spleen in order to regulate the stomach to relieve vomiting. The combination of Pinellia Rhizome(半夏, Banxia) and Fresh Ginger (生姜, Shengjiang) is good at treating vomiting caused by cold dampness attacking the stomach.

Pinellia Rhizome (半夏, Banxia) and Fresh Ginger (生姜, Shengjiang) are also more effective for removing phlegm and stopping cough. Pinellia Rhizome (半夏, Banxia) mainly dries dampness and removes phlegm; Fresh Ginger (生姜, Shengjiang) mainly warms the lung to remove evil fluid. The combination of Pinellia Rhizome(半夏, Banxia) and Fresh Ginger (生姜, Shengjiang) improves the treatment of cough due to cold-lung. If Dried Ginger (干姜, Ganjiang) substitutes for Fresh Ginger (生姜, Shengjiang), it has stronger functions of warming the lung and dispersing the evil fluid.

2. 天南星, Tiannanxing

English name: Jackinthepulpit Tuber

Pharmaceutical name: Rhizoma Arisaematis

Botanical name: Arisaema consanguineum Schott, A. amurense Maxim., A. heterphyllum Bl., or A. japonicaum Bl. Many other plants of this genus are also used for this herb.

天南星

Properties and tastes: bitter, sour, warm, poisonous.

Meridian tropism: lung, liver, and spleen

Functions: 1. dry dampness and remove phlegm

2. expel the wind and relieve convulsion

3. detumescentify and relieve pain (for external use)

4. antitumor effect

5. tranquilize the mind

Indications: 1. phlegm, damp-phlegm, cold-phlegm, cough and profuse phlegm, feeling of fullness in the chest

2. dizziness due to wind-phlegm

3. apoplexy——numbness of hands and feet, hemiplegia, deviation of eye and mouth

4. epilepsy, tetanus

5. carbuncle and dermapostasis, multiple abscess, scrofula and subcutaneous nodule, traumatic injury, snake-bite (for external use)

6. cervix carcinoma

7. swelling pain due to rheumatoid arthritis

Dosage: 5～9g of fried Jackinthepulpit Tuber (制南星, Zhinanxing). Proper amount of crude Nanxing for external use.

Contraindication: Use cautiously for women during pregnancy. Generally, crude Jackinthepulpit Tuber (天南星, Tiannanxing) is not used for oral medication.

Combinations: 1. add Sanqi Root (三七, Sanqi), Japanese Thistle Herb or Root (大蓟, Daji)——onset of paralysis caused by apoplexy

2. add Centipede (蜈蚣, Wugong), Dan-shen Root (丹参, Danshen)——hemiplegia caused by cerebral apoplexy.

3. add Scorpion (全蝎, Quanxie), Centipede (蜈蚣, Wugong)——tetanus.

4. add Scorpion (全蝎, Quanxie), Silkworm with Batrytis Larva (白僵蚕, Baijiangcan)——epilepsy

5. add Baikal skullcap Root (黄芩, Huangqin), Pinellia Rhizome (半夏, Banxia)——cough due to heat-phlegm, profuse and yellow phlegm

6. add Pinellia Rhizome (半夏, Banxia),

Cassia Bark (肉桂, Rougui)——coughing due to cold-phlegm, profuse phlegm and short breath

7. add Pinellia Rhizome(半夏,Banxia),Divaricate Saposhnikovia Root (防风, Fangfeng)——dizziness, epilepsy, spasm of hands and feet, apoplexy, tetanus

8. add Bamboo Shavings (竹茹, Zhuru), Grassleaf Sweetflag Rhizome(菖蒲,Changpu)——dizziness and apoplexy, deviation of eye and mouth, hemiplegia, spasm and infantile convulsions

9. add Tangerine Peel(橘皮,Jupi), Pinellia Rhizome(半夏,Banxia)——cough, profuse and thin phlegm, congestion of the chest, and greasy coating of the tongue induced by stagnation of phlegm-dampness

10. add Inula Flower (旋覆花, Xuanfuhua)——stubborn phlegm and asthma as well as numbness of the extremities

Prescription: Phlegm Removing Decoction(导痰汤,Daotan Tang)

Notes: Jackinthepulpit Tuber(天南星,Tiannanxing) is divided into processed and unprocessed from Jackinthepulpit Tuber(天南星, Tiannanxing). The processed Nanxing is made from crude Jackinthepulpit(生南星 Shengnanxing). The unprocessed Jackinthepulpit Tuber(天南星,Tiannanxing) is poisonous, so it can not be used for oral medication. It can also be used externally to dissipate blockage and relieve pain in order to treat carbuncle, cellulitis, subcutaneous nodules and dermapostasis. It is in recent years found that this herb is effective as an antitumor, mainly used for the carcinoma of the cervix.

Both Jackinthepulpit Tuber (天南星, Tiannanxing) and Pinellia Rhizome(半夏, Banxia) can dry dampness to relieve phlegm, but Jackinthepulpit Tuber (天南星,Tiannanxing) is especially useful for the removal of obstructions in meridians or collaterals and used primarily for apoplexy; Pinellia Rhizome(半夏,Banxia) enters the gastrointestinal tract and is used primarily for vomiting and hiccups. Pinellia Rhizome (半夏, Banxia) also disperses abdominal masses and regulates the functions of the stomach because of its sour and bitter tastes; whereas Nanxing relieves swelling and dissipates blockage.

Arisaema With Bile(胆南星, Dannanxing) is a product stirred by Jackinthepulpit Tuber(天南星, Tiannanxing) prepared with bovine bile. It is bitter and cool. It clears heat-phlegm and calms the endopathic wind to arrest convulsions. It is used for convulsions and spasms caused by heat-phlegm and apoplexy as well as epilepsy. The dosage is 2 ~6g.

The propertics of Jackinthepulpit Tuber (天南星, Tiannanxing) of Arisaema With Bile(胆南星,Dannanxing) are antagonistic. Jackinthepulpit Tuber(天南星, Tiannanxing) is bitter, sour and warm. It mainly dries dampness to remove phlegm and expel wind. Arisaema With Bile (胆南星, Dannanxing) is bitter, cool and moist. It is not dry, so it does not damage the yin. It mainly eliminates phlegm, arrests convulsion and clears heat. It is mainly used for convulsions due to heat-phlegm.

3. 白附子, Baifuzi

English name: Giant Typhonium Rhizome

Pharmaceutical name: Rhizoma Typhonii Gigantei seu Radix Aconiti Coreani

Botanical name: Typhonium giganteum Engl. or Aconitum coreanum (Levl.) Raipaics.

When writing prescriptions the former is usually called Yu Bai Fu and the latter Guan Bai Fu.

Properties and tastes: sour, sweet, warm; poisonous.

Meridian tropism: stomach, liver

Functions: 1. dry dampness and remove phlegm

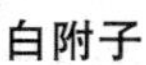
白附子

2. expel the wind and relieve spasm

3. detoxicate and scatter blockage

4. relieve pain and itching

5. antibiotic of bacteriostatic felycobacterium tuberculosis

Indications: 1. phlegm stagnation syndrome——apoplexy, infantile convulsions, epilepsy, phlegm syncope

2. facial paralysis

3. tetanus

4. migraine

5. multiple abscess and subcutaneous nodule——chronic lymphadenitis, tuberculosis of the lymphnodes. The fresh Giant Typhonium Rhizome (白附子, Baifuzi) can be pounded for application

6. snake-bite——for external application

7. arthritis due to wind, cold and dampness——joints ache, dysfunction of flexion and extension

8. eczema on the scrotum

Dosage: 3 ~ 6g. Proper amount for external use. Put the plaster on the affected area.

Contraindication: It may not be used in case of there is internal wind due to yin or blood deficiency, up stirring of the liver and during pregnancy. Generally, the crude herb is not used for oral medication.

Combinations: 1. add Jackinthepulpit Tuber (天南星, Tiannanxing), Pinellia Rhizome (半夏, Banxia)——apoplexy, stagnation of phlegm

2. add Scorpion (全蝎, Quanxie), Silkworm with Batrytis Larva (白僵蚕, Baijiangcan)——deviation of eye and mouth

3. add Jackinthepulpit Tuber (天南星, Tiannanxing), Tall Gastrodia Rhizome (天麻, Tianma), Divaricate Saposhnikovia Root (防风, Fangfeng)——tetanus

4. add Dahurian Angelica Root (白芷, Baizhi), Szechwan Lovage Rhizome (川芎, Chuanxiong)——migraine

5. add Doubleteeth Pulbescent Angelica Root (独活, Duhuo), Chinese Clematis Root (威灵仙, Weilingxian)——arthritis due to wind, cold and dampness

6. add Puncturevine Caltrop Fruit (刺蒺藜, Cijili), Rhizome or Root of Forbes Notopterygium (羌活, Qianghuo)——eczema on the scrotum

Prescription: Powder for Treating Face Distortion (牵正散, Qianzheng San)

Notes: Giant Typhonium Rhizome (白附子, Baifuzi) is sour, warm, dry and poisonous. It is ascending and dispersing, so it can lead the other herbs tend to ascend. It is useful for expelling the wind of the head and face. It expels wind-phlegm and dispels cold-dampness. Treating excessive wind-phlegm of the head and face is its main functions. It is usually used for facial hemiparalysis due to apoplexy, migraine, headaches due to phlegm syncope. It is also used to treat symptoms of apoplexy and accumulation of phlegm, aphasia and spasms due to tetanus.

BothGiant Typhonium Rhizome (白附子, Baifuzi) and Jackinthepulpit Tuber (天南星, Tiannanxin) are important main herbs to treat wind-phlegm. But Giant Typhonium Rhizome (白附子, Baifuzi) ascends and mainly expels the excessive wind-phlegm of the head and the face; Jackinthepulpit Tuber(天南星, Tiannanxin) expels wind-phlegm to arrest convulsion and is used mainly for apoplexy and accumulation of phlegm, infantile convulsions and tetanus. When compared with Prepared Daughter Root of Commom Monkshood(附子, Fuzi), Giant Typhonium Rhizome(白附子, Baifuzi) is sour, warm and drying. It ascends and especially enters the Upper-jiao. It is used to treat symptoms of wind evil of the head and the face, accumulation of wind-phlegm and dysphasia. Prepared Daughter Root of Commom Monkshood(附子, Fuzi) is sour and hot. It enters the Lower-jiao to warm the kidney-yang, recuperate depleted yang and rescue the patient from collapse.

4. 白芥子, Baijiezi

English name: White Mustard Seed

Pharmaceutical name: Semen Sinapis Albae

Botanical name: Brassica alba (L.) Boiss.

Properties and tastes: sour, warm.

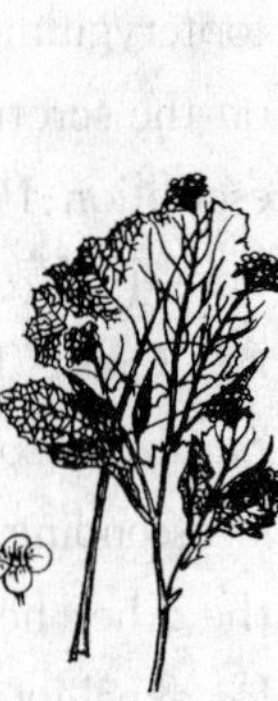

白芥子

Meridian tropism: lung, stomach.

Functions: 1. warm the lung and expel phlegm

2. promote qi circulation and disperse blockage

3. remove obstruction of the meridians to relieve pain

Indications: 1. cough and asthma——used for stagnation of cold-phlegm, cough and asthma, profuse phlegm, feeling of fullness in the chest, hypochondriac pain

2. pain or numbness of limbs and joints due to obstruction of meridians by phlegm-dampness

3. chronic cellulitis, multiple absceses, subcutaneous nodules

4. exudative pleurisy

5. acute or chronic infantile bronchitis, pneumonia

6. facial paralysis

Dosage: 3～9g. Do not decoct this herb for a long time. Proper amount is for external use. The powder of this herb is mixed with vinegar for external application.

Contraindication: External application causes vesiculation. Do not use it where there is an ulcer in the digestive tract, bleeding and dermal sensitivity, chronic coughing due to lung deficiency, or yin deficiency with fire. Do not use excessively, or it may cause gastroenteritis

Combinations: 1. add Perilla Seed(苏子, Suzi), Radish Seed(莱菔子, Laifuzi)——cough and asthma, profuse and thin expectoration, expecially for deficient cough of old men or deficient people

2. add Kansui Root(甘遂, Gansui), Peking Euphorbia Root(大戟, Daji)——feeling of fullness in the chest and hypochondriac pain due to stagnation of phlegm retention in the chest and diaphragm

3. add Myrrh(没药, Moyao), Common Aucklandia Root(木香, Muxiang)——pain or numbness of shoulders, arms, limbs and joints

4. add Antler Glue(鹿角胶, Lujiaojiao), Cassia Bark(肉桂, Rougui)——chronic cellulitis

Prescriptions: 1. Decoction of Three Kinds of Seed for the Aged(三子养亲汤, Sanziyangqin Tang)

2. Decoction of Prepared Rehmannia, Cinnamon Bark and Ephedra Combination(阳和汤, Yanghe Tang)

Notes: Zhu Zhenheng(朱震亨) said: "If

phlegm exists under the hypochondrium and the space between skin and pleurodiaphragm, only White Mustard Seed(白芥子,Baijiezi) can reach it."Li Shizhen(李时珍)said that"this herb promotes qi circulation and eliminates phlegm, warms the Middle-jiao and promotes digestion, relieves pain and subdues swelling and eliminates turbid evils." In recent years, this herb has been used for pleurisy, for it can remove hydrops of the thoracic cavity.

White Mustard Seed(白芥子, Baijiezi) and Jackinthepulpit Tuber (天南星, Tiananxing) all enter into meridians and collaterals to treat invisible sputum. But White Mustard Seed(白芥子, Baijiezi) promotes qi circulation and dissipates blockage, so it is used to treat symptoms such as joint obstruction and pain due to wind-phlegm stagnation of meridians and collaterals, and chronic cellulitis; Jackinthepulpit Tuber(天南星, Tiananxing) expels the wind and eliminates sputum, so it is used to treat spasm due to wind-phlegm and hemiplegia.

Both White Mustard Seed(白芥子, Baijiezi) and Perilla Seed(苏子, Suzi) can treat asthma and cough due to cold-phlegm. But White Mustard Seed(白芥子, Baijiezi) is warm and dry and good for entering into meridians and collaterals in order to eliminate phlegm between the skin and the pleurodiaphragm; Perilla Seed(苏子, Suzi) descends qi and eliminates phlegm and is good for treating asthma and dyspnea due to cold-phlegm.

5. 桔梗, Jiegeng

English name: Balloonflower Root

Pharmaceutical name: Radix Platycodi Grandiflori

Botanical name: Platycodon grandiflorum (Jacq.) A. DC.

桔 梗

Properties and tastes: bitter, sour, medium.

Meridian tropism: lung.

Functions: 1. promote the dispersing function of the lung, relieve sore-throat

2. expel phlegm and evacuate pus

3. relieve cough

4. anti-inflammatory

5. tranquilize, relieve pain and reduce fever

6. inhibit gastric juice secretion, anti-gastric ulcer

7. reduce blood sugar

8. reduce blood-lipid

Indications: 1. cough——cough with profuse phlegm, difficulty in spitting, chest congestion. Not matter whether the cough is due to exterior, interior, cold or heat evil, this herb can all be used.

2. pulmonary abscess——chest pain, cough and hemoptysis, yellow and sticky phlegm, for example, pulmonary abscess

3. sorethroat, hoarseness——tonsillitis, pharyngitis, laryngitis, etc.

4. uroschesis, constipation or dysentery and tenesmus

Dosage: 3～9g. Fried Balloonflower Root(桔梗, Jiegeng) is good for moistening the lungs and expelling phlegm.

Contraindication: Contraindicated in case of hemoptysis due to yin deficiency with fire and reversed upward flow of qi.

Combinations: 1. add Thinleaf Milkwort Root (远志, Yuanzhi), Common Coltsfoot Flower (款冬花, Kuandonghua)——exopathic cough, difficulty in spitting

2. add Medicine Terminalia Fruit (诃子,

Hezi) Licorice Root (甘草, Gancao)——hoarseness and chronic laryngitis, tuberculosis of larynx

3. add Snakegourd Fruit (瓜蒌, Gualou), Coix Seed (薏苡仁, Yiyiren)——pulmonary abscess, phlegm with pus blood

4. add Bitter orange (枳壳, Zhiqiao)——qi stagnation, phlegm obstruction, chest congestion. Usingthe combination of two, one ascends, the other descends and both of them regulate movement of qi

5. add Mulberry Leaf (桑叶, Sangye), Chrysanthemum Flower (菊花, Juhua)——wind-heat attacking the lung, itchy painful throat, dry mouth

6. add Fineleaf Schizomepeta Herb (荆芥, Jingjie), Wild Mint (薄荷, Bohe), Licorice Root (甘草, Gancao)——common cold, cough with profuse phlegm, acute tonsillitis, acute pharyngitis, acute laryngitis

7. add Membranous Milkvetch Root (黄芪, Huangqi), Chinese Thorowax Root (柴胡, Chaihu), Licorice Root (甘草, Gancao)——collapse of Middle-jiao qi, prolapse of the uterus, prolapse of the rectum

8. add Dandelion (蒲公英, Pugongying), Tokyo Violet Herb (紫花地丁, Zihuadiding)——skin and external diseases

9. add Membranous Milkvetch Root (黄芪, Huangqi), Apricot Seed (杏仁, Xingren), Tendrilleaf Fritillary Bulb (贝母, Beimu)——chronic bronchitis

Prescription: Decoction of Balloonflower Root and Licorice Root (桔梗甘草汤, Jiegenggancao Tang)

Notes: Balloonflower Root (桔梗, Jiegeng) is sour for dispersion and bitter for purgation. This herb disperses the lung qi and regulates diaphragm qi. It also has the function of expelling phlegm. It can be used to treat cough and a great deal of phlegm whether caused by lung-cold or lung-heat. In addition, the herb is also used to treat pulmonary abscess for it can discharg epus. Because Balloonflower Root (桔梗, Jiegeng) can direct other herbs ascending, it is used as a conductant herb for treating Upper-jiao diseases, especially for discomfort of the chest, diaphragm and throat.

Both Balloonflower Root (桔梗, Jiegeng) and Apricot Seed (杏仁, Xingren) enter into the lung meridian, but Balloonflower Root (桔梗, Jiegeng) mainly disperses lung qi and relieves phlegm; while Apricot Seed (杏仁, Xingren) mainly descends lung-qi and relieves cough and asthma. They work well together to treat dysfunction of the lung to disperse and descend due to cold-evil stagnating in the lung, manifested as cough, asthma, chest fullness and nasal obstruction.

In addition, Balloonflower Root (桔梗, Jiegeng) treats dysentery, for it can purge intestinal stagnation; while Apricot Seed (杏仁, Xingren) treats constipation, for it loosens the bowel to relieve constipation.

6. 旋覆花, Xuanfuhua

English name: Inula Flower

Pharmaceutical name: Flos Inulae

Botanical name: Inula britanica L., I. Brittanica L. var chinesis (Rupr.) Reg., or less commonly I. Linariaefolia Turcz.

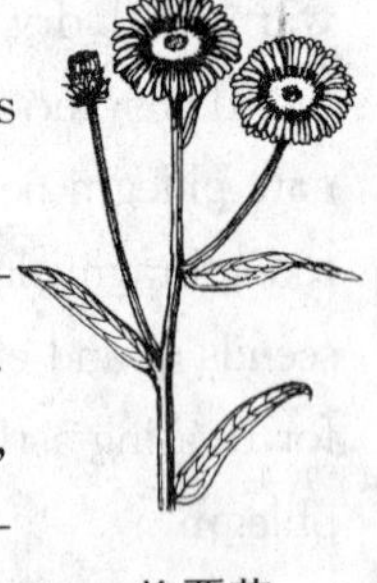
旋覆花

Properties and tastes: bitter, sour, salty, slightly warm.

Meridian tropism: lung, spleen, stomach, and large intestine.

Functions: 1. remove phlegm and induce diuresis

2. descend qi and prevent vomiting

Indications: 1. stagnation of phlegm and evil fluid in the lungs——cough with profuse expectoration, chest congestion, hypochondriac pain

2. hiccup, vomiting

3. gastrointestinal neurosis

Dosage: 3 ~ 9g, decoct it after it is wrapped with a gauze-sack.

Contraindication: Do not use where there is yin deficiency with dry cough, body deficiency and diarrhoea.

Combinations: 1. add Fresh Ginger (生姜, Shengjiang), Pinellia Rhizome(半夏, Banxia), Manchurian Wildginger Herb (细辛, Xixin)——cough due to cold-phlegm

2. add Balloonflower Root(桔梗, Jiegeng), White Mulberry Root-bark(桑白皮, Sangbaipi), Rhubarb (大黄, Dahuang)——the excessive syndrome of cough due to heat-phlegm

3. add Hematite(代赭石, Daizheshi), Ginseng(人参, Renshen)——spleen and stomach qi deficiency, vomiting, eructation due to reversed upward flow of phlegm-dampness, abdominal mass and fullness

Prescription: Decoction of Inula and Red Ochre(旋覆代赭汤, Xuanfu Daizhe Tang)

Notes: Inula Flower (旋覆花, Xuanfuhua) dominates in eliminating phlegm, with descending qi, resolving hard mass and inducing diuresis. In ancient times, it was said: "all flowers ascend, only Inula Flower(旋覆花, Xuanfuhua) descends."

Both Inula Flower(旋覆花, Xuanfuhua) and Pinellia Rhizome(半夏, Banxia) can expel phlegm, dissipate blockage, regulate the stomach and relieve vomiting. Inula Flower (旋覆花, Xuanfuhua) is usually combined with Pinellia Rhizome (半夏, Banxia) to treat cough and asthma due to phlegm retention, vomiting and eructation due to cold-damp attacking the stomach.

Inula Flower(旋覆花, Xuanfuhua) is used when there is a great deal of sticky phlegm which does not easily expectorate, fluid retention in chest and abdomen, hypochondriac pain and fullness, vomiting and eructation due to water-damp evil attacking the stomach, for it descends qi, dissipates blockage and induces diuresis; Pinellia Rhizome (半夏, Banxia) is used for substantial and thin phlegm which is easy to expectorate, for it dries dampness and removes phlegm.

7. 白前, Baiqian

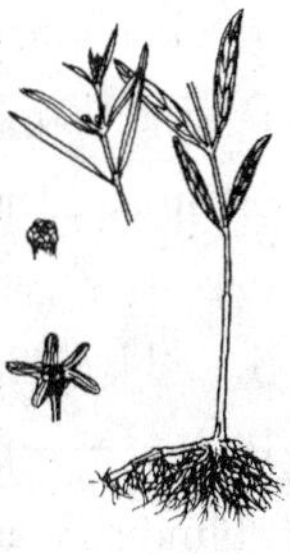

English name: Willowleaf Swallowwort Rhizome

Pharmaceutical name: Radix et Rhizoma Cynanchii Stautoni

Botanical name: Cynanchum stautoni (Decne.) Schltr. Ex Levl., or less often C. glaucescens (Decne.) Hand.-Mazz.

白 前

Properties and tastes: sour, bitter, and slightly warm.

Meridian tropism: lung

Functions: 1. expel phlegm

2. descend qi and relieve cough

Indications: 1. the syndromes of cough, asthma and profuse phlegm——It is used to treat syndromes of obstruction of the lung qi manifested as profuse phlegm and difficulty in cough, reversed upward flow of qi and dyspnea

2. cough due to exopathic wind cold

Dosage: 3~9g. The fried herb with Honey(蜂

蜜, Fengmi) is good for moistening the lungs to relieve cough.

Contraindication: Use cautiously where there is gastropathy.

Combinations: 1. add Tatarian Aster Root (紫苑, Ziyuan)——obstruction of the lung qi, profuse phlegm and difficulty in cough, reversed upward flow of qi and dypsnea mainly due to cold evil

2. add White Mulberry Root-bark (桑白皮, Sangbaipi), Chinese Wolfberry Root-bark (地骨皮, Digupi)——obstruction of the lung qi, profuse phlegm and asthma mainly due to heat evil

3. add Fineleaf Schizomepeta Herb (荆芥, Jingjie), Balloonflower Root (桔梗, Jiegeng), Tangerine Peel (陈皮, Chenpi——cough due to exopathic wind cold

4. add Tatarian Aster Root (紫苑, Ziyuan), Peking Euphorbia Root (大戟, Daji)——asthma, edema, whooping in the throat of excessive syndrome

5. add Sessile Stemona Root (百部, Baibu)——prolonged cough, cough due to pulmonary tuberculosis

Prescription: Cough Powder (止嗽散, Zhisou San)

Notes: Willowleaf Swallowwort Rhizome (白前, Baiqian) is bitter, sour and slightly warm. It is good at descending qi. If qi descends, phlegm retention vanishes and cough stops naturally. It is known as "the major herb of pulmonary cough." With proper combination, it can be used to treat Lung qi stagnation, cough and profuse phlegm, chest fullness and dyspnea no matter whether it is caused by cold or heat evil. In ancient documents, there were two conflicting ideas, one is Willowleaf Swallowwort Rhizome (白前, Baiqian) "can tonify the lung", the other is "it can not tonify the lung." Actually, Willowleaf Swallowwort Rhizome (白前, Baiqian) disperses and descends qi and doesn't have tonifying property. So most of the later generations advocate that chronic cough due to lung deficiency can not be treated by this herb. In addition, clinical practice indicates that this herb has a strong phlegm-removing function which stimulates the stomach slightly. If patients have stomach disease, the dosage should not exceed 6g. So use it cautiously. If when the dosage exceeds 10g, it may cause nausea and vomiting.

Willowleaf Swallowwort Rhizome (白前, Baiqian)'s origin is similar to Blackend Swallowwort Root (白薇, Baiwei)'s. But they are different in property. Willowleaf Swallowwort Rhizome (白前, Baiqian) enters into the lung meridian, descends qi and eliminates phlegm; Blackend Swallowwort Root (白薇, Baiwei) enters into the liver meridian, clears away heat from blood, and reduces fever.

Both Willowleaf Swallowwort Rhizome (白前, Baiqian) and Balloonflower Root (桔梗, Jiegeng) can eliminate phlegm. But Willowleaf Swallowwort Rhizome (白前, Baiqian) mainly descends the lung qi, because of its taste. It is used for fullness of the chest and diaphragm, asthma, dyspnea, whooping in the throat. Balloonflower Root (桔梗, Jiegeng) mainly disperses lung qi. It is used for cough, nosal obstruction, chest fullness and sore throat. It is also used for cough and asthma and profuse phlegm due to dysfunction of the lung to disperse and descend fullness in the chest and diaphragm.

Both Willowleaf Swallowwort Rhizome

(白前,Baiqian) and Whiteflower Hogfenel Root(前胡,Qianhu) can descend qi and eliminate phlegm. They have a mutual reinforcing function when treating cough due to wind evil and phlegm. But Whiteflower Hogfenel Root (前胡, Qianhu) is slightly cold. It also expels wind and relieves exterior syndrome. It mainly treats exterior syndrome due to wind heat. Willowleaf Swallowwort Rhizome(白前,Baiqian) is slightly warm. It is only used for lung qi stagnation, profuse phlegm, asthma and dyspnea.

8. 前胡,Qianhu

English name: Whiteflower Hogfenel Root

Pharmaceutical name: Radix Peucedani

Botanical name: Peucedanum praeruptorum Dunn or P. Decurisivum(Miq.)Maxim.

前 胡

Properties and tastes: bitter, sour, and slightly cold.

Meridian tropism: lung.

Functions: 1. descend qi and expel phlegm
2. disperse wind heat.
3. dilate coronary artery
4. inhibit influenza virus
5. relieve pain, tranquilize

Indications: 1. cough and asthma——wind heat attacking the lung, dysfunction of the lung qi to descend, reversed upward flow of qi, asthma and cough, profuse and yellowish phlegm, or thirst
2. the syndrome of external wind heat——cyclic fever, expectoration, headache

Dosage: 6～9g

Contraindication: Do not use where there is yin deficiency with dry cough, cold saliva and cough.

Combinations: 1. add Pinellia Rhizome(半夏, Banxia), Apricot Seed(杏仁, Xingren), Tangerine Peel(橘皮, Jupi)——obstruction by phlegm with qi, discomfort of chest and diaphragm, abdominal mass, chest congestion, vomiting, anorexia
2. add White Mulberry Root-bark(桑白皮, Sangbaipi), Tendrilleaf Fritillary Bulb(贝母, Beimu)——lung heat, phlegm obstruction, cough with thick phlegm, dypsnea, chest congestion
3. add Wild Mint(薄荷, Bohe), Great Burdock Achene(牛蒡子, Niubangzi)——exopathic wind heat, profuse phlegm, cough, sorethroat
4. add Tatarian Aster Root(紫苑, Ziyuan), Lily Bulb(百合, Baihe)——tuberculosis of the lung
5. add Willowleaf Swallowwort Rhizome(白前, Baiqian)——onset of cough, difficulty in spitting

Notes: Whiteflower Hogfenel Root (前胡, Qianhu) descends qi, removes phlegm, disperses wind heat. It is the best herb for exopathic wind heat, especially for cough due to stagnation of wind heat in the lung. So Li Shizhen(李时珍) called it "the principal herb for treating phlegm-qi."

In addition, modern pharmacological research indicates that this herb dilates the coronary arteries. It does not affect the heart beat, cardiac contractility and blood pressure. So it is believed that this herb is a strong alternative expander of the coronary arteries.

Both Whiteflower Hogfenel Root(前胡, Qianhu) and Apricot Seed(杏仁, Xingren) can disperse and descend the lung qi. But Whiteflower Hogfenel Root(前胡, Qianhu) is cool in property. It mainly descends and purges the lung heat. It is used for asthma due to stagnation of phlegm-heat. Apricot Seed(杏仁,Xingren)is warm in property. It mainly descends qi, relieves cough and asthma. It is used for asthma due to its wind cold attacking the lung.

Whiteflower Hogfenel Root(前胡,Qianhu) and Chinese Thorowax Root(柴胡,Chaihu) are known as"two-Hu". Doctors believe that they have similar functions. In fact, Whiteflower Hogfenel Root(前胡,Qianhu) enters into the lung-meridian, dominates descent, mainly descends qi and eliminates heat and phlegm; Chinese Thorowax Root(柴胡, Chaihu) enters into liver and gallbladder meridian, mainly ascends liver yang qi and expels exopathogens between the interior and exterior layers. For treatment of wind heat syndrome with cough, fullness and pain of chest and diaphragm, they are always used together.

9. 瓜蒌, Gualou

English name: Snakegourd Fruit

Pharmaceutical name: Fructus Trichosanthis

Botanical name: Trichosanthes kirilowii Maxim. Or T. Uniflora Hao

瓜 蒌

Properties and tastes: sweet, cold.

Meridian tropism: ung, stomach, and large intestine.

Functions: 1. quench the lung heat and remove phlegm

2. promote circulation of qi to relieve the chest

3. ablate boils and dissipate blockage

4. loosen the bowel to relieve constipation

5. dilate coronary artery

6. reduce blood lipid

7. bacteriostasis

8. anticancer

Indications: 1. cough due to lung-heat, thick phlegm difficult to expectorate

2. obstruction in the chest, accumulation of pathogens in chest

3. coronary atherosclerotic cardiopathy, angina pectoris due to obstruction of turbid phlegm

4. constipation with dryness

5. pulmonary abscess, appendicitis, swelling pain due to mastadenitis

6. tracheitis with suffocation, pulmonary asthma

Dosage: use the whole plant 9~18g, use the peel of Snakegourd Fruit(瓜蒌, Gualou): 6~12g, for seed of Snakegourd Fruit(瓜蒌, Gualou) 9~15g.

Contraindication: Incompatible with Prepared Daughter Root of Commom Monkshood(附子, Fuzi).

Do not use it where there is spleen deficiency with diarrhea, damp phlegm and cold phlegm.

Combinations: 1. add Licorice Root (甘草, Gancao)——sore throat

2. add Apricot Seed(杏仁, Xingren), Balloonflower Root(桔梗, Jiegeng)——accumulation of phlegm-heat, cough and dyspnea

3. add Tendrilleaf Fritillary Bulb(贝母, Beimu), Pinellia Rhizome(半夏, Banxia)——chronic bronchitis

4. add Dandelion(蒲公英, Pugongying), Frankincense(乳香, Ruxiang)——acute mastadenitis

5. add Longstament Onion Bulb(薤白, Xiebai), Pinellia Rhizome(半夏, Banxia)——obstruction in the chest, so much

pain leading to difficulty in sleeping cough

6. add Coptis Rhizome(黄连, Huanglian), Pinellia Rhizome(半夏, Banxia)——accumulation of pathogens in the chest manifested as fullness and tenderness

7. add Heartleaf Houttuynia Herb(鱼腥草, Yuxingcao), Reed Rhizome (芦根, Lugen)——pulmonary abscess manifested as vomiting of blood with pus

8. add Hemp Seed(火麻仁, Huomaren), Bitter Orange(枳壳, Zhiqiao)—constipation due to dry intestine

9. add Hemp Seed(火麻仁, Huomaren), Chinese Angelica Root(当归, Danggui)——constipation due to blood deficiency

Prescriptions: 1. Decoction of Trichosanthis Allii Macrostemi and Rhizoma Pinelliae(瓜蒌薤白半夏汤, Gualou Xiebai Banxia Tang)

2. Decoction for Mild Phlegm——heat Syndrome in the Chest(小陷胸汤, Xiaoxianxiong Tang)

Notes: In the clinic, this herb is divided into Snakegourd seed (瓜蒌仁, Gualouren), Snakegourd peel(瓜蒌皮, Gualoupi) and the whole of Snakegourd fruit. Snakegourd peel (瓜蒌皮, Gualoupi) is good for clearing the lungs; resolving phlegm, promoting the flow of qi to treat the chest oppression; Snakegourd seed is good for moistening the bowels; while the whole of Snakegourd fruit clears away heat in the lung and stomach to remove phlegm and dissipate blockage in the Upper-jiao, loose dryness syndrome of the large intestine to relieve constipation in the Lower-jiao. Its indications are extensive. *Transactions of Famous Physicians* (《名医别录》, Mingyibielu) said: " Snakegourd Fruit(瓜蒌, Gualou) treats obstruction in the chest, soothes the face". *Records of the Discerning of Herbals* (《本草思辨录》, Bencaosibianlu) said: "Snakegourd Fruit(瓜蒌, Gualou) is good at inducing phlegm downward, so it may treat obstruction of qi in the chest." Experimental studies indicate that Snakegourd Fruit(瓜蒌, Gualou) CAH dilate coronary artery, increasing the blood volume of arteria coronaria, antihypoxia and hyperlipemia. It also has an antibacterial function for many bacilli and antitumor. Clinically, it is widely used for coronary atherosclerotic cardiopathy, pulmonary infection and gastritis.

10. 贝母, Beimu

English name: Tendrilleaf Fritillary Bulb

Botanical name: Fritillariae, Bulbus

Properties and tastes: Sichuan Tendrilleaf Fritillary Bulb (川贝母, Chuanbeimu): bitter, sweet, slightly cold

贝 母

Zhejiang Tendrilleaf Fritillary Bulb(浙贝母, Zhebeimu): bitter, cold

Meridian tropism: lung, heart

Functions: 1. Sichuan Tendrilleaf Fritillary Bulb(川贝母, Chuanbeimu): quench the lung heat to remove phlegm, moisten the lungs and relieve cough, dissipate blockages, relieve swelling

2. Zhejiang Tendrilleaf Fritillary Bulb(浙贝母, Zhebeimu): quench the lung heat to remove phlegm, dissipate phlegm retention, relieve swelling

Indications: 1. chronic cough due to lung-deficiency, dry cough due to yin-deficiency——scanty sputum, dry throat bloody phlegm. Sichuan Tendrilleaf Fritillary Bulb(川贝母,

Chuanbeimu) is used to treat the said syndromes

2. cough due to wind heat, phlegm heat and dryness heat——Zhejiang Tendrilleaf Fritillary Bulb (浙贝母, Zhebeimu) is used to treat thick, yellowish phlegm

3. Both Sichuan Tendrilleaf Fritillary Bulb (川贝母, Chuanbeimu) and Zhejiang Tendrilleaf Fritillary Bulb (浙贝母, Zhebeimu) are used to treat the syndromes of multiple abscess, goiter, mastadenitis, pulmonary abscess, and other external diseases

4. tyryoma, tuberculosis lymphatic ganglion of lymph——Zhejiang Tendrilleaf Fritillary Bulb (浙贝母, Zhebeimu) is preferable

Dosage: 3～9g. Grind into powder, and take the powder after mixing it with water, 1～1.5g per dose

Contraindication: Incompatible with Prepared Daughter Root of Commom Monkshood (附子, Fuzi). Do not use where there is cold phlegm and damp phlegm

Combinations: 1. add Sichuan Tendrilleaf Fritillary Bulb (川贝母, Chuanbeimu), Coastal Glehnia Root, and Fourleaf Ladybell Root (沙参, Shashen), Dwarf Lilyturf Root (麦冬, Maidong)——chronic cough due to lung deficiency, scanty sputum, dry throat

2. add Zhejiang Tendrilleaf Fritillary Bulb (浙贝母, Zhebeimu), Mulberry Leaf (桑叶, Sangye), Great Burdock Achene (牛蒡子, Niubangzi)——cough due to exopathic wind heat or accumulation of phlegm fire

3. add Zhejiang Tendrilleaf Fritillary Bulb (浙贝母, Zhebeimu), Figwort Root (玄参, Xuanshen), Oyster Shell (牡蛎, Muli)——multiple abscess

4. add Zhejiang Tendrilleaf Fritillary Bulb (浙贝母, Zhebeimu), Dandelion (蒲公英, Pugongying), Snakegourd Root (天花粉, Tianhuafen)——skin and external disease, mastadenitis

5. add Zhejiang Tendrilleaf Fritillary Bulb (浙贝母, Zhebeimu), Heartleaf Houttuynia Herb (鱼腥草, Yuxingcao) and Coix Seed (薏苡仁, Yiyiren)——pulmonary abscess

Notes: Tendrilleaf Fritillary Bulb (贝母, Beimu) has two variants-Sichuan Tendrilleaf Fritillary Bulb (川贝母, Chuanbeimu) and Zhejiang Tendrilleaf Fritillary Bulb (浙贝母, Zhebeimu). Sichuan and Zhejian Beimu all quench the lung and remove phlegm to stop cough. All can be used for cough due to phlegm heat. But Sichuan Tendrilleaf Fritillary Bulb (川贝母, Chuanbeimu) is cold and sweet, and has the function of moistening the lung. It is often used for chronic cough due to the lung deficiency. Zhejiang Tendrilleaf Fritillary Bulb (浙贝母, Zhebeimu) is very bitter and cold, and has a stronger effect in clearing away the heat and dissipating blockage. It is mainly used for cough due to exopathogenic wind heat or stagnation of phlegm fire.

Both herbs have the effect of clearing away heat to dispel the accumulation of sores, abscesses and scrofula. But Zhejiang Tendrilleaf Fritillary Bulb (浙贝母, Zhebeimu) is better than Sichuan Tendrilleaf Fritillary Bulb (川贝母, Chuanbeimu).

11. 天竹黄, Tianzhuhuang

English name: Tabasheer

Pharmaceutican name: Concretio Silicea Bambusae

Botanical name: Bambusa textilis McClure

Properties and tastes: sweet, cold

Meridian tropism: heart, liver, and gall bladder

Functions: 1. quench the lung heat to remove phlegm

2. clear away heart heat and arrest convulsio

3. relieve pain, anti-inflammation

Indications: 1. spasm due to phlegm heat——infantile convulsion and epilepsy, coma due to febrile disease

天竹黄

2. apoplexy and phlegm stagnation

Dosage: 3～6g.

Combinations: 1. add Tumeric Root-tuber(郁金, Yujin), Cape Jasmine Fruit(栀子, Zhizi), Silkworm with Batrytis Larva(白僵蚕, Baijiangcan)——convulsion due to phlegm－heat

2. add Arisaema with Bile (胆南星, Dannanxing——apoplexy and syncope

Notes: This herb clears away heart and lung heat, breaks through phlegm obstruction to induce resuscitation. It is good at arresting convulsion and checking endogenous wind. It is often used for infantile convulsion due to phlegm heat and fever, asthma, and insomnia. It has a better effect in adult's cerebral apoplexy, aphasis.

Tabasheer(天竹黄, Tianzhuhuang) and Bamboo Juice(竹沥, Zhuli) are similar in function. All can break through phlegm obstruction to induce resuscitation, They are all used for accumulation of phlegm heat in the lung and cerebral apoplexy, and accumulation of phlegm. But Bamboo Juice(竹沥, Zhuli), quickly reaches meridians and collaterals. The property of cold and smooth are stronger. It is good at breaking through phlegm obstruction and inducing resuscitation, often used for asthma and coma due to phlegm heat and cerebral apoplexy with phlegm accumulation; Tabasheer(天竹黄, Tianzhuhuang) clears away heart heat and reduces fever. It has the effect of calming the nervousness due to fright, so it is often used for infantile convulsion.

Both Tabasheer(天竹黄, Tianzhuhuang) and Arisaema With Bile(胆南星, Dannanxing) can clear away heat, break through phlegm obstruction and arrest convulsion. For infantile fever, asthma, coma and convulsion due to phlegm heat in the lung, the two herbs are often used together. But Tabasheer(天竹黄, Tianzhuhuang) has a stronger effect for calming nervousness due to fright, arresting convulsion and tranquilizing the mind. Arisaema With Bile(胆南星, Dannanxing) clears away heat and breaks through phlegm obstruction with greater strength.

12. 竹茹, Zhuru

English name: Bamboo Shavings

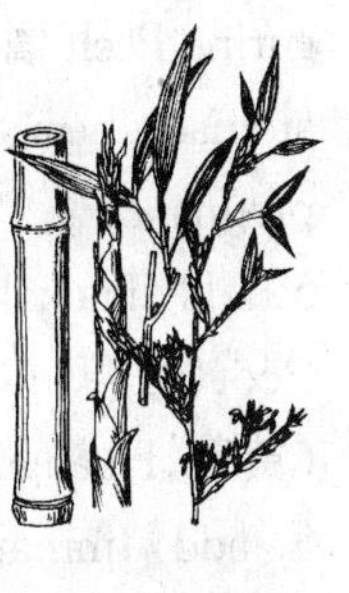

竹茹

Pharmaceutical name: Caulis Bambusae in Taeniis

Botanical name: Phyllostachys nigra(Lodd.)Munro var. henonis (Mitf.) Stapf ex Rendle, Bambusa breviflora Munro, or Sinocalamus beechelyanus (Munro)McClure var. pubescens P. F. Li.

Properties and tastes: sweet, slightly cold

Meridian tropism: lung, stomach

Functions: 1. remove heat phlegm

2. relieve restlessness and prevent vomiting

3. remove heat from the blood to arrest bleeding

4. bacteriostasis

Indications: 1. cough due to lung heat, expectorate yellowish and thick phlegm

2. disturbance of phlegm fire, restlessness
3. vomiting due to stomach heat, vomiting due to stomach deficiency with heat or pregnancy
4. hematemesis, epistaxis, massive or incessant metrorrheagia due to blood heat

Dosage: 6～9g

Contraindication: Do not use where there is spleen and stomach deficiency

Combinations: 1. add Coptis Rhizome(黄连, Huanglian), Pinellia Rhizome(半夏, Banxia)——obstruction of damp-heat in the stomach, vomiting, abdominal congestion
2. add Tangerine Peel(橘皮, Jupi), Pinellia Rhizome(半夏, Banxia)——accumulation of phlegm and heat, restlessness, vomiting
3. add Baikal skullcap Root(黄芩, Huangqin), Snakegourd Fruit(瓜蒌, Gualou)——cough due to lung heat, expectorate thick-yellowish phlegm
4. add Cape Jasmine Fruit(栀子, Zhizi) Tangerine Peel(橘皮, Jupi)——vomiting due to stomach heat, acute gastritis, vomit during pregnancy
5. add Tuckahoe(茯苓, Fuling), Licorice Root(甘草, Gancao), Baikal skullcap Root (黄芩, Huangqin)——restlessness, fever
6. add Immature Bitter Orange(枳实, Zhishi), Tangerine Peel(橘皮, Jupi), Pinellia Rhizome(半夏, Banxia)——disturbance of phlegm heat, palpitation due to fright, fidgeting of deficiency type
7. add Ginseng(人参, Renshen), Tangerine Peel(橘皮, Jupi), Fresh Ginger(生姜, Shengjiang)—hiccup due to stomach deficiency, chest congestion and abdominal mass

Prescription: Decoction for Warming Gallbladder(温胆汤, Wendan Tang)

Notes: This herb clears away heat phlegm, and relieves restlessness to stop vomiting. It is often used for insomnia and restlessness due to phlegm heat, vomiting due to stomach heat, in addition to treating phlegm due to lung heat.

Bamboo Shavings (竹茹, Zhuru) and Pinellia Rhizome(半夏, Banxia) all have the functions of removing phlegm, stopping vomiting, and tranquilizing the mind. For restlessness, dizziness and blurred vision, vomiting and belching, they have a coordinating effect, but Bamboo Shavings(竹茹, Zhuru) is cool and moist. It can treat heat phlegm and vomiting, and belching due to stomach heat. It is also good at relieving mental stress and regulating qi of the diaphragm to relieve restlessness. It has the best curative effect for treating irritability, postnatal restlessness of deficiency type headache, and fullness in the heart. Pinellia Rhizome(半夏, Banxia) is sour, warm and dry, it can treat vomiting and belching due to cold phlegm and damp phlegm. Because this herb is sour and dispersing, bitter and descending, it scatters blockage to relieve the feeling of fullness. For food indigestion and disgusting, vomiting, it has the best curative effect.

13. 竹沥, Zhuli

English name: Bamboo Juice

Pharmaceutical name: Succus Bambusae

Botanical name: Phyllostachys nigra(Lodd.) Munro bar. Heonis (Mitf.) Stapf ex Rendle.

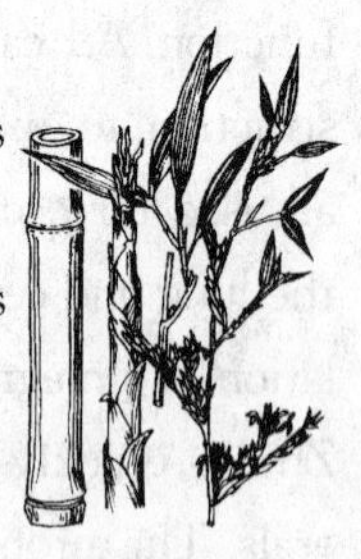
竹 沥

Properties and tastes: sweet, cold.

Meridian tropism: heart, lung, and stomach

Functions: 1. quench the lung heat and remove

phlegm

2. arrest convulsion and induce resuscitation

3. relieve cough

Indications: 1. syndrome of lung heat and phlegm accumulation, manifested as cough, chest congestion, thick and yellowish phlegm, yellowish and greasy tongue coating, slippery and rapid pulse

2. syndrome of apoplectic phlegm——apoplectic coma, profuse phlegm

3. encephalitis B, epidemic encephalitis——high fever and coma, vomiting, spasm. Drink Bamboo Juice(竹沥, Zhuli) incessantly.

4. infantile convulsion and epilepsy

5. schizophrenia

Dosage: 30～50g, take it after mixing it with water.

Contraindication: It's cold and slippery in property. It is contraindicated in patients with cough due to cold, and diarrhea due to spleen deficiency.

Combinations: 1. add Snakegourd Fruit(瓜蒌, Gualou), Loquat Leaf(枇杷叶, Pipaye)——profuse sputum and cough due to lung heat

2. add Juice of Fresh Ginger(生姜汁, Shengjiangzhi)——apoplexy, with coma, profuse sputum

3. add Scorpion(全蝎, Quanxie)——epilepsy

4. add Chlorite-Schist(礞石, Mengshi)——schizophresis

Notes: It has the best curative effect for cough with thick sputum caused by heat evil, and also can treat syndromes caused by accumulation of phlegm heat disturbing the mind. It is suitable for coma due to cerebral apoplexy, infantile convulsion and manic-depressive psychosis. Bamboo Juice (竹沥, Zhuli) has the power to remove phlegm throughout the body. It can decend phlegm from the vertex, break through phlegm from the chest and diaphragm, disperse phlegm from the extremities, dispel phlegm from the viscera and bowels as well as the meridians and collaterals, and remove the phlegm between the cortex and membrance. Therefore, it's the most effective for resolving heat phlegm.

Bamboo Juice (竹沥, Zhuli) and Fresh Ginger (生姜, Shengjiang) juice are both good for eliminating phlegm. They are often used together in clinical treatment for the symptoms caused by heat phlegm accumulated in the lung, the apoplexy due to stagnation of phlegm, and manic-depressive psychosis due to heat phlegm. Zhu Danxi(朱丹溪) said that"Bamboo Juice(竹沥, Zhuli) is good for removing heat phlegm. The meridians and collaterals can not be dredged without Fresh Ginger(生姜, Shengjiang) juice". Bamboo Juice(竹沥, Zhuli) is very cold and slippery in property. It is just suitable for heat phlegm, and can easily damage the stomach and cause diarrhea. Fresh Ginger (生姜, Shengjiang) juice can warm the middle-jiao and replenish the stomach. It is often used for poor appetite caused by deficiency of the stomach vomiting, and hiccup caused by cold fluid. It's also often used for the syndromes of cold phlegm and damp phlegm.

14. 海蛤壳, Haigeqiao

English name: Clam Shell

Pharmaceutical name: Concha Cyclinae Sinensis

Botanical name: Cyclinae Sinensis, Concho

Properties and tastes: salty, cold

Meridian tropism: lung, stomach

Functions: 1. quench lung heat to remove phlegm
2. resolve hard lumps
3. promote urination to relieve edema
4. relieve hyperacidity and pain
5. astringe dampness to treat wounds(external use)

海哈壳

Indications: 1. lung heat, thick phlegm uneasy to expectorate, cough, asthma
2. goiter, multiple abscess, subcutaneous nodule——mainly used to treat hyperthyroidism, tuberculosis of lymphatic ganglions
3. dropsy, urine retention
4. stomachache, acid regurgitation——mainly used to treat gastroduodenal bulbar ulcer(calcining usage)
5. burn, scald, eczema, etc.

Dosage: 9～15g the powder of Giant Gecko (蛤蚧, Gejie) schould be wrapped in a small cloth-sack before decoction

Contraindication: Do not use where there is lung deficiency with cold, deficiency of Middle-yang.

Combinations: 1. add Pumice (海浮石, Haifushi), Willowleaf Swallowwort Rhizome (白前, Baiqian), White Mulberry Root-bark (桑白皮, Sangbaipi)——asthma and cough due to heat-phlegm
2. add Natural Indigo(青黛, Qingdai), Cape Jasmine Fruit (栀子, Zhizi), Snakegourd Fruit (瓜蒌, Gualou)——accumulation of phlegm fire, hypochondriac pain
3. add Seaweed(海藻, Haizao), Kelp(昆布, Kunbu)——goiter, subcutaneous nodule
4. add Talc(滑石, Huashi), Oriental Waterplantain Rhizome(泽泻, Zexie)——dropsy, urine retention
5. add Calcined Concha Arcae(煅瓦楞子, DuanWalengzi)——stomachache, acid regurgitation

Notes: It is salty in flavor, and cold in property. It can soften and dissolve hard mass with the salty flavor, and clear away the lung heat and remove phlegm by the cold property. It can promote urination as well. Therefore, it is suitable for treating stubborn phlegm like gelatin which is difficult in expectoration, chest pain and hypochondrial pain due to the stagnation of the phlegm and fire, goiter and subcutaneous nodule.

Clam Shell (海蛤壳, Haigeqiao) and Pumice (海浮石, Haifushi) are similar in property, flavor and functions. Clam Shell (海蛤壳, Haigeqiao) can not only clear away and descend the heat phlegm, but also improve the activities of qi. It is usually used for cough, pain in the chest due to the stagnation of heat phlegm and qi, Pumice(海浮石, Haifushi) can eliminate thick phlegm which is difficult to expectorate.

Clam Shell(海蛤壳, Haigeqiao) and Ark shell(瓦楞子, Walengzi) both have the effects of eliminating thick phlegm and restricting gastric acid. The former is cold in property, and often used for cough due to lung heat. The latter is medium in property, and is applied to the treatment of all kinds of stagnation of phlegm. The former has the function of inducing diuresis to alleviate edema, the latter has the function of resolving blood stasis, dissipating blockage and ablating masses.

15. 海藻, Haizao

English name: Seaweed
Pharmaceutical name: Herba Sargassii
Botanical name: Sargassum fusiforme (Harv.) Setch. or S. Pallidum (Turn.) C. Ag.

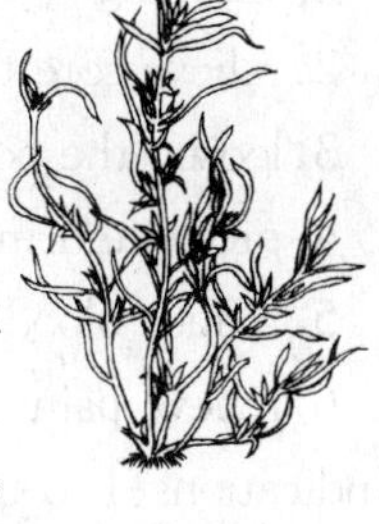
海 藻

Properties and tastes: salty, cold.

Meridian tropism: liver, stomach, and kidney

Functions: 1. remove phlegm and resolve the hard lumps

2. promote urination to relieve edema

Indications: 1. goiter——such as hyperplasia of thyroid, thyroid enlargement, thyroma

2. scrofula abscess——such as tuberculosis of lymphnode, lymphnoditis

3. hepatosplenomegaly

4. testicle enlargement

5. flaccidity of lower limbs, dropsy and edema

Dosage: 9～15g.

Combinations: 1. add Kelp(昆布, Kunbu), Tendrilleaf Fritillary Bulb(贝母, Beimu), Green Tangerine Peel(青皮, Qingpi)——goiter

2. add Common Selfheal——Fruit-spike(夏枯草, Xiakucao), Weeping Forsythia Capsule(连翘, Lianqiao), Figwort Root(玄参, Xuanshen)——scrofula

3. add Turtle Carapace(鳖甲, Biejia), Oyster Shell(牡蛎, Muli), Peach Seed(桃仁, Taoren)——hepatosplenomegaly

4. add Szechwan Chinaberry Fruit(川楝子, Chuanlianzi), Fennel Fruit(小茴香, Xiaohuixiang), Hawthorn Fruit (山楂, Shanzha)——testicle enlargement

5. add Common Floweringquince Fruit(木瓜, Mugua), Perilla Leaf(苏叶, Suye)——edema in cases of beriberi

Prescription: Jangerine Seed Pill(橘核丸, Juhe Wan)

Notes: Seaweed(海藻, Haizao) is rich in iodine. It has a curative effect for thynoma due to iodine deficiency. It's also used for hyperthyroidism, thyroiditis, emphnoditis and orchiopathy. Seaweed(海藻, Haizao) and Clam Shell(海蛤壳, Haigeqiao) both are salty in flavor and cold in property. They have the effects of resolving hard masses and dissipating phlegm and inducing diuresis to alleviate edema. However, Seaweed(海藻, Haizao) is acts on the liver meridian, has the strong effect of resolving hard lumps. It is suitable for goiter, scrofula, pain of the testicles, and swollen hepato-splenomegaly. Clam Shell(海蛤壳, Haigeqiao) is acts on the lung meridian, has a better effect for clearing away and lowering heat phlegm, and it is used primarily for cough and chest pain due to fire phlegm.

16. 昆布, Kunbu

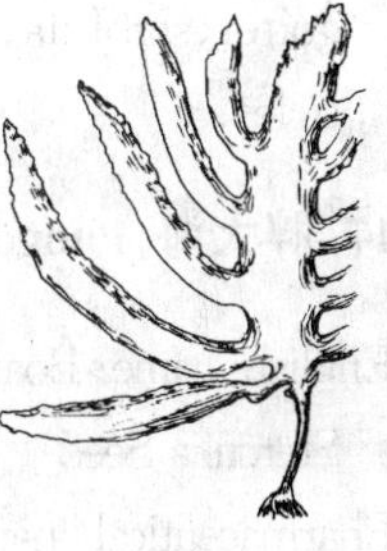
昆 布

English name: Kelp

Pharmaceutical name: Thallus Algae

Botanical name: Laminaria japonica Aresch., Ecklonia kurome Okam., or Undaria painnatifida(Harv.)Sur.

Properties and tastes: salty, cold.

Meridian tropism: liver, stomach, kidney

Functions: 1. remove phlegm and resolve the hard lumps

2. promote urination to relieve edema

3. reduce blood lipid

4. antitumor

5. reduce blood pressure

Indications: 1. goiter, scrofula——such as thyroid enlargement and adenoma, tuberculosis of lymphnode

2. cirrhosis, hepatosplenomegaly

3. testicle enlargement

4. edema in case of beriberi

5. hypertension

Dosage: 9～15g.

Combinations: 1. add Common Selfheal Fruit-spike(夏枯草, Xiakucao), Oyster Shell(牡蛎, Muli), Figwort Root(玄参, Xuanshen)——chronic tuberculosis of lymphnode, goiter due to iodine deficiency, cirrhosis

2. add Ricepaperplant Pith(通草, Tongcao), White Mulberry Root-bark(桑白皮, Sangbaipi)——edema, in case of beriberi, oliguria

Notes: Li Dongyuan(李东垣) said that the herb is"salty in flavor AHD can resolve hard mass. It is an excellent for dissolving a goiter which is like a stone. It is similar to Seaweed(海藻, Haizao) in function."In order to strengthen the curative effect it's often used with Seaweed(海藻, Haizao) to treat goiter, scrofula, swollen and pain in the testicles.

17. 胖大海, Pangdahai

English name: Boat-fruited Sterculia Seed

Pharmaceutical name: Semen Sterculiae Scaphigerae

Botanical name: Sterculia scaphigera Wall.

胖大海

Properties and tastes: sweet, cold

Meridian tropism: lung, large intestine

Functions: 1. promote the dispersing function of the lung

2. relieve sore throat and hoarseness
3. loosen the bowel to relieve constipation
4. promote urination
5. reduce blood pressure
6. relieve pain

Indications: 1. cough due to phlegm heat
2. hoarseness due to lung heat, sore throat
3. acute tonsillitis
4. constipation due to heat accumulation——accompanied by headache, conjunctival congestion, mild fever

Dosage: 3～5 pieces.

Combinations:

1. add Balloonflower Root(桔梗, Jiegeng), Cicada Slough(蝉衣, Chanyi)——hoarseness due to lung heat, cough due to phlegm heat

2. add Rhubarb(大黄, Dahuang), Chrysanthemum Flower(菊花, Juhua)——constipation due to accumulation of heat accompanied by headache, and conjunctival congestion

Notes: It is applied to treat obstruction of lung qi, cough caused by heat phlegm and hoarseness caused by heat evil attacking the lung. It is mostly used alone and drunk as common tea, and also used with other drugs. It is also used orally alone as a beverage by soaking it in water to obtain the juice for treating constipation caused by accumulated heat. For severe cases, it should be used together with purgative herbs.

Appendix: Other Drugs For Removing Phlegm

Name	Properies and tastes	Meridian tropism	Functions	Indications	Dosage	Contraindication
Chinese Honeylocusy Fruit (皂荚, Zaojia)	sour, warm, mild, poisonous	Lung, large intestine	Expel phlegm, induce resuscitation, scatter mass, subdue swelling	Phlegm accumulation in the chest, a sthenia syndrome of coma, carbuncle, (for external use), constipation	1.5~6g, Parching into brown. Swallow 0.6~1.5g.	It is forbidden for cases with qi and yin deficiency and pregnancy
Pumice (浮海石, Fuhaishi)	salty, cold	Lung	Quench lung-heat, remove phlegm, resolve the hard mass	Coughing due to phlegm-heat, coughing due to lung-heat, multiple abscess, subcutaneous nodule, stranguria complicated by hematuria, or stranguria with stone.	6~9g	
Chlorite-Schist (礞石, Mengshi)	sweet, salty, medium	Lung, liver	Descend qi, expel phlegm soothe the liver, arrest convulsion	Stubborn phlegm, coughing, asthma, convulsion due to phlegm-heat, epilepsy	6~9g	Do not use for qi deficiency, spleen-deficiency, chronic infantile convulsion and in pregnancy
Rhizome of Airpotato Yan(黄药子, Huangyaozi)	bitter, cold, poisonous	Lung, liver	Scatter blockage, ablate goiter, remove heat, detoxicate, cool blood to stop bleeding, relieve cough and asthma	Goiter, wound swelling, inflammation of the throat, snake bite, tumor, hemorrhagic diseases.	9~15g	Excessive dosage or taking for a long time may cause vomitting, diarrhea, abdominal pain, as well as influence on Liver function Taking it for a long-term also causes loss of hair
Bile of Pig Gall (猪胆汁, Zhudanzhi)	bitter, cold	Liver, gall bladder, lung, large intestine	quenchs the lung-heat, removes phlegm, removes heat, detoxicate, relieve cough and asthma, normalize the secretion from gallbladder, anti-bacteria	Cough due to lung-heat, whooping cough, conjunctival congestion, swelling pain, pharyngitis, jaundice, dysentery, skin and external disease, constipation of heat accumulation	6~9g	
India Rorippa Herb or Flower (蔊菜, Hancai)	Sour, bitter, medium	Lung, liver	Expel phlegm to relieve coughing, remove heat, detoxicate, remove dampness to treat jaundice	Cough due to cold or heat evil, sore-throat, carbuncle, skin and external disease, jaundice due to damp-heat, influenza, bronchitis, pneumonia	9~30g	

Name	Properies and tastes	Meridian tropism	Functions	Indications	Dosage	Contraindication
Grosvenor Momordica Fruit(罗汉果, Luohanguo)	sweet, slightly cold	Lung, large intestine	Moisten the lungs to relieve cough, promote the production of body fluid to quench thirst	Cough due to lung-heat or lung-dryness, whooping cough, fluid-injury due to summer-heat, constipation	15~30g	
Water Chestnut (荸荠, Biqi)	sweet, slightly cold	Lung, stomach, large intestine	Remove phlegm, ablate stagnation, remove heat, promote the production of the body fluid, improve eyesight, treat cataracta	Cough due to phlegm-heat, subcutaneous nodule, multiple abscess, fluid-injury and thirst due to febrile disease, constipation, conjunctival congestion due to liver-heat, cataracta or external oculopathy	30~90g	
Medicinal Changium Root (明党参, Mingdangshen)	sweet, slightly bitter, slightly cold	Lung, liver	Moisten the lungs to relieve cough, nourish the stomach and mediate the middle-jiao	Cough due to lung-heat or yin-deficiency, body fluid disorder and thirst due to stomach-heat, anorexia, vomit and hiccup	6~9g	Deficiency of the spleen and stomach
Hen Egg's Inner Shell Membrance (凤凰衣, Fenghuangyi)	sweet, medium	Lung	Moisten the lungs to relieve cough	Chronic coughing due to lung deficiency, loss of voice due to chronic cough, diphtheria, cataract	3~6g	

Chapter 12
Drugs for Relieving Cough and Asthma

Definition: Drugs which can relieve or stop coughing or asthma are called cough-asthma relieving drugs.

Functions: This class of drugs has functions of relieving cough and asthma. Most of them can also expel phlegm. Some of them have the functions of ventilating the lung and relieving exterior syndrome; regulating and descending qi, moistening the lung and nourishing yin; quenching the lung-heat.

Indications: Cough and asthma caused by internal or external injury.

Classification: According to its properties and mechanism, this type of drugs can be divided into the following sorts of drugs: dispersing lung, moistening lung, quenching lung, warming lung, descending qi, astringing lung and purging lung.

Cautions: 1. Cough due to onset of measles: promote the dispersing function of the lung and expel evil, don't astringe the lung to relieve cough.

2. Asthma due to productive phlegm: firstly, expel phlegm or select those drugs which can expel phlegm to relieve cough and asthma.
3. Distinguish the nature of asthma, asthma due to kidney deficiency should be treated by tonifying the kidney.

4. According to cold, heat, phlegm and dryness of asthma, select the corresponding drugs and combines with lung-warming drugs, heat-clearing drugs, phlegm-removing drugs and lung-moistening drugs.

Phlegm, cough and asthma are related in pathogenesis. The symptoms among them are complicated. Asthma is usually complicated by phlegm, while phlegm is the main cause of asthma. So they are discussed together.

Asthma results from adverse upward flow of qi. Phlegm results from retention of fluid. Therefore, phlegm, cough and asthma are diseases caused by retention of fluid in body. Fluid disease is treated by treating qi. In ancient times, there was a theory which stated "phlegm disease is not treated by treating phlegm, qi should be regulated before treating phlegm." We must know this princile.

If fluid disease lasts a long time, this induces the prolonged disease to enter the collaterals and involve the blood system. The method of promoting blood circulation and removing obstruction of collaterals must be used.

1. 杏仁, Xingren

English name: Apricot Seed

Pharmaceutical name: Semen Pruni Armeniacae

Botanical name: Prunus armentiaca L. var. ansu Maxim. or P. Armeniaca L.

Properties and tastes: bitter, slightly warm, and slightly poisonous

Meridian tropism: lung, large intestine

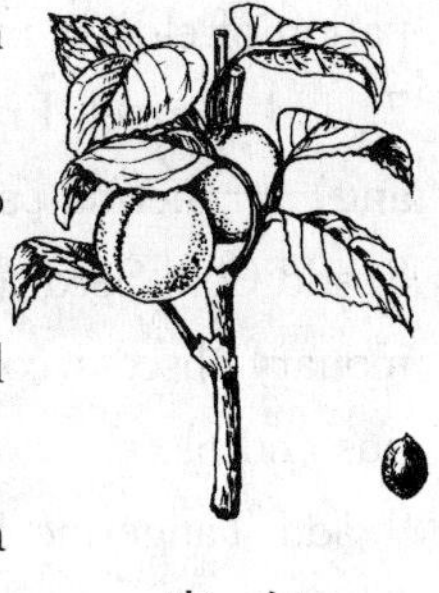
杏 仁

Functions: 1. relieve cough and asthma

2. loosen the bowel to relieve constipation

Indications: 1. asthma and cough——used for several kinds of asthma with different combinations

2. dryness of intestine and constipation——this herb is moist and oily, used for constipation caused by fluid deficiency in the large intestine

Dosage: 3～9 g.

Contraindication: slightly poisonous. Do not overtake or take for a long time. Use the herb cautiously with children.

Combinations: 1. add Balloon flower Root (桔梗, Jiegeng)——common cold, and cough with much phlegm. It is also used for the onset of dysentery

2. add Mulberry Leaf (桑叶, Sangye), Chrysanthemum Flower (菊花, Juhua)——common cold due to wind heat, cough with yellowish phlegm

3. add Ephedra (麻黄, Mahuang), Licorice Root (甘草, Gancao)——common cold due to wind cold, cough with whitish phlegm

4. add Mulberry Leaf (桑叶, Sangye), Coastal Glehnia Root, and Fourleaf Ladybell Root (沙参, Shashen)——cough caused by dry-heat evil, little sputum and difficulty in spitting

5. add Ephedra (麻黄, Mahuang), Gypsum (石膏, Shigao)——asthma and cough caused by pneumonia

6. add Hemp Seed (火麻仁, Huomaren), Chinese Angelica Root (当归, Danggui)——constipation caused by dry intestine: for example, constipation after childbirth, consti-

pation of elderly men

7. add Fennel Fruit (小茴香, Xiaohuixiang)——hernia pain

8. add Coix Seed(薏苡仁, Yiyiren)——pulmonary abscess, cough and spit phlegm with pus and blood

9. add Tangerine Peel(橘红, Juhong)——dyspnea caused by stagnation of phlegm and dampness in the lung, discomfort of chest and diaphragm, indigestion, and constipation

10. add Sichuan Tendrilleaf Fritillary Bulb (川贝母, Chuanbeimu)——cough due to lung deficiency or phlegm heat by the method of combination of moisture with descent

Prescriptions: 1. Decoction of Ephedra, Apricot, Gypsum and Licorice (麻杏石甘汤, Maxingshigan Tang)

2. Ephedra Decoction (麻黄汤, Mahuang Tang)

Notes: Apricot Seed(杏仁, Xingren) can perform the function of lowering the adverse flow of qi to relieve asthma. With other drugs Apricot Seed(杏仁, Xingren) can treat cough and asthma caused by wind cold or wind heat. *Seeking Truth of Herbals* (《本草求真》, Benchaoquzhen) recorded that "Apricot Seed(杏仁, Xingren) can not only disperse wind cold, but also lower the adverse flow of qi to relieve asthma. The pungence in its flavor can disperse the pathological factors; its bitter flavor can lower the adverse flower of qi; moisten property and relax the bowels; Warm property can remove phlegm." Bitter Apricot Seed(苦杏仁, Kuxingren) hydrolyzed by enzyme can produce hydrocyanic acid which can perform a calming effect for the respiratory center, can result in intoxication when absorbed through the intestines, so Bitter Apricot Seed(苦杏仁, Kuxingren) can be used clinically only after processing.

Both Apricot Seed (杏仁, Xingren) and Ephedra(麻黄, Mahuang) belong to the lung meridian and can treat cough and asthma caused by wind cold attacking the lung cooperatively. Ephedra(麻黄, Mahuang) tends to disperse the wind cold to promote the flow of lung qi to allay asthma; Apricot Seed (杏仁, Xingren) tends to lower the flow of qi to relieve cough. One for dispersing, the other for lowering, they can regulate the flow of lung qi to relieve cough and asthma. In addition, Ephedra (麻黄, Mahuang) can disperse lung qi to induce diuresis and reduce edema caused by attacking wind; Apricot Seed(杏仁, Xingren) can regulate flow of qi and remove pathological factors to treat the damp-warm syndrome.

There are differences in the functions between Bitter Apricot Seed(苦杏仁, Kuxingren) Sweet Apricot Seed(甜杏仁, Tianxingren). Bitter Apricot Seed(苦杏仁, Kuxingren) is characterized by bitterness in its flavor and tends to lowering the flow of adverse qi, which is good for treating cough and asthma; while Sweet Apricot Seed(甜杏仁, Tianxingren) tends to moisten and treats mostly chronic cough due to lung qi deficiency. Both of them can treat constipation due to loss of body fluid.

2. 百部, Baibu

English name: Sessile Stemona Root

Pharmaceutical name: Radix Stemonae

Botanical name: Stemona sessilifolia (Miq.) Franch. Et Sav., S. Japonica(BL.) Miq., or S. Tuberosa Lour.

Properties and tastes: sweet, bitter, and neutral

Meridian tropism: lung

Functions: 1. moisten the lungs and relieve cough

2. destroy dermatozoon and relieve itching

3. effect of inhibiting germs

百 部

Indications: 1. cough——for short-term or prolonged cough, whooping cough, and cough caused by pulmonary tuberculosis

2. oxyuriasis, head and body lice, urticaria, dermatitis, scabies(Externally used)

Dosage: 6～9 g. Appropriate dosage for exteral use. The processed herb with Honey(蜂蜜, Fengmi) has the strong function of moistening the lung to relieve cough, It is useful for prolonged cough, dry cough, cough due to pulmonary tuberculosis and whooping cough.

Combinations: 1. add Fineleaf Schizomepeta Herb(荆芥, Jingjie), Balloonflower Root(桔梗, Jiegeng), Licorice Root (甘草, Gancao)——onset of cough

2. add Chinese Magnoliavine (五味子, Wuweizi), Medicine Terminalia Fruit (诃子, Hezi)——prolonged cough

3. add Dried Ginger (干姜, Ganjiang), Pinellia Rhizome(半夏, Banxia)——cough caused by cold evil

4. add Baikal skullcap Root (黄芩, Huangqin), Bamboo Shavings (竹茹, Zhuru)——cough caused by heat evil

5. add willowleaf Swallowwort Rhizome(白前, Baiqian), Tendrilleaf Fritillary Bulb(贝母, Beimu), Coastal Glehnia Root, and Fourleaf Ladybell Root (沙参, Shashen)——whooping cough

6. add Baikal skullcap Root (黄芩, Huangqin), Dan-shen Root (丹参, Danshen)——pulmonary tuberculosis, tuberculosis of lymphnode

Prescription: Cough Powder(止嗽散, Zhisou San)

Notes: Sessile Stemona Root(百部, Baibu) is characterized by sweetness in flavor, moist in property and bitter in flavor by which it is descending in property, without hot or cold properties. It can perform the function of moistening the lung to lower the adversed flow of qi and relieve cough, as well as poisoning and expelling parasites. It is a good drug for cough caused by tuberculosis of the lung. It can treat cough no matter if it is acute or chronic, cold or hot. It is good at treating chronic and deficient cough. Commonly it is used in the clinic for chronic or uncurative cough due to whooping cough, tuberculosis and chronic tracheitis. For pinworm, Sessile Stemona Root(百部, Baibu) 30g daily is simmered with water to get the decoction 30 ml for entention-enema at 9～10 o' clock pm, for five days. For external use the production made of 20% Sessile Stemona Root(百部, Baibu) soaking with alcohol is good for relieving itching caused by urticaria, dermatitis, tinea corporis, or by mosquito and other insectbites.

Sessile Stemona Root (百部, Baibu) is similar to Cochinchinese Asparagus Root(天门冬, Tianmendong). Both of them can treat lung disorders and have anthelmintic function according to Dr Li Shizhen(李时珍). Sessile Stemona Root (百部, Baibu) with moistening and without dryness in property can treat all of the syndromes of phlegm and cough. However Cochinchinese Asparagus Root (天门冬, Tianmendong) with sweet and cold, as well as stick and greasy in property, it can only treat cough due to dry heat and yin exhaustion. It is not suitable to treat cough and asthma due to fluid retention and phlegm stagnation.

Both Sessile Stemona Root(百部,Baibu) and Common Coltsfoot Flower(款冬花,Kuandonghua) are moistening without dryness in property, and can treat any type of cough. Common Coltsfoot Flower(款冬花,Kuandonghua) is good at treating cough and asthma characterized by phlegm retention caused by cold evil attacking the lung, because it tends to pungent in flavour and warm in property and having the effect of dispersing. Sessile Stemona Root(百部,Baibu) tends to be sweet in flavor and moistening in property. It is not as warm as Common Coltsfoot Flower(款冬花,Kuandonghua) in property. It is good at performing anthelmintic functions. It is suitable to treat chronic cough or cough caused by tuberculosis. Modern pharmacological research indicates that Common Coltsfoot Flower(款冬花,Kuandonghua) focuses on sedation; Sessile Stemona Root(百部,Baibu) focuses on antibiotics and anti-inflammation, and has a sedation function as well.

3. 紫菀, Ziyuan

English name: Tatarian Aster Root

Pharmaceutical name: Radix Asteris Tatarici

Botanical name: Aster tataricus L.

Properties and tastes: bitter, sweet, and slightly warm

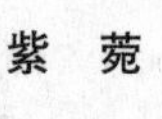

紫 菀

Functions: 1. remove phlegm and relieve cough 2. inhibit germ

Indication: Cough with phlegm——whether the cough is acute or chronic, cold or heat, deficient or excessive, such as acute or chronic bronchitis, pulmonary tuberculosis.

Dosage: 6～9g

Combinations: 1. add Ephedra(麻黄,Mahuang), Apricot Seed(杏仁,Xingren) Manchurian Wildginger Herb(细辛,Xixin)——asthma and cough due to fluid evil, chest congestion, unable to lie flat, cough or dyspnea caused by abnormal rising of lung qi, with sounds in the throat

2. add Cochinchinese Asparagus Root(天门冬,Tianmendong), Baikal skullcap Root(黄芩,Huangqin), White Mulberry Root-bark(桑白皮,Sangbaipi)——chronic cough mainly due to heat-evil, even vomit pus and blood

3. add Balloonflower Root(桔梗,Jiegeng), Fineleaf Schizomepeta Herb(荆芥,Jingjie)——phlegm stagnation, common cold with cough and profuse phlegm due to cold wind

4. add Common Anemarrhea Rhizome(知母,Zhimu), Sichuan Tendrilleaf Fritillary Bulb(川贝母,Chuanbeimu), Ass-hide Glue(阿胶,Ajiao)——prolonged cough caused by lung deficiency, hemoptysis

5. add Tangerine Peel(橘红,Juhong)——all kinds of cough especially for cough due to pulmonary tuberculosis

6. add Perilla Seed(苏子,Suzi)——asthma and cough, difficulty in spitting

7. add Ass-hide Glue(阿胶,Ejiao)——chronic cough due to lung deficiency, with bloody sputum and hemoptysis

Prescription: Cough Powder(止嗽散,Zhisou San)

Notes: It's warm and moist in property and it can resolve phlegm without dryness. It has a good effect on stopping a cough and is very suitable to treat cough due to an adverse flow of qi with unsmooth expectoration as well as chronic cough with bloody expectoration due to lung deficiency.

Both Tatarian Aster Root(紫苑,Ziyuan) and Common Coltsfoot Flower(款冬花, Kuandonghua) have a gentle action. They can be used together for any type of cough no matter it belongs to cold or heat, deficient or excessive. Howeve, Tatarian Aster Root(紫苑, Ziyuan) focuses on promoting the flow of qi and it has the actions in both qi and blood systems. It is good at treating the syndrome of wind cold evil lighting the lung manifested as a stiff and full sensation in the chest and hypochondriac region, unsmooth expectoration and bloody expectoration. Common Coltsfoot Flower(款冬花, Kuandonghua) is gentler than Tatarian Aster Root(紫苑,Ziyuan) in promoting the flow of qi, is good at stopping cough by moistening the lung, and is very suitable to treat a serious cough. Current research shows that Tatarian Aster Root(紫苑, Ziyuan) focuses on resolving phlegm, Common Coltsfoot Flower(款冬花, Kuandonghua) focuses on relieving cough.

4. 款冬花, Kuandonghua

English name: Common Coltsfoot Flower

Pharmaceutical name: Flos Tussilagi Farfarae

Botanical name: Tussilago farfara L.

Properties and tastes: sour, slightly bitter, warm

款冬花

Meridan tropism: lung

Functions: 1. moisten the lungs and descend qi
2. relieve cough and remove phlegm

Indication: Cough with much phlegm——whether acute or chronic, cold or heat, deficient or excessive, especially for cough with a great deal of much phlegm caused by lung cold and cough caused by lung deficency with bloody sputum.

Dosage: 6～9 g. The processed herb with Honey(蜂蜜, Fengmi) is good for moistening the lung.

Contraindication: Use cautiously where there is severe hemoptysis and pulmonary abscess.

Combinations: 1. add Chinese Magnoliavine (五味子, Wuweizi), Pinellia Rhizome(半夏, Banxia)——damp phlegm, cough, asthma, thin and much sputum
2. add Tatarian Aster Root(紫苑, Ziyuan), Common Anemarrhea Rhizome(知母, Zhimu)——chronic coughing and dyspnea, phlegm with blood
3. add Apricot Seed(杏仁, Xingren), Tendrilleaf Fritillary Bulb(贝母, Beimu)——sudden cough
4. add White Mulberry Root-bark(桑白皮, Sangbaipi)——for cough caused by lung heat, yellow phlegm
5. add Balloonflower Root(桔梗, Jiegeng), Coix Seed(薏苡仁, Yiyiren)——cough caused by pulmonary abscess, stick phlegm
6. add Lily Bulb(百合, Baihe)——prolonged cough caused by lung deficiency, phlegm with blood

Notes: It is an important drug for treating cough by warming the lung. It is usually applied in combintion with Tatarian Aster Root(紫苑, Ziyuan) in order to improve the effect for treating asthma and cough because it is warm in property, it is suitable to treat a cold cough characterized by thin sputum. If it is applied properly, in coordination with other drugs, it can be used to treat various types of cough. *Compendium of Materia*

Medica (《本草纲目》, Bencaogangmu) said that "Common Coltsfoot Flower(款冬花, Kuandonghua) is characterized as warm without dryness, moisture without cold, and dispersing without descending in property. As a result it is suitable for treating any type of cough which belongs to the lung whether caused by deficiency, excess, cold or heat."

5. 苏子, Suzi

English name: Perilla Seed

Pharmaceutical name: Fructus Perillae Frutescentis

Botanical name: Perilla frutescens (L.) Britt. Var crispa (Thunb.) Hand.-Mazz. or P. frutescens (L.) Britt. var. acuta (Thunb.) Kudo

苏 子

Properties and tastes: sour, warm

Meridian tropism: lung, large intestine

Functions: 1. relieve cough and asthma
2. descend qi and remove phlegm
3. loosen the bowel to relieve constipation

Indications: 1. cough, asthma with a great deal of phlegm
2. constipation of drynes

Dosage: 6~9 grams

Contraindication: Use cautiously where there is prolonged cough caused by qi deficiency, asthma caused by Yin deficiency, diarrhea caused by spleen deficiency.

Combinations: 1. add Perilla Stem(苏梗, Sugeng), Apricot Seed(杏仁, Xingren)——cough and constipation caused by phlegm and qi stagnation
2. add Pinellia Rhizome(半夏, Banxia)——cough caused by reversed upward flow of qi and a great deal of phlegm
3. add Radish Seed(莱菔子, Laifuzi)——chest and abdominal distention, phlegm-asthma and stagnation of food
4. add White Mulberry Root-bark(桑白皮, Sangbaipi)——cough caused by lung heat, edema and abdominal distention.
5. add Hemp Seed (火麻仁, Huomaren)——constipation by dryness
6. add Coptis Rhizome (黄连, Huanglian)——vomiting with pregnancy, restlessness
7. add Tangerine Peel(橘皮, Jupi), Chinese Angelica Root(当归, Danggui), Largehead Atractylodes Rhizome(白术, Baizhu)——threatened abortion
8. add Apricot Seed(杏仁, Xingren), Balloonflower Root(桔梗, Jiegeng)——common cold due to wind cold, cough with thin phlegm
9. add Tatarian Aster Root (紫苑, Ziyuan)——bronchitis, difficulty in spitting, feeling of fullness and distention in the chest and diaphragm
10. add Wrinkled Gianthyssop Herb(藿香, Huoxiang)——common cold due to wind cold in summer, abdominal pain with vomiting and diarrhea

Prescription: Decoction of Three Kinds of Seed for the Aged(三子养亲汤, Sanziyangqin Tang)

Notes: It can perform the functions of relieving cough and asthma and lowering the adverse flow of qi to remove phlegm. It is very suitable to treat cough and asthma characterized by profuse phlegm and feeling of stuffiness and fullness in the chest and diaphragm region. Because it contains grease with moisture in property, it can moisten intestines to loose the bowels.

Both Perilla Seed (苏子, Suzi) and

Ephedra(麻黄, Mahuang) are important drugs to relieve asthma and can perform concerted function to treat cold phelgm, asthma and cough. Perilla Seed(苏子,Suzi) is characterized by resolving phlegm and lowering the adversed flow of qi to calm down asthma and is suitable to treat acute asthma with excessive phlegm due to cold phlegm accumulation in the lung. Ephedra (麻黄, Mahuang) is characterized by dispersing wind cold, promoting the flow of the lung qi to allay asthma, is suitable to treat asthma and cough due to wind cold evil tightening the lung.

6. 桑白皮, Sangbaipi

English name: Bark of Mulberry Root

Pharmaceutical name: Cortex Mori Albae Radicis

Botanical name: Morus Alba L.

桑白皮

Properties and tastes: sweet, cold

Meridian tropism: lung

Functions: 1. purge lung and relieve asthma
2. promote urination to relieve edema
3. reduce blood pressure
4. tranquilize, relieve pain, anti-convulsion
5. inhibit germs
6. anti tumor

Indications: 1. cough and asthma caused by lung-heat——be effective in treatment of cough, yellowish phlegm, fever caused by acute trachitis, pneumonia, excessive syndrome of edema
2. excessive syndrome of edema——edema, urine retention, distention and fullness, rapid respiration, etc.
3. hypertension——due to hyperactivity of liver yang

Dosage: 9 ~ 15 g of the Honey(蜂蜜, Fengmi)——processed herb to moisten the lung and relieve coughing. The crude herb purges the lung and promotes urination to relieve edema.

Contraindication: If the cough is caused by cold lung, do not use this herb.

Combinations: 1. add Chinese Wolfberry Root-bark(地骨皮, Digubi)——cough caused by lung heat, asthma due to reversed upward flow of qi, thick and sticky sputum, body-heat and thirst
2. add Loquat Leaf(枇杷叶, Pipaye), Baikal skullcap Root(黄芩, Huangqin)——pulmonary emphysema complicated by inflammation and cough-asthma due to acute bronchitis
3. add Plantain Seed(车前子, Cheqianzi)——edema of lower body, urine retention
4. add Areca Peel(大腹皮, Dafupi), Tuckahoe(茯苓, Fuling)——edema, disuria, abdominal distention and fullness
5. add Barbary Wolfberry Fruit(枸杞子, Gouqizi)——diabetes
6. add Rhizome or Root of Forbes Notopterygium(羌活, Qianghuo), Abalone Shell(石决明, Shijueming)——hypertension

Prescriptions: 1. Powder for Expelling Lung Heat(泻白散, Xiebai San)
2. Decoction of Peel of Five Drugs(五皮饮, Wupi Yin)

Notes: It can perform the functions of clearing the lung and inducing diuresis. It is suitable to treat edema due to acute nephritis, dysuria combined with upper respiratory tract infection. It is said that in ancient times, "it can not resolve the excessive syndrome of the lung without White Mulberry Root-bark

(桑白皮,Sangbaipi)".

Both White Mulberry Root-bark (桑白皮, Sangbaipi) and Pepperweed Seed or Flixweed Tansymustard Seed (葶苈子, Tinglizi) have the effects of removing heat from the lung and promoting diuresis to relieve asthma, reducing edema and relieving the fullness sensation in the body. Both of them are often used cooperatively for a fullness sensation and asthma, as well as scanty urination and swelling of the face caused by water retention in the lung. White Mulberry Root-bark (桑白皮, Sangbaipi) focuses on removing heat from the lung and is suitable to treat cough and asthma with yellow sputum; Pepperweed Seed or Flixweed Tansymustard Seed (葶苈子, Tinglizi) focuses on removing heat from the lung and promoting diuresis. It is suitable to treat asthma with a fullness sensation and on symptoms caused by excessive phcegm.

7. 葶苈子, Tinglizi

English name: Pepperweed Seed or Flixweed Tansymustard Seed

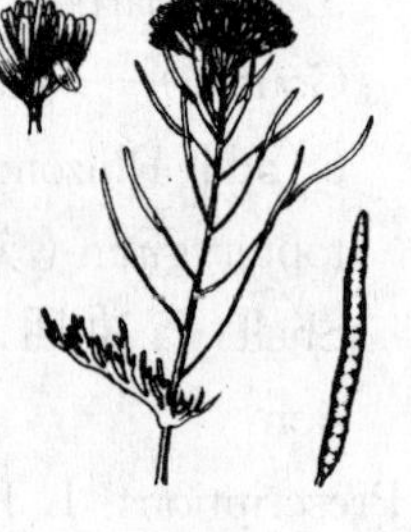
葶苈子

Pharmaceutical name: Semen Tinglizi

Botanical name: Lepidium apetalum Willd., or L. virginicum L., or Descurainia sophia (L.) Schur, or Drapa nemorosa L.

Properties and tastes: bitter, sour, and very cold

Meridian tropism: lung, urinary bladder

Functions1. purge lung and relieve asthma

2. promote urination to relieve edema

3. strenghen the heart

Indications: 1. excessive syndromes of phlegm retention, cough and dyspnea

2. edema, urine retention

3. chronic cor pulmonale complicated by heart failure

4. osmotic pleurisy, hydrops of thoracic cavity

Dosage and Usage: 3～9 g. Large amounts are as much as 30g

Contraindication: Do not use where there is edema due to spleen deficiency, dyspnea due to lung deficiency. Do not use for a long time.

Combinations: 1. add Chinese Date (大枣, Dazao)——cough with a great deal of phlegm, dyspnea, edema of body and face, urine retention etc.

2. add Fourstamen Stephania Root (防己, Fangji), Rhubarb (大黄, Dahuang)——edema, the excessive syndrome of urine retention

3. add Apricot Seed (杏仁, Xingren), Rhubarb (大黄, Dahuang), Mirabilite (芒硝, Mangxiao)——hydrops of thoracic cavity

4. add Prepared Daughter Root of Common Monkshood (附子, Fuzi), Membranous Milkvetch Root (黄芪, Huangqi)——pulmonary disease, heart failure, edema, asthma

Prescription: Decoction of Lepidium and Jujube for Removing Phlegm from Lung (葶苈大枣泻肺汤, Tingli Dazao Xiefei Tang)

Notes: It can perform the functions of not only clearing heat evil of the lung, eliminating sputum and relieving asthma, but also inducing diuresis to reduce edema dyspnea. It is good at treating cough with profuse sputum, inability to lie flat due to dyspnea, and generalized edema.

Pepperweed Seed or Flixweed Tansymustard Seed (葶苈子, Tinglizi) and Ephedra (麻

黄,Mahuang)can relieve asthma,and induce diuresis. Pepperweed Seed or Flixweed Tansymustard Seed(葶苈子,Tinglizi)is characterized as bitter in flavor, cold in property, and good at eliminating evil. It has strong effect to clear heat in the lung as well as induce diuresis, is suitable to treat dyspnea caused by accumulation of phlegm and water in the lung, and hydrops in the chest and abdomen. Ephedra(麻黄,Mahuang)is characterized as pungent, bitter in flavor, warm in property and good at promoting the flow of lung qi to dispel wind cold evil, is suitable to treat cough and asthma caused by wind cold evil tightening the lung, as well as acute edema caused by failure to disperse and descend the lung qi. Modern research indicates that Pepperweed Seed or Flixweed Tansymustard Seed(葶苈子,Tinglizi)focuses on tonifying the heart to induce diuresis. Ephedra(麻黄,Mahuang)focuses on relieving bronchospasm to relieve asthma, as well as inducing diuresis.

8. 枇杷叶,Pipaye

English name: Loquat Leaf

Pharmaceutical name: Folium Eriobotryae Japonicae

Botanical name: Eriobotrya japonica(Thunb.) Lindl.

Properties and tastes: bitter, cold

Meridian tropism: lung, stomach

枇杷叶

Functions: 1. remove phlegm and relieve cough

2. regulate the stomach and check the upward adverse flow of qi

3. clear stomach heat and prevent vomit

Indications: 1. cough and asthma, thick sputum

2. stomach heat and thirst, vomiting and hiccup

Dosage and Usage: 9～15g. Wrapped in a piece of cloth before decoction. The Honey(蜂蜜, Fengmi)-processed herbs are better for treatment of lung diseases, the ginger-processed herbs are better for treatment of gastric diseases.

Combinations:

1. add Whiteflower Hogfenel Root(前胡, Qianhu), Mulberry Leaf (桑叶, Sangye)——common cold, cough due to wind heat

2. add White Mulberry Root-bark(桑白皮, Sangbaipi), Coastal Glehnia Root, and Fourleaf Ladybell Root (沙参, Shashen)——cough and asthma caused by dry heat, little sputum, difficulty in spitting

3. add White Mulberry Root-bark(桑白皮, Sangbaipi), Apricot Seed(杏仁, Xingren), Dutchmanspipe Fruit (马兜铃, Madouling)——cough and asthma caused by lung heat, profuse and yellow phlegm.

4. add Heartleaf Houttuynia Herb(鱼腥草, Yuxingcao), Dandelion(蒲公英, Pugongying), Honeysuckle Flower(金银花, Jinyinhua)——stagnation of phlegm-heat in the lung, cough caused by itching of throat

5. add Honey-frued Tatarin Aster Root(炙紫苑, Zhiziyuan), Common Coltsfoot Flower(款冬花, Kuandonghua)——prolonged cough and phlegm-asthma

6. add Dwarf Lilyturf Root(麦冬, Maidong), Bamboo Shavings(竹茹, Zhuru), Reed Rhizome(芦根, Lugen)——stomach heat and thirst, vomiting and hiccup

7. add Pinellia Rhizome(半夏, Banxia), Lalang Grass Rhizome(白茅根, Baimaogen), Bamboo Shavings(竹茹, Zhuru)——vomiting caused by stomach heat.

8. add Gypsum (生石膏, Shengshigao), Dwarf Lilyturf Root (麦门冬, Maimendong)——cough caused by dry lung, dry throat, phlegm with blood

Prescription: Decoction for Relieving Dryness of the Lungs (清燥救肺汤, Qingzaojiufei Tang)

Notes: Loquat Leaf (枇杷叶, Pipaye) can perform the function of purging heat with its bitter flavor and the actions of descending. It can not only clear away the lung qi in order to relieve cough, but also check upward adverse flow of stomach qi in order to prevent vomiting. It can be applied to treat cough, vomiting and hiccups caused by wind heat and dry heat. As a result, it is a commonly used herb to relieve cough and prevent vomiting. There is a lot of hair on the back of the Loquat Leaf (枇杷叶, Pipaye) leading to the difficulty in filtering and irritating the throat causing an itching sensation, so it should be wrapped in a piece of gauze for decocting. The stir-baked herb is suitable for relieving cough and removing phlegm, the unprepared one for regulating the stomach and preventing vomiting.

Both Loquat Leaf (枇杷叶, Pipaye) and Willowleaf Swallowwort Rhizome (白前, Baiqian) are good at descending lung qi. However, Loquat Leaf (枇杷叶, Pipaye) is cool and humidifying in property. It is suitable for a cough with difficulty in expectoration, dyspnea due to heat, or dryness attacking the lung. Willowleaf Swallowwort Rhizome (白前, Baiqian) is slightly warm and dry in property. It is suitable to treat a stuffy sensation in the chest, dyspnea with wheezing in the throat due to external evils invading the lung resulting in abundant expectoration. Loquat Leaf (枇杷叶, Pipaye) has the function of clearing away stomach heat and preventing vomiting and hiccups.

Both Loquat Leaf (枇杷叶, Pipaye) and Pinellia Rhizome (半夏, Banxia) can treat the diseases which belong to the lungs and stomach, but they are different in property. Loquat Leaf (枇杷叶, Pipaye) can quench lung heat in order to relieve cough and remove phlegm. It is good for cough caused by phlegm-heat and dryness of the lung. Pinellia Rhizome (半夏, Banxia) can treat the lung diseares by regulating the spleen. It is good for drying dampness and removing phlegm. It is mostly used for the syndrome of cough with dyspnea caused by damp-phlegm. Loquat Leaf (枇杷叶, Pipaye) can treat stomach disorders by clearing away and descending the stomach heat in order to prevent vomiting and relieve thirst. Pinellia Rhizome (半夏, Banxia) also can treat stomach disorders by removing sputum and fluid in order to regulate the stomach, prevent vomiting and hiccups. That is to say, the former is called humidifying in property, the latter is warm and drying in property. The former focuses on clearing away and descending the lung and stomach qi, the later focuses on eliminating dampness and resolving phlegm.

9. 马兜铃, Madouling

English name: Dutchmanspipe Fruit

Pharmaceutical name: Fructus Aristolochiae

Botanical name: Aristolochia debilis Sieb. et Zucc. Of A. contorta Bge.

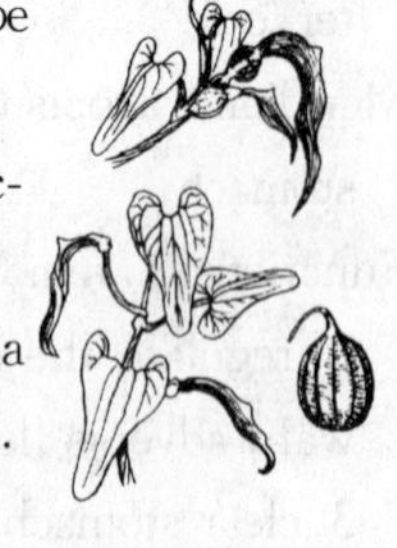
马兜铃

Properties and tastes: bitter, slightly sour, cold

Meridian tropism: lung, large intestine

Functions: 1. quench the lung heat to remove phlegm

2. relieve cough and asthma

3. reduce blood pressure

4. anticancer

Indications: 1. cough with profuse sputum and chronic cough due to lung deficiency

2. swelling pain and bleeding of hemorrhoids

3. hypertension——due to hyperactivity of liver yang, dizziness and a flushed face

Dosage: 3 ~ 9g. Quantum satis for external use.

Contraindication: Excessive dosage may cause vomiting. Do not use where there is cold of deficient type, dyspnea, diarrhea due to spleen deficiency.

Combinations: 1. add White Mulberry Root-bark(桑白皮, Sangbaipi), Baikal skullcap Root(黄芩, Huangqin), Apricot Seed(杏仁, Xingren)——heat-cough with profuse sputum

2. add Apricot Seed(杏仁, Xingren), Great Burdock Achene(牛蒡子, Niubangzi), Ass-hide Glue (阿胶, Ejiao)——asthma and cough due to lung deficiency with heat

3. add Ass-hide Glue(阿胶, Ejiao), Bletilla Rhizome (白及, Baiji)——cough, phlegm mixed with blood

4. add Japanese Pagodatree Flower(槐花, Kuihua), Garden Burnet Root (地榆, Diyu)——swelling pain and bleeding of hemorrhoids

5. add Baikal skullcap Root (黄芩, Huangqin), Common Selfheal Fruit-spike (夏枯草, Xiakucao), Gambirplant Hooked stem and Branch(钩藤, Gouteng)——hypertension due to hyperactivity of the liver yang

Notes: Dutchmanspipe Fruit(马兜铃, Madouling) is bitter and sour in flavor, cold in property. It can perform the function of clearing away heat and lowering the lung qi, as well as scattering and discharging heat. It is mainly characterized by quenching and lowering the adverse flow of lung qi. As a result, it is applied for cough with phlegm and dyspnea caused by retention of heat with dryness in the lung. Modern pharmacological research revealed that Dutchmanspipe Fruit(马兜铃, Madouling) can perform a constant function of lowering high blood pressure as well as tranquilize the mind and relieve clinical symptoms. It can achieve a successful curative effect in the early stage of essential hypertension. In addition, it also can be applied to treat acute filthy disease, hernia, carbuncle, cellulitis, furuncle, abscess, favus of the scalp, and snake bite by oral administration or external use.

Both Dutchmanspipe Fruit (马兜铃, Madouling) and Loquat Leaf (枇杷叶, Pipaye) are quenching and descending heat in nature and can be applied for cough caused by lung heat. However, Dutchmanspipe Fruit(马兜铃, Madouling) is cold in property, good at quenching lung heat, suitalbe to treat cough and hemoptysis caused by lung heat and dry heat, and excessive fire due to yin deficiency. Loquat Leaf (枇杷叶, Pipaye) focuses on descending qi, removing phlegm and relieving cough. It is suitable to treat cough, adverse rising of lung qi, difficulty in expectoration and vomiting, hiccups, and thirst caused by stomach heat. It's power is not as strong as Dutchmanspipe Fruit(马兜铃, Madouling) for clearing away heat; but it is more advanced in eliminating phlegm and relieving cough than Dutchmanspipe Fruit(马兜铃,Madouling).

10. 白果, Baiguo

English name: Ginkgo Seed

Pharmaceutical name: Semen Ginkgo

Botanical name: Ginkgo biloba L.

Properties and tastes: sweet, bitter, astringent, neutral mild poisonous

白 果

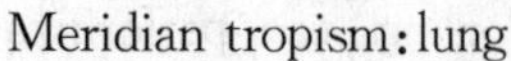

Meridian tropism: lung

Functions: 1. astringe the lung to relieve asthma

2. induce astringency to cure leukorrhea

Indications: 1. asthma and cough with profuse sputum

2. leukorrhea

3. frequent urine, enuresis

Dosage: 6～9g

Contraindication: Excessive dosage and eating crude herb cause poisoning. Use cautiously where there is cough with thick phlegm.

Combinatons:

1. add Ephedra(麻黄, Mahuang), Licorice Root(甘草, Gancao)——asthma, cough

2. add Baikal Skullcap Root(黄芩, Huangqin), White Mulberry Root-bark(桑白皮, Sangbaipi)——phlegm-dyspnea due to lung heat, rapid respiration

3. add Lotus Seed(莲子, Lianzi), Peper(胡椒, Hujiao)——deficiency of Lower-jiao deficiency, thin leukorrhea

4. add Chinese Corktree Bark(黄柏, Huangbai), Gordon Euryale Seed(芡实, Qianshi)——leukorrhea due to damp-heat

5. add Sevenlobed Yam Rhizome(萆薢, Bixie), Sharpleaf Galangal Fruit(益智仁, Yizhiren)——white and turbid leukorrhea

Prescription: Antiasth Matic Decoction(定喘汤, Dingchuan Tang)

Notes: It's astringent in property with the effect of inducing astringency, acting on the lung meridian. It can treat asthma and cough by controlling lung qi and stop profuse leukorrhea by astringing dampness. It is more suitable to treat asthma and cough with profuse phlegm which tends to be heat in property.

Both Ginkgo Seed(白果, Baiguo) and Chinese Magnoliavine(五味子, Wuweizi) can astringe the lung qi to stop asthma and cough. Ginkgo Seed(白果, Baiguo) focuses on astringing the lung to stop asthma, and mainly treat asthma and cough characterized by profuse phlegm caused by heat retained in the lung; Chinese Magnoliavine(五味子, Wuweizi) focuses on astringing the lung to stop cough, which tends to be warm in property and is suitablc to treat long standing cough due to lung deficiency as well as cough and asthma characterized by profuse phlegm caused by cold retained in the lung. Both of them can treat the diseases that belong to the lower warmer. Ginkgo Seed(白果, Baiguo) performs the function of inducing astringency to stop profuse leukorrhea and is mainly used to treat profuse leukorrhea caused by excessive dampness. Chinese Magnoliavine(五味子, Wuweizi) controls the energy of the lower warmer and nourishes kindney yin and is often used to treat seminal emission, frequency of urintion and down diarrhea caused by kidney deficiency. In addition, Chinese Magnoliavine(五味子, Wuweizi) can also function to promote the production of body fluid and astringe the heart qi to treat morbid thirst, hyperhidiosis, anxiety and insomnia caused by injury of both qi and yin. Li Shizhen(李时珍) reported about the toxic reaction of Ginkgo Seed (白果, Baiguo) that "overeating causes an over astringing function manifested as abdominal distension, and syncope". There are several records about the toxic reaction from Ginkgo Seed(白果, Baiguo), the lowest toxic dose for children is 7 pills, for adults 40. The toxic reaction includes vomiting, coma, lethargy, fear, convulsion, vague mind, fever, dyspnea respiration, blue-purple complexion, myosis or platycoria, asthenocoria, and abdominal pain, diarrhea, etc. A few cases manifested as complete flaccid paralysis or slight paralysis of the lower extremities with anaphia and analgesia. Most of the patients can achieve recovery by taking orally the decoction of Licorice Root (甘草, Gancao) 60g, or Ginkgo Seed (白果壳, Baiguoqiao) 30g as well as Musk (麝香, Shexiang) 1g infused in warm boiled water. In addition, Ginkgo Seed (白果叶, Baiguoye) is sweet and bitter in flavor, astringent and medium in property. It can astringe the lung qi, relieve asthma, and relieve pain. In the last few years, researchers revealed that flavonol component of the herb can expand coronary arteries and the cerebral arteries, promote cardiocerebral circulation, decrease serum cholesterol, and relax the bronchus. It has achieved the successful curative effect to treat coronary heat disease, angina pectoris, hypertension hyperlipemia and cerebrovascular spasm, etc. There are production such as 6911 tablet, Ginkgo Leaf flavone aglycone tablet, the dosage is 3～6g.

Appendix: Other Drugs For Relieving Cough And Asthma

Name	Properties and tastes	Meridian tropism	Functions	Indications	Dosage	Contraindication
Japanese Ardisia Herb(矮地茶, Aidicha)	bitter, medium	Lung, liver	Relieve cough, remove phlegm, promote urination to relieve edema, remove blood stasis	All sorts of cough, jaundice due to damp-heat, traumatic injury, artharalgia, abnormal amenorrhea, abdomial pain, acute and chronic nephritis	9～30g	A few people have gastrointestinal reaction
Datura Flower (洋金花, Yangjinhua)	pungent, warm, poisonous	Heart, lung, spleen	Relieve cough and asthma, expel the wind to relieve pain, relieve spasm and convulsion, anesthetic effect	Asthma cough due to cold-phlegm, stomachache, abdominal pain, arthritis, epilepsy, recurrence of convulsive seizures in asthenic infants, traumatic injury	0.3～0.6g	This herb has hypertoxicity actions. The Dosage should be controlled strictly. Do not use where there is heat-cough with thick phlegm, uneasily expectorated, heart disease, hypertension, during pregnancy, galucoma

Name	Properties and tastes	Meridian tropism	Functions	Indications	Dosage	Contraindication
Funneled Physochlaine Root (华山参, Huashanshen)	sweet, slightly bitter, hot, poisonous	Lung	Relieve asthma and cough	Asthma and cough due to cold-phlegm	0.3～0.9g	Containing alkaloid of hyoscyamine. Do not use for galucoma.
Stalactite (钟乳石, Zhongrushi)	sweet, warm	Lung, kidney, stomach	Warm the lung to relieve asthma, benefit the kidney and restore yang to improve inspiration by attracting qi downward, improve lactation	Cold-asthma, phlegm-asthma due to pulmonary tuberculosis,, cold and pain due to yang deficiency, impotence, frequent seminal emission, hypogalactia, pregnant calcipriva	9～15g	High fever and excessive asthma do not use the herb. Using the herb for a long time may cause stomach stone

PART Ⅵ
Drugs for Mental Diseases

Mental drugs refer to drugs, which can act on the central nervous system and have the function of tranquilizing to relieving spasm and inducing resuscitation. In the clinic, they can be used for the treatment of unconsciousness, palpitation, insomnia, dizziness, coma, and manic-depressive psychosis. The three kinds of drugs can supplement each other according to their different functions.

Chapter 13
Tranquilizing Drugs

Definition: A drug, which has the function of calming the mind, is called a tranquilizing drug.

Functions: Tranquilizing drugs come primarily from mineral drugs or seeds drugs. Mineral drugs are heavy in quality and descending in nature. Therefore, they have the function of tranquilization with heavy material. As seed drugs are smooth in quality and invigorating in nature, they function to tranquilize the mind by nourishing the heart.

Indications: Tranquilizing drugs are mainly used in the treatment of dysphoria, palpitation, insomnia, dreamful sleep, infantile convulsion, epilepsy and manic-depressive psychosis caused by heart qi deficiency, heart blood deficiency, flaring heart fire or other reasons.

Notes: 1. Drugs which have the function of tranquilization with heavy material and tranquilizing the mind by nourishing the heart can be applied separately to the syndromes of deficiency and excess.

2. Material drugs, if taken in balls or powder, can cause impairment of the stomach and consumption of qi. As a result, they should be temporarily taken at the discretion by combining with the drugs for nourishing the stomach and invigorating the spleen. In addition, since some of the drugs are toxic, they must be used cautiously.

1. 朱砂, Zhusha

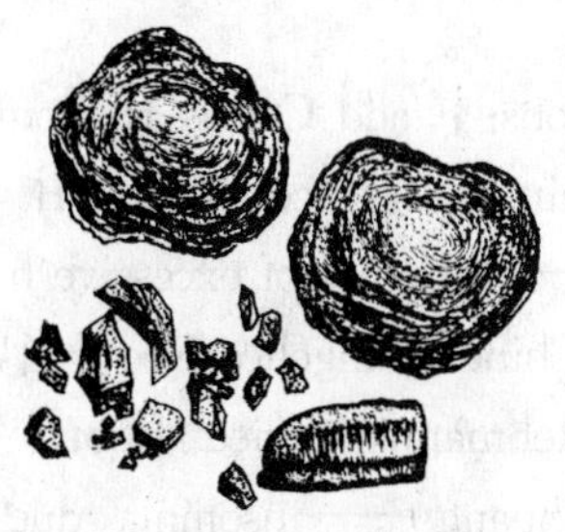

朱 砂

English name: Cinnabar

Pharmaceutical name: Cinnabaris

Properties and tastes: sweet, cold, and toxic

Meridian tropism: heart

Functions: 1. relieve palpitation and tranquilize the mind

2. clear away heat and toxic material

3. kill insects and restrain the reproduction of bacteria (for external use)

Indications: 1. restlessness caused by excessive heat, fire of deficiency type, blood deficiency, and phlegm heat in combination with other of drugs. Most suitable for dysphoria, palpitation and insomnia due to flaring-up of heart fire

2. high fever, dysphoria, coma and delirium due to febrile disease or accumulation of phlegm heat in the interior, and epilepsy

3. carbuncle, cellulitis, skin and external diseases (for oral medication or external use)

4. inflammation of throat and aphthosis

Dosage: 0.3 ~ 1g. Ground into powder and taken with water, or made into balls or powder. Externally used in appropriate dosage.

Contraindication: The drug contains more than 80% mercury, therefore, overdosage should be avoided for oral medication so as to avoid mercury poisoning. Those suffering from hepatic and renal failure must be cautious in use of the drug. Clacking is prohibited, because it can separate out mercury that is hypertoxic.

Combinations: 1. add Coptis Rhizome (黄连, Huanglain), Licorice Root (甘草, Gancao)——syndromes of excessive heart-fire

2. add Chinese Angelica Root (当归, Danggui), Rehmannia Dried Root (生地黄, Shengdihuang)——insomnia due to deficiency of heart blood

3. add Magnetite (磁石, Cishi), Medicated Leaven (神曲, Shenqu)——epilepsy

4. add Sulfur (雄黄, Xionghuang)——skin and external diseases (for external use)

5. add Borneol (冰片, Bingpian)——throat inflammation, and aphthosis

Prescription: Cinnabaris Tranquilizing Pill (朱砂安神丸, Zhushaanshen Wan)

Notes: Cinnabar (朱砂, Zhusha), sweet in taste, cold in nature and heavy in mass, is a key drug in calming the mind and clearing away fire, arresting convulsion and tranquilizing the mind. It can be used to treat such syndromes as restlessness, an irritable feverish sensation in the chest and palpitation and insomnia caused by flaring-up of heart fire. It can also be combined with other kinds of drugs to treat vexation, palpitation and insomnia caused by deficiency syndromes.

Both Cinnabar (朱砂, Zhusha) and Coptis Rhizome (黄连, Huanglian) can be used to treat restlessness, insomnia and dysphoria due to excessive heart fire as they are both able to clear away heart fire, so as to tranquilize the mind. Manic-depressive psychosis and epilepsy caused by phlegm-heat are treated with Cinnabar (朱砂, Zhusha) more effectively as it is capable of tranquilizing the mind, as well as clearing phlegm. Coptis Rhizome (黄连, Huanglian) is usually used for dysphoria and coma or abnormal flow of the blood caused by pathogenic heat attacking the blood stage and the ying stage of epidemic febrile diseases as it is superior in purging pathogenic fire, clearing away heat and eliminating pathogenic heat from the blood.

2. 磁石, Cishi

English: Magnetite

Pharmaceutical name: Magnetitum

Properties and tastes: salty, cold

Meridian tropism: liver, heart, and kidney

磁 石

Functions: 1. tranquilize the mind

2. calm the liver and check exuberance of yang

3. improve audition and eyesight

4. relieve asthma by attracting qi downward

5. tonify blood

Indications: 1. dysphoria, palpitation, insomnia, dizziness and headache caused yin deficiency and hyperactivity of yang, and epilepsy or neurosism

2. tinnitus, deafness and blurring vision due to yin deficiency of liver and kidney, such as cataract, optic neuritis

3. asthma due to kidney-deficiency

4. iron-deficiency anemia

Dosage: 9 ~ 30g. Made into balls or powder from 1g to 3g each time.

Contraindication: It is difficult to digest the drug after swallowing it. If made into balls or powder, it can not be taken more. Those suffering from weakness of the spleen and stomac must be cautious when using the drug.

Combinations: 1. add Cinnabar (朱砂, Zhusha)——dysphoria, palpitation, insomnia, dizziness, headache, epilepsy and cataract due to deficiency of yin and hyperactivity of yang

2. add Prepared Rhizome of Adhesive Rehmannia (熟地黄, Shdihuang), Asiatic Cornelian Cherry Fruit (山茱萸, Shanzhuyu), Chinese Magnoliavine (五味子, Wuweizi)——deafness, tinnitus and blurring vision due to yin deficiency of the liver and kidney

3. add Cinnabar(朱砂, Zhusha), Cassia Seed (决明子, Juemingzi) Tuber Fleeceflower Root(何首乌, Heshouwu)——poor vision

4. add Hematite(代赭石, Daizheshi), Chinese Magnoliavine(五味子, Wuweizi)——asthma due to deficiency of the kidney

5. add Abalone Shell (石决明, Shijueming)——dizziness, heaviness in the head and high blood pressure due to hyperactivity of liver yang

Notes: Magnetite (磁石, Cishi) is one of the tranquilizers. All the diseases that can be cured by Magnetite (磁石, Cishi) are the ones caused by deficiency of the liver and kidney and upward floating of insufficienct yang, "Dysphoria may be cured with weighty sedatives." As pointed out by Li Shizhen(李时珍), "Magnetite(磁石, Cishi) can cure various diseases of the kidney so as to improve eye sight and hearing."

BothMagnetite (磁石, Cishi) and Hematite(代赭石, Daizheshi) are the drugs for checking exuberance of yang, relieving convulsion and easing mental strain. It is used for the treatment of dizziness, tinnitus and headache due to the adverse rising of the liver yang, also for infantile convulsion and epilepsy caused by upward floating of yang to disturb the mind. Nevertheless, Magnetite (磁石, Cishi) tends to protect yin, and relieves the upward floating of yang, it is applicable to such syndromes because of insufficiency of yin or upward floating of yang. Red ochre is suitable not only for the syndromes stated above, but for vomiting, belching and shortness of breath which occur due to adverse rising of qi attacking the lung and stomach as well as it serves a particular function of reducing reversed qi and subduing liver fire. It can also eliminate pathogenic heat from the blood, to arrest bleeding, and thus to treat the syndromes of bleeding due to excessive heat.

3. 琥珀, Hupo

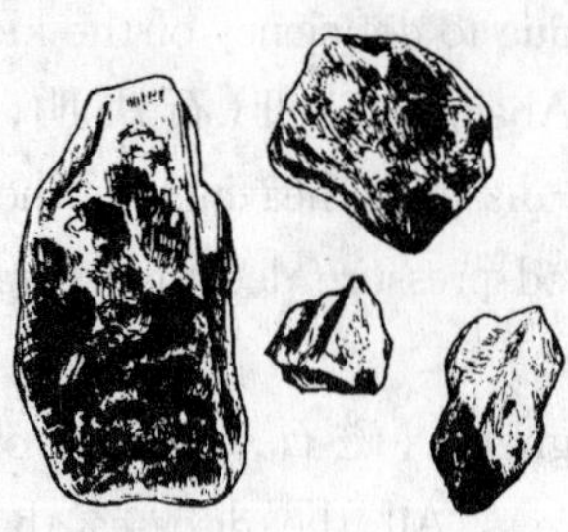

琥 珀

English name: Amber

Pharmaceutical name: Succinum

Properties and tastes: sweet, medium

Meridian tropism: liver, heart, and urinary bladder

Functions: 1. arrest convulsion and tranquilize the mind

2. remove blood stasis

3. induce diuresis for treating stranguria

4. astringe the wounds and promote tissue regeneration (for external use)

Indications: 1. palpitation and insomnia

2. infantile convulsion and epilepsy

3. amenorrhea due to stagnation of blood, and abdominal mass with pain

4. swollen scrotum, labial blood swell of the vulva or blood stasis in the womb

5. stranguria complicated by hematuria, stranguria caused by the passage of urinary stone, stranguria caused by evil heat, oliguria and uroschesis urinary infection and stone

6. cataracta and poor vision

7. angina pectoris

8. prolonged ulcer

Dosage: 1.5 ~ 3g. Ground into powder and taken with water. Unsuitable for a decoction. Stop at once after the cure. It should not be taken for a long time.

Contraindication: Those suffering from interior heat due to yin deficiency. These with frequency of urine must be advised not to use this drug.

Combinations: 1. add Cinnabar (朱砂, Zhusha), Scorpion (全蝎, Quanxie)——infantile convulsion and epilepsy

2. add Spine Date Seed (酸枣仁, Suanzaoren), Cinnabar (朱砂, Zhusha)——palpitation, insomnia and dreaminess

3. add Chinese Angelica Root (当归, Danggui), Zedoray (莪术, Ezhu)——amenorrhea due to stagnation of blood

4. add Sanchi Root (三七, Sanqi)——angina pectoria (taken in powder)

5. add Plantain Seed (车前子, Cheqianzi)——blood urine

6. add Christina Loosetrife Herb (金钱草, Jinqiancao), Akebia Stem (木通, Mutong)——stone and infection in urinary system

7. add Cinnabar (朱砂, Zhusha)——restless mind and paroxysmal auricular fibrillation

Notes: Amber (琥珀, Hupo), sweet and medium in taste and warm in nature. It relieves convulsion and induces resuscitation, and usually used to treat the diseases manifested as palpitation due to fright, or severe palpitation. It is particularly effective for palpitation and insomnia occurring in those who are suffering from coronary heart disease or apoplexy. If it is taken alone without being combined with other drugs, a more effective treatment will be achieved for the swollen scrotum, hematoma of the vulva or hematometra and hematuria.

Amber(琥珀,Hupo)is a fossil resin(hydrocarbon), which comes from pine resin that has been preserved in the earth's crust for centuries. It is capable of acting on blood stage and relieves masses and promotes diuresis. Combined with drugs pungent in flavor and warm in nature, it has the ability to promote the circulation of blood and remove blood stasis. Therefore, it can be used to eliminate blood stasis and mass in the abdomen due to accumulation. It has the function of promoting urination in a combination of drugs to drain dampness. It can be used in the treatment of five types of stranguria and retention of urine. Combined with mineral, metals or shells for use as a sedative or to tranquilize the mind. It can be employed to treat infantile convulsion and epilepsy.

Amber(琥珀,Hupo)and Cinnabar(朱砂, Zhusha)can both be used as a sedatives and tranquilizers, but Amber(琥珀, Hupo) can also remove blood stasis from the heart, and Cinnabar(朱砂,Zhusha)also can clear away excessive heart fire. Therefore, if they are used together to treat palpitation, insomnia and epilepsy, they will be highly effective. In addition, Amber(琥珀,Hupo)can resolve blood stasis to regulate the meridians, remove pathogenic accumulation and diminish stagnation and promote diuresis. If used externally, it can astringe the ulcer to stop bleeding, treat prolonged unhealed ulcers and the traumatic hemorrhage. As Cinnabar (朱砂,Zhusha)serves the function of detoxication and expelling parasites, it is a good remedy for skin and external diseases, pyogenic infections and scabies.

Amber(琥珀, Hupo) and Tuckahoe(茯苓,Fuling)have the functions of tranquilizing the mind and calming the fear. Therefore, it is usually used in the treatment of palpitation, severe palpitation, insomnia, dreaminess, infantile convulsion and mania. Nevertheless, since Amber(琥珀, Hupo) is able to act on the blood stage and is inclined to purge pathogenic fire, it is a commonly used remedy for restlessness due to hyperactivity of yang or excessive heart fire. But when compared with Amber(琥珀,Hupo), poria is inclined to invigorate qi. So it is applicable for mental disturbances (diseases) due to water retention attacking the heart or deficiency of heart qi. As for the promotion of urination, Amber(琥珀, Hupo) can be used to treat stranguria with urinary obstruction in the urethra, and hematuria caused by retention of damp heat in the interior, and accumulation of qi and blood in the body. It can remove blood stasis and promote urination, while poria can tonify qi and remove dampness. It is usually used to treat swelling and dysuria due to deficiency of qi.

4. 龙骨, Longgu

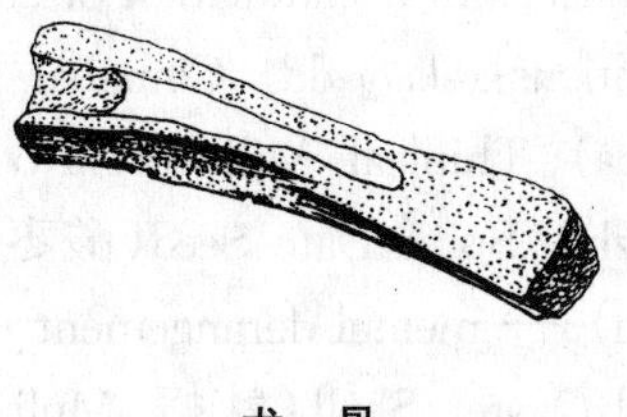

龙 骨

English name: Dragon's Bone
Pharmaceutical name: Os Draconis
Botanical name: Dragon's Bone
Properties and tastes: sweet, astringent and slightly cold
Meridian tropism: liver, heart and kidney
Functions: 1. calm the liver and check exuberance of yang

2. tranquilize the mind
3. induce astringency
4. reduce blood pressure

Indications: 1. hyperactivity of liver yang manifested as irritability, dizziness, high blood pressure, etc.
2. mental diseases manifested as dysphoria, palpitation, insomnia, infantile convulsion and manic-depressive psychosis, such as neurosism, and schizophrenia etc.
3. severe diarrhea manifested as frequent seminal emission, profuse leukorrhea, sweating due to deficiency, massive metrorrhagia, hematemesis, epistaxis, hematochezia, hematuria, prolonged diarrhea, and prolonged dysentery.
4. moist ulcer, eruption with itching, skin and external diseases, and prolonged ruptured abscess (for external use)

Dosage: 15 ~ 30g. Decocted first and proper dose for external use. Calcined for inducing astringency and freshly used for other purposes.

Contraindication: The drug is prohibited for those suffering from uncured severe diarrhea and concurrent accumulation of damp heat.

Combinations: 1. add Cinnabar (朱砂, Zhusha), Thinleaf Milkwort Root (远志, Yuanzhi), Spine Date Seed (酸枣仁, Suanzaoren)——mental derangement
2. add Oyster Shell (牡蛎, Muli), Gordon Euryale Seed (芡实, Qianshi)——frequent seminal emission, and premature ejaculation due to kidney deficiency
3. add Oyster Shell (牡蛎, Muli), Common Yam Rhizome (山药, Shanyao)——leukorrhea with bloody discharge, and menorrhagia
4. add Tangerine Peel (橘皮, Jupi), Tumeric Root-tuber (郁金, Yujin)——hypochondriac pain and concurrent hepatosplenomegaly
5. add Oyster Shell (牡蛎, Muli), Gambirplant Hooked stem and Branch (钩藤, Gouteng), Twotooth Achyranthes Root (牛膝, Niuxi)——high blood pressure and neurosism due to deficiency of yin and hyperactivity of yang
6. add Combined Spicebush Root (乌药, Wuyao), Mantis Egg-case (桑螵蛸, Sangpiaoxiao)——enuresis
7. add Oyster Shell (牡蛎, Muli), Asiatic Cornelian Cherry Fruit (山茱萸, Shanzhuyu), Chinese Magnoliavine (五味子, Wuweizi)——sweating due to deficiency
8. add White Peony Root (白芍药, Baishaoyao), Hematite (代赭石, Daizheshi), Tortoise Shell and Plastron (龟版, Guiban)——vertigo with feeling of fullness in the head, or tinnitus with vertigo, dysphoria, insomnia, palpitation due to fright, and numbness of limbs due to deficiency of yin and hyperactivity of yang, and up-stirring of liver wind

Prescriptions: 1. Decoction Ramulus Cinnamomi with Dragon's Bone and Oyster Shell (桂枝加龙骨牡蛎汤, Guizhijia Longgu Muli Tang)
2. Decoction of Bupleurum, plus Os Draconis, Concha Ostreae (柴胡加龙骨牡蛎汤, Chaihujia Longgu Muli Tang)

Notes: Dragon's Bone (龙骨, Longgu) is sweet and astringent in taste and weighty in mass, with the particular function of calming the mind and subduing hyperactivity. It is used for tranquilization because of its being weighty in mass, and for arrest exhaustion of qi because of its being astringent in taste. Any syndrome induced by deficient yin causing predominant yang and upward floating of yang-qi can be cured with it. The calined Dragon's Bone(龙骨, Longgu) is an important drug for eliminating dampness to heal ulcers. If levigated and applied externally, it is suitable for damp ulcer and prurigo as well as prolonged healing of ulcers. As stated in *Seeking Truth of Herbals* (《本草求真》, Bencaoquzhen) "Dragon's Bone(龙骨, Longgu) serves the same function as Oyster Shell(牡蛎, Muli), but Oyster Shell (牡蛎, Muli) is able to act on the kidney, for it is salty and astringent in taste, and as a result it can soften hard mass, resolve phlegm and clear away heat. This belongs to the category of sweet with astringents acting on the liver to stop exhaustion of qi and control bleeding with astringents, relieving convulsion and tranquilizing the mind."

Dragon's teeth(龙齿, Longchi) is specially used to tranquilize the mind, and its dosage is the same as Dragon's Bone(龙骨, Longgu).

Dragon's Bone(龙骨, Longgu) has been chiefly used to treat infantile rickets and senile osteoporosis in recent years.

5. 酸枣仁, Suanzaoren

English name: Spine Date Seed

Pharmaceutical name: Semen Ziziphi Spinosae

Botanical name: Ziziphus jujuba var. spinosa

Properties and tastes: sweet, sour, medium

Meridian tropism: liver, heart

酸枣仁

Functions: 1. tranquilize the mind by nourishing the heart

2. astringe to arrest sweating

3. tranquilize to induce sleep

4. relieve pain and lower fever

5. reduce blood pressure and resist arrhythmia

Indications: 1. dysphoria manifested as palpitation, severe palpitation, insomnia and amnesia

2. spontaneous perspiration and night sweating due to lowered body resistance and weak constitution

Dosage: 9 ~ 18g. Ground into powder and swallowed (1.5g to 3g each time before sleeping).

Contraindication: Pregnant women should not use the drug, because it may cause excitement of the uterus.

Combinations: 1. add Oyster Shell (牡蛎, Muli), Largehead Atractylodes Rhizome(白术, Baizhu)——spontaneous perspiration, and night sweating due to lowered body resistance and weak constitution

2. add Chinese Angelica Root(当归, Danggui), White Peony Root (白芍药, Baishaoyao)——insomnia and palpitation due to blood deficiency of heart and liver

3. add Common Anemarrhea Rhizome (知母, Zhimu), Tuckahoe(茯苓, Fuling)——vexation, vertigo and hyperhidrosis

4. add Dang-shen Root(党参, Dangshen), Chinese Angelica Root(当归, Danggui)——insomnia due to deficiency of heart and spleen

5. add Rehmannia Dried Root (生地黄, Shengdihuang), Figwort Root(玄参, Xuanshen)——insomnia, palpitation, amnesia, dry mouth and throat, reddened tongue with thin fur due to deficiency of heart and kidney, deficiency of yin, and hyperactivity of yang

6. add Cape Jasmine Fruit(栀子, Zhizi)——dysphoria, dreaminess and insomnia due to flaring-up of heart fire

7. add Thinleaf Milkwort Root（远志，Yuanzhi）——insomnia, palpitation and timidness due to breakdown of the normal physiological coordination between the heart and the kidney

Prescriptions: 1. Semen Ziziphi Spinosae Decoction(酸枣仁汤,Suanzaoren Tang)

2. Decoction for Invigorating the Spleen and Nourishing the Heart(归脾汤,Guipi Tang)

Notes: Spine Date Seed(酸枣仁,Suanzaoren) is considered to be a key drug used for insomnia with deficient dysphoria. Therefore, it is mainly employed to treat palpitation and insomnia induced by deficiency of the blood resulting in failure to nourish the heart or flaring-up of deficiency fire. It is mostly used in the modern clinics for the treatment of insomnia due to neurosis and climacteric syndrome. Li Shizhen(李时珍) said: "this drug can be used to treat insomnia due to deficiency of gallbladder qi, morbid thirst and deficient sweating; however, if taken in its crude state, it can be used to treat insomnia due to gallbladder heat." However, this is not always true. It has been proved clinically and experimentally that whether taken after being prepared or in its crude state, it always serves the function of relieving mental strain. If it is fried to such an extent that all its oil is lost, its function of tranquilizing the mind will be no longer achieved.

6. 柏子仁, Baiziren

English name: Chinese Arborvitae Seed

Pharmaceutical name: Semen Biotae Orientalis

Botanical name: Biota orientalis(L.)Endl.

Properties and tastes: sweet, medium

Meridian tropism: heart, kidney, and large intestine

Functions: 1. tranquilize the mind by nourishing the heart

2. lubricate the bowel to relieve constipation

柏子仁

Indications: 1. fidgeting of deficiency type, insomnia, palpitation due to fright and severe palpitation mainly caused by deficiency of heart yin and incoordination between the heart and the kidney

2. constipation due to dryness of the intestines

Dosage: 9～18g.

Contraindication: Those suffering from diarrhea and abundant expectoration must be cautious in their use of the drug.

Combinations: 1. add Spine Date Seed(酸枣仁, Suanzaoren)——fidgeting of deficiency type, insomnia, palpitation due to fright and severe palpitation

2. add Ginseng(人参, Renshen), Oyster Shell(牡蛎, Muli), Chinese Magnoliavine(五味子, Wuweizi)——vexation, insomnia and night sweating

3. add Apricot Seed(杏仁, Xingren), Hemp Seed(火麻仁, Huomaren)——constipation due to dryness of the intestines

Prescription: Mindeasing Tonic Bolus of Semen Biotae(柏子养心丸, Baiziyangxin Wan)

Notes: Li Shizhen(李时珍) said: " Chinese Arborvitae Seed(柏子仁, Baiziren) is medium in nature, (Neither cold nor dry used for reinforcing due to its sweetness in taste and moistening due to its acridness). It can dispel the pathogenic factors from heart and kidney, tonify the stomach and invigorate the spleen due to its fragrante in smell."

Both Chinese Arborvitae Seed(柏子仁,

Baiziren) and Spine Date Seed(酸枣仁, Suanzaoren) are main drugs normally used to nourish the heart and tranquilize the mind, they have a better therapeutic effect on palpitation and severe palpitation, insomnia and dreaminess caused by blood deficiency. But Chinese Arborvitae Seed(柏子仁, Baiziren) serves particularly well to nourish the heart as it is humidifying in nature and it can tonify the kidney and loosen the bowel. Spine Date Seed(酸枣仁, Suanzaoren) tends to act on the liver. In addition to being used in the treatment of insomnia and deficient dysphoria, it can also arrest sweating.

7. 远志, Yuanzhi

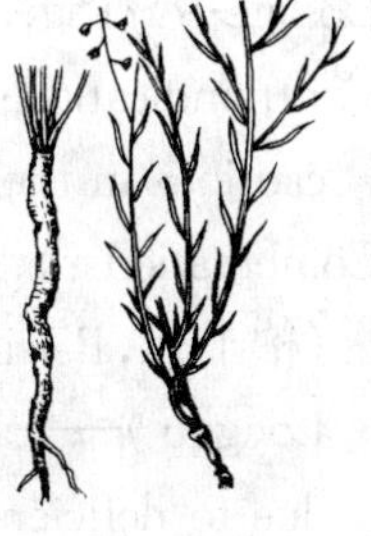
远 志

English name: Thinleaf Milkwort Root

Pharmaceutical name: Radix Polygalae Tenuifoliae

Botanical name: Polygala tenuifolia Willd.

Properties and tastes: bitter, sour, and slightly warm

Meridian tropism: heart, kidney, and lung

Functions: 1. relieve mental stress by calming the heart

2. tranquilize the mind and relieve convulsion

3. induce resuscitation by dispelling phlegm

4. detumescentify

Indications: 1. dysphoria especially caused by incoordination between the heart and the kidney manifested as palpitation due to fright, insomnia and amnesia

2. stagnation of phlegm in the heart manifested as mental confusion, vague mind, epilepsy induced by terror

3. cough with abundant expectoration which may be difficult to spit due to retention of phlegm or exopathy

4. carbuncle, cellulitis, furuncle, acute mastadenitis, and breast fibrosarcoma

Dosage: 3～9g. Proper dose for external use. Freshly taken for dispelling phlegm and prepared with Honey(蜂蜜, Fengmi) for tranquilizing the mind.

Contraindication: Those suffering from ulcer and gastritis must be cautious in their use of the drug.

Combinations: 1. add Spine Date Seed(酸枣仁, Suanzaoren), Lily Bulb(百合, Baihe)——neurosism, tachycardia, palpitation, dyspnea, insomnia, vertigo and amnesia

2. add Tendrilleaf Fritillary Bulb(贝母, Beimu), Bamboo Shavings(竹茹, Zhuru)－difficult expectoration

3. add Grassleaf Sweetflag Rhizome(石菖蒲, Shichangpu)——dizziness, dysphoria, vexation, insomnia, hypomnesis, or plain

4. add Grassleaf Sweetflag Rhizome(石菖蒲, Shichangpu), Tumeric Root-tuber(郁金, Yujin), Arisaema With Bile(胆南星, Dannanxing)——unconsciousness, complexion and dementia infantile convalsion auditus depression, and poor vision due to accumulation of phlegm in the heart

5. add Apricot Seed(杏仁, Xingren)——cough with abundant expectoration due to stagnation of phlegm

6. add Tall Gastrodia Rhizome(天麻, Tianma), Scorpion(全蝎, Quanxie), Pinellia Rhizome(半夏, Banxia)——epilepsy

7. add Tuckahoe(茯苓, Fuling), Spine Date Seed(酸枣仁, Suanzaoren)——neurosism, fidgeting of deficiency type and insominia after illness

Prescription: Pills to smoothe the mind(安神定志丸, Anshendingzhi Wan)

Notes: Thinleaf Milkwort Root(远志,

Yuanzhi) is used to treat various kinds of mental diseases and unconsciousness. It is especially applicable to those caused by turbid phlegm disturbing the heart because of its function of relieving mental stress and tranquilizing. It can be ground into powder and taken with wine alone, or used for superficial application after being infused in the treatment of carbuncle and pyogenic infections.

Thinleaf Milkwort Root(远志, Yuanzhi) and Tuckahoe(茯苓, Fuling) both serve the function of relieving mental strain and improving intelligence. Tuckahoe (茯苓, Fuling)is able to tonify the heart and kidney, expel stagnation, eliminate phlegm and induce resuscitation; Poria is able to nourish the heart and spleen, nourish qi, promote urination and remove dampness. If they are combined, they can be used to treat syndromes breakdown of the normal physiological coordination between the heart and the kidney. Tuckahoe(茯苓, Fuling) is suitable to the syndromes due to overthinking or phlegm accumulated in the heart. Poria, however, is most applicable to the syndromes caused by insufficiency of the heart and the spleen or water retention attacking the heart. With the treatment of cough and hyperphlegm, Thinleaf Milkwort Root (远志, Yuanzhi) tends to relieve stagnation to dissipate phlegm. It is applicable to such a syndrome as difficult expectoration due to thick phlegm. Poria is able to nourish qi and promote urination, applicable to such a syndrome as easy expectoration with excessive, thin and clear phlegm.

8. 合欢皮, Hehuanpi

English name: Silktree Albiziae Bark

Pharmaceutical name: Cortex Albiziae Julibrissin

Botanical name: Albiizzia julibrissin Durazz.

Properties and tastes: sweet, medium

Meridian tropism: liver, heart

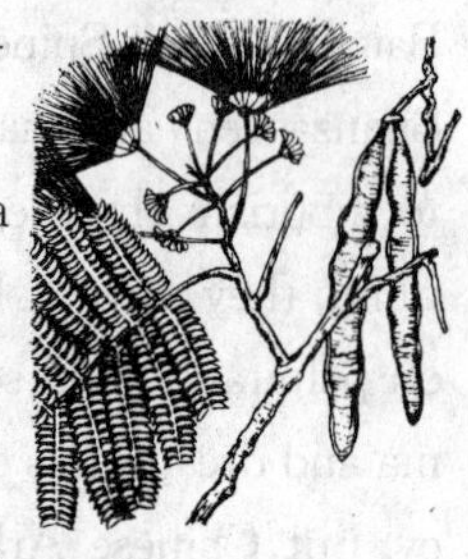
合欢皮

Functions: 1. alleviate mental depression
2. promote blood circulation to detumescentify
3. promote reunion of fractured bones

Indications: 1. palpitation, vexation, amnesia and insomnia due to stagnation of liver qi
2. traumatic injury and fracture
3. carbuncle, cellulitis, skin and external diseases

Dosage: 9～15g.

Contraindication: Pregnant women must be cautious in their use of the drug.

Combinations: 1. add Chinese Arborvitae Seed (柏子仁, Baiziren), Dragon's Bone(龙骨, Longgu)——anger, depression, fidgeting due to deficiency type, amnesia and insomnia due to mental depression
2. add Chinese Angelica Root(当归, Danggui), Sappan Wood(苏木, Sumu)——fracture
3. add Dandelion(蒲公英, Pugongying), Indian Chrysanthemum Flower (野菊花, Yejuhua)——carbuncle, cellulitis, skin and external diseases

Notes: Silktree Albiziae Bark (合欢皮, Hehuanpi) serves to disperse stagnated liver qi to smooth the liver and to tranquilize the mind. It is used primarily to treat such syndromes as anger, depression, deficient dysphoria, amnesia and insomnia induced by emotional hurt. It is effective if used alone, but it is mild in nature and not powerful, so it is necessary to take it in a large dosage and for a long period of time, to obtain such results as "tranquilizing five zang organs, harmonizing the mind and making people happy and free from depression." This is probably related with its action of tranquilization and the ability to induce sleep. Besides, Silktree Albizia Immature Flower(合欢花, Hehuanhua) is identical in nature, taste and action with Silktree Albiziae Bark (合欢皮, Hehuanpi), but it is mild in nature and not potent. Its dosage is 6～9g.

9. 灵芝, Lingzhi

English name: Lucid Ganoderma

Pharmaceutical name: Ganoderma Lucidum Seu Japonicum

Botanical name: Ganoderma lucidum (Leyss. ex Fr.) Karst

灵 芝

Properties and tastes: sweet, medium

Meridian tropism: liver, heart, and lung

Functions: 1. nourish the heart to calm the mind

2. relieve cough and asthma

3. invigorate qi and nourish blood

4. tranquilize

5. improve physical immunity

Indications: 1. deficiency of heart and spleen manifested as palpitation, amnesia, insomnia, dreaminess, physical tiredness, and poor appetite

2. phlegm manifested as cough and asthma, with a profuse cold feeling and clear expectoration, insomnia, poor appetite, tiredness, and chronic asthma of branches

3. poor appetite and tiredness due to deficiency of spleen and stomach, soreness of waist, vertigo, and deficiency of energy due to deficiency of liver and kidney, coronary heart disease, angina pectoris, chronic hepatitis, hyperlipemia, hypertension, and leukopenia

Dosage: 3～15g. Taken in powder each time from 1.5g to 3g. At present many forms of processed Lucid Ganoderma(灵芝, Lingzhi) have been sold in the market.

Notes: It is stated in *Shennong' Herbal Classic* (《本经》, Benjing) that Lucid Ganoderma(灵芝, Lingzhi) chiefly serves primarily to relieve deafness, promote circulation of qi to normalize all the joints, protect vitality, replenish vital essence and qi, strengthen the tendon and the bone and improve the color of facial skin. Modern studies show that its pharmacological action is demonstrated in various aspects and it has been clinically employed to treat many kinds of diseases of different systems, including cancer. But further study is needed in order to give a fair evaluation of its pharmacological action.

10. 紫石英, Zishiying

English name: Fluorite Ore

Pharmaceutical name: Fluoritum

Properties and tastes: sweet, warm

Meridian tropism: liver, heart, lung, and kidney

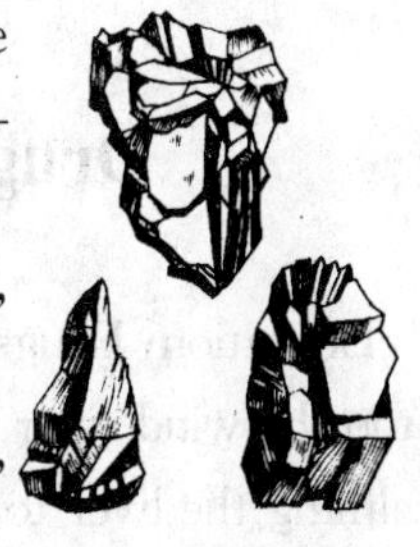
紫石英

Functions: 1. tranquilize the heart to calm the frightened

2. warm the lung to relieve asthma

3. warm the kidney to invigorate uterus

Indications: 1. mental diseases: palpitation due to fright, severe palpitation, dysphoria, epilepsy and spasm

2. cough with asthma due to lung-cold: aversion to cold, abundant thin cold expectoration, asthma

3. deficiency cold of Lower-jiao: sterility, massive metrorrhagia and profuse leukorrhea due to cold in the uterus, soreness of waist, impotence and spermatorrhoea due to deficiency of the kidney

Dosage: 9 ~ 15g. Broken into pieces and decocted first.

Contraindication: Contraindicated in cases of hyperactivity of fire due to yin deficiency and asthma due to lung heat.

Combinations: 1. add Dragon's Bone(龙骨, Longgu), Oyster Shell (牡蛎, Muli), Mirabilita Crystal (寒水石, Hanshuishi)——spasm due to phlegm-heat

2. add Desertliving Cistnache(肉苁蓉, Roncongrong), Ginseng (人参, Renshen)——deficiency of Lower-jiao

3. add Arabic Coery Shell (紫贝齿, Zibeichi)——palpitation due to fright, insomnia, dreaminess, and hypertension

4. add Abalone Shell (石决明, Shijueming)——headache, feeling of fullness in the head, dizziness and high blood pressure due to hyperactivity of liver yang

5. add Iron Scales (生铁落, Shengtieluo)——manic-depressive psychosis, epilepsy and hypertension

6. add Magnetite (磁石, Cishi)——dizziness, tinnitus and hypertension in case of deficiency due to water failing to nourish wood

Notes: Fluorite Ore (紫石英, Zishiying) is warm and moist in nature, has the function of tranquilization sedatives, warming and invigorating. It can be used to hinder adverse rising qi of Chong meridian and improve pulse.

Zhang Bingcheng(张炳成)remarked that Fluorite Ore(紫石英, Zishiying) is able to act on the blood stage of the heart and the liver, warm the uterus, and adversely hinder adverse rising qi of Chong meridian. In addition, it can produce a moistening effect and have property of supplement, so it is most suitable for women's sterility due to deficiency and cold of Chong meridian.

Chapter 14
Drugs for Calming the Liver to Stop the Wind

Definition: Drugs for calming the liver to stop the wind refer to drugs which function as calming the liver to stop the wind or checking the exuberance of yang to tranquilize.

Functions: These kinds of drugs separately serve the function of relieving convulsion by calming the liver wind and checking exuberance of yang to tranquilize. Modern research shows that these drugs play an important part in tranquilizing, relieving infantile convulsion, reducing fever and stopping pain.

Indications: Infantile convulsion and spasm due to stirring up of liver wind, dizziness caused by hyperactivity of the liver yang.

Notes: 1. These drugs mainly come from animal drugs. It is well said that the drugs made by shells or insects separately serve the function of checking the exuberance of yang and stopping the wind.

2. Most of the drugs one-sidedly have the

characteristic of coldness, but somewarm-dryness. Chronic infantile convulsion due to deficiency of spleen is unsuitably treated with the drugs cold in nature. Drugs warm and drying in nature should be cautiously used in treatment of blood deficiency and yin insufficiency.

1. 羚羊角, Lingyangjiao

English name: Antelope Horn

Pharmaceutical name: Cornu Antelopis

Properties and tastes: salty, cold

Meridian tropism: liver, heart

羚羊角

Functions: 1. calm the liver and check exuberance of yang
2. relieve convulsion by stopping the wind
3. improve sight by removing the liver heat
4. clear away heat and toxic material
5. induce sleep by tranquilizing
6. stop pain by clearing away heat
7. reduce blood pressure

Indications: 1. convulsion and spasm due to stirring up of the liver wind
2. high fever coma, delirium and mania of epidemic febrile disease
3. high blood pressure due to hyperactivity of liver yang
4. conjunctival congestion with swelling pain, headache with photophobia, poor vision, and glaucoma caused by flaming-up of the liver fire
5. primary thrombocytopenic purpura

Dosage: 1～3g in powders or pills taken directly or used in decoction. 0.3～0.5g each dose.

Contraindication: Contraindicated in case of chronic infantile convulsion due to spleen deficiency.

Combinations: 1. add Gambirplant Hooked stem and Branch(钩藤, Gouteng), Chrysanthemum Flower(菊花, Juhua), Rehmannia Dried Root(生地黄, Shengdihuang)——convulsion due to febrile disease
2. add Chrysanthemum Flower(菊花, Juhua), Abalone Shell(石决明, Shijueming)——dizziness due to high blood pressure
3. add Cassia Seed(决明子, Juemingzi), Baikal skullcap Root(黄芩, Huangqin), Chinese Gentian Root(龙胆草, Longdancao)——headache and conjunctival congestion due to excess of liver fire
4. add Gypsum(石膏, Shigao), Buffalo Horn(水牛角, Shuiniujiao)——coma, delirium and high fever due to epidemic febrile disease
5. add Plantain Seed(车前子, Cheqianzi), Figwort Root(玄参, Xuanshen), Common Anemarrhea Rhizome(知母, Zhimu)——glaucoma
6. add Rehmannia Dried Root(生地黄, Shengdihuang), Lalang Grass Rhizome(白茅根, Baimaogen), Ass-hide Glue(阿胶, E-jiao)——primary thrombocytopenic purpura

Prescription: Decoction of Cornu Antelopis and Ramulus Uncariaecum Uncis(羚角钩藤汤, Lingjiao Gouteng Tang)

Notes: Antelope Horn(羚羊角, Lingyangjiao) functions as clearing away liver fire, removing toxic heat, and produces a good effect on relieving convulsion by calming the liver to stop the wind. It is a key drug that can be used for treating convulsion and spasm of hands and feet caused by febrile disease. In clinic, two principles should be followed: firstly it is applicable to treat spasm and coma due to high fever, and more serious spasm of hands and feet caused by excessive heat in liver meridian generating wind. Secondly, it can be taken temporarily to treat dizziness due to hyperactivity of liver yang, conjunctival congestion with swelling pain and headache caused by excessive liver fire, which are more serious but can not be treated with other common drugs.

Both Antelope Horn (羚羊角, Lingyangjiao) and Buffalo Horn (水牛角, Shuiniujiao), salty in taste and cold in nature, act on the blood stage in the liver and heart meridian to detoxicate, cool blood, tranquilize and stop the wind. Therefore, they are also combined with each other to treat coma, delirium and spasm due to warm-heat pathogen going into Ying blood and stages. Antelope Horn (羚羊角, Lingyangjiao) can predominantly act on the liver meridian, and function as removing liver fire and calming liver wind to treat spasm due to liver heat generating wind. It may not be necessarily used for coma without spasm and high fever. Buffalo Horn (水牛角, Shuiniujiao) acts on the heart meridian first, and its function is to clear up heart heat, and cool blood. Therefore, it is frequently used for coma, delirium, eruption and hemorrhage due to pathogens entering into pericardium.

Since Antelope Horn (羚羊角, Lingyangjiao) and Gambirplant Hooked Stem and Branch (钩藤, Gouteng) serve the function of calming the liver to stop the wind and clearing away heat to arrest convulsion, spasm due to excessive heat can be treated with their combination. They are also used for headache, conjunctival congestion and dizziness due to heat in the liver meridian and hyperactivity of liver yang. In addition, as Antelope Horn (羚羊角, Lingyangjiao), cold in nature and salty in taste, acts on blood stage with the function of cooling liver to stop the wind and activating blood circulation to detoxicate, it is applicable to treat eruption, measles, coma and delirium caused by blood heat and excessive pathogens. Since Gambirplant Hooked Stem and Branch (钩藤, Gouteng) has the function of expelling the pathogenic factor, it can be commonly used for headache and conjunctival congestion due to exogenous wind heat.

Goat Horn (山羊角, Shanyangjiao) can substitute material to Antelope Horn (羚羊角, Lingyangjiao), with a similar but weak function. It is necessary to relatively increase the dosage, about 9～15g.

2. 石决明, Shijueming

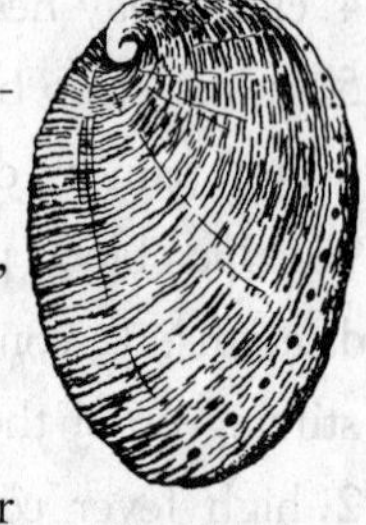
石决明

English name: Abalone Shell
Pharmaceutical name: Concha Haliotidis
Properties and tastes: salty, bitter
Meridian tropism: liver
Functions: 1. calm the liver and check exuberance of yang

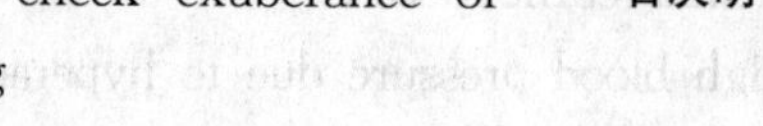

2. improve sight by removing the liver heat
3. neutralize gastric acid

Indications: 1. dizziness and high blood pressure in either deficient or excessive cases due to hyperactivity of liver yang,
2. eye diseases: conjunctival congestion with swelling pain due to liver fire, external oculopthy due to wind heat, and xenophthalmia due to liver deficiency
3. epigastralgia due to hyperhydrochloria
4. hemorrhage due to trauma (for external

use)

Dosage: 15～30g. It should suitably be broken into pieces and decocted first. It functions at calming the liver, checking exuberance of yang, and removing liver heat to improve sight when it is used in crude form. Its function is getting weaker to calm the liver by calcining, but has astringency.

Contraindication: This drug is contraindicated in cases of poor appetite and loose stool due to deficiency of the spleen and the stomach.

Combinations: 1. add Fluorite Ore(紫石英, Zishiying)——dizziness and high blood pressure due to hyperactivity of liver-yang

2. add Magnetite(磁石, Cishi)——high blood pressure

3. add Antelope Horn(羚羊角, Lingyangjiao)——spasm due to liver heat

4. add Coptis Rhizome(黄连, Huanglia n)——conjunctival congestion due to liver heat

5. add Cassia Seed(决明子, Juemingzi)——eye diseases due to liver heat, and high blood pressure

Notes: As Abalone Shell(石决明, Shijueming) is the principal drug with the function of cooling and calming the liver, and liver has its specific body opening in the eye, the drug is predominantly used to treat eye diseases, (i. e. cataracta and external oculopathy.) Zhang Xichun(张锡纯) says: "this drug can be a key remedy for encephalemia with headache and dizziness, which is commonly caused by flaming-up of liver qi and liver fire complicated by blood, since it has the function of cooling and calming the liver."

3. 牡蛎, Muli

English name: Oyster Shell

Pharmaceutical name: Concha Ostreae

Properties and tastes: salty, astringent, and slightly cold

Meridian tropism: liver, kidney

牡 蛎

Functions: 1. calm the liver and check exuberance of yang

2. soften and resolve the hard lumps

3. induce astringency

4. alleviate stomachache by relieving gastric hyperacidity

5. immunologic enhancement

Indications: 1. dysphoria, palpitation, insomnia, dizziness and tinnitus due to hyperactivity of liver yang

2. stirring-up of endopathic wind of deficiency type: spasm of hands and feet due to yin deficiency of liver and kidney or consumption of yin caused by febrile disease

3. scrofula, subcutaneous nodule, thyroid enlargement

4. abdominal masses, and hepatosplenomegaly

5. profuse leukorrhea, massive metrorrhagia

6. frequent seminal emission, spermatorrhoea, premature ejaculation

7. night sweat due to tuberculosis, spontaneous perspiration, enuresis and frequency of urine

8. stomachache with acid regurgitation due to gastric and duodenal ulcer

9. rickets

Dosage: 15～30g. It can be decocted first and or used in its crude form. When being calcined, it is only used for inducing astringency.

Contraindication: It is prohibited for excessive damp heat.

Combinations: 1. add Dragon's Bone(龙骨,

Longgu), Spine Date Seed(酸枣仁, Suanzaoren), Thinleaf Milkwort Root (远志, Yuanzhi)——dysphoria, palpitation, insomnia, dizziness, and tinnitus due to yin deficiency resulting in hyperactivity of liver fire

2. add Ephedra Root (麻黄根, Mahuanggen), Membranous Milkvetch Root(黄芪, Huangqi)——night sweat due to consumption

3. add Ass-hide Glue(阿胶, Ejiao), Himalayan Teasel Root(续断, Xuduan)——body fluid profuse leukorrhea, massive metrorrhagia

4. add Chinese Thorowax Root(柴胡, Chaihu), Green Tangerine Peel(青皮, Qingpi), Common Selfheal Fruit-spike(夏枯草, Xiakucao)——chronic hepatitis, and hepatomegaly with pain

5. add Figwort Root(玄参, Xuanshen), Common Selfheal Fruit-spike(夏枯草, Xiakucao)——tuberculosis of lymph nodes

6. add Dan-shen Root(丹参, Danshen), Turtle Carapace(鳖甲, Biejia)——hepatosplenomegaly

7. add Dragon's Bone(龙骨, Longgu), Gordon Euryale Seed(芡实, Qianshi)——frequent seminal emission, and premature ejaculation due to kidney deficiency

8. add Dragon's Bone(龙骨, Longgu), Twotooth Achyranthes Root(牛膝, Niuxi), Gambirplant Hooked Stem and Branch(钩藤, Gouteng)——vexation, susceptibility of anger, vertigo, feeling of qi and blood rushing up to the head, insomnia, and palpitation due to yin deficiency of liver and kidney, and hyperactivity of liver yang. (generally found in those suffering from high blood pressure)

9. add Figwort Root(玄参, Xuanshen), Rehmannia Dried Root(生地黄, Shengdihuang), White Peony Root(白芍药, Baishaoyao)——night thirst, fever and dysphoria due to yin deficiency

10. add Membranous Milkvetch Root(黄芪, Huangqi), White Peony Root(白芍药, Baishaoyao)——sweating due to debility

11. add Tortoise Shell and Plastron(龟版, Guiban), Turtle Carapace(鳖甲, Biejia)——stirring up of liver wind in febrile disease and spasm of hands and feet

12. add Swordlike Atractylodes Rhizome(苍术, Cangzhu)——rickets due to vitamin D deficiency in children

13. add Lobed Kudzuvine Root(葛根, Gegei)——high blood pressure with wiry pulse

Prescriptions: 1. Decoction of Three Jia for Restoring Pulse(三甲复脉汤, Sanjiafumai Tang)

2. Tranqilizing Liver-wind Decoction(镇肝息风汤, Zhenganxifeng Tang)

Notes: Oyster Shell(牡蛎, Muli) and Dragon's Bone(龙骨, Longgu) have the functions of calming the liver to check exuberance of yang and inducing astringency, and are always combined with each other. Nevertheless, Dragon's Bone(龙骨, Longgu) is inclined to treat palpitation, insomnia, epilepsy induced by terror, and manic-depressive psychosis because of its predominant function of tranquilization, and is commonly combined with tranquilizing drugs, such as Thinleaf Milkwort Root(远志, Yuanzhi), Spine Date Seed(酸枣仁, Suanzaoren) etc. Oyster Shell(牡蛎, Muli) can be used to treat not only spasm of the hands and feet due to febrile disease damaging yin with the function of stopping the wind to arrest convulsion in combination of Tortoise Shell and Plastron(龟版, Guiban) and Turtle Carapace

(鳖甲,Biejia) but also scrofula and subcutaneous nodule with another function of resolving masses. Moreover, in recent years it is also used for hepatosplenomegaly in the clinic.

4. 珍珠, Zhenzhu

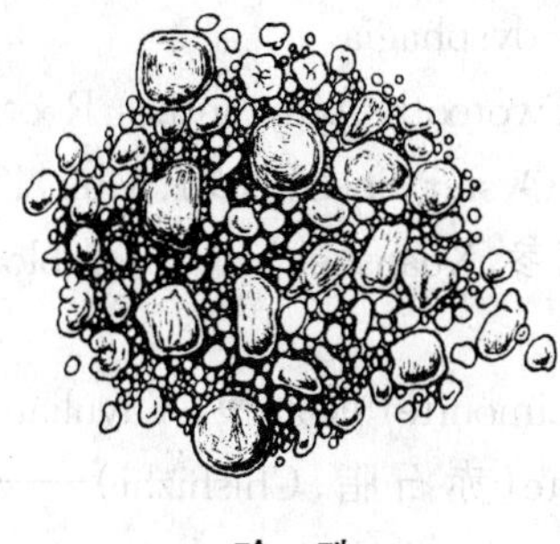

珍 珠

English name: Pearl
Pharmaceutical name: Magarita
Properties and tastes: sweet, salty, cold
Meridian tropism: liver, heart
Functions: 1. calm the frightened by tranquilizing
2. remove nebula by clearing away liver fire
3. astringe and promote tissue regeneration
Indications: 1. palpitation, epilepsy, and acute infantile convulsion
2. conjunctival congestion, pterygium, catarcta and external oculopathy (for external use)
3. ulcerative stomatitis, sore throat with rottenness, unhealed ulcerative sores, eczema, scald (for external use)
Dosage: 0.3～1g. It is mainly applicable in powder and bolus, and used externally in just the right amount.
Combinations: 1. add Honey (蜂蜜, Fengmi)——neurosism, palpitation and insomnia. (Taken after mixing it with another decoction)
2. add Amber (琥珀, Hupo), Jackinthepulpit Tuber (天南星, Tiannanxing)——epilepsy
3. add Cinnabar (朱砂, Zhusha)——acute infantile convulsion (taken after mixing it with other liquid)
4. add Amber (琥珀, Hupo), Borneol (冰片, Bingpian)——eye diseases (for external use)
5. add Elephant Hide (象皮, Xiangpi)——unhealed sore (for external use)
6. add Cow-Bezoar (牛黄, Niuhuang)——sore throat and toothache (sprayed on to affected part)
7. add Gypsum (石膏, Shigao)——infantile convulsion and contracture of hand and feet
8. add Garden Burnet Root (地榆, Diyu)——cataracta and external oculopathy
Notes: The drug acts on heart and liver meridians, and functions to relieve palpitation and improve sight, so it is a key remedy for mental diseases and eye diseases. It is ground into powder to treat unhealed ulcerative sores heal and skin erosion by injury. Use externally.

5. 代赭石, Daizheshi

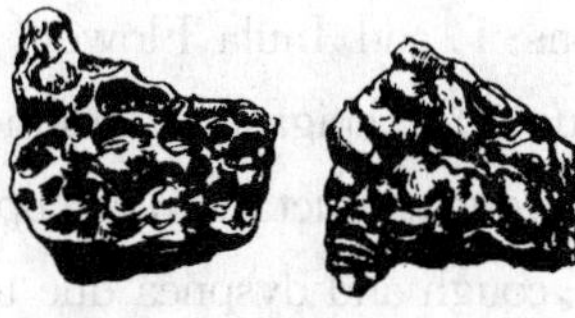

代赭石

English name: Hematite
Pharmaceutical name: Haematitum
Properties and tastes: bitter, cold
Meridian tropism: liver, heart
Functions: 1. calm the liver and check exuberance of yang
2. check upward adverse flow of qi with heavy material
3. tonify blood to remove heat from the

blood

4. arrest bleeding by astrigency

Indications: 1. high blood pressure, vertigo and tinnitus due to hyperactivity of liver yang

2. vomiting, hiccup, eructation, and feeling of fullness in the stomach due to adverse rising of the stomach qi

3. adverse upward flow of qi resulting in dyspnea and dyspnea of excess type due to deficiency of both lung and kidney

4. syndrome characterized by hemorrhage due to blood heat: hematemesis, epistaxis, and massive metrorrhagia

5. auditory vertigo

6. iron-deficiency anemia

Dosage: 9～30g. It is pounded into pieces and decocted first. It can be used in its crude form for calming the liver and checking upward adverse flow of qi. It is calcined for arresting bleeding.

Contraindication: Pregnant women and those suffering from qi collapse due to deficiency of spleen must be prohibited from use of the drug. It is not good to take this for a long period of time.

Combinations: 1. add Inula Flower(旋覆花, Xuanfuhua)——epigastric fullness and rigidity, frequent eructation, hiccup, nausea, vomiting, cough and dyspnea due to stagnation of phlegm in the interior

2. add White Peony Root(白芍药, Baishaoyao), Lalang Grass Rhizome(白茅根, Baimaogen)——hematemesis and epistaxis

3. add Dang-shen Root(党参, Dangshen), Asiatic Cornelian Cherry Fruit(山茱萸, Shanzhuyu)——adversed upward flow of qi resulting in dyspnea due to deficiency of both lung and kidney

4. add Achyranthis Root(怀牛膝, Huainiuxi)——dizziness due to hyperactivity of liver yang

5. add Perilla Seed(苏子, Suzi), Apricot Seed(杏仁, Xingren)——dyspnea of excess type

6. add Dang-shen Root(党参, Dangshen) and Chinese Angelica Root(当归, Danggui)——dysphagia

7. add Twotooth Achyranthes Root(牛膝, Niuxi), Oyster Shell(牡蛎, Muli), Figwort Root(玄参, Xuanshen)——high blood pressure

8. add Limonite(禹余粮, Yuyuliang), Red Halloysite(赤石脂, Chishizhi)——massive metrorrhagia, dizziness

9. add Rhubarb(大黄, Dahuang)——alienation caused by lochioschesis, and hypochondriac pain after child birth

Prescriptions: 1. Decoction of Inula and Red Ochre(旋覆代赭汤, Xuanfu Daizhe Tang)

2. Tranqilizing Liver wind Decoction(镇肝息风汤, Zhenganxifeng Tang)

Notes: Hematite(代赭石, Daizheshi), coming from red iron ore, is heavy in mass. Thus it is primarily used to check upward adverse flow of qi, dispel phlegm and prevent vomiting. Additionally, Hematite(代赭石, Daizheshi), cold natured, can have the function of cooling blood and astrigency to arrest bleeding. Consequently it can be used in treatment of hematemesis. Zhang Xichun (张锡纯) said: "Hematite(代赭石, Daizheshi) is the most effective drug for checking upward adverse flow of stomach qi. However, hematemesis can be best treated by checking upward adverse flow of stomach-qi."

Both Hematite(代赭石, Daizheshi) and Inula Flower(旋覆花, Xuanfuhua) have the function of checking upward adverse flow of lung or stomach qi, stopping vomiting and belching, and relieving asthma. Hematite(代赭石, Daizheshi) can be used to remove liver heat and check upward adverse flow of qi, and Inula Flower(旋覆花, Xuanfuhua) can expel phlegm by descending qi and abate abdominal mass by removing water retention. Therefore, they can be combined together for treating stagnation of phlegm in the interior, epigastric fullness and rigidity, eructation, regurgitation, vomiting, and dyspnea. But Hematite(代赭石, Daizheshi) is commonly used for the diseases caused by hyperactivity of liver yang and bleeding due to liver fire. Inula Flower(旋覆花, Xuanfuhua) can be best used to treat dyspnea due to accumulation of phlegm, feeling of stuffiness in the chest due to accumulation of phlegm, and edema and abdominal fullness due to water retention.

6. 钩藤, Gouteng

English name: Gambirplant Hooked Stem and Branch

Pharmaceutical name: Ramulus Uncariae Cum Uncis

Botanical name: Uncaria rhyncholphylla (Miq.) or U. Sinensis(Oliv.) Havil.

钩 藤

Properties and tastes: sweet, slightly cold

Meridian tropism: liver, pericardium

Functions: 1. relieve convulsion and spasm

2. calm the liver by clearing away the heat

3. reduce blood pressure

4. tranquilize

Indications: 1. infantile convulsion and tetanus due to up-stirring of liver

2. feeling of fullness in the head, headache, high blood pressure and dizziness due to liver heat

3. morbid night crying of babies

4. headache, conjunctival congestion and measles without eruption due to the invasion of exterior pathogenic wind heat

Dosage: 9～15g. It is not suitable to be decocted longer.

Combinations: 1. add Honeysuckle Flower(金银花, Jinyinhua), Wild Mint(薄荷, Bohe), Earth Worm (地龙, Dilong)——infantile convulsion with fever, spasm of limbs

2. add Mulberry Leaf (桑叶, Sangye), Chrysanthemum Flower (菊花, Juhua), White Peony Root (白芍药, Baishaoyao)——dizziness due to high blood pressure

3. add Scorpion(全蝎, Quanxie), Centipede (蜈蚣, Wugong)——intractable headache, facial hemiparalysis, prosopalgia and facial nerve spasm

4. add Twotooth Achyranthes Root(牛膝, Niuxi)——dizziness, feeling of fullness in the head, headache hemianesthesia, tiredness, hypertension and cerebral vascular spasm due to hyperactivity of liver yang

5. add Wild Mint (薄荷, Bohe)——dizziness, feeling of fullness in the head and headache due to the invasion of exterior pathogenic wind heat or stirring up of interior wind

6. add Gypsum (石膏, Shigao), Tuckahoe (茯苓, Fuling)——more serious hyperactivity of liver yang with flushed face, conjunctival congestion, vexation with irritability, yellow tongue, and wiry and rapid pulse

Prescription: Decoction of Gastrodia and Uncaria(天麻钩藤饮, Tianma Gouteng Yin)

Notes: Gambirplant Hooked stem and Branch (钩藤, Gouteng), acting on liver meridian, can be used to cool blood, calm the wind and reduce fever. As a result, stopping the wind and clearing heat can cure infantile convulsion, spasm, vertigo and dizziness. And this drug has a good effect on treatment of high blood pressure especially due to liver heat and hyperactivity of yang. Though both Gambirplant Hooked stem and Branch(钩藤, Gouteng) and Chrysanthemum Flower (菊花, Juhua) have the function of calming the liver to stop the wind, Gambirplant Hooked stem and Branch(钩藤, Gouteng) can emphatically be used for relieving convulsion and spasm by stopping the wind. Therefore, it can be a general remedy for dizziness, infantile convulsion and spasm due to fire and wind stirring up each other. But since Chrysanthemum Flower(菊花, Juhua) has the chief function of dispelling wind to remove heat, it can be used for treating the invasion of exogenous wind heat manifested as headache, conjunctival congestion and dizziness.

7. 天麻, Tianma

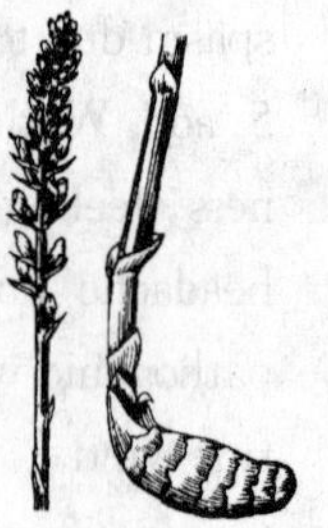

English name: Tall Gastrodia Rhizome

Pharmaceutical name: Rhizoma Gastrodiae Elatae

Botanical name: Gastrodia elata Bl.

天 麻

Properties and tastes: sweet, medium

Meridian tropism: liver

Functions: 1. relieve convulsion and spasm

2. calm the liver and check exuberance of yang

3. expel wind dampness and alleviate pain by removing obstruction in the meridians

4. reduce blood pressure

5. tranquilize, arrest infantile convulsion and relieve pain

Indications: 1. spasm due to high fever, acute and chronic infantile convulsion spasm caused by tetanus, and epilepsy

2. vertigo with headache and high blood pressure due to hyperactivity of liver yang or up stirring of wind phlegm

3. numbness and pain in shoulders, back and limbs due to pathogenic wind dampness

4. apoplectic sequelae: numbness of limbs, paralysis of limbs and facial paralysis

5. neuralgia: sciatica, prosopalgia, supraorbital neuralgia, and angioneurotic headache

6. neurosism, Meniere's disease

Dosage: 3～9g.

Combinations: 1. add Silkworm with Batrytis Larva(白僵蚕, Baijiangcan), Scorpion(全蝎, Quanxie), Fineleaf Schizomepeta Herb (荆芥, Jingjie)——facial paralysis

2. add Chinese Angelica Root(当归, Danggui), Rhizome or Root of Forbes Notopterygium (羌活, Qianghuo), Twotooth Achyranthes Root(牛膝, Niuxi)——numbness of limbs

3. add Gambirplant Hooked stem and Branch(钩藤, Gouteng)——infantile convulsion due to high fever

4. add Largeleaf Gentian Root(秦艽, Qinjiao)——numbness and paralysis of limbs or chronic rheumatic arthritis due to wind-cold-dampness

5. add Earth Worm(地龙, Dilong), Szechwan Lovage Rhizome (川芎, Chuanxiong)——migraine due to liver wind and phlegm dampness

6. add Baikal skullcap Root (黄芩, Huangqin), Common Selfheal Fruit-spike (夏枯草, Xiakucao), Twotooth Achyranthes Root (牛膝, Niuxi)——dizziness and headache due to high blood pressure

7. add Pinellia Rhizome(半夏, Banxia), Tuckahoe(茯苓, Fuling), Largehead Atractylodes Rhizome(白术, Baizhu)——hemiplegia due to apoplexy and abundant expectoration

8. add Jackinthepulpit Tuber(天南星, Tiannanxing), Divaricate Saposhnikovia Root(防风, Fangfeng)——tetanus

9. add Scorpion(全蝎, Quanxie), Silkworm with Batrytis Larva(白僵蚕, Baijiangcan)——irritating syndrome in cerebral nerve caused by epidemic encephalitis, and encephalitis B

Prescription: Decoction of Gastrodia and Uncaria(天麻钩藤饮, Tianma Gouteng Yin)

Notes: Tall Gastrodia Rhizome(天麻, Tianma) and Gambirplant Hooked stem and Branch (钩藤, Gouteng) function at relieving convulsion and spasm, calming the liver and checking exuberance of yang, and are used for infantile convulsion and spasm due to hyperactivity of liver yang. They can also combined to treat the diseases. Gambirplant Hooked stem and Branch(钩藤, Gouteng) is sweet in taste and cold in nature, with the function of clearing away liver heat. Therefore, it is most suitably used for infantile convulsion and spasm belonging to heat syndrome. Tall Gastrodia Rhizome(天麻, Tianma), medium in nature, can especially calm the liver to stop the wind, but it can not clear away heat. It can be used to treat infantile convulsion and spasm due to either cold or heat. In addition, Tall Gastrodia Rhizome(天麻, Tianma) can play an important role in expelling wind dampness evil, relieving pain, and clearing and activating the meridians and collaterals. Therefore, it can be used for treating pain due to pathogenic wind dampness and apoplectic sequelae. However, Gambirplant Hooked stem and Branch(钩藤, Gouteng) is also used for diseases due to exopathic wind heat, since it can dispel wind and reduce heat. Tall Gastrodia Rhizome(天麻, Tianma) was known as Chijian(赤箭) in ancient times.

8. 刺蒺藜, Cijili

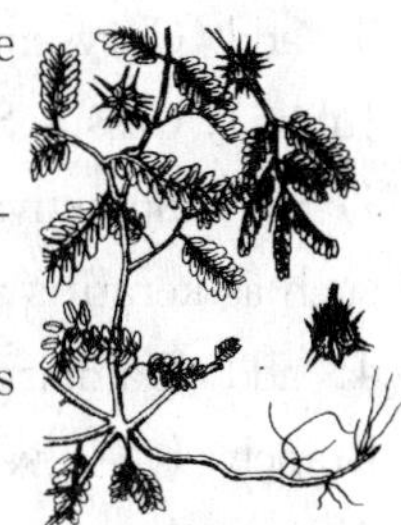

刺蒺藜

English name: Puncturevine Caltrop Fruit

Pharmaceutical name: Fructus Tribuli

Botanical name: Ttibulus terrestris L.

Properties and tastes: bitter, acrid, medium

Meridian tropism: liver

Functions: 1. calm the liver and check exuberance of yang

2. relieve a depressed liver

3. dispel wind and arrest itching

4. expel wind to improve sight

Indications: 1. headache, vertigo and high blood pressure due to hyperactivity of liver yang

2. discomfort in the chest and hypochondrium, irregular menstruation, galactostasis due to liver qi stagnation, and hepatitis with hypochondriac pain

3. skin itching: rebulla with itching, chronic eczema, neurodermatitis, vitiligo and verruca vulgaris

4. eye diseases: conjunctival congestion with tears and cataracta due to pathogenic wind heat

Dosage: 6～9g.

Contraindication: Pregnant women must be cautious when using the drug.

Combinations: 1. add Chinese Thorowax Root

(柴胡,Chaihu), Green Tangerine Peel(青皮, Qingpi)——discomfort in chest and hypochondrium, and galactostasis dut to liver qi stagnation

2. add Cicada Slough(蝉蜕,Chantui), Silkworm with Batrytis Larva(白僵蚕, Baijiangcan), Szechwan Lovage Rhizome(川芎, Chuanxiong)——rebulla with itching and vitiligo

3. add Chrysanthemum Flower(菊花, Juhua), Cassia Seed(决明子, Juemingzi)——conjunctival congestion with tears, such as keratitis and acute conjunctivitis

4. add Gambirplant Hooked Stem and Branch(钩藤, Gouteng), Twotooth Achyranthes Root(牛膝, Niuxi)——high blood pressure resulting in vertigo and headache due to hyperactivity of liver yang

5. add Prepared Tuber Fleeceflower Root(制首乌, Zhishouwu)——headache, dizziness, insomnia, hypomnesis, and itching due to over thinking, blood deficiency and hyperactivity of the liver

6. add Silkworm with Batrytis Larva(白僵蚕, Baijiangcan)——facial pigmentation, nervous headache and prosopalgia

7. add Cicada Slough(蝉蜕, Chantui), Divaricate Saposhnikovia Root(防风, Fangfeng)——neurodermatitis, urticaria and chronic eczema

8. add Sanchi Root(三七, Sanqi)——coronary heart disease with angina pectoris

Notes: Puncturevine Caltrop Fruit(刺蒺藜, Cijili) has the function of eliminating blood stasis and expelling liver-wind, and is considered a key drug for improving sight by calming wind in ancient times. *Seeking Truth of Herbals* (《本草求真》, Bencaoquzhen) also says: "It is effectively used to treat conjunctival congestion with swelling and vitiligo with itching of the whole body due to hyperactivity of wind because of its function as dispelling liver wind." Additionally and clinically those suffering from vitiligo must be cautious when using drug since it is liable to decrease the number of white blood cells in long-term use. This drug is also termed Puncturevine Caltrop Fruit(刺蒺藜,Cijili).

9. 决明子, Juemingzi

English name: Cassia Seed

Pharmaceutical name: Semen Cassiae Torae

Botanical name: Cassia tora L.

Properties and tastes: sweet, bitter, salty, slightly cold

Meridian tropism: liver, kidney, large intestine, stomach

决明子

Functions: 1. calm the liver and check exuberance of yang

2. remove liver heat to improve sight

3. lubricate the bowel to relieve constipation

4. reduce blood pressure and serum cholesterol

Indications: 1. headache and vertigo due to hyperactivity of liver yang, and high blood pressure

2. eye diseases: conjunctival congestion, blurred vision and photophobia due to flaming-up of the liver heat, pathogenic wind heat of liver meridian or deficiency of liver and kidney. In the clinic, it is used for treating glaucoma, night blindness and neuratrophia

3. constipation due to collection of heat or dryness in the large intestine, and habitual constipation

4. hyperlipidemia, arteriosclerosis, and high

blood pressure

Dosage: 9～15g. It is unsuitably decocted for a long time for relaxing the bowels. It infused, it can be used for reducing blood pressure.

Contraindication: Contraindicated in those suffering from loose stool due to spleen deficiency and hypotension.

Combinations: 1. add Chrysanthemum Flower (菊花, Juhua), Shrub Chastetree Fruit (蔓荆子, Manjingzi), Common Scouring Rush Herb (木贼, Muzei)——acute conjunctivitis

2. add Barbary Wolfberry Fruit (枸杞子, Gouqizi), Flatstem Milkvetch Seed (沙苑子, Shayuanzi)——diminution of vision due to yin deficiency of liver and kidney

3. add Belvedere Fruit (地肤子, Difuzi)——glaucoma and night blindness

4. add Abalone Shell (石决明, Shijueming)——high blood pressure

5. add Chinese Angelica Root (当归, Danggui)——constipation due to dryness in the large intestine

6. add Szechwan Lovage Rhizome (川芎, Chuanxiong)——headache

7. add Common Selfheal Fruit-spike (夏枯草, Xiakucao)——eye-ball pain due to hyperactivity of liver yang

Notes: As Cassia Seed (决明子, Juemingzi) and Common Selfheal Fruit-spike (夏枯草, Xiakucao) have the function of removing liver heat to improve sight, they can be used together to treat eye diseases caused by liver heat. However, Common Selfheal Fruit-spike (夏枯草, Xiakucao) chiefly functions at removing liver heat, and dispersing the stagnation. As a result, it is the key drug for treating goiter. In addition, since the function of Cassia Seed (决明子, Juemingzi) is to lubricate the bowel to relieve constipation, it is a perfect drug for treating constipation due to dryness in the intestine. As Cassia Seed (决明子, Juemingzi) and Abalone Shell (石决明, Shijueming) have the function of removing liver heat to improve sight, they are usually used together to treat dizziness, conjunctival congestion with swelling pain due to hyperactivity of liver heat or liver fire. However, Abalone Shell (石决明, Shijueming), salty-tasted, cold-natured and heavy-massed, can have the chief function of calming the liver and checking exuberance of yang, and concurrently replenishing liver yin. Since Cassia Seed (决明子, Juemingzi) is bitter-tasted, and cold-natured, it emphatically has the function of removing liver heat and dispeling wind. It is mainly used for excessive fire in the liver meridian. It is the seed of a herbal plant. In order to distinguish it from Abalone Shell (石决明, Shijueming), which is a kind of shell, it is also named Cassia Seed (决明子, Juemingzi).

10. 全蝎, Quanxie

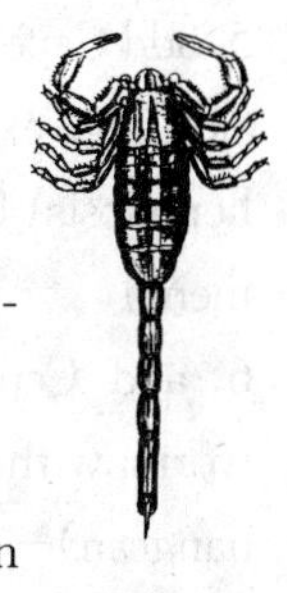
全 蝎

English name: Scorpion

Pharmaceutical name: Buthus Martensi

Properties and tastes: acrid, medium, and poisonous

Meridian tropism: liver

Functions: 1. relieve convulsion and spasm

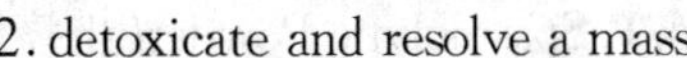

2. detoxicate and resolve a mass

3. remove obstruction in the meridians to relieve pain

4. reduce blood pressure

Indications: 1. convulsion and spasm: chronic and acute infantile convulsion, facial paralysis, tetanus, and epilepsy

2. skin and external diseases, scrofula tuber-

culosis, osteoarticular tuberculosis, thromboangiitis obliterans, and etc.

3. intractable headache and pain due to pathogenic wind dampness

Dosage: 3～6g. It can be swallowed as pounded powder. 0.6g～1g per dose. It must have the proper quantity for external use.

Contraindication: As the drug is poisonous, it cannot be used excessively. Pregnant women and those suffering from diseases due to blood deficiency generating wind must be cautious in use of the drug.

Combinations: 1. add Centipede (蜈蚣, Wugong), Prepared Jackinthepulpit Tuber (制南星, Zhinanxing)——tetanus

2. add Silkworm with Batrytis Larva (白僵蚕, Baijiangcan)——facial paralysis

3. add Tall Gastrodia Rhizome (天麻, Tianma), Gambirplant Hooked Stem and Branch (钩藤, Gouteng)——infantile convulsion

4. add Dang-shen (党参, Dangshen), Tall Gastrodia Rhizome (天麻, Tianma)——chronic infantile convulsion due to spleen deficiency

5. add Cape Jasmine Fruit (栀子, Zhizi)——skin and external diseases, and scrofula tuberculosis (for external application as ointment)

6. add Centipede (蜈蚣, Wugong), Silkworm with Batrytis Larva (白僵蚕, Baijiangcan)——intractable headache and pain due to pathogenic wind dampness

Prescriptions: 1. Spasmolytic Powder (止痉散, Zhijing San)

2. Powder for Treating Face Distortion (牵正散, Qianzheng San)

Notes: Scorpion (全蝎, Quanxie) has the good function of relieving convulsion and spasm. Li Dongyuan (李东垣) called it "the key drug for treating convulsion". *Amplified Materia Medica* (《本草衍义》, Bencaoyanyi) says: "It is even more indispensable for treating infantile convulsion." As a result, it is always used to treat spasm and convulsions in the clinic. Additionally, it functions at detoxicating and resolving a mass, and removing obstruction in the meridians to relieve pain, therefore, it is commonly used for skin and external diseases and bi-syndromes. Szechwan Lovage Rhizome (川芎, Chuanxiong) is another name for Scorpion (全蝎, Quanxie).

11. 蜈蚣, Wugong

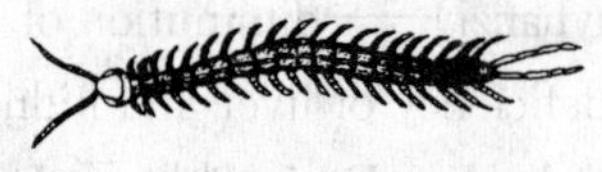

蜈 蚣

English name: Centipede

Pharmaceutical name: Scolopendra Subspinipes

Properties and tastes: acrid, warm, and poisonous

Meridian tropism: liver

Functions: 1. relieve convulsion and spasm

2. detoxicate and resolve a mass

3. remove obstruction in the meridians to relieve pain

4. inhibit mycobacterium, tuberculosis and has some anticancer activity

5. restrain convulsion (stronger than Scorpion (全蝎, Quanxie) for this function)

Indications: 1. same as Scorpion (全蝎, Quanxie)

2. bite of viper and toxic swelling

3. liver cancer, stomach cancer and esophagal cancer

4. maxillofacial lymphnoditis

Dosage: 1～3g. It can be swallowed as pounded powder. 0.6g～1g per time. It must be in proper quantity for external use as pounded powder or for external application with the oil that the drug has been immersed in.

Contraindication: As the drug is poisonous, it cannot be used excessively more. Pregnant women and those debilitated must be contraindicated in use of the drug.

Combinations: 1. add Prepared Jackinthepulpit Tuber(制南星, Zhinanxing), Divaricate Saposhnikovia Root(防风, Fangfeng)——tetanus

2. add Scorpion(全蝎, Quanxie)——acute infantile convulsion, tetanus, apoplexy, epilepsy with spasm, skin and external diseases, toxic swelling, scrofula, and other pain

3. add Scorpion(全蝎, Quanxie), Ground Beetlé(土鳖虫, Tubiechong)——bone tuberculosis

4. add Prepared Licorice Root(炙甘草, Zhigancao)——impotence

Prescription: Spasmolytic Powder(止痉散, Zhijing San)

Notes: Since Centipede(蜈蚣, Wugong) and Scorpion(全蝎, Quanxie) have the function of relieving convulsion and spasm, detoxicating and resolving a mass, and removing obstruction in the meridians to relieve pain, they are the key drugs for treating convulsion. In addition, they are always used together to further relieve convulsion and spasm. Nevertheless, Scorpion(全蝎, Quanxie), medium in nature, has a little weaker function in relieving convulsion and spasm. Moreover, owing to its comparatively weak toxicity, its function in eliminating toxic material and resolving a mass is not as good as Centipede(蜈蚣, Wugong). Centipede(蜈蚣, Wugong), fierce in strength, drying in nature and good at travelling, has the stronger function of relieving convulsion and spasm. It can produce a good effect on counteracting toxic material to treat skin and external diseases, and removing obstruction in the meridians to relieve pain due to its drastic toxicity. Furthermore, Centipede(蜈蚣, Wugong) is usually used for hemorrhoid, erysipelas etc. Earth Worm(地龙, Dilong) or White Mulberry Root-bark(桑白皮, Sangbaipi) can be used to detoxicate, if overdose results in poisoning. Centipede(蜈蚣, Wugong) is also named Tianlong(天龙) or Baizu(百足).

12. 白僵蚕, Baijiangcan

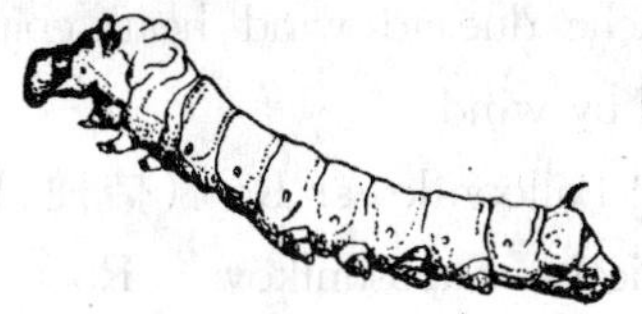

白僵蚕

English name: Silkworm with Batrytis Larva

Pharmaceutical name: Bombyx Batryticatus

Properties and tastes: salty, acrid, medium

Meridian tropism: liver, lung

Functions: 1. relieve convulsion and spasm

2. dispel wind to relieve pain

3. detoxicate and resolve a mass

Indications: 1. convulsion and spasm: acute infantile convulsion due to phlegm heat, chronic infantile convulsion due to spleen deficiency, epilepsy, tetanus, paralysis due to apoplexy

2. headache, conjunctival congestion, throat inflammation and toothache due to wind heat or liver heat

3. scrofula, subcutaneous nodule, skin and external diseases and mumps

4. rebulla with itching

Dosage: 3～9g. 1～1.5g in powder each time.

Contraindication: Contraindicated in those suffering from the diseases due to blood deficiency without wind.

Combinations: 1. add Scorpion(全蝎, Quanxie), Tall Gastrodia Rhizome(天麻, Tianma), Arisaema With Bile(胆南星, Dannanxing)——infantile convulsion due to excessive phlegm-heat

2. add Scorpion(全蝎, Quanxie), Giant Typhonium Rhizome(白附子, Baifuzi)——facial paralysis, facial muscular twitch of apoplexy

3. add Fineleaf Schizomepeta Herb(荆芥, Jingjie), Mulberry Leaf(桑叶, Sangye)——headache due to wind heat, epiphora induced by wind

4. add Balloonflower Root(桔梗, Jiegeng), Divaricate Saposhnikovia Root (防风, Fangfeng)——pain in throat due to wind heat

5. add Common Selfheal Fruit-spike(夏枯草, Xiakucao), Weeping Forsythia Capsule (连翘, Lianqiao)——scrofula, subcutaneous nodule, furuncle, and erysipelas

6. add Cicada Slough(蝉蜕, Chantui), Wild Mint(薄荷, Bohe)——rebulla with itching

7. add Coptis Rhizome (黄连, Huanglian)——numbness and swelling of tongue

8. add Dahurian Angelica Root (白芷, Baizhi)——superciliary arch pain leukorrhea, and chloasma

9. add Earth Worm(地龙, Dilong)——prolonged headache, infantile convulsion due to high fever, facial paralysis, and prosopalgia

Notes: Silkworm with Batrytis Larva(白僵蚕, Baijiangcan) is weaker than Scorpion(全蝎, Quanxie) and more inferior than Centipede (蜈蚣, Wugong) in relieving convulsion and spasm, detoxicating and resolving mass and relieving pain. However, since this drug has the character of eliminating phlegm damp to expel liver wind, it is the better remedy for diseases caused by wind phlegm, and also can be slightly suitable to treat conjunctival congestion and sore throat due to wind heat and rubella with itching.

13. 地龙, Dilong

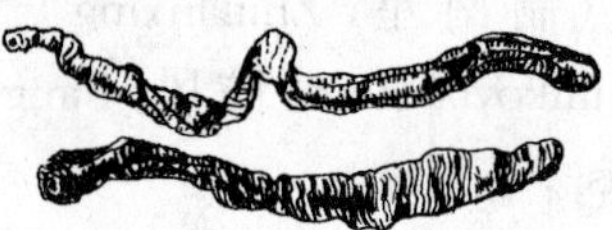

地 龙

English name: Earth Worm

Pharmaceutical name: Lumbricus

Properties and tastes: salty, cold

Meridian tropism: liver, spleen, and bladder

Functions: 1. remove heat to stop wind

2. relieve asthma

3. remove obstruction in the meridians

4. promote urination

5. dilate blood vessels and reduce blood pressure

6. dilate bronchi

Indications: 1. high fever with infantile convulsion, manic-depressive psychosis

2. dyspnea and cough due to lung heat, bronchial asthma belonging to heat syndrome, Whooping cough

3. Bi-syndrome manifested as red and swollen joints with heat pain and limited movement, such as rheumatic and rheumatoid arthritis

4. oliguria due to accumulation of heat in the urinary bladder

5. high blood pressure due to hyperactivity of liver yang

6. apoplexy sequela

7. pain with hematoma due to injuries from falls, fractures, contusions and strains

Dosage: 6～12g. Take fresh drug 10～20g. Grind into powder and take it orally from 1g～2g. Used moderately and externally

Contraindication: Those suffering from diseases due to deficiency and cold must be cautious in use of the drug.

Combinations: 1. add Silkworm with Batrytis Larva(白僵蚕, Baijiangcan)——prolonged headache due to accumulation of wind phlegm in the meridians and collaterals, facial paralysis, prosopalgia, convulsion, dyspnea and rale

2. add Apricot Seed(杏仁, Xingren)——bronchitis and asthma

3. add Arisaema With Bile(胆南星, Dannanxing)——pain in joints with limited movement due to attack of pathogenic wind dampness

4. add Common Selfheal Fruit-spike(夏枯草, Xiakucao), Gambirplant Hooked Stem and Branch(钩藤, Gouteng)——high blood pressure

5. add Plantain Seed(车前子, Cheqianzi), Akebia Stem(木通, Mutong)——oliguria due to accumulation of heat in the urinary bladder

6. add Gypsum(生石膏, Shenshigao)——high fever and spasm due to epidemic febrile disease

7. add Membranous Milkvetch Root(黄芪, Huangqi), Chinese Angelica Root(当归, Danggui)——hemiplegia due to apoplexy

8. add Twotooth Achyranthes Root(牛膝, Niuxi), Christina Loosetrife Herb(金钱草, Jinqiancao)——stranguria from urolithiasis caused by the passage of urinary stone

9. add Peach Seed(桃仁, Taoren), Cassia Bark(肉桂, Rougui)——pain due to traumatic injury

10. add Tall Gastrodia Rhizome(天麻, Tianma), Largehead Atractylodes Rhizome(白术, Baizhu)——wind phlegm headache

Prescription: Decoction Invigorating Yang for Recuperation(补阳还五汤, Buyanghuanwu Tang)

Notes: Earth Worm(地龙, Dilong) is earthworm, cold in nature, and a tendency of its function is descending, purgative and also travelling. Li Shizhen(李时珍) said: " A cold-natured drug can treat any disease due to pathogenic heat. As its function in the human body tends to descend, purge and travel, it can promote urination and treat foot diseases by removing obstruction in the meridians and collaterals. "As a result, Earth Worm(地龙, Dilong) is a proper remedy for asthma, spasm and oliguria caused by pathogenic heat. When used in cold syndrome, it should be combined with hot-natured drugs. This drug is weaker than Scorpion(全蝎, Quanxie) or Centipede(蜈蚣, Wugong) in relieving spasm. Those suffering from weakness of the stomach must be cautious in use of the drug, since the drug is cold in nature and stinking in smell.

As both Earth Worm(地龙, Dilong) and Arisaema With Bile(胆南星, Dannanxing) have the function of removing heat to arrest convulsions, they can treat high fever, dysphoria, spasm and cough with asthma due to flaming of heart fire resulting in scorching the essence of the lung. Nonetheless, since Earth Worm(地龙, Dilong) has stronger function in removing heat to calm the liver, it is mainly used in treating cough and asthma due to lung heat and madness due to excessive heat. Furthermore, as Arisaema With Bile(胆南星, Dannanxing) better functions at dispelling wind, resolving phlegm and arresting convulsion, it can predominantly treat cough, asthma and spasm due to accumulation of phlegm and heat in the lung. In the treatment of apoplexy, Earth Worm(地龙, Dilong)'s function is inclined to remove obstruction in the meridians, it can therefore be used in treating hemiplegia. In addition, Arisaema With Bile(胆南星, Dannanxing)'s action lays particular stress on dispelling wind and resolving phlegm, it is a frequent remedy for coma due to phlegm heat hence.

Appendix:

Name	Properties and tastes	Meridian tropism	Functions	Indications	Dosage	Contraindication
Nacre (珍珠母, Zhenzhumu)	Salty, cold	Liver, Heart	calm the liver to check exuberance of yang, improve eye sight by removing liver heat, tranquilize with heavy material, and induce astringency (external use)	Headache with dizziness, manic-depressive psychosis due to hyperactivity of liver yang, infantile convulsion, palpitation, insomnia, blurring vision due to liver deficiency, conjunctival congestion due to liver heat, and damp ulcer with itching	15~30g. Broken into pieces and decoct first. Used externally with proper dosage.	
Hawksbill Carapace (玳瑁, Daimao)	Sweet, salty, cold	Heart, liver	arrest spasm and convulsion by calming the liver, clear away heat and toxic material, resolve pathogenic accumulation. (to clear away heat and toxic material, same as Xi jiao)	high fever with dysphoria, acute infantile convulsion and apoplexy due to epidemic febrile disease, smallpox, and ulcer.	3~6g. Put into ball or powder, or ground into juice with water	
Arabic Cowry Shell (紫贝齿, Zibeichi)	Salty, medium	Liver	calm the liver to check exuberance of yang, improve sight by removing liver-heat, tranquilize and allay excitement.	Infantile high fever with convulsion, vexation and insomnia due to yin deficiency and hyperactivity of yang, conjunctival congestion with swelling pain due to liver fire	9 ~ 15g. Broken into pieces and decoct first.	
Dogbame Herb (罗布麻, Luobuma)	Sweet, bitter, slightly cold	Liver, heart	clear away heat to calm the liver, exert a tonic effect on the heart to induce diuresis, and reduce blood pressure	High blood pressure, heart failure, cardiac and renal edema	3~9g.	

Name	Properties and tastes	Meridian tropism	Functions	Indications	Dosage	Contraindication
Iron Scales (生铁落, Shengtieluo)	Slightly sweet, medium	Liver, heart	check hyper-function of the liver and relieve convulsion	Madness due to phlegm heat	30～60g.	

Chapter 15
Drugs for Inducing Resuscitation

Definition: A drug which is sour in taste, fragrant in smell and travelling throughout all the body, and functions at restoring consciousness is called an inducing-resuscitation drug.

Functions: restoring consciousness, clearing and activating the meridians and collaterals, and relieving pain (Modern research indicates that this kind of drug can thrill the central nerve system.)

Indications: Mainly used in Bi-syndrome manifested as coma, delirium and convulsion due to retention of pathogenic heat in the pericardium or accumulation of phlegm in the interior, and onset of fainting due to apoplexy or other factors.

In recent years, drugs for inducing resuscitation combined with drugs for warming the Middle-jiao to stop pain and for promoting qi and blood circulation are used to treat coronary heart disease, angina pectoris, and achieve the good result.

Cautions:

Resuscitation inducing drugs can be used for Bi-syndrome resulting in fainting, but not for collapse syndrome. Prostration syndrome is divided into heat-prostration syndrome and cold-prostration syndrome, therefore, drugs must be cautiously chosen.

Resuscitation inducing drugs can temporarily be used in emergency and superficiality, they are unsuitable to be taken for a long time in order to avoid consuming primordial qi.

Resuscitation inducing drugs are fragrant in smell and volatilize easily, most of them are put in bolus and powder, very few can be put in decoction.

1. 麝香, Shexiang

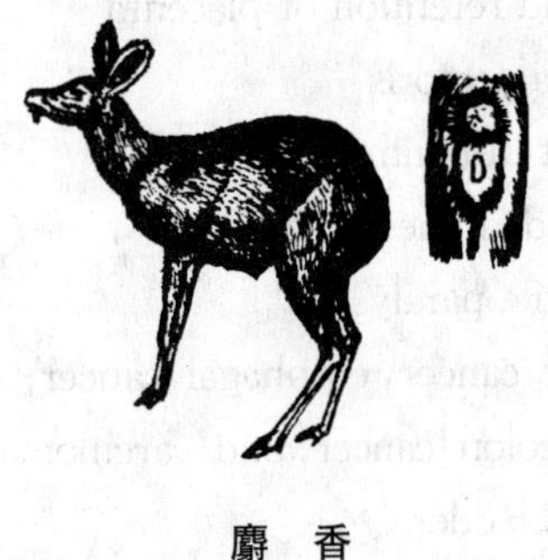

麝 香

English name: Musk

Pharmaceutical name: Secretio Moschus Moschiferi

Properties and tastes: sour, warm

Meridian tropism: heart, spleen

Functions: 1. induce resuscitation and restore consciousness

2. promote blood circulation to remove obstruction

3. alleviate pain
4. induce contraction of the uterus to expedite child delivery
5. excite the central nervous system
6. increase volume of blood flow in the coronary artery, elevate blood pressure, increase frequency of respiration
7. to resist tumors

Indications: 1. Bi-syndrome resulting in coma: epidemic febrile disease with retention of pathogenic heat in pericardium, epilepsy, heat-stroke and acute infantile convulsion
2. apoplectic coma: sudden onset of faint, loss of consciousness, and wheezing confusion due to phlegm heat which obstruct the heart
3. traumatic injury with pain(for oral medication or external use)
4. throat inflammation, carbuncle, cellulitis, subcutaneous nodule and mammary cancer (for oral medication or external use)
5. amenorrhea due to blood stasis, abdominal mass, and retention of placenta
6. angina pectoris
7. throat inflammation
8. wind dampness syndrome
9. infantile paralysis
10. liver cancer, esophagal cancer, stomach cancer, colon cancer, and carcinoma of the urinary bladder

Dosage: 0.06～0.1g. Only put into bolus and powder.

Contraindication: Pregnant women are contraindicated in use. Those have high blood pressure must be cautious in their use of the drug.

Combinations: 1. add Cassia Bark (肉桂, Rougui)——retention of dead fetus, retention of placenta, or dystocia due to blood stasis caused by cold
2. add Cow-bezoar(牛黄, Niuhuang)——coma, delirium and clonic convulsion due to febrile disease
3. add Dragon's Blood(血竭, Xuejie)——traumatic injury with pain
4. add Toad Skin Secretion Cake (蟾酥, Chansu)——carbuncle, skin and external diseases, and cellulitis
5. add Giant Typhonium Rhizome(白附子, Baifuzi), Arisaema With Bile(胆南星, Dannanxing)——apoplectic coma
6. add Common Aucklandia Root (木香, Muxiang), Peach Seed(桃仁, Taoren)——angina pectoris
7. add Common Burreed Rhizome (三棱, Sanleng), Zedoray(莪术, Ezhu)——tumor, amenorrhea, dysmenorrhea due to blood stasis
8. add Cow-bezoar(牛黄, Niuhuang), Pearl (珍珠, Zhenzhu)——throat inflammation

Prescription: Bezoare Pill for Resurrection(安宫牛黄丸, Angong Niuhuang Wan)

Notes: Musk (麝香, Shexiang), fragrant in smell and travelling around the body, can clear any orifice and remove the obstruction in meridians or collaterals, consequently, it is the key drug in the treatment of unconsciousness. It is always contained in many Chinese patent medicines with the function of inducing resuscitation, such as Bezoare Pill for Resurrection(安宫牛黄丸, Angong Niuhuang Wan), Bolus of Precious Drugs (至宝丹, Zhibao Dan), Resina Liquidambaris Orientails Bolus (苏合香丸, Suhexiang Wan). Li Shizhen(李时珍) said: " Why is the drug used as a guide in the treatment of the diseases caused by pathogenic wind, stagnation of qi and blood stasis, pain, epilepsy, and abdominal mass with obstruction in meridians and collaterals, and orifices unable to work? Modern research shows that the drug can excite the central nervous system. As a result, it is always the first-aid remedy for unconsciousness. In addition, since Musk(麝香, Shexiang) has the function of promoting blood circulation, detumescentifying and relieving pain, it is widely used in the treatment of traumatic injury, carbuncle, skin and external diseases, and cellulitis, not only oral medication but external use. If a small amount of it is put into all corresponding prescriptions, curative effect will increase. For this reason, Musk(麝香, Shexiang) is still considered a key drug in the orthopedic department of Chinese Medicine.

Musk(麝香, Shexiang) and Cow-bezoar (牛黄, Niuhuang) function as inducing resuscitation, so they can be remedies for coma due to febrile disease, apoplexy and mental confusion due to phlegm. However, Musk (麝香, Shexiang) emphasizes restoring consciousness so it can be used for cold or heat Bi-syndrome. As Cow-bezoar (牛黄, Niuhuang) is inclined to clear away heart heat, expel phlegm and calm the frightened, it is only used in coma, manic-depressive psychosis and epilepsy due to excessive heat and accumulation of phlegm.

The granular of Musk(麝香, Shexiang) is of high quality and well known as Danymen zi, while the powder from it is called Yuancunxiang(元寸香) or Cunxiang(寸香).

2. 冰片, Bingpian

English name: Borneol

Pharmaceutical name: Borneol

Botanical name: Dryobalanops aromatica Gaertn.

Properties and tastes: sour, bitter, and slightly cold

Meridian tropism: heart, spleen, and lung

Functions: 1. induce resuscitation and restore consciousness

2. clear away heat to relieve pain

3. restrain bacteries proliferation

4. start labor

冰 片

Indications: 1. Bi-syndrome resulting in coma: epidemic febrile disease with retention of pathogenic heat in pericardium, heat-stroke, acute infantile convulsion, apoplexy and epilepsy due to stagnation of phlegm heat in the interior

2. skin and external diseases (for external use)

3. throat inflammation, ulcerative stomatitis, and swelling pain in gum

4. conjunctival congestion, blurring vision (for external use)

5. acute or chronic otitis media suppurativa (for external use)

6. angina pectoris

Dosage: 0.03～0.1g. Only put into bolus or powder. Proper amount for external use.

Contraindication: Pregnant women must be cautious in use of the drug.

Combinations: 1. add Musk (麝香, Shexiang)——coma and clonic convulsion due to febrile disease

2. add Cinnabar(朱砂, Zhusha), Mirabilite (芒硝, Mangxiao)——throat inflammation, and ulcerative stomatitis (for external use)

Prescriptions: 1. Bezoare Pill for Resurrection (安宫牛黄丸, Angong Niuhuang Wan)

2. Resina Liquidambaris Orientails Bolus(苏合香丸, Suhexiang Wan)

Notes: Since Borneol(冰片, Bingpian) has the function of clearing away heat to relieve pain for external use, it is a common drug used in the department of ophthalmology and department of laryngology. Take the treatment of conjunctival congestion for example, it is immediately effective to put drops into eyes with the drug only. Both Borneol(冰片, Bingpian) and Musk(麝香, Shexiang) are sour in taste, fragrant in smell and travel around the body, functions as inducing resuscitation. Nonetheless, Borneol (冰片, Bingpian) is weaker than Musk(麝香, Shexiang) and only gives assistance to Musk(麝香, Shexiang) in treatment. Borneol(冰片, Bingpian) and Musk(麝香, Shexiang) can treat skin and external diseases due to toxic heat. However, Musk(麝香, Shexiang)'s function emphasizes to promote blood circulation to remove obstruction in meridians. Furthermore, Borneol(冰片, Bingpian)'s function is inclined to remove stagnated fire and detumescentify to relieve pain.

3. 苏合香, Suhexiang

English name: Storesin

Pharmaceutical name: Styrax Liquidis

Botanical name: Liquidambar orientalis Mill.

苏合香

Properties and tastes: sour, warm

Meridian tropism: heart, spleen

Functions: 1. induce resuscitation and restore consciousness

2. eliminate turbid evils to relieve pain

3. improve volume of blood flow in coronary artery and lower oxygen consumption of myocardium

Indications: 1. cold Bi-syndrome: apoplexy and phlegm syncope manifested as onset of fainting, black face and cold extremities

2. feeling of stuffiness in chest and abdomen with cold pain, colic caused by ascaris

3. angina pectoris

4. motor paralysis, and spasm of muscle and tendon

Dosage: 0.3～1g. The drug is better put into bolus, but not into decoction.

Contraindication: The drug is not to be taken for Bi-syndrome and prostration due to yin deficiency and excessive fire.

Combinations: 1. add Musk(麝香, Shexiang), Clove Flower-bud(丁香, Dingxiang), Benzoinum(安息香, Anxixiang)——apoplexy and phlegm syncope

2. add Sandalwood(檀香, Tanxiang), Borneol(冰片, Bingpian), Frankincense(乳香, Ruxiang)——angina pectoris

Prescription: Resina Liquidambaris Orientails Bolus(苏合香丸, Suhexiang Wan)

Notes: Storesin(苏合香, Suhexiang), sour in taste, warm in nature and extremely fragrant in smell, is inclined to eliminate turbidity and induce resuscitation. Therefore, it is a good remedy for Bi-syndrome manifested as onset of fainting due to apoplexy, stagnation of phlegm and qi stagnation. Nevertheless, as Bi-syndrome is divided into cold and heat Bi-syndrome, Bi-syndrome can be treated in a cold or warm manner. The drug, warm in nature and travelling through the body to eliminate turbid evil, can be suitably used for cold Bi-syndrome manifested as onset of fainting due to apoplexy, phlegm syncope and stagnation of qi, but unsuitably for heat Bi-syndrome and prostration syndrome. In recent years, it is widely used in the treatment of angina pectoris, with a good result. *New Compilation of*

Materia Medica (《本草从新》, Bencaocongxin) said: " Persons at present time use Resina Liquidambaris Orientails Bolus(苏合香丸, Suhexiang Wan) without limit, who don't know that drugs fragrant in smell can dispel genuine qi. If taken it frequently, those who suffer from minor illness can become more serious and individuals suffer from serious illness may die immediately. Only those with excessive qi and strong constitutions can temporarily take one or two bolus, otherwise, it should be deeply prohibited. These inmarks are still said in modern time.

Storesin(苏合香, Suhexiang) and Musk (麝香, Shexiang), sour in taste, warm in nature and fragrant in smell, have the function of inducing resuscitation. In the treatment of unconsciousness due to apoplexy or phlegm stagnation belonging to cold Bi-syndrome, they can be combined with each other in order to strengthen the function of restoring consciousness. But Storesin(苏合香, Suhexiang) has the better function of eliminating turbid evil and expelling phlegm, so it is the best remedy for syncope due to turbid evil attacking the human body or coma caused by apoplexy and abundant expectoration. Musk(麝香, Shexiang) is stronger than Storesin(苏合香, Suhexiang) in the function of inducing resuscitation. Moreover, it has the function of travelling around the body and removing obstruction in meridians and collaterals. Therefore, it is also commonly used in the treatment of swelling pain due to stagnation of blood and qi.

4. 石菖蒲, Shichangpu

English name: Grassleaf Sweetflag Rhizome

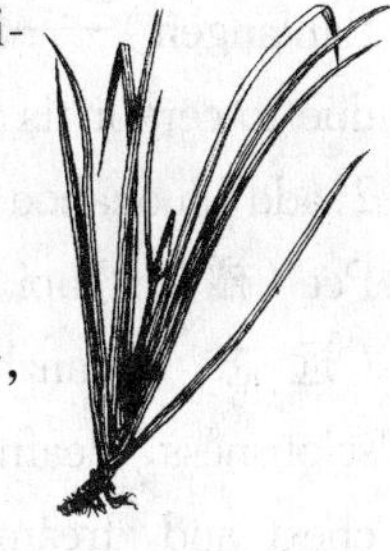
石菖蒲

Pharmaceutical name: Rhizoma Acori Graminei

Botanical name: Acorus gramineus Soland.

Properties and tastes: sour, bitter, warm

Meridian tropism: heart, stomach

Functions: 1. induce resuscitation and restore consciousness
2. resolve dampness to regulate the stomach
3. promote intelligence and auditus
4. tranquilize the mind
5. relieve spasm and stop infantile convulsion
6. relieve cough and expel phlegm

Indications: 1. unconsciousness: retention of damp evil in seven orifices, such as coma due to damp-warm, manic-depressive psychosis, epilepsy, and senile dementia
2. retention of dampness in the Middle-jiao, fullness in chest and abdomen with pain, bitter and sticky taste, and anorexia
3. toxic dysentery, and enteritis
4. coma due to pulmonary encephalopathy, cerebritis, cirrhosis of liver and cerebral hemorrhage
5. disturbance of mind manifested as hypomnesis, insomnia, tinnitus and deafness, and child mental defect
6. chronic bronchitis and bronchial asthma
7. hoarseness due to edema of vocal fold and laryngitis

Dosage: 6～9g. Fresh drug must be doubled in use.

Contraindication: The drug is unsuitable for those with yin deficiency, blood deficiency, spermatorrhoea and hyperhidrosis.

Combinations: 1. add Honeysuckle Flower(金银花, Jinyinhua), Indigwoad Root(板蓝根,

Banlangen)——fever, coma and delirium due to cerebritis

2. add Tuckahoe(茯苓, Fuling), Tangerine Peel(橘皮, Jupi), Thinleaf Milkwort Root (远志, Yuanzhi)——temporary unconsciousness, deafness, oppressed feeling in chest and dreaminess due to retention of damp-phlegm in the interior

3. add Wrinkled Gianthyssop Herb(藿香, Huoxiang), Officinal Magnolia Bark(厚朴, Houpo), Tangerine Peel(橘皮, Jupi)——feeling of stuffiness and choking in chest and poor appetite due to stagnation of phlegm in the Middle-jiao

4. add Tumeric Root-tuber(郁金, Yujin), Bamboo Shavings(竹茹, Zhuru), Pinellia Rhizome(半夏, Baixia)——coma due to retention of phlegm evil in seven orifices, such as pulmonary encephalopathy

5. add Honeysuckle Flower(金银花, Jinyinhua), Dandelion(蒲公英, Pugongying)——toxic dysentery

6. add Ginseng(人参, Renshen), Tuckahoe (茯苓, Fuling)——prolonged dysentery

7. add Cow-bezoar(牛黄, Niuhuang), Arisaema With Bile(胆南星, Dannanxing)——coma due to encephalitis B and epidemic encephalitis

8. add Dragon's Bone(龙骨, Longgu), Oyster Shell(牡蛎, Muli)——epilepsy

9. add Thinleaf Milkwort Root (远志, Yuanzhi), Trotoise Shell and Plastron(龟版, Guiban)——dysphoria, insomnia, amnesia, and five kinds of retardation

10. add Tumeric Root-tuber(郁金, Yujin)——obstruction of qi in the chest and angina pectoria

11. add Thinleaf Milkwort Root (远志, Yuanzhi)——amnesia, dementia and unconsciousness after apoplexy

Prescriptions: 1. Pills to smoothe the mind(安神定志丸, Anshendingzhi Wan)

2. Rhizoma Acori Graminei and Radix Curcumae Decoction(菖蒲郁金汤, Changpu Yujin Tang)

Notes: Grassleaf Sweetflag Rhizome(石菖蒲, Shichangpu), fragrant in smell, has the function of inducing resuscitation, clearing away obstruction in seven orifices and concurrently invigorating the spleen to eliminate dampness. It is the proper remedy for psychological and mental symptoms complicated with dampness syndrome manifested as abundant expectoration, choking sensation in the chest, loss of appetite, and greasy coating.

PART Ⅶ
Other drugs

Besides the drugs mentioned above, there are other drugs that remove food stagnation, expel parasites, drugs for external use, and drugs that induce vomiting.

As traditionally used drugs are seldom applied now adays in the clinic, they are not discussed.

Chapter 16
Drugs for Improving Appetite and Digestion and Removing Food Stagnation

Definition: Drugs, which are principally used to improve appetite and digestion and remove food stagnation, are known as drugs for removing food stagnation.

Functions: These drugs can remove stagnated food. They also have the functions of inducing appetite and digestion and regulating the stomach. Very few drugs can restore the normal functions of the spleen in transporting and distributing nutrients. Modern studies indicate that most drugs of this class promote gastrointestinal peristalsis, increase digestive juice, which help digestion.

Application: They are indicated for abdominal distension, eructation, acid regurgitation, nausea, vomiting, irregular bowel movements due to indigestion and food retention. They are also effective for deficiency of the spleen and the stomach, indigestion, abdominal masses and infatile malnutrition.

1. 山楂, Shanzha

English name: Hawthorn Fruit

Pharmaceutical name: Fructus Crataegi

Botanical name: Crataegus pinnatifida Bge. var major N. E. Br. or C. cuneata Sieb. et Zucc.

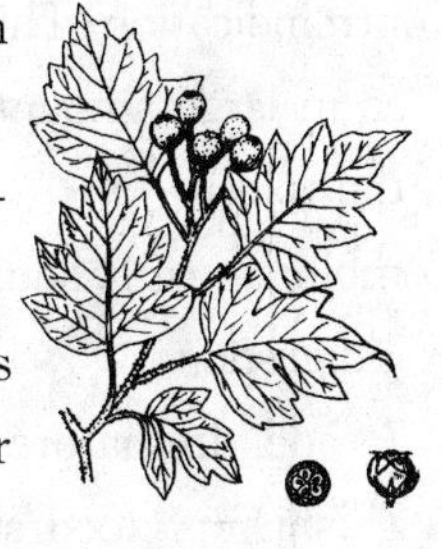
山 楂

Properties and tastes: sour, sweet, and slightly warm

Meridian tropism: spleen, stomach, and liver

Functions: 1. improve digestion, remove retention of food

2. promote blood circulation and resolve blood stasis

3. stop diarrhea and dysentery

4. promote eruption

5. strengthen the heart, antiarrhythmia, in-

crease volume of the blood flow of coronary artery

6. expand blood vessels, reduce blood pressure

7. reduce blood lipid, and serum cholesterol

8. bacteriostatic function

9. contract uterine

Indications: 1. indigestion and retention of food manifested as indigestion, anorexia, abdominal distention, abdominal pain and diarrhea

2. female blood stasis syndrome——dysmenorrhea due to blood stasis, postpartum abdominal pain, lochiorrhea and amenorrhea

3. hernial distending pain

4. acute bacillary dysentery, enteritis

5. measles without adequate eruption——due to stagnation of blood and qi complicated by food retention

6. hypertension, hyperlipemia, angina pectoris of coronary heart disease

Dosage: 9～15g, large dosage much as 30g.

Contraindication: This drug should not be taken in large amounts in case of deficiency of the spleen.

Combinations: 1. add Malt(麦芽, Maiya)——indigestion

2. add Immature Bitter Orange (枳实, Zhishi)——food stagnation, abdominal distention

3. add Motherwort Herb (益母草, Yimucao)——postpartum abdominal pain, dysmenorrhea

4. add Lychee Seed(荔枝核, Lizhihe)——hernial, distending pain

5. add Dan-shen Root(丹参, Danshen)——hypertension, hyperlipemia, coronary heart disease

6. add Chicken Gizzard Membrane(鸡内金, Jineijin) and Medicated Leaven (神曲, Shenqu)——diarrhea due to food stagnation

7. add Aucklandia Root(木香, Muxiang), Bitter Orange (枳壳, Zhiqiao)——acute bacillary dysentery

8. add Cattail Pollen(蒲黄, Puhuang), India Madder Root (茜草, Qiancao)——hepatosplenomegaly

9. add Coptis Root(黄连, Huanglian), Honeysuckle Flower(金银花, Jinyinhua)——dysentery with bloody stool

10. add Prunella Spike(夏枯草, Xiakucao), Chrysanthemum Flower(菊花, Juhua)——hypertension, dizziness and vertigo

Prescription: Pill for Promoting Digestion(保和丸, Baohe Wan)

Notes: Hawthorn Fruit (山楂, Shanzha) can promote the secretion of gastric acid, and gastric digestive ferment. So it may help digestion. It is an important drug for removing food stagnation. Therefore, Zhu Zhenheng(朱震亨), an ancient physician said: "Hawthorn Fruit(山楂, Shanzha) can remove food stagnation effectively." Zhang Xichun (张锡纯), an ancient physician pointed out: "if Hawthorn Fruit (山楂, Shizha) adds sweet adjuvant drug, it removes blood stasis but does not injury new blood, it regulates qi of diaphragm but does not injure healthy trends." So today clinics often use it to promote qi circulation and for blood stasis with the constipation syndrome. Since it has the effect of removing food stagnation, Hawthorn Fruit(山楂, Shanzha) is used for diarrhea, measles, cardiovascular disease and gynopathy.

Annotation on Shennong's Herbal Classic (《本草经疏》, Bencaojingshu) sum up its effect saying that it removes food and drink, invigorates the spleen and stomach, promotes qi circulation, and ablates blood-stasis. So children and woman in delivery are likely to eat it.

2. 神曲, Shenqu

English name: Medicated Leaven
Pharmaceutical name: Massa Fermentata
Properties and tastes: sweet, pungent, warm
Meridian tropism: spleen, stomach
Functions: 1. improve digestion and regulate the stomach
2. activate the spleen and regulate the function
Indications: 1. indigestion and retention food of the Middle-jiao——abdominal distention, loss of appetite, borborygmus, diarrhea
2. help metal herbs to be absorbed easily
Dosage: 6～15g.
Contraindication: It should not be used in the case of hyperhydrochdoria.
Combinations: 1. add Chicken Gizzard Membrane(鸡内金, Jineijin)——indigestion and food retention, anorexia
2. add Tuckahoe(茯苓, Fuling)——damp retention in the Middle-jiao, nausea, vomiting, diarrhea, etc.
3. add Swordlike Atractylodes Rhizome(苍术, Cangzhu)——food retention, diarrhea due to deficiency of the spleen yang
4. add Tangerine Peel(陈皮, Chenpi)——stagnated food, vomiting, nausea, chest congestion and abdominal distension
5. add Areca Seed(槟榔, Binlang)——infantile dyspepsia and malnutrition, abdominal distension
6. add Howthorn Fruit (山楂, Shanzha)——stagnated meat
7. add Wrinkled Gianthyssop Herb(藿香, Huoxiang)——stagnated food with common cold
Prescription: Pill for Promoting Digestion(保和丸, Baohe Wan)
Notes: For Medicated leaven(神曲, Shenqu) takes a large amount of wheat flour, bran, almond paste, red bean powder, fresh Sweet Wormwood(鲜青蒿, XianQinghao), fresh Achene of Siberian Cocklebur(鲜苍耳, Xiancanger) and fresh Culrage Body fluid(鲜辣蓼汁, Xianlaliaozhi) which mix together for fermentation, playing the effect of invigorating stomach and promoting digestion. It is good at digesting retentions of millet(unhusked rice) and alcohol. It should add Radish Seed(莱菔子, Laifuzi), Immature Bitter Orange(枳实, Zhishi), and other drugs which have function of promoting qi circulation when there is food stagnation, gastric cavity and stomach distending. It adds drug for invigorating the spleen and tonifying qi in cases of astheria spleen and stomach.

3. 麦芽, Maiya

English name: Malt
Pharmaceutical name: Fructus Hordei Vulgaris
Botanical name: Hordeum vulgare L.
Properties and tastes: sweet, neutral
Meridian tropism: spleen, stomach, and liver

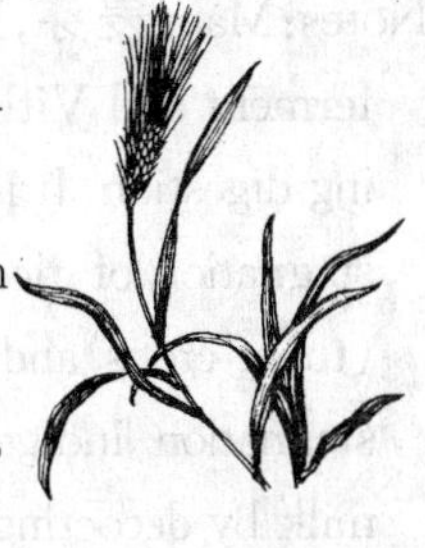
麦芽

Functions: 1. improve digestion and invigorate the stomach
2. smooth depressed liver, stop milk secretion
3. reduce blood sugar
4. bacteriostatic function
Indications: 1. indigestion and retention of food——dyspepsia, loss of appetite, abdominal distention, infantile vomiting of milk due

to dyspepsia

2. stagnation of liver qi——distention in the chest and hypochondrium, eructation

3. breast distending pain due to stop of milk secretion or milk stagnation, lactorrhea

4. superficialmycotic infection

Dosage: 9～15g; Large dosage can be as much as 30～120g. For smoothing depressed liver qi and stopping milk secretion, the unprepared herb is better with a large dosage.

Contraindication: It should not be prescribed for breast-feeding women.

Combinations: 1. add Medicated Leaven (神曲, Shenqu)——food retention and indigestion

2. add Dried Ginger (干姜, Ganjiang)——food indigestion due to stomach cold

3. add Largehead Atractylodes Rhizome (白术, Baizhu)——indigestion due to deficiency of the spleen, loss of appetite

4. add Cyperus Tuber (香附, Xiangfu)——stagnation of liver qi

Notes: Malt (麦芽, Maiya) contains a digestive ferment and VitB. It has the effect of helping digestion. It is good at digesting the food stagnation of rice, wheat flour, potato, taro (tuber crops) and starch. It is used for milk stagnation indigestion leading to vomiting milk by decocting when taken alone. It contributes the stagnation of the liver qi syndrome. Adding Chinese Thorowax Root (柴胡, Chaihu), Nutgrass Galingale Rhizome (香附, Xiangfu) etc, they are used for stagnation of liver qi with food stagnation indigestion.

In addition, Rice Sprout (谷芽, Guya) and Malt (麦芽, Maiya) all have the effect of digesting food stagnation and invigorating the spleen. But Rice Sprout is not better than Malt (麦芽, Maiya), it places its emphasis on nourishing the stomach. Milt places its emphasis on digesting food stagnation. The two used together can strengthen the effect and their dosage is 9～15g.

4. 莱菔子, Laifuzi

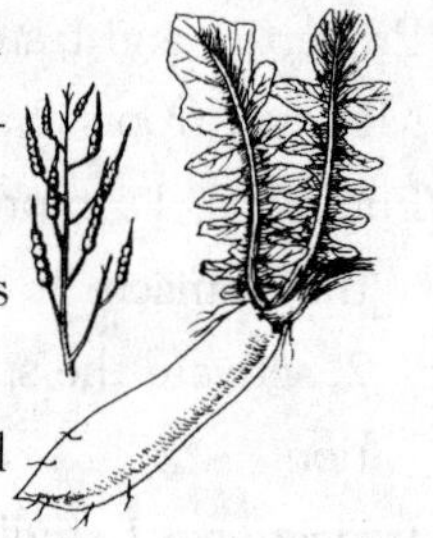

English name: Radish Seed

Pharmaceutical name: Semen Raphani Sativi

Botanical name: Raphanus sativus L.

Properties and tastes: acid and sweet, neutral.

莱菔子

Meridian tropism: spleen, stomach, and lung.

Functions: 1. improve digestion and relieve fullness

2. descend qi and resolve phlegm

3. anti-inflammation, bacteriostatic function, relieve pain

4. reduce blood pressure

Indications:

1. retention of indigested food and stagnation of qi-abdominal distension, ructation with fetid odor and acid regurgitation or abdominal pain, diarrhea with tenesmus, etc.

2. cough and dyspnea-especially for retention of excessive phlegm and saliva with food retention

3. constipation, intestinal obstruction——ascaris intestinal obstruction, adhesive ileus obstipation, senile constipation and infantile constipation

4. hyperosteogeny pain

5. hypertension

Dosage: 6～9g

Contraindication: Radish seed (莱菔子, Laifuzi) tends to cause consumption of qi, therefore it should not be used in cases of deficiency of qi and without retention of food and phlegm. It should not be used with Ginseng (人参,Renshen).

Combinations: 1. add Medicated Leaven (神曲, Shenqu)——retention of indigested food

2. add Pinellia Rhizome(半夏,Banxia)——retention of indigested food, frequent eructation

3. add Weeping Forsythia Capsule (连翘, Lianqiao)——retention of indigested food with fever

4. add Perilla Seed (苏子, Suzi)——retention of excessive phlegm and saliva, cough and dyspnea

5. add Rhubarb(大黄,Dahuang), Common Aucklandia Root(木香,Muxiang)——constipation, intestinal obstruction

6. add Suberect Spatholobus Stem(鸡血藤, Jixuiteng)——hyperosteogeny pain

7. add Chinese Honeylocust Fruit(皂荚,Zaojia)——phlegm qi and dyspnea

Prescriptions: 1. Decoction of Three Kinds of Seed for the Aged (三子养亲汤, Sanziyangqin Tang)

2. Pill for Promoting Digestion (保和丸, Baohe Wan)

Notes: Radish Seed (莱菔子,Laifuzi) is an important drug for expelling phlegm and regulating qi. Zhu zhenheng (朱震亨) said: "Radish Seed (莱菔子, Laifuzi) treating phlegm has the effect like pushing down the walls." Li Shizhen(李时珍) said: "The function of Radish Seed(莱菔子,Laifuzi) is good at regulating qi, the raw drug can raise, and the cooked drug can descend." Raising may vomit wind phlegm, eliminate wind cold, having a wound and rash, descending may relieve asthma and cough, regulate diarrhea and tenesmus, stop pain due to disorder of qi. They are functions of requlating qi. "It is excessive syndrome that this drug treats. It should combine with regulating qi drugs when food stagnation doesn't remove. It should be used in combination with purgative drugs when there is constipation and intestinal obstruction. It should be used in combination with drugs for removing blood stasis and tonifying the kidney when there is osteoproliferation. It should be used in combination with phlegm removing and cough relieving drugs when there is cough, asthma, and reversed upward flow of qi and wheezy phlegm. Used in combination with qi tonifying and spleen invigorating drugs for the person with deficient qi. But don't combine with Ginseng (人参, Renshen) because it may dispel medicinal effect of Ginseng(人参,Renshen).

Radish Seed(莱菔子,Laifuzi) and White Mustard Seed(白芥子,Baijiezi), all have an effect of removing phlegm. It may be used to treat phlegm asthma cough. But White Mustard Seed (白芥子,Baijiezi) is medium in property, it is good at entering the viscera, and it regulates qi circulation of the lung. It is used for the stomach and large intestine to relieve fullness and remove food stagnation. It is all used for cold or heat syndrome. White Mustard Seed (白芥子, Baijiezi) is acrid, warm and very dry, tending to penetrate through meridians. It is good at breaking through excessive phlegm obstruction between skin and membrane. It only uses a cold drug as if it treats phlegm asthma and cough.

5. 鸡内金,Jineijin

English name: Chicken Gizzard Membrane

Pharmaceutical name: Engithelium Corneum Gigeraiae Galli

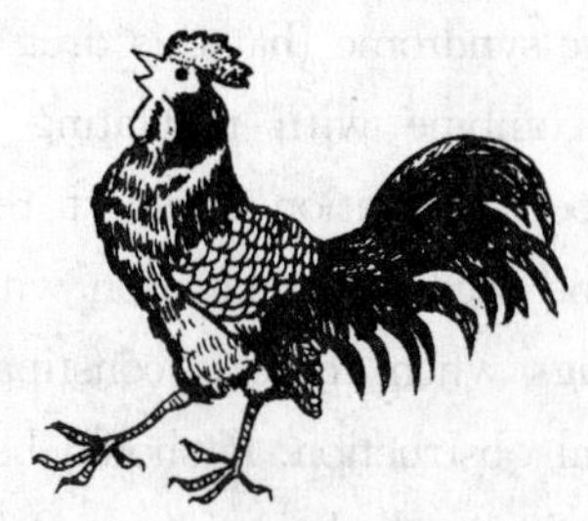
鸡内金

Properties and tastes: sweet, meutral

Meridian tropism: spleen, stomach, small intestine and urinary bladder

Functions: 1. activate the spleen to improve digestion

2. treat spontaneous emission

3. promote urination, lithagogue effect

Indications: 1. dyspepsia, retention of food, infantile dyspepsia and malnutrition

2. child enuresis and adult frequency of urination, polyuria at night

3. frequent seminal emission due to deficiency of the body

4. urolithiasis, gallbladder lithiasis

Dosage: 3～9g. 1.5～3g of its powder is infused for an oral use, the therapeutic effect will be better than that of the decoction form.

Combinations: 1. add Dan-shen Root (丹参, Danshen)——stomachache, anorexia, hepatosplenomegaly, anorexia due to radiatation treatment of cancer, etc.

2. add Medicated Leaves(神曲, Shenqu)——dyspepsia, abdominal distension, vomiting, diarrhea

3. add Mirabilite (芒硝, Mangxiao)——urolithiasis

4. add Turmeric Root-tuber(郁金, Yujin), Christina Loosetrife Herb(金钱草, Jinqiancao)——gallbladder lithiasis, lithiasis of urinary system

5. add Sharpleaf Galangal Fruit (益智仁, Yizhiren), Mantis Egg-case(桑螵蛸, Sangpiaoxiao)——infantile enuresis, adult frequency of urination

6. add Gordon Euryale Seed(芡实, Qianshi) Lotus Seed(莲肉, Lianrou) and Dodder Seed (菟丝子, Tusizi)——seminal emission

7. add Turtle Carapace (鳖甲, Biejia)——hepatosplenomegaly

Notes: The Chicken Gizzard Membrane(鸡内金, Jineijin) has strong effect of digesting food stagnation. It is used to treat stagnation like flesh stagnation, milk stagnation, millet stagnation and the other stagnation. This drug is always used to treat milk and food stagnation in children, thin body with big abdomen and blue muscle, abdominal mass stagnation and malnutrition. Zhang Xichun(张锡纯), an ancient physician, used its function of digesting stagnation "to treat abdominal mass, nodules of breast, abdominal masses and restore menstruation." which are original experience.

Chapter 17
Anthelmintics

Definition: Drugs that have a major effect in expelling or poisoning parasites are called anthelmintics.

Functions: Drugs of this class can poison,

numb, or expel parasites in the body. A part of this class can invigorate the spleen and regulate the stomach, and remove stagnation.

Application: Anthelmintics are indicated for parasites in the intestinal tract such as ascariasis, enterobiasis, cestodiasis ancylostomiasis and fasciolopsiasis, etc. A part of anthelmintics can also expel or poison parasites, such as schistosomiasis and trichomonasis vaginalis. In addition, some of these drugs can treat infantile malnutrition and indigestion.

Cautions: 1. Anthelmintics should be used or supplemented with other types of suitable drugs according to specific parasites, whether the patient's constitution is strong or weak, or wether the condition is acute. If the disease is a deficiency of the spleen and stomach, drugs for strengthening spleen and regulating the stomach should be prescribed.

2. Use on an empty stomach.

3. If anthelmintics do not have the effects of a purgation, purgatives should be given to help expelling the parasites.

4. If anthelmintics are quite poisonous, the dosage and administration must receive careful attention, not to avoids poisoning or damaging genuine-qi. Administer special caution for pregnant women, the aged, or weak.

5. For patients with fever and severe abdominal pain, temporarily suspend use of the drug until symptoms relax.

1. 使君子, Shijunzi

English name: Rangooncreeper Fruit

Pharmaceutical name: Fructus Quisqualis Indicae

Botanical name: Quisqualis Indica L.

Properties and tastes: sweet, warm.

Meridian tropism: spleen, stomach.

Functions: 1. expel parasites and remove stagnation of food

2. antifungus

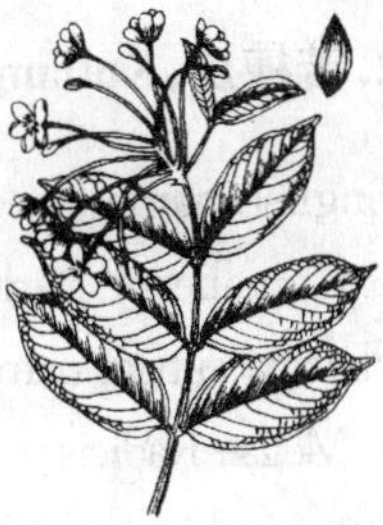

Indications: 1. ascarisis, enterobiasis and trichomonasis vaginalis

2. infantile malnutrition

使君子

Dosage: 9 ~ 15g. The stir-baked drug for swallow after chewing is 6 ~ 9g, give children, 1 ~ 1.5g per day for each year of age with the total not exceeding 20g. When using anthelmintics, on an empty stomach, take one time per day, for three days.

Contraindication: If it is taken in large amounts or taken with hot tea, it may give rise to reactions like hiccupping, dizziness, vomitting, diarrhea, etc. So large amounts of tea should be avoided when this drug is used.

Combinations: 1. add Szechwan Chinaberry Bark (苦楝皮, Kulianpi)——ascariasis and enterobiasis

2. add Chicken Gizzard Membrane (鸡内金, Jineijin), Medicated Leaven (神曲, Shenqu)——infantile malnutrition

Prescription: Fattening Baby Pill (肥儿丸, Feier Wan)

Notes: Rangooncreeper Fruit (使君子, Shijunzi) is sweet in taste and warm in property. This herb can kill worms, strengthen the spleen and treat infantile malnutrition. It is a major herb for poisoning and expelling ascarid. If it is taken in large amounts, it may give rise to reactions like hiccupping, etc, which will disappear spontaneously after quitting the herb. If necessary, take orally Clove Flower-bud (丁香, Dingxiang) or Licorice Root (甘草, Gancao).

2. 苦楝皮, Kulianpi

English name: Szechwan Chinaberry Bark

Pharmaceutical name: Cortex Meliae Radicis

Botanical name: Melia azedarach L. or M. toosendan Sieb. et Zucc.

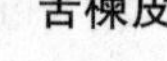

苦楝皮

Properties and tastes: bitter, cold, and poison.

Meridian tropism: liver, spleen and stomach.

Functions: 1. poison and expel parasites

2. treat tinea

3. antifungus

Indications: 1. ascariasis, enterobiasis, ancylostomiasis. It can be used to treat infantile ascaris, intestinal obstruction, ascariasis of biliary tract

2. trichomonasis vaginalis

3. tinea, scabies, eczema itching (external use)

Dosage: 6～9g. Use 15～30g if it is fresh.

Contraindication: This drug is poisonous, it should not be taken in large amounts or taken over a long period of time. It should be given caustiously to patients with deficiency of the spleen and stomach. It should not be prescribed to those with heart, liver, and kidney diseases.

Combinations: 1. add Rangooncreeper Fruit (使君子, Shijunzi), Areca Seed (槟榔, Binlang)——abdominal pain due to parasites

2. add Sessile Stemona Root (百部, Baibu), Smoked Plum (乌梅, Wumei)——enterobiasis

3. add Areca Seed (槟榔, Binlang)——ancylostomiasis

Notes: Szechwan Chinaberry Bark (苦楝皮, Kulianpi) is bitter in taste, cold in property and is poisonous. It is best used to treat ascariasis, and enterobiasis ancylostomiasis. The effect of this herb is better and more dependable than Rangooncreeper Fruit (使君子, Shijunzi). Toosendanin (川楝素, Chanliansu) is the main composition of this herb which excites intestinal muscle, therefore, it is not necessary to take with purgative herbs when expelling worms. In addition, it can treat tinea, and dry dampness. It can be used externally for scabies, and tinea.

3. 槟榔, Binlang

English name: Areca Seed

Pharmaceutical name: Semen Arecae Catechu

Botanical name: Areca catechu L.

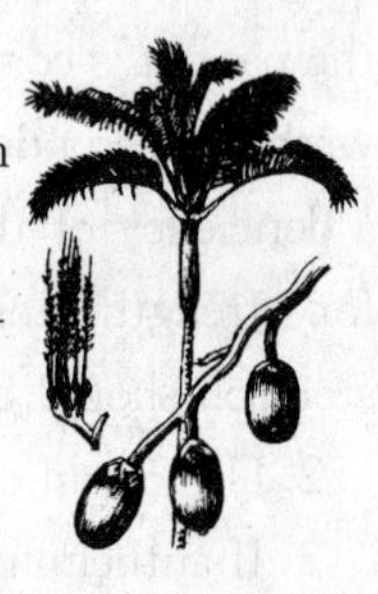

槟榔

Properties and tastes: acid, bitter, warm.

Meridian tropism: stomach and large intestine.

Functions: 1. expel parasites

2. laxative effect

3. promote qi circulation to remove stagnation

4. induce diuresis to alleviate edema

5. regulate function of gallbladder to remove calculus

6. increase intestinal peristalsis (excite M choline)

7. prevent attack of malaria

Indications: 1. parasitosis in the intestinal tract——expel and poison cestodiasis, fasciolopsiasis, ancylostomiasis, ascariasis, enterobiasis, etc. Expelling cestodiasis is its main function

2. dyspepsia——food retention and indigestion, abdominal distention, constipation.

Best used for food retention with qi stagnation. It also treats dysentery with tenesmus

3. edema of excessive type, swelling pain due to beriberi

4. malaria cyclic fever

5. gallbladder lithiasis

6. cholelithiasis

Dosage: 6 ~ 15g. It is used alone in treating cestodiasis and fasciolopsiasis with the dosage as much as 60 ~ 120g. To remove food stagnation, stir - baked preporction is better. The raw or unprepared herb is used for other purposes. Proper dosage for external use.

Contraindication: It is not suitable in the cases of deficiency of the spleen with loose stool.

Combinations: 1. add Pharbitis Seed(牵牛子, Qiannuzi)——many kinds of parasitosis in the intestinal tract, such as ascariasis, cestodiasis, and ancylostomiasis

2. add Cushaw Seed(南瓜子, Nanguazi)——cestodiasis

3. add Common Aucklandia Root(木香, Muxiang), Green Tangerine Peel(青皮, Qingpi)——food retention and stagnation of qi marked by abdominal distension, consitipation or dysentery with tenesmus

4. add Medicinal Evodia Root(吴茱萸, Wu zhuyu), Tangerine Peei(陈皮, Chenpi)——pain of beriberi

5. add Common Floweringquince Fruit(木瓜, Mugua), Fourstamen Stephania Root (防己, Fangji)——edema of beriberi

6. add Dang-shen Root(党参, Dangshen), Green Tangerine Peel(青皮, Qingpi), Tangerine Peel(陈皮, Chenpi)——intestinal paralysis after surgery

7. add Officinal Magnolia Bark(厚朴, Houpo), Caoguo(草果, Caoguo)——mountainous evil air, damp-toxin.

8. add Pokeberry Root(商陆, Shanglu), Oriental Waterplantain Rhizome(泽泻, Zexie)——edema of excess type

9. add Areca Peel(大腹皮, Dafupi)——dispelling ascites, for treatment of abdominal fullness and distension, tympanites, edema, oliguria due to stagnation of qi and water. It's also used for eructation with fetid odor, abdominal distention due to food stagnation

10. add Charred Hawthorn Fruit(焦山楂, Jiaoshancha)——abdominal distension and pain due to indigestion

11. add Rhubarb(大黄, Dahuang), Tumeric Root-tuber(郁金, Yujin)——gallbladder lithiasis

12. add Sweet Wormwood(青蒿, Qinghao)——malaria

Prescription: Decoction with Direct Effect on Mogum(达原饮, Dayuan Yin)

Notes: Areca Seed(槟榔, Binlang) can treat many kinds of parasitosis in the intestinal tract, such as astoaisis, fasciolopsiasis, ancylostomiasis, ascariasis, and enterobiasis. Its purgative function can help discharge the parasites. It is best used to treat cestodiasis and expel poison pork tapeworm. It has been used with Cushaw Seed(南瓜子, Nanguazi) to strengthen the effect to destroy tapeworm. Eye drops produced by Areca Seed(槟榔, Binlang) have effects of reducing miosis and intraocular pressure of glaucoma.

It is a good herb for mintic and has the function of relieving diarrhea, scattering qi blockage, promoting qi circulation and urination. *Compendium of Materia Medica* (《本草纲目》, Bencaogangmu) said: "Areca Seed(槟榔, Binlang) treats dysentery with tenesmus, heart and abdominal pain, difficulty in urination and constipation, phlegm qi, asthma, malaria, prevents subtropical disease."

Zhang Bingcheng (张秉成) explained: "descending qi is the major function. It could be used for all diseases of viscera qi stagnation. Removing phlegm and dispersing water due to qi descent; removing food stagnation due to scattering qi blockage." So, descending qi and scattering qi blockage are Areca Seed (槟榔, Binlang)'s major functions.

Appendix: 大腹皮, Dafupi

English name: Areca Peel

Pharmaceutical name: Pericarpium Arecae Catechu

Botanical name: Areca catechu L.

Properties and tastes: bitter, slightly warm

Meridian tropism: spleen, stomach and small intestine

大腹皮

Functions: 1. promote qi circulation to alleviate stagnation in the Middle-jiao

2. induce diuresis to alleviate edema

Indications: 1. abdominal distension——abdominal distension and fullness, dyschesia, vomiting due to stagnation of qi in the stomach and intestine

2. edema——edema of light type, especially subcutaneous dropsy

Dosage: 3~15g

Contraindication: It sould not be used in disease with qi deficiency.

Combinations: 1. add Officinal Magnolia Bark (厚朴, Houpo), Wrinkled Gianthyssop Herb stem (藿香梗, Huoxianggeng)——abdominal distension and fullness due to stagnation of qi and retention of dampness, pyrexias malaria

2. add Areca Seed (槟榔, Binlang)——ascites, abdominal distension, edema of legs, dysuria, abdominal distension and fullness due to stagnation of qi and food retention

3. add Common Floweringquince Fruit (木瓜, Mugua) Perilla Leaf (紫苏, Zisu)——edema and fullness of beriberi due to dampness stagnation

4. add White Mulberry Root-bark (桑白皮, Sangbaipi)——dropsy, dysuria

5. add Officinal Magnolia Bark (厚朴, Houpo), Capillary Wormwood Herb (茵陈蒿, Yinchenhao)——chronic hepatitis, abdominal distension and fullness due to indigestion, dyschesia

Prescriptions: 1. Herbal Agastachis Powder for Restoring Healthy Energy (藿香正气散, Huoxiangzhengqi San)

2. Decoction of Peel of Five Drugs (五皮饮, Wupi Yin)

Notes: Areca Peel (大腹皮, Dafupi) is Areca Seed (槟榔, Binlang)'s peel, it has the same major functions as Areca Seed (槟榔, Binlang). Howevre it can not descend qi. It can excite the spleen to promote urination. It is used for promoting qi circulation to resolve dampness. Together with aromatic herbs, it can resolve dampness. It can treat edema by promoting urination. It can be used with bland drugs to induce diuresis.

4. 南瓜子, Nanguazi

English name: Cushaw Seed

Pharmaceutical name: Semen Cucurbitae Moschatae

Botanical name: Cucurbita moschata Duch.

Properties and tastes: sweet, neutral

Meridian tropism: stomach, large intestine

Functions: anthelmintic function

Indications: cestodiasis, ascariasis, and schistosomiasis

Dosage: 60～120g

Combinations: add Areca Seed (槟榔, Binlang)——ascariasis, cestodiasis, schistosomiasis of acute and advanced stage, especially for those who are not preferable to the treatment of antimonials.

南瓜子

Notes: Cushaw Seed (南瓜子, Nanguazi) can kill parasitosis, if it is used alone. If it is used together with Areca Seed (槟榔, Binlang), its action against tapeworms can be strengthened, Cushaw Seed (南瓜子, Nanguazi) 60～120g (unprepared with husk), ground into fine powder, mix with cold boiled water: two hours later, the decoction of 60～120g Areca Seed (槟榔, Binlang) is administered orally and 15g Mirabilite (芒硝, Mangxiao) infusion follows another half hour later to help discharge the parasites. In addition, It can also treat schistosomiasis and promote lactation.

Appendix: Other Anthelmintics

Name	Properties and tastes	Meridian tropism	Functions	Indications	Dosage	Contraindication
Hairvein Agrimonia Herb (鹤草芽, Hecaoya)	bitter, stringing and cool	Liver, small intestine and large intestine	Anthelmintic function, purgation	An important drug for expelling and poisoning cestodiasis. Also for vaginal trichomoniasis and dysentery.	Not for decoction. 30～50g for adults. 0.7～0.8g per kilogram for children. Ground into powder and swallow on an empty stomach in the morning.	A slight nausea and vomiting after taking the drug.
Stone-like Omphalia (fungus) (雷丸, Leiwan)	bitter, cold, slightly poisonous	Stomach and large intestine	Anthelmintic function	Cestodiasis, hookworm, ascariasis	6～15g for pill and powder. 12～18g of powder for cestodiasis, three times a day, take 3 days.	
Common Carpesium Fruit (鹤虱, Heshi)	bitter, pungent, medium slightly poisonous	Spleen and stomach	Anthelmintic function	Many kinds of parasitosis in the intestinal tract.	6～15g	Reactions of dizziness, nausea, tinnitus and abodiminal pain which can be disappeared themselves.
Grand Torreya Seed (榧子, Feizi)	medium and sweet	Lung and large intestine	Anthelmintic function, moisten lung to relieve cough	Many kinds of parasitosis in the intestinal tract, cough due to lung-dryness	30～50g	Don't use in condition of phlegm and cough due to lung-heat. It is not proper to take with Mung bean (绿豆, Lüdou)

Name	Properties and tastes	Meridian tropism	Functions	Indications	Dosage	Contraindication
Bigfruit Elm Fruit (芜荑, Wuyi)	pungent, bitter and warm	Spleen and stomach	Anthelmintic function, remove accumulation	Abdominal pain due to parasite, diarrhea due to infantile malnutrition. External use for tinea and malignant boil.	3～9g for pill and powder.	Not used for deficient spleen, stomach
Male Fern Rhizome (贯众, Guanzhong)	bitter and little cold	Liver and spleen	Anthelmintic function, clear away heat, detoxicate and stop bleeding	Many kinds of parasitosis in the intestinal tract, cold of wind-heat, skin eruption, mumps, bleeeding due to blood heat.	9 ～ 15g. Parching into charcoal for stop bleeding. Unprepared use for others.	It is not proper to use in cases of yin deficiency with interior heat and deficiency cold of spleen and stomach. The drug produced in the north-east China is poisonous. Don't use it for women in pregnancy, infants and digestive ulcer patients. Do not eat oily food when the drug is used.

Chapter 18
Drugs for External Use

Definition: Drugs which are mainly used externally are called drugs for external use.

Function: These drugs have the functions of eliminating toxic material, subduing swelling, promoting pus discharge, promoting tissue regeneration, killing worms and relieving itching, etc.

Indications: They can be use for skin infections, scabies, tinea, traumatic injury, insect and poisonous snakebite, disease of the five sense organs, etc.

As the above mentioned diseases occur in different part of the body. The application methods of the drugs for external use are various, such as plaster, external application, fumigation, insufflation, nasal drip and eye drip, etc. Some drugs can be used internally. But pharmacological actions between internal use and external use are quite different. Special attentin must be paid to this fact.

Notes: Quite a few drugs in this group have toxicity. They should be used with caution. On one hand, pay attention to processing and dispensing methods; on the other hand, strictly controlled the dosage to prevent poisoning.

In addition, some drugs are difficult to be classified, so they are listed at the end of this chapter.

1. 硫黄, Liuhuang

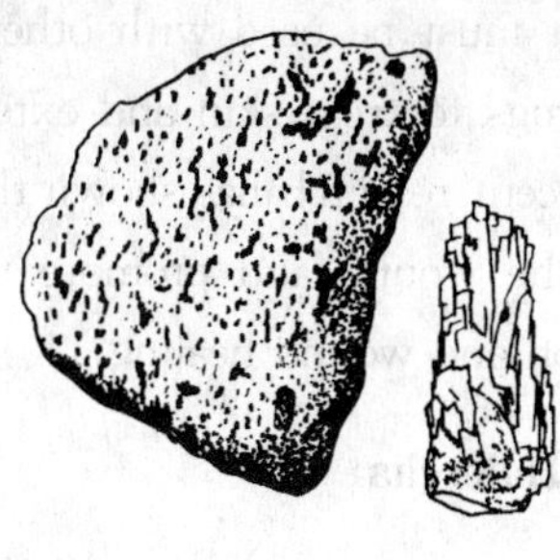

硫 黄

English name: Sulfur

Pharmaceutical name: Sulphur

Properties and tastes: sour, warm, and poisonous

Meridian tropism: kidney, large intestine

Functions: 1. external use for eliminating toxic material, killing worms, relieving itching

2. internal use for tonifying fire, strengthening yang and relaxing bowels

3. relieve cough and expel phlegm

Indications: 1. scabies, tinea, eczema, itching

2. nephritis due to yang-deficiency of the spleen and the kidney

3. asthma due to deficiency of the kidney yang, failure in receiving qi such as chronic obstructive emphysema

4. impotence-insufficiency of the kidney yang, complicated by frequent urination, cold and pain of the loins and legs, etc.

5. deficient cold constipation

Dosage: Proper amount for external use, it is ground into powder then scattered on the affected areas; or mixed with oil or smoked. Internal use 1～3g, used in pill or powder

Contraindication: It is not advisable for yin deficiency with fire, and women in pregnancy.

Combinations: 1. add Prepared Daughter Root of Commom Monkshood (附子, Fuzi), Cassia Bark (肉桂, Rougui)——cold asthma

2. add Hairy Antler (鹿茸, Lurong), Malaytea Scurfpea Fruit (补骨脂, Buguzhi)——impotence due to kidney yang deficiency

3. add Pinellia Rhizome (半夏, Banxia)——constipation of deficiency-cold type

Notes: Its external use is for killing worms, relieving itching due to scabies, tinea, and eczema. For example, In *A Handbook of Prescriptions for Emergencies* (《肘后方》, Zhouhoufang), Sulfur (硫黄, Liuhuang) is ground into powder, mixed with seasame oil and applied externally to treat scabies. *General Collection for Holy Relief* (《圣济总录》, Shengjizonglu) recorded that use it with efflores cence carbon, ninium, then grind them into powder, mix the powder with oil, then apply it externally to treat wet-tinea. For treatment of labial or scrotum itching, use Sulfur (硫黄, Liuhuang) 3g, smoke it by fire for one hour per time, one time per day or every two days.

Li Shizhen (李时珍) said: "Sulfur (硫黄, Liuhuang) was characterized by pure-yang and it is very hot in property, used for tonifying the fire of gate of life. It can regulate the large intestine." It is used in Black Tin Pill (黑锡丹, Heixi Dan) to treat deficient cold of the Lower-jiao, and improve inspiration by attracting the kidney qi downward. It is used in Pill of Pinellia Rhizome and Sulfur (半硫丸, Banliu Wan) to activate yang and expel turbidity for treating deficient constipation of the old.

2. 炉甘石, Luganshi

English name: Calamine

Pharmaceutical name: Smithsonitum

Properties and tastes: sweet, medium

Meridian tropism: liver, stomatch

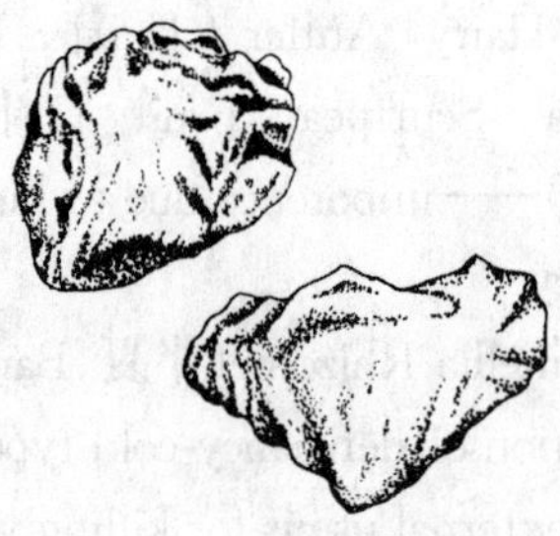

炉甘石

Functions: 1. eliminate toxic material, improve eyesight, relieve nebula

2. astringe dampness, promote tissue regeneration and wound healing

Indications: 1. eye disease——conjunctival congestion, nebula, marginal blepharitis, pterygium dryness sensation in the eye, photophobia and delacrimation(eye drip)

2. skin disease——unhealed ulcer, skin eczema, cracked nipple(external use)

Dosage: Proper amount for external use, grind into powder to sprinkle over affected eye, refine powder with water to drip the eye.

Combinations: 1. add Mirabilite(芒硝, Mangxiao)——sudden conjunctival congestion(eye drip)

2. add Cuttle Bone(海螵蛸, Haipiaoxiao)——eye diseases(ground into powder, eye drip)

3. add Acacia Catechu(孩儿茶, Haiercha)——wound of valvae(powder, mixed with sesame oil)

4. add Clam Shell(海蛤壳, Haigeqiao)——pruritus valvae(ground into powder, external use)

6. add Ophicalcite(花蕊石, Huaruishi), Mirabilita Crystal(寒水石, Hanshuishi)——cracked nipple(ground into powder)

Notes: Calamine(炉甘石, Luganshi) is a major drug that treats eye diseases and itching skin. Its medicinal effect is gentle. The effect of eliminating toxic material is not strong. It must be used with other detoxicating drugs to treat skin and external diseases. Recent research has shown that it can protect the wound and promote tissue regeneration and wound healing.

3. 孩儿茶, Haiercha

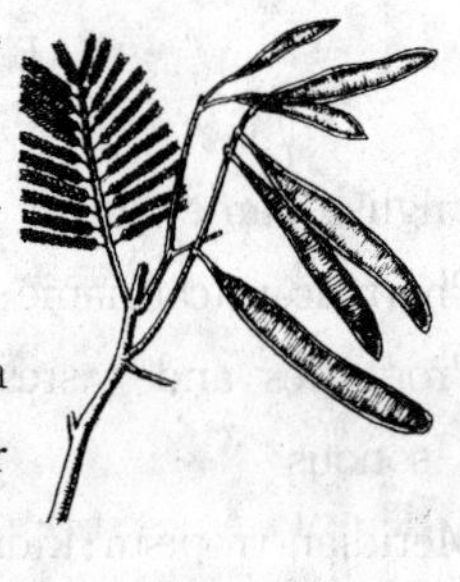

孩儿茶

English name: Acacia Catechu

Pharmaceutical name: Acacia seu Uncaria

Botanical name: Acacia catechu(L.) Willd. Or Uncaria gambier Roxb.

Properties and tastes: bitter, astringent, cold

Meridian tropism: lung

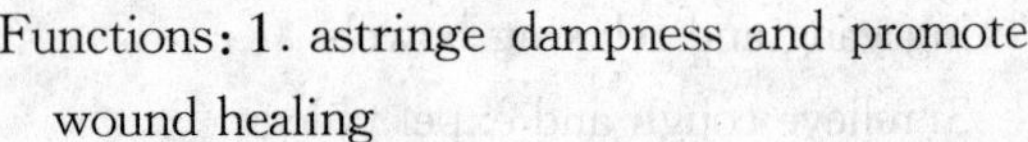

Functions: 1. astringe dampness and promote wound healing

2. promote tissue regeneration, arrest bleeding

3. quench the lung heat, remove phlegm

4. promote the production of the body fluid and relieve cough

5. astringe the intestine to correct diarrhea

6. promote blood circulation to help treat the wound

Indications: 1. skin and external diseases——moist ulcer with drainage, carbuncle and cellulitis, unhealed ulcer, malnutrition involving the teeth, aphthosis, chancre, wound of valvae, swelling and pain of hemorrhoid (Extenal use)

2. blood diseases——hematemesis, epistaxis, hematochezia, metrorrhagia and metrorrhagia, traumatic hemorrhage

3. cough and asthma due to lung heat

4. impairment of the body fluid, thirst due

to heat during summer months

5. infantile dyspepsia, diarrhea and dysentery.

6. digestive tract ulcer.

7. chyluria

8. traumatic injury, swelling and pain

Dosage: Proper dosage for external use, grind it into powder and apply the powder on the affected area, or mix it with rice wine for external application. Intenal use for 0.1～1g in pill or powder.

Combinations: 1. add Dragon's Blood(血竭, Xuejie), Frankincense(乳香, Ruxiang), Myrrh(没药, Moyao)——skin and external diseases resistant to healing(ground into powder for external use)

2. add Borax(硼砂, Pengsha)——ulcerative gingivitis, aphthosis(divided equally then applied on)

3. add Pearl(珍珠, Zhenzhu) and Borneol(冰片, Bingpian)——chancre(ground into powder for external application)

4. add Calcining Dragen's Bone(煅龙骨, Duanlonggu), Dragon's Blood(血竭, Xuejie), Bletilla Rhizome(白及, Baiji)——bleeding of traumatic injury(ground into powder for external application)

5. add Calcining Dragen's Bone(煅龙骨, Duanlonggu), Borneol(冰片, Bingpian)——moist ulcer, fluid discharge(external use)

6. add Snakegourd Fruit(瓜蒌, Gualou)——cough due to lung heat

7. add Dwarf Lilyturf Root(麦门冬, Maimendong)——impairment of the body fluid, thirst due to summer heat

8. add Sanchi Root(三七, Sanqi)——injury hemorrhage

9. add Red Halloysite(赤石脂, Chishizhi)——diarrhea and dysentery

Notes: Acacia Catechu(孩儿茶, Haiercha) is bitter, astringent, and cold. It can be used externally or internally. External use for astringing dampness and relieving boils, relieving pain and arresting bleeding indicated for unhealed ulcer, pus, injury bleeding, aphthae in children, ulcerative gingivitis, and chancre.

Internal use for quenching the lung heat in Upper-jiao, removing phlegm and promoting the production of body fluid, indicated for cough due to lung heat, thirst due to summer heat and bleeding.

4. 斑蝥, Banmao

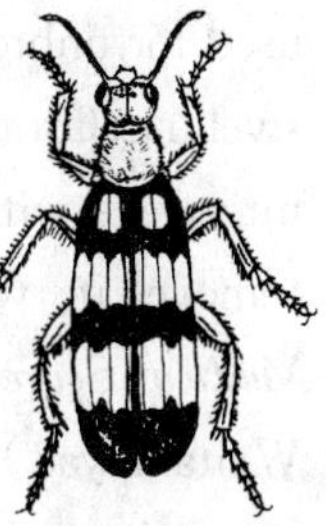

English name: Large Blister Beetle

Pharmaceutical name: Mylabris

Botanical name: Mylabris phalerata Pallas

斑蝥

Properties and tastes: pungent, cold, and very poisonous

Meridian tropism: large intestine, small intestine, liver, and kidney

Functions: 1. eliminate toxic material and corrode boils

2. scatter blood stasis and scatter blockage

Indications:

1. wound and tinea——carbuncle, cellulitis, syphilis, obstinate tinea, multiple abscess and scrofula, neurodermatitis, common wart, ect.

2. abnormal amenorrhea due to blood stasis, abdominal mass

3. carcinoma——best for primary liver carcinoma, it is also used for cancer of the rectum, and cancer of the colon, cancer of the esophagus

Dosage: Proper amount for external use, it is

ground into powder then applied on in order to induce blister, or soaked in wine or in vingar then spread on. Internal use: 0.03～0.06g in pill or powder.

Combinations: 1. add Alum (白矾, Baifan), Natural Indigo(青黛,Qingdai)——multiple abscess, scrofula, and fissure (ground into powder, spill the dry powder on the wound) 2. add Peach Kernel (桃仁, Taoren), Rhubarb(大黄,Dahuang)——amenorrhea

Notes: It is very poisonous. External use for inducing blistering and red skin and boils. Renzhai's *Straightforward Prescriptions* (《仁斋直指方》, Renzhaizhizhifang): "It is used for unbroken carbuncle and cellulitis's swelling. Ground into powder, then pounded into paste with garlic. Apply to the wound, remove it when the skin swells." *The Medical Secrets an official* (《外台秘要》, Waitaimiyao): "It is used for obstinate tinea, the powder of the baked herb mixed with Honey (蜂蜜, Fengmi) can be applied." *A Comprehensive Summary of Chinese Medical Prescriprions* (《医方大成论》, Yifangdachenglun): "Take 21 pieces of Large Blister Beetle (斑蝥, Banmao), add one-spoon glutinous rice, bake three times, discard Large Blister Beetle (斑蝥, Banmao), grind rice into powder, take after being mixed with cold water on empty stomah. Recently, it has been used for different kinds of carcinmoa." *Chinese Materia Medica Dictionaly* (《中药大辞典》, Zhongyaodacidian) says: "For treatment of liver cancer, stomach cancer, scratch a hole on an egg, put in 1～3 pieces of Large Blister Beetle(斑蝥, Banmao) which do not have the head, feet and wing, roast the egg, then discard Large Blister Beetle (斑蝥, Banmao), eat the egg, one egg every day." In recent years, internal use of cantharidin for treating liver cancer; external use of alcohol preparation of Large Blister Beetle (斑蝥, Banmao) for neurodematitis, etc. All obtain good curative effects.

Large Blister Beetle (斑蝥, Banmao) is used to induce blisters. It is used to treat facial paralysis, infantile asthma, and wind damp arthritis. Soak it in wine before it is externally to treat alpecia areata.

5. 毛茛 Maogen

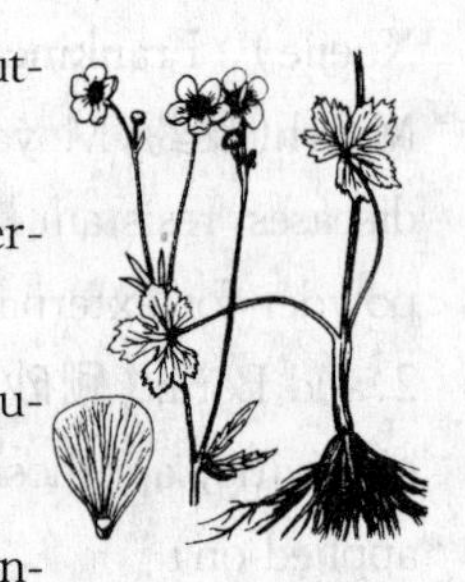
毛 茛

English Name: Japanese Buttercup Herb

Pharmaceutical name: Herba Ranunculi Japonici

Botanical name: Ranunculus japonicus Thunb.

Properties and tastes: pungent, warm, havepoisonous

Meridian tropism: not known

Functions: 1. induce blistering

2. relieve pain

3. prevent attack of malaria

4. relieve asthma

5. corrode boils, remove pus, counteract toxic material and kill worms

Indications: 1. It is cold moxibustion in traditional Chinese medicine in which common fresh ranunculus japonicus thunb can be pounded into paste for topical application on the affected part or acupoint. This can induce blisters with the effects of expelling wind dampness evil, removing obstruction of meridians and relieving pain. Indicated for many types of pain due to wind-cold-dampness and injury, toothache, migraine, conjunctivitis, also for asthma, bronchitis of gasp and malaria as it has the actions of relieving asthma and preventing an attack.

2. wound, multiple abscess, scrofula, tinea, leprosy

Dosage: Proper amout for external use. Fresh herb is pounded into paste or dry drug is ground into powder for application. Applied on the affected part or place on the acupoints. After blistering, the small blisters one stabbed and broken, the biglers are stabbed to discharge water. Make sure to manipulate asepticly and protect surface of wound.

Contraindication: atilize aseps is use casguly in patients wivh derional sevs tioily. Not for internal use.

Notes: *Renew of Herbal Medicine* (《本草推陈》, Bencaotuichen) said: "Many herbs are used externally but have internal curative effects in traditional Chinese medicine. The effect of Japanese Buttercup Herb (毛莨, Maogen) is the most remarkable. It is easy to apply and widely used. Japanese Buttercup Herb(毛莨, Maogen) is mainly for external use. Apply it on the affected part or acupoint. The therapeutic effect is developed directly or indirectly. The function of inducing blisters newly processed Japanese Buttercup Herb(毛莨, Maogen) is very powerful, but it won't induce blisters if it is used 3 days later.

6. 大蒜, Dasuan

English name: Garlic Bulb

Pharmaceutical name: Bulbus Alli Sativi

Botanical name: Allium sativum L.

Properties and tastes: pungent, warm

Meridian tropism: spleen, stomach, and lung

Functions: 1. detumescentify and eliminate toxic material

2. kill worms

3. broad-spectrum antiseptic effect

4. relieve dysentery

5. anticarcinoma

6. reduce blood lipid and blood pressure

7. enhance body immunity

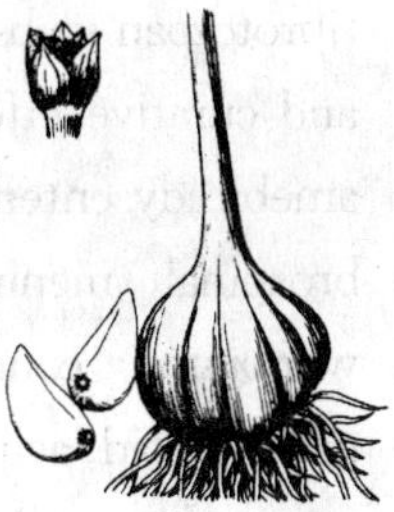

大蒜

Indications: 1. carbuncle, furuncle, scabies, tinea (cut into slices to spread on or pound into paste for external application)

2. infiltrative pulmonary tuberculosis, whooping cough

3. diarrhea, dysentery (treat and prevent)

4. ancylostomiasis, enterobiasis, trichomoniasis vaginalis, amebic vaginitis.

5. prevent hyperlipemia

6. advanced stage carcinoma

7. prevent and cure plumbism

8. prevent and cure influenza, epidemic encephalitis, and encephalitis B.

Dosage: Proper amount for external use, 3～5 pieces for internal use. Eat fresh garlic or boil it into decoction for use.

Contraindication: It should be used cautiously in cases of hyperactivity of fire due to yin deficiency, eye diseases, disease of tougue, throat, mouth, and teeth. It should not be applied for a long time because it makes the skin red and hot. Enema is not suitable for women during pregnancy.

Notes: Garlic Bulb (大蒜, Dasuan) is warm in property, and strong in taste. It is like a warm tonic to in vigorate the spleen, promote kidney and regulate five viscera through all orifices. It is a clearing herb, because it can detumescentify, and kill worms and relieve dysentery. The function of this herb is abstruse.

Garlic Bulb (大蒜, Dasuan) contains a large amount of antiseptic, antifungal and antiprotozoan substances. It has preventable and curative effects of bacillary dysentery, amebic dysentery, influenza, epidemic cerebrospinal meningome, lobar preumonia, whooping cough, diphtheria, typhoid, paratyphoid, acute appendicitis, otitis media suppurativa, trichomonal vaginitis, amebic vaginits, tinea scalp and oxyuriasis.

7. 蛇床子, Shechuangzi

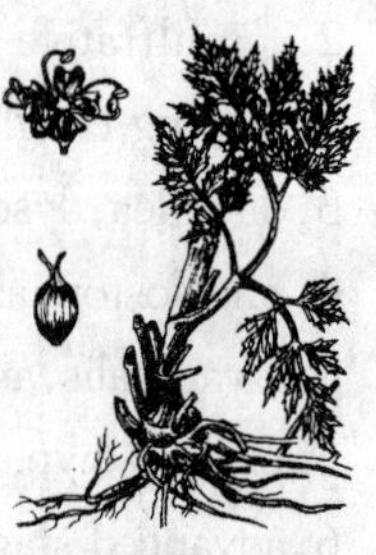
蛇床子

English name: Common Cnidium Fruit

Pharmaceutical name: Semen Cnidii Monnieri

Botanical name: Cnidium monnieri(L.)Cusson

Properties and tastes: pungent, bitter, warm.

Meridian tropism: kidney

Functions: 1. dry dampness and kills worms

2. expel cold and expel the wind

3. warm the kidney to strengthen yin

4. relieve asthma.

5. antifungus, antivirus

Indications: 1. disease due to kidney yang deficiency——impotence, sterility due to cold in the uterus, complicated by aversion to cold, cold limbs, valvae trichomonasis vaginalis, and valvae tine

2. leukorrhagia of cold dampness——profuse and thin leukorrhagia, cold of valvae

3. pain in the loins due to dampness——heavy and pain in the loins, and heavy on a cloudy day with rain

4. various infections on the body surface——eczema, exudative boils, scabies, tinea, tinea capitis

Dosage: internal use 3～9g, external use 15～30g

Contraindication: Exuberance of fire due to yin deficiency or heat dampness in the Lowerjiao should not be used internally.

Combinations: 1. add Chinese Magnoliavine (五味子, Wuweizi), Dodder Seed(菟丝子, Tusizi)——impotence, sterility due to cold in uterus

2. add Asiatic Comelian Cherry Fruit(山茱萸, Shanzhuyu), Chinese Magnoliavine(五味子, Wuweizi), Plantain Seed(车前子, Cheqianzi)——leucorrhagia of cold dampness

3. add Chinese Taxillus Twig(桑寄生, Sangjisheng), Eucommia Bark(杜仲, Duzhong), Largeleaf Gentian Root(秦艽, Qinjiao)——pain in the waist due to cold dampness

4. add Alum(白矾, Baifan)——pruritus valvae, eczema of scrotum(decoction for fumigation and washing)

5. add Chinese Corktree Bark(黄柏, Huangbai)——trichomonasis vaginalis made into suppository and put into vagina

6. add Chinese Corktree Bark(黄柏, Huangbai), Lightyellow Sophora Root(苦参, Kushen)——obstinate tinea, eczema (ground into powder, applied on after being mixed with oil)

Notes: The nature of Common Cnidium Fruit (蛇床子, Shechuangzi) is acid, bitter and warm. It can dry dampness. The function of Common Cnidium Fruit (蛇床子, Shechuangzi) may warm kidney to reinforce yang. It treats the various syndromes of yang asthenia and cold dampness. It may be used orally and externally. *A New Book of Materia Medica* (《本草新编》, Bencaoxinbian) said: "The nature of Common Cnidium Fruit(蛇床子, Shechuangzi) is very wonderful, the internal and external use may all be effective, but it is better for external use." *Transactions of Famous Physicians* (《名医别录》, Mingyibielu) said: "the function of it is warming the Middle-jiao to descend qi. It makes the woman uterine organ hot. It causes male priapism. It makes the color of face become good and the women pregnant." It is thus clear that Common Cnidium Fruit(蛇床子, Shechuangzi) is taken as a yang-strengthening drug. It may be fumigated and washed or as suppository. It can dry dampness, destroy parasites and relieve itching. It may treat the scrotum eczema. Normally the dosage for this drug is 15g to lavage vagina by decoction. Or using 30g of this drug, Chinese Corktree Bark(黄柏, Huangbai) 30g with glycerin taken as matrix to be made into suppositories of 2g's weight. Treat trichomonas vaginitis by putting one into the vagina everyday. This drug is also used to treat skin disease of scab and damp wound and so on. Besides external use, it may also be used oral administration.

8. 蟾酥, Chansu

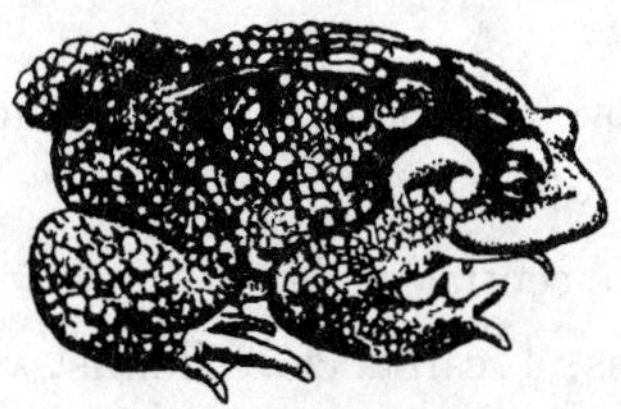

蟾 酥

English name: Toad Skin Secretion Cake

Pharmaceutical name: Secretio Bufonis

Properties and tastes: pungent, sweet, warm, poisonous

Botanical name: Bufo bufo gargarizans Cantor

Meridian tropism: heart

Functions: 1. eliminate toxic material, reduce swelling

2. anesthesia and alleviating pain

3. induce resuscitation and eliminate turbid evils

4. strengthening the heart

5. raising blood pressure

6. excite breathing

7. increase blood cell and resist radiation

8. resist carcinoma

9. improve immunity

10. promote urination, relieve congh, remove phlegm and relieve asthma

Indications: 1. carbuncle, cellulitis, skin infections, multiple abscess, scrofula, (external or internal use)

2. sore throat such as scarlet fever, acute throat trouble, tonsillitis and laryngopharyngitis

3. carcinoma——lung cancer, liver cancer, breast gland cancer, skin cancer and white blod cell disease

4. local anaesthesia to relieve pain——toothache, oral cavity and nasal cavity operation

5. coma due to acute filthy disease, abdominal pain, vomiting and diarrhea (smell it to sneeze)

Dosage: Proper amount for external use. Oral use for 0.015~0.03g in pill or powder.

Contraindication: Large dosage would be poisonous, do not use large dosage. This drug can contract the uterus, so pregnant women should not use it.

Combinations: 1. add Black Nightshade Herb (龙葵, Longkui)——liver cancer

2. add Spreading Hedyotis Herb(白花蛇舌草, Baihuasheshecao), Indian Mockstrawberry Herb (蛇莓, Shemei)——intestinal cancer

3. add Twig and Leaf of Fortune Plumyew (三尖杉, Sanjianshan), Glabrous Sarcandra Herb(肿节风, Zhongjiefeng)——leukemia

4. add Sulfur(雄黄,Xionghuang),Borax(硼砂,Pengsha),Licorice Root(甘草,Gancao)——toothache(local use)

5. add Common Monkshood' sMother Root(川乌,Chuanwu),Kusnezoff Monkshood Root(草乌,Caowu),Jackinthepulpit Tuber(天南星,Tiannanxing),Pinellia Rhizome(生半夏,Shengbanxia)——local anaesthesia,also for pain due to malignant tumor

6. add Musk(麝香,Shexiang)——inducing resuscitation and restoring consciousness,eliminating turbid evils and relieving pain, treat throat inflammation,acute filthy disease, abdominal pain, coma, infantile dyspepsia

7. add Musk(麝香,Shexiang),Ginseng(人参,Renshen),Sanchi Root(三七,Sanqi)——sinus syndrome

Prescription: Pill of Six Mirraculous Drugs(六神丸,Liushen Wan)

Notes: The Toad Skin Secretion Cake(蟾酥,Chansu) can be used in many aspects. It is used just a small amount but with remarkable effect. It is used for emergency treatment with pills or powder. The ancient people called it"assault toxic and disperse toxic", "inducing resuscitation, avoid evil, search evil", "pass through various places of twelve regular channels, viscera, tormogen, muscular interstice, joint and other places". It is thus clear that it is good at capturing and opening sowder. It is used for apoplectic coma and a sthenia syndrome. Modern time preparation injecta of the Dried Venom of Toads is used to treat circulation system disease and respiratory failure.

In addition, the Toad Skin(蟾皮,Chanpi) has acid taste, slightly cold property and is slightly poisonous. Its function is clearing away heat and detoxicating, dispelling water and removing distension. It is indicated for ulcer swelling toxic, infantile malnutrition, abdominal distension. It may be stuck in affected part by exodermis of fresh toad cake. Modern man uses it to treat cough with excessive phlegm or malignant tumour (cancer). Use 3~9g for oral administration, appropriate amount for external use, dried drug is for externally applied by levigation. Now it is made into injection for intravenous perfusion.

9. 马钱子, Maqianzi

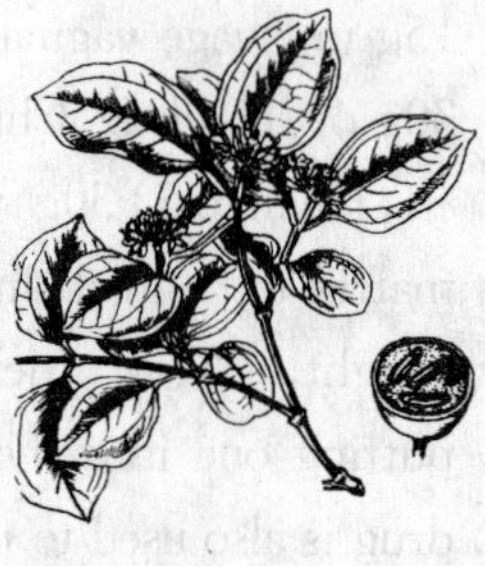

English name: Nux Vomica

Pharmaceutical name: Semen Strychnotis

Botanical name: Strychnos nux vomica L. or S. Wallichiana

马钱子

Properties and tastes: bitter, cold, and very poisonous

Meridian tropism: liver, spleen

Functions: 1. detumescentify and scatter blockage

2. remove obstruction in the collaterals and relieve pain

3. excite central nerve

Indications: 1. carbuncle, cellulitis, wound(external use)

2. sweeling pain of traumatic injury, arthritis, muscular constricture, paralysis.

3. myasthenia gravis and facial paralysis.

Dosage: Proper amount for external use. Internal use for 0.3~0.6g in pills and powder after processing.

Contraindication: The toxicity is reduced after processing. This drug can not be used internally for a long time or given in large doses. It sould not be prescribed to pregnant women. Be cautious when it is applied on mucous membrane of mouth.

Combinations:

1. add Liquorice(甘草, Gancao)——numbness of extremeties, hemiplegia

2. add Earth Worm (地龙, Dilong)——paralysis of respiratory muscle

Notes: Nux Vomica (马钱子, Maqianzi) contains strychnine of alkaloid etc. Over taking may lead to chemical poisoning. It makes nervous centralis first excited and then paralysis. It may lead to suffocation and death from catalepsy or respiratory paralysis. This drug must be processed for oral taking. Zhang Xichun(张锡纯) said: its poison is very strong, …its effect is removing obstruction from meridians and its strong effect can pass through the joints. So it is much move effective than other drugs. Generally the poisonous drugs treat disease, whether they are poison or drugs, their usage, dosage and preparation make a difference.

Nux Vomica (马钱子, Maqianzi) is also called Fanmubie(番木鳖, Fanmubie). Momordica Cochinchinensis(木鳖子, Mubiezi) is also called Tumubie(土木鳖, Tumubie). Do not confuse the two drugs. Momordica Cochinchinensis seed are bitter and slightly sweet in taste, and warm in property, and it is poisonous. It has the function of detumescentifying, scattering blockage and counteracting toxic material. It treats the carbuncle or abscess, furuncle, scrofula, hemorrhoids, prolapse of rectum, tinea and wound, arthritis pain, traumation etc. Proper amount is used for external use, grind it into powder for oral taking or grind the drug into juice for washing. It is 0.5～1g for oral taking in pills and powder. It is forbidden for pregnant women and the people who are weak.

10. 露蜂房, Lufengfang

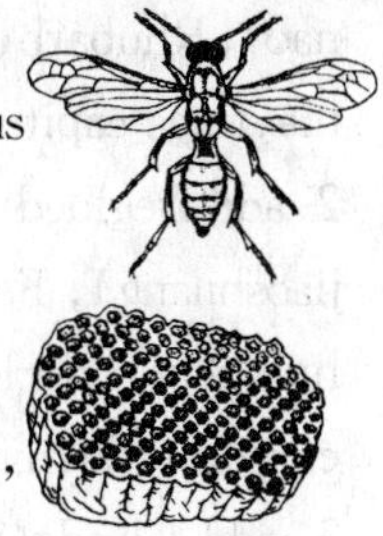

English name: Vasps Nest

Pharmaceutical name: Nidus Vespae

Botanical name: Polistes mandarinus Saussure

Properties and tastes: sweet, medium, poisnous

Meridian tropism: stomach, liver

露蜂房

Functions: 1. combat poison with poison

2. expel wind to relieve pain

3. destroy dermatozoon to relieve itching

4. antitumor

Indications: 1. carbuncle, cellulitis and wound——This herb can be used no matter hour long the duration is. This herb is especially good at treating mastadenitis

2. pruritus obscinate itching due to rubella, tinea. Add this herb based on the differentiation of symptoms and signs

3. pain due to arthritis caused by wind dampness——swelling of joints, even deformation. Add this herb to help enhance curative effect

4. multiple abscess and scrofula——sinus of scrofula with pus(external use)

5. cancer——oral administration compound prescription, treat carcinoma of breast, barynx, nasopharynx, lymphogenous metastasis, liver and stomach

6. pharyngitis, toochache, swelling pain of the tongue, external use to stop pain

Dosage: Appropriate amount for external use. 3～9g for oral administration, take decoction 1～2g per time, twice every day. It is used in pills and powder.

Contraindication: qi and blood deficiency are

not suitable

Combinations: 1. add Charred Human Hair(血余炭, Xueyutan), Camphor(樟脑, Zhangnao), Rhubarb(大黄, Dahuang)——ecthyma, tinea capitis, and scald

2. add Deglued Antler Powder(鹿角霜, Lujiaoshuang), Fennel Fruit(小茴香, Xiaohuixiang)——leukorrhea that failed to be cured by astringent drugs

3. add Cicada Slough(蝉蜕, Chantu)——itching of skin(divided equally, mixed with wine)

4. add Dried Alum(枯矾, Kufan)——itching of tinea(applied after being mixed with vinegar)

5. add Szechwan chinaberry Fruit(川楝子, Chuanlianzi), Green Tangerine Peel(青皮, Qingpi)——multiple abscess, scrofula, mastadenitis, breast carcinoma

6. add Scorpion(全蝎, Quanxie), Gecko(守宫, Shougong), Silkworm with Batrytis Larva(白僵蚕, Baijiangcan)——cancer

7. add Scorpion(全蝎, Quanxie), Centipede(蜈蚣, Wugong), Ground Beetle(土鳖虫, Tubiechong)——arthritis, osteomyelitis

8. add Gambirplant Hooked Stem and Branch(钩藤, Gouteng)——cough, manifested as red face, dyspnea, and tears while coughing intermittent

Notes: Nidus vespae(露蜂房, Lufengfang) is a poison that is used to combat poison. *Herbals for Easy Approaching* (《本草便读》, Bencaobiandu) said: "It has a function of treating suppurative osteomyelitis, mammary carcinoma etc. Remove them with it if the poisonous root affect viscera. *The Newly-revised Materia Medica* (《新修本草》, Xinxiubencao) and *Compendium of Materia Medica* (《本草纲目》, Bencaogangmu) record that the drug may treat "impotence". The drug seems to have the effect of tonifying the kidney and warming yang. Our ancestors were careful with oral use of this drug. It is often burnt into ash and ground into powder for external application. But modern man's experience proves that is has not been found toxic and hos no side effects in clinic with large oral dose(6～12g every day for decoction, 2～4g for powder every day.)

11. 丝瓜络, Sigualuo

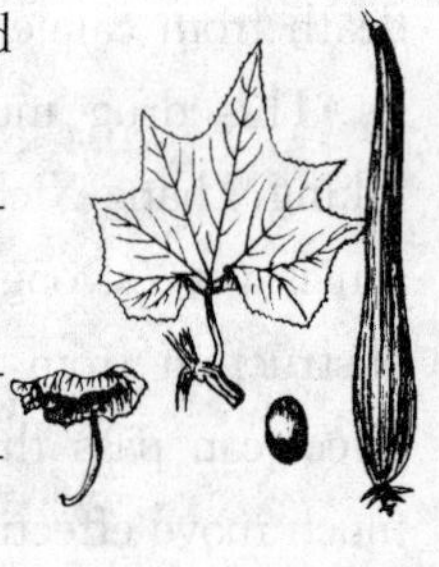

English name: Towel Gourd Vegetable Sponge

Pharmaceutical name: Fasciculus Vascularis Luffae

Botanical name: Luffa cylindrica(L.)or L. acutangula Roxb.

丝瓜络

Properties and tastes: sweet, neutral

Meridian tropism: lung, stomach, and liver

Functions: 1. detoxicate and remove phlegm

2. expel the wind to remove obstruction of collaterals

3. remove phlegm to relieve cough

4. stimulate and improve lactation

5. arrest bleeding

Indications: 1. carbuncle and skin wounds

2. arthritis due to wind dampness, muscular constricture

3. hypochondric pain

4. distending pain of women's breast, hypogalactia

5. coughing due to phlegm heat

6. hematochezia, massive and incessant metrorrhagia(backed until carbonized)

Dosage: internal use: 9～15g, decoct it or burn it into ash and grind into powder. Appropriate amount for external use.

Combinations: 1. add Mulberry Twig(桑枝, Sangzhi)——appoplexy, hemiplegia, muscular constricture

2. add Snakegourd Fruit (瓜蒌, Gualou)——coughing and chest pain

Notes: The nature of Towel Gourd Vegetable Sponge(丝瓜络, Sigualuo) is mild in effect. It has the function of removing obstruction of meridians, activating blood circulation, removing phlegm and guiding qi downward, but mainly dredging meridians. It is often used in a compound prescription in clinic.

12. 血竭, Xuijie

English name: Dragon's Blood

Pharmaceutical name: Sanguis Draconis

Botanical name: Daemonorops draco Bl.

Properties and tastes: sweet, salty, medium

血 竭

Meridian tropism: heart, liver

Functions: 1. for external use: arrest bleeding, promote tissue regeneration and wound healing

2. for oral use: promote blood circulation to relieve pain

Indications: 1. for external use: traumatic bleeding, chronic skin sores and swelling pain of hemorrhoid

2. for oral use: amenorrhea due to blood stasis, dysmenorrhea, alienation caused by lochioschesis after child birth, swelling pain due to blood stasis. It is also used for hemorrhage of the upper digestive tract and chronic rheumatic arthritis

Dosage: Proper amount for external use. Grind into powder and sprinkle over affeced area. 1～15g for oral medication used in powder.

Contraindication: Don't take this drug if there is no blood stasis. Women during pregnancy and in menstruation period, are forbidden to use this drug.

Combinations: 1. add Myrrh (没药, Moyao)——blood stasis in the abdomen, alienation caused by lochioschesis after child-birth

2. add Minium(铅丹, Qiandan)——syphilis for many years (powder for external liniment)

3. add Sanchi Root(三七, Sanqi)——coronary atheroslerotic cardiopathy and angina pectoris

Notes: The function of Dragon's Blood(血竭, Xuejie) is similar to that of labanotus and Myrrh(没药, Moyao), but it is mild, it is good at both internal and external use. So clinical doctors all like using it. *Essentials of Materia Medica* (《本草备要》, Bencaobeiyao) said: "Dragon's Blood (血竭, Xuejie) acts on the heart, liver and blood-stage, it is good at removing blood stasis. If it is used to stop pain and promote tissue regeneration the drug can stop pain by activating blood and can promote tissue vegeneration by removing blood stasis."

13. 樟脑, Zhangnao

English name: Camphor

Pharmaceutical name: Camphora

Botanical name: Cinnamomum camphora(L.) Presl

Properties and tastes: acid, hot, and poisonous

Meridian tropism: heart, spleen

樟 脑

Functions: 1. remove dampness to kill dermatozoon

2. warm to relieve pain

3. restore consciousness and eliminate turbid evils

4. antiseptic effect

Indications: 1. itching due to sarcoptidosis

2. skin and external diseases, swelling and pain of damp and worm area, forstbite (external use)

3. traumatic injury and toothache (external use)

4. aching due to acute filthy disease caused by cold－dampness and turbid evils

Dosage: Proper amounts for external use

0.1～0.2g for oral administration used in powder or melted in wine.

Contraindication: Don't use in condition of qi and yin deficiency, heat evils in the body. Women during pregnancy are forbidden to use. This herb is poisonous, take cautions when it is used orally.

Combinations: 1. add Borax (硼砂, Pengsha)——bed sores (melt in alcohol for external application)

2. add Alumen (明矾, Mingfan), Mirabilite (芒硝, Mangxiao)——itching of anus (add water for demibain)

Notes: Camphor (樟脑, Zhangnao) has the function of clearing the nasal passage and dispersing cold damp. It may lead to respiratory failure and death (7～15g for oral taking and 4g for muscular injection). Therefore it has little use for oral taking. Its dosage is not even large for external use to treat skin ulcers in order to avoid stimulated pain.

14. 瓦楞子, Walengzi

English name: Ark Shell

Pharmaceutical name: Concha Arcae

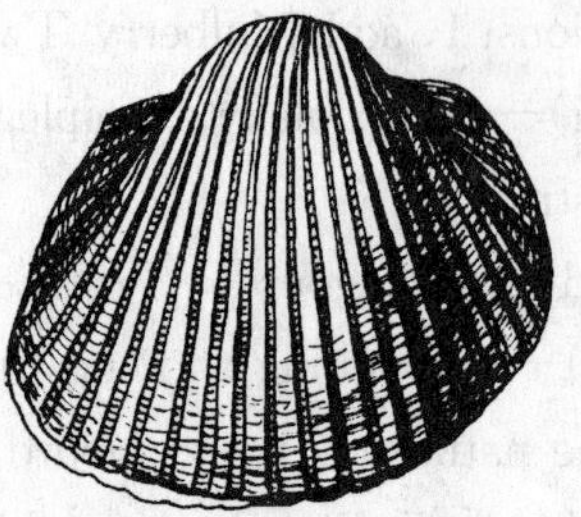

瓦楞子

Botanical name: Arca granosa Linnaeus, Arac subcrenata Lischke

Properties and tastes: salty, medium

Meridian tropism: lung, stomach, liver

Functions: 1. expel phlegm and remove stasis

2. resolve the hard lumps

3. relieve hyperacidity to relieve pain

Indications: 1. multiple abscess and scrofula, goiter

2. abdominal masses (This herb is used for hepatosplenomegaly and tumor of the digestive tract in recent years)

3. stubborn phlegm and chronic coughing

4. stomachache and acid regurgitation. This herb is used to treat gastroduodenal ulcer in recent years.

Dosage: 9～30g, It should be decocted for a long time. 1～3g per time in pill or powder. The unprocessed herb is suitable for eliminating phlegm and scattering blockage; the calcined herb is suitable for relieving hyperaciding to relieve pain.

Combinations: 1. add Common Selfheal Fruitspike (夏枯草, Xiakucao), Tendrilleaf Fritillary Bulb (贝母, Beimu)——multiple abscess and scrofula

2. add Zedoray (莪术, Ezhu), Common Burreed Rhizome (三棱, Sanleng)——hepetosplenomegaly

3. add Cuttle Bone (乌贼骨, Wuzeigu), Tangerine Peel (橘皮, Jupi)——stomachache

and acid regurgitation

4. add Licorice Root(甘草, Gancao)——gastroduodenal ulcer

Notes: Ark Shell(瓦楞子, Walengzi) can soften hard mass with salty. It may clear all phlegmatic retention, blood retention, qi stagnation. It has weak power when using it alone. Put it in prescription for the disease to use.

15. 守宫, Shougong

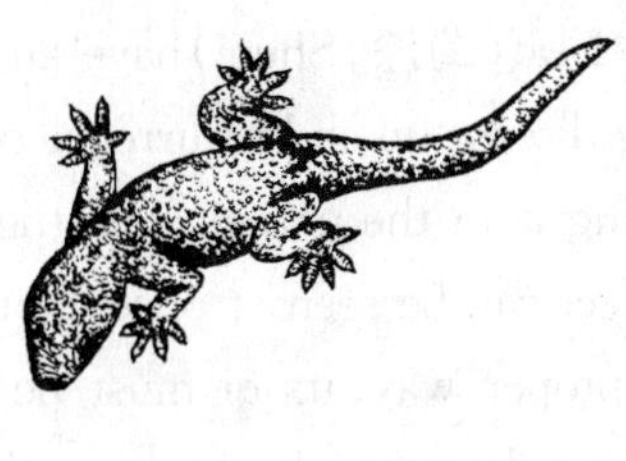

守 宫

English name: Gecko

Properties and tastes: salty, cold, and slightly poisonous

Meridian tropism: liver, stomach, and spleen

Functions: 1. scatter blockage and detoxicate

2. expel the wind to remove obstruction of collaterals

3. relieve pain and arrest convulsion

4. inhibit tuberculomyces

5. antitumor

Indications: 1. multiple abscess, scrofula, subcutaneous noelules——internal use for unbroken abscess; external use for broken abscess. For treatment of sinus of abscess, insert tail of live Gecko(守宫, Shougong) into the bottom of sinus in order to induce drainage. For treatment of other tuberculous sores, it also has effects of detoxication, eliminating the rooten, scattering blockage and subduing swelling.

2. carbuncle and skin wounds(external use)

3. various tumors, especially for the digestive system tumor and malignant lymphoma

4. arthritis due to wind dampness

5. lockjaw and opisthotonus of tetanus, muscular constricture

6. infantile convulsion due to phlegm heat

Dosage: appropriate amounts for external use; 3～6g for oral decoction; 1～2g for pulverization and pill or powder

Contraindication: Although this herb is slightly poisonous, the side-effect does not occurred in oral medication

Combinations: 1. add Centipede(蜈蚣, Wugong)——tuberculous sores

2. add Toad(蟾蜍, Chanchu), Black Nightshade Herb(龙葵, Longkui)——hepatocarcinoma

3. add Glabrous Sarcandra Herb(肿节风, Zhongjiefeng), Centipede (蜈蚣, Wugong)——carcinoma of stomach

4. add Umbellate Pore Fungus(猪苓, Zhuling), Tokin Sophora Root(山豆根, Shandougen)——pulmonary carcinoma

5. add Frankincense(乳香, Ruxiang), Myrrh(没药, Moyao), Opium Poppy Pericarp(罂粟壳, Yingsuqiao)——hand and feet paralysis, migratory pain.

6. add Cinnabar(朱砂, Zhusha), Musk(麝香, Shexiang)——infantile convulsion due to heart deficiency

Notes: Gecko(守宫, Shougong) can expel wind and arrest convulsion penetrate tendons to collaterals, combat poison for poison, arrest couvulsion and relieves epilepsy, its function is as Centipede(蜈蚣, Wugong), Scorpion (全蝎, Quanxie), but it has cold property. It can treat multiple abscess, skin and external disease for oral taking or external use, particularly wound ulceration pain or ruptured leading to fistula. Modern research has shown that Gecko(守宫, Shougong) has an effect of antitubercular and anticancer.

16. 常山, Changshan

English name: Antifebrile Dichroa Root

Pharmaceutical name: Radix Dichorae Febrifugae

Botanical name: Dichora febrifuga Lour.

Properties and tastes: acrid, bitter, cold, poisonous

常 山

Meridian tropism: lung, heart, and liver

Functions: 1. vomit phlegmatic saliva

2. prevent attack of malaria

3. reduce fever

4. antitumor

Indications: 1. malaria——Antifebrile Dichroa Root (常山, Changshan) has good effect on alternate breaking out of chill and fever in all sorts of malaria

2. phlegmatic accumulation in the chest——fullness and distending pain of chest and diaphragm due to phlegmatic saliva accumulation in the chest and diaphragm

Dosage: 6～9g The crude herb is preferable for vomiting, the alcohol baked herb is preferable for preventing attacks of malaria

Contraindication: use caustiously where there is body deficiency

Combinations: 1. add Licorice Root (甘草, Gancao)——vomiting due to phlegmatic saliva in the chest

2. add Areca Seed (槟榔, Binlang)——malaria

Preseription: Drink of Seven Kinds of Treasure for Preventing the Attack of Malaria (截疟七宝饮, Jienueqibao Yin)

Notes: Root of Antipyretic Dichroa (常山, Changshan) is seldom used as emetic. It gets a curative effect for fever caused by exogenous disease and cold heat complex as in malaria.

The spear and spray of Root of Antipyretic Dichroa is called ramulus dichroae. Its taste and effect is as well as those of Root of Antipyretic Dichroa, but its power is better than Root of Antipyretic Dichroa. Its dosage is 3 ～ 6g, *Compendium of Materia Medica* (《本草纲目》, Bencaogangmu) said: Antifebrile Dichroa Root (常山, Changshan) and Antifebrile Dichroa Branchlet and Leaf (蜀漆, Shuqi) have an effect of holding disease up and recurrence of malaria …, Using it in the proper way, the miraculous effect can be seen at once. Not using it in the proper way, its qi must be injured. Using raw drug may lead to vomiting of reversed qi. It has slow flow of qi by using the drug, which is decocted or fried with wine. Using small dosage doesn't lead to vomiting.

17. 皂角刺, Zaojiaoci

English Name: Chinese Honeylocust Spine

Pharmaceutical name: Spina Gleditsiae

Botanical name: Gleditsia sinensis Lam.

Properties and tastes: acid, warm

皂角刺

Meridian tropism: liver, stomach

Functions: 1. relieve swelling and promote pus discharge

2. expel the wind and destroy dermatozoon

Indications: 1. the beginning of carbuncle and cellulitis, unbroken pus and woman's mastadenitis

2. acute tonsillitis

3. leprosy, obstinate tinea

Dosage: 3～9g

Contraindication: Donot use for patients with broken carbuncle and cellulitis.

Combinations: 1. add Honeysuckle Flower(金银花, Jinyinhua), Licorice Root(甘草, Gancao)——the beginning of carbuncle and cellulitis

2. add Membranous Milkvetch Root(黄芪, Huangqi), Frankincense(乳香, Ruxiang)——unbroken wound, carbuncle.

3. add Siberian Cocklebur Fruit(苍耳子, Cangerzi)——leprosy

4. add Densefruit Pittany Root-bark(白鲜皮, Baixianpi)——itching due to obstinate tinea

5. add Pangolin Scales(穿山甲, Chuanshanjia)——unbroken carbuncle and cellulities

Prescritption: Powder for Promoting Pus Discharge(透脓散, Tounong San)

Notes: The nature of Chinese Honeylocust Spine(皂角刺, Zaojiaoci) is acid, dispersing and warm. Its property is comparatively sharp, it has an effect of detumescentifying and evacuating pus. It is used for carbuncle or abscess, and swelling toxie. It can remove the ripe carbuncle. It is often used in surgical departments.

Appendix: chemical components of externally used mineral drugs

Realgar(雄黄, Xionghuang)——arsenic sulfide(As_S)

Auripigmentum(雌黄, Cihuang)——arsenic trisulfide(As_2S_3)

Arsenolite Ore(砒石, Pishi)——arsenic trioxide(As_2O_3)

Calomeas(轻粉, Qingfen)——mercurous chloride(Hg_2Cl_2)

Mercuric Oxide－Mixture(升药, Shengyao)——mercuric oxide(HgO)

Minium(铅丹, Qiandan)——oxide of lead(Pb_3O_4 or $2PbO \cdot PbO_2$)

Lithargyrum(密陀僧, Mituoseng)——lead oxide(PbO)

Borax(硼砂, Pengsha)——$Na_2B_4O_7 \cdot 10H_2O$

Alumen(白矾, Baifan)——hydrous potassium aluminum sulfate($KAl(SO_4)_2 \cdot 12H_2O$)

Melanterite(皂矾, Zaofan)——ferrous sulfate($FeSO_4 \cdot 7H_2O$)

Calix(石灰, Shihui)——quicklime is calcium oxide(CaO) dried lime is calcium hydroxide($Ca(OH)_2$)

Nitrum(火硝, Huoxiao)——potassium nitrate(KNO_3)

Sal-ammoniac(硇砂, Naosha)——Sal Ammoniaci(白硇砂, Bainaosha) mainly contains ammonium chloride(NH_4Cl)

Chalcanthnium(胆矾, Danfan)——hydrous copper sulfate($CuSO_4 \cdot 5H_2O$)

Appendix: Other Drugs For External Use

Name	Properties and tastc	Meridian tropism	Functions	Indications	Dosage	Contraindication
Red Orpiment (雄黄, Xionghuang)	acid, bitter, warm, poisonous	Heart, liver, kidney	Counteract toxic substance, dry dampness, destroy worms, expel phlem, prevent attack of malaria, arrest convulsion	Carbuncle, cellulitis, furuncle, scabies, snake-bike, syphilis, leprosy, malaria, asthma, infantile convulsion, tetanus, tumor	0.15~0.3g used in pill or powder. Proper amount for external use	Do not use with pregnant women and in cases of blood-yin deficiency It can not be calcined. Don't exceed dosage or take it for a long time. The poisoning symptoms are vomiting and diarrhea (arsenic poisoning)
Arsenolite Ore(砒石, Pishi)	Acid, very hot. Poisonous	Lung, liver	Corrode boils, destroy worms, remove phlegm, relieve asthma, prevent attack of malaria.	Similar as Red Orpiment (雄黄, Xionghuang). Harmful to body. Seldom used internally. Used for carcinoma of skin, cervix, penis, etc. Internal used only for refractory asthma due to cold-phlegm and chronic malaria	Internal use: 1~4mg per time used in pill or powder, proper. amount for external use.	The applied area should not be large. Don't use for a long time, otherwise it may cause poisoning. Don't use in cases of bleeding of wound surface and damage of skin.
Mercuros Chloride (轻粉, Qingfen)	Acid, cold, poisonous	Liver, kidney	Counteract detoxic substance, destroy worms, induce diuresis, relax the bowels	Festered skin and external diseause, syphils, scabies, itching, rosacea, furuncle of prickly heat, edema and tympanites	Internal use: 0.06 ~ 0.15g, less than twice per day. Used in pill or powder. Don't be used in decoction. Proper amount for external use.	This herb is intensively poisonous, internal use should be cautious. Don't use in pregnancy or deficient people. Don't exceed dosage or take for a long time.
Mercuric Oxide-Mixture (升药, Shengyao)	Acid, hot, very poisonous	Lung, spleen	Remove toxic substances, pus and slough	Much pus of ulcerative carbuncle, cellulitis, anadequate discharge of pus, removal of slough, nonregeneration of flesh.	Little amount for external use, ground into refined powder. Rub with the powder or mix the powder, or stain the slender roll of medicated paper with powder Often combined with Calcined Gypsum (石膏, Shigao)	Very poisonous, generally not for internal use. Don't use in the places of mucous membrane and joints. Avoid using it if wound surface is big.

Name	Properties and taste	Meridian tropism	Functions	Indications	Dosage	Contraindication
Minium (铅丹, Qiandan)	Acid, slightly cold, poisonous	Liver, heart	External use: remove toxic substances, astringe dampness, promote regeneration of tissue. Internal use: eliminate phlegm, relieve convulsion, counteract toxic substances, prevent attack of malaria	External use: skin and external diseases, eczema, tinea, tinea unguium, moist and rotten of toe's gap due to tinea, bromnidrosis. internal use: infantile convulsion, epilepsy and malaria	Proper amount for external use. Internal use: 0.3 ~ 0. 6g per time. Used in pill or powder, or take after being ground into powder.	Pregnant women and deficient people do not take this herb and don't take for a long time or exceed dosage for it is Poisonous. Don't use it for a long time or over a big area externally.
Litharge (密陀僧, Mituoseng)	Salty, acid, medium poisonous	Liver, spleen	Counteract the toxic substances, destroy worms, induce astringence	Much pus of skin and external diseases, eczema, bromhidrosis, rosacea, tinea versicolor	Proper amount for external use. Sprinkle over the affected area after being ground into powder or mixed with oil seldom used internally	
Borax (硼砂, Pengsha)	Salty, sweet, cool	Lung, stomach	External use: clear away heat to detoxicate, subdue suelling, internal use clear lung-heat and remove phlegm	External use: sorethroat, aphthae, conjunctival congestion, nebula, pterygium, internal use: cough due to phlegm-heat.	Proper amount for external use. internal use: 1. 5 ~ 3g. in pill or powder.	Use cautiously for internal use
Alum (白矾, Baifan)	Sour, cold	Lung, liver, spleen, stomach, large intestine	Detoxicate and destroy worms, dry dampness and relieve itching, arrest bleeding, induce astringency, relieve diarrhea, clear away heat to remove phlegm, normalize the functions of gallbladder, reduce blood lipid.	Skin and external diseases, scabies, eczema, itching, vomit blood, traumatic bleeding, chronic diarrhea and dysentery, epilepsy, phlegm syncope, jaundice due to damp-heat, hyperlipemia.	Proper amount for external use. internal use: 1 ~ 3g in pill or powder	Deficient people don't use.
Malachite Ore(皂矾, Zaofan)	Sour, astringent cool	Liver, spleen	Detoxicate and astringe sores, dry dampness, kill worms, tonify blood	Festered skin and external diseases, scabies, itching, pharyngitis, aphthae, marginal blepharitis, iron-deficiency anemia, hookworm disease.	Proper amount for external use, internally used in pill or powder, 0.3 ~ 0.6g per time if not for decoction, twice or three times every day	Large dosage may induce vomiting, abdominal pain, diarrhea, vertigo, etc. Stomachache and hematemesis patients don't use, don't take together with tea.

Name	Properties and tastc	Meridian tropism	Functions	Indications	Dosage	Contraindication
Calix (石灰, Shihui)	Acid, warm, poisonous	Liver, spleen	Induce astringency and dry dampness, detoxicate and corrode biols, kill worms, relieve itching, arrest bleeding	Scald, carbuncle, cellutitis, erysipelas, mutiple abscess, mutiple abscess, scrofula, subcutaneous nodule, syphilis, wart, clavus, eczema, itching, scabies, traumatic bleeding	Proper amount for external use, don't use internally.	
Nitrum (火硝, Huoxiao)	Bitter, salty, cold, poisonous	Heart, liver	Counteract toxic substances, subdue swelling, induce diuresis and purgation, scatter masses.	Carbuncle, wound, conjunctival congestion, pharyngitis, stranguria, vesical calculus, jaundice (together with Malachite Ore (皂矾, Zaofan)), cholera morbus, pain due to acute filthy disease, tumor	Proper amount for external use. internal use: 1. 3 ~ 3g, usually used in pill or powder	Deficient people and pregnant women do not use
Sal-ammoniac (硇砂, Naosha)	Salty, bitter, acid, warm	Liver, spleen, stomach	Scatter blood-stasis, corrode boils, ablate masses, resolve the hard lumps.	Large carbuncle, mutiple abscess and scrofula, pharyngitis, nebula, wart, polypus, snake-bite, swelling pain, abdominal masses, dysphagia, regurgitation of food from stomach, tumor	Proper amount for external use, internally used in pill or powder, 0. 3 ~ 1g per time, less than 2g every day.	Don't exceed dosage for internal use, deficiency people and pregnant women don't use
Blue Vitriol (胆矾, Danfan)	Sour, acid, cold, poisonous	Liver, gall bladder	Internal use for inducing vomiting, external use for detoxication, astringe dampness, corrode boils	Productive wind-phlegm, pharyngitis, epilepsy, aphthae, ulcerative gingivitis, marginal blepharitis, unfestered carbuncle.	0. 1 ~ 0. 3g take after being melted in decoction. Proper amount for external use.	
Leaf of Cottonrose (芙蓉叶, Furongye)	Acid, medium	Lung, liver	Remove heat from blood, detoxicate, subdue swelling to relieve pain	Carbuncle and cellulitis, erysipelas, scald, traumatic injury	Poper amount for external use.	
Chaulmoogratree Seed (大风子, Dafengzi)	Acid, hot, big poisonous	Liver, spleen, kidney	Expels the wind, dry dampness, counteract toxic substances, kills worms	Leprosy	Proper amount for external use 0.3 ~ 1g per time for internal use	This herb has intensive poison. It is seldom used except for leprosy

Name	Properties and tastc	Meridian tropism	Functions	Indications	Dosage	Contraindication
Shrubalthea Bark (木槿皮, Mujinpi)v	Sweet, bitter, cool	Large intestine, liver, spleen	Clear away heat and detoxicate, remove dampness, kills worms, relieve itching and arrest bldding	External use for scabies itching, prolapse of rectum, traumatic bleeding; both internal and external used for leukorrhea, dysentery due to damp-heat, hemotochzia	Proper amount for external use. Internal use: 3～9g	
Golden Larch Bark (土荆皮, Tujingpi)	Acid, bitter, warm, poisonous	Not clear	Dry dampness to relieve itching, kill worms to treat tinea	All sorts of tinea, eczema	Proper amount for external use. Applied externally after being soaked in wine.	Not used internally
Chinese Stellera Root(狼毒, Langdu)	Bitter, acid, medium, poisonous	Liver, spleen, lung	Counteract toxic substances, scatter blockage, kill worms, remove water retention by hydragogue	Multiple abscess and scrofula (tuberculosis of lymph), scabies, psoriasis, abdominal pain due to stagnation of phlegm, food and worms, edema, abdominal distention, tumor	Internal use: 0.5～3g. Proper amount for external use	This herb has the same origin as Knoxia Root (大戟, Daji), so it can't be used together with Liquorice (甘草, Gancao). It is poisonous, the dosage should be controlled strictly.
Colophony (松香, Songxiang)	Bitter, sweet, warm	Liver, spleen, lung	Dry dampness, kill worms remove toxic substances, promote regeneration of tissue, expel the wind and relieve pain.	Scabies, itching, large carbuncle, pain due to arthralgia-syndrome, thromboangiitis and psoriasis	Proper amount for external use 3～9g per time for internal use. Used in pill or powder or taken after being soaked in wine.	Don't use in cases of heat-syndrome
Elephant Hide(象皮, Xiangpi)	Sweet, salty, warm	Spleen, lung	Arrest bleeding, promote regeneration of tissue, astringe sores	Traumatic bleeding, non-healing of wounds	Proper amount for external use	It's improper for carbuncles with pus toxic or for suppurative incised wound.
Cera Chinensis (虫白蜡, Chongbaila)	Sweet, warm	Liver, lung	Astringe to arrest bleeding, promote regeneration of tissue, relieve pain, tonify deficiency, moisten the lung	Bleeding due to incised wound, non-healing of large carbuncle(external use), hematuria, hematochezia (internal use), chronic cough due to lung deficiency, phlegm with blood. It is a raw material making paste, ointment and pill.	3～9g for internal use. Proper amount for external use.	Don't use if carbuncle and cellulitis don't fester or have festered with thick pus.

Name	Properties and tastc	Meridian tropism	Functions	Indications	Dosage	Contraindication
Muskmelon Fruit Pedicel (瓜蒂, Guadi)	Bitter, cold, poisonous	Stomach	Induce vomiting, expel damp-heat, anti-tumor	Heat phlegm, jaundice, headache. Its preparation is used for carcinoma of liver	2.5～5g. Used in pill or powder is 0.1～0.15g. A small amount for external use.	Don't use in condition of deficient condition, loss of blood.

References

Reference Ⅰ　Classification of Herbal Medicines

Flower Herbs

Honeysuckle Flower
（金银花，Jinyinhua）
Clove Flower-bud
（丁香，Dingxiang）
Fineleaf Schizonepeta Herb
（荆芥穗，Jinjiesui）
Biond Magnolia Flower-bud
（辛夷，Xinyi）
Chrysanthemum Flower
（菊花，Juhua）
Lilac Daphne Flower-bud
（芫花，Yuanhua）
Hindu Lotus Stamen
（莲须，Lianxu）
Safflower
（红花，Honghua）
Japanese Pagodatree Flower
（槐花，Huaihua）
Inula Flower
（旋覆花，Xuanfuhua）
Common Coltsfoot Flower
（款冬花，Kuandonghua）
Rugose Rose Flower
（玫瑰花，Meiguihua）
Silktree Albizia Immature Flower
（合欢花，Hehuanhua）
Pale Butterflybush Flower
（密蒙花，Mimenghua）
Plum Flower Bud
（绿萼梅，Lvemei）
Chinese Rose Flower
（月季花，Yuejihua）
Datura Flower
（洋金花，Yangjinhua）
Chinese Trumpetcreeper Flower
（凌霄花，Lingxiaohua）

Leaf Herbs

Bamboo leaf
（竹叶，Zhuye）
Indigowoad Leaf
（大青叶，Daqingye）
Common Perilla Leaf
（苏叶，Suye）
Mulberry Leaf
（桑叶，Sangye）
Senna Leaf
（番泻叶，Fanxieye）
Argy Wormwood Leaf
（艾叶，Aiye）
Taiwan Beautybetter Leaf
（紫珠，Zizhu）
Hindu Lotus Leaf
（荷叶，Heye）
Chinese Arborvitae Leafy Twig
（侧柏叶，Cebaiye）
Japanese Felt Fern Leaf
（石韦，Shiwei）
Loquat Leaf
（枇杷叶，Pipaye）

Branch, Stem and Wood Herbs

Honeysuckle Stem
（忍冬藤，Rendongteng）
Ephedra
（麻黄，Mahuang）
Gambirplant Hooked Stem and Branch
（钩藤，Gouteng）
Cassia Twig
（桂枝，Guizhi）
Chinese Tamarish Twig
（西河柳，Xiheliu）
Common Scouring Rush Herb
（木贼，Muzei）
Desertliving Cistanche
（肉苁蓉，Roucongrong）
Dendrobium Herb
（石斛，Shihu）
Suberect Spatholobus Stem
（鸡血藤，Jixueteng）
Bamboo Shavings
（竹茹，Zhuru）
Rosewood
（降香，Jiangxiang）
Fortune Windmillpalm
（棕榈炭，Zonglutan）
Chinese Starjasmine Stem
（络石藤，Luoshiteng）
Mulberry Twig
（桑枝，Sangzhi）
Sandalwood
（檀香，Tanxiang）
Sappan Wood
（苏木，Sumu）
Chinese Taxillus Twig
（桑寄生，Sangjisheng）
Songaria Cynomorium Herb
（锁阳，Suoyang）
Akebia Stem
（木通，Mutong）
Ricepaperplant Pith
（通草，Tongcao）

Bark Herbs

Chinese Corktree Bark
（黄柏，Huangbai）
Largeleaf Chinese Ash Bark
（秦皮，Qinpi）
Tree Peony Bark
（牡丹皮，Mudanpi）
Densefruit Pittany Root-bark
（白鲜皮，Baixianpi）
Chinese Wolfberry Root-bark
（地骨皮，Digupi）
Cassia Bark
（肉桂，Rougui）
Eucommia Bark
（杜仲，Duzhong）
Tree of Heaven Ailanthus Bark
（椿皮，Chunpi）
Cortex Acanthopanacis Radicis
（五加皮，Wujiapi）
Officinal Magnolia Bark
（厚朴，Houpo）
White Mulberry Root-bark
（桑白皮，Sangbaipi）
Silktree Albiziae Bark
（合欢皮，Hehuanpi）
Szechwan Chinaberry Bark
（苦楝皮，Kulianpi）

Resin Herbs

Chinese Eaglewood Wood
（沉香，Chenxiang）
Frankincense
（乳香，Ruxiang）
Myrrh
（没药，Moyao）
Storesin
（苏合香，Suhexiang）

Dragon's Blood
（血竭，Xuejie）

Root Herbs

Baikal Skullcap Root
（黄芩，Huangqin）
Coptis Rhizome
（黄连，Huanglian）
Indigwoad Root
（板蓝根，Banlangen）
Lightyellow Sophora Root
（苦参，Kushen）
Rehmannia Dried Root
（生地黄，Shengdihuang）
Red Peony Root
（赤芍药，Chishaoyao）
Chinese Pulsatilla Root
（白头翁，Baitouweng）
Tonkin Sophora Root
（山豆根，Shandougen）
Prepared Daughter Root of Common Monkshood
（附子，Fuzi）
Incised Notopterygium Rhizome and Root
（羌活，Qianghuo）
Dahurian Angelica Root
（白芷，Baizhi）
Chinese Ligusticum Rhizome
（藁本，Gaoben）
Root of Sinkiang Arnebia
（紫草，Zicao）
Chinese Thorowax Root
（柴胡，Chaihu）
Lobed Kudzuvine Root
（葛根，Gegen）
Kansui Root
（甘遂，Gansui）
Peking Euphorbia Root
（大戟，Daji）
Pokeberry Root
（商陆，Shanglu）
Ginseng
（人参，Renshen）
Tangshen Root
（党参，Dangshen）
Heterophylla Falsestarwort Root
（太子参，Taizishen）
American Ginseng Root
（西洋参，Xiyangshen）
Membranous Milkvetch Root
（黄芪，Huangqi）
Chinese Gentian Root
（龙胆草，Longdancao）
Licorice Root
（甘草，Gancao）
Medicinal Indian-mulberry Root
（巴戟天，Bajitian）
Himalayan Teasel Root
（续断，Xuduan）
Chinese Angelica Root
（当归，Danggui）
Prepared Rhizome of Adhesive Rehmannia
（熟地黄，Shoudihuang）
Tuber Fleeceflower Root
（何首乌，Heshouwu）
White Peony Root
（白芍药，Baishaoyao）
Coastal Glehnia Root, and Fourleaf Ladybell Root
（沙参，Shashen）
Dwarf Lilyturf Root
（麦门冬，Maimendong）
Cochinchinese Asparagus Root
（天门冬，Tianmendong）
Ephedra Root
（麻黄根，Mahuanggen）
Common Aucklandia Root
（木香，Muxiang）
Combined Spicebush Root
（乌药，Wuyao）

Turmeric Root－tuber
(郁金, Yujin)
Common Burreed Rhizome
(三棱, Sanleng)
Dan－shen Root
(丹参, Danshen)
Sanchi Root
(三七, Sanqi)
Chinese Clematis Root
(威灵仙, Weilingxian)
Fourstamen Stephania Root
(防己, Fangji)
Largeleaf Gentian Root
(秦艽, Qinjiao)
Willowleaf Swallowwort Rhizome
(白前, Baiqian)
Whiteflower hogfenel Root
(前胡, Qianhu)
Sessile Stemona Root
(百部, Baibu)
Tatarian Aster Root
(紫苑, Ziyuan)
Thinleaf Milkwort Root
(远志, Yuanzhi)
Antifebrile Dichroa Root
(常山, Changshan)
Balloonflower Root
(桔梗, Jiegeng)
Siberian Solomonseal Rhizome
(黄精, Huangjing)
Snakegroud Root
(天花粉, Tianhuafen)
India Madder Root
(茜草, Qiancao)
Starwort Root
(银柴胡, Yinchaihu)

Rhizome Herbs

Nutgrass Galingale Rhizome
(香附, Xiangfu)
Doubleteeth Pulbescent Angelica Root
(独活, Duhuo)
Oriental Waterplantain Rhizome
(泽泻, Zexie)
Common Anemarrhea Rhizome
(知母, Zhimu)
Glabrous Greenbrier Rhizome
(土茯苓, Tufuling)
Blackberrylily Rhizome
(射干, Shegan)
Dried Ginger
(干姜, Ganjiang)
Lesser Galangal Rhizome
(高良姜, Gaoliangjiang)
Pinellia Rhizome
(半夏, Banxia)
Fresh Ginger
(生姜, Shengjiang)
Divaricate Saposhnikovia Root
(防风, Fangfeng)
Shunk Bugbane Rhizome
(升麻, Shengma)
Largehead Atractylodes Rhizome
(白术, Baizhu)
Common Yam Rhizome
(山药, Shanyao)
East Asian Tree Fern Rhizome
(狗脊, Gouji)
Common Cruculigo
(仙茅, Xianmao)
Siberian Solomonseal Rhizome
(黄精, Huangjing)
Fragrant Solomonseal Rhizome
(玉竹, Yuzhu)
Szechwan Lovage Rhizome
(川芎, Chuanxiong)
Yanhusuo
(延胡索, Yanhusuo)
Turmeric Rhizome
(姜黄, Jianghuang)

Zedoray
(莪术, Ezhu)
Giant Knotweed Rhizome
(虎杖, Huzhang)
Garden Burnet Root
(地榆, Diyu)
Sevenlobed Yam Rhizome
(萆薢, Bixie)
Jackinthepulpit Tuber
(天南星, Tiannanxing)
Lalang Grass Rhizome
(白茅根, Baimaogen)
Bletilla Rhizome
(白及, Baiji)
Swordlike Atractylodes Rhizome
(苍术, Cangzhu)
Tall Gastrodia Rhizome
(天麻, Tianma)
Grassleaf Sweetflag Rhizome
(石菖蒲, Shichangpu)
Rhubarb
(大黄, Dahuang)
Hindu Lotus Rhizome-node
(藕节, Oujie)
Reed Rhizome
(芦根, Lugen)
Giant Typhonium Rhizome
(白附子, Baifuzi)

Bulb Herbs

Lily Bulb
(百合, Baihe)
Longstament Onion Bulb
(薤白, Xiebai)
Garlic Bulb
(大蒜, Dasuan)
Tendrilleaf Fritillary Bulb
(贝母, Beimu)

Seed Herbs

Great Burdock Achene
(牛蒡子, Niubangzi)
Prepared Soybean
(淡豆豉, Dandouchi)
Hemp Seed
(火麻仁, Huomaren)
Boat-fruited Sterculia Seed
(胖大海, Pangdahai)
Rangooncreeper Fruit
(使君子, Shijunzi)
Mongolian Snakegourd Seed
(瓜蒌仁, Gualouren)
Bushcherry Seed
(郁李仁, Yuliren)
Pharbitis Seed
(牵牛子, Qianniuzi)
Croton Seed
(巴豆, Badou)
Walnut
(胡桃仁, Hutaoren)
Flatstem Milkvetch Seed
(沙苑子, Shayuanzi)
Dodder Seed
(菟丝子, Tusizi)
Common Fenugreek Seed
(胡芦巴, Huluba)
Malaytea Scurfpea Fruit
(补骨脂, Buguzhi)
Tuber Onion Seed
(韭子, Jiuzi)
Glossy Privet Fruit
(女贞子, Nuzhenzi)
Lotus Seed
(莲子, Lianzi)
Hindu Lotus Plumule
(莲子心, Lianzixin)
Black Sesame
(黑芝麻, Heizhima)
Lychee Seed
(荔枝核, Lizhihe)
Peach Seed

（桃仁，Taoren）
Cowherb Seed
（王不留行，Wangbuliuxing）
Coix Seed
（薏苡仁，Yiyiren）
Plantain Seed
（车前子，Cheqianzi）
Japanese Climbing Fern Spores
（海金沙，Haijinsha）
Rice Bean
（赤小豆，Chixiaodou）
White Mustard Seed
（白芥子，Baijiezi）
Apricot Seed
（杏仁，Xingren）
Perilla Seed
（苏子，Suzi）
Pepperweed Seed or Flixweed Tansymustard Seed
（葶苈子，Tinglizi）
Spine Date Seed
（酸枣仁，Suanzaoren）
Chinese Arborvitae Seed
（柏子仁，Baiziren）
Cassia Seed
（决明子，Juemingzi）
Malt
（麦芽，Maiya）
Radish Seed
（莱菔子，Laifuzi）
Cushaw Seed
（南瓜子，Nanguazi）
Common Cnidium Fruit
（蛇床子，Shechuangzi）
Nut－vomitive Poisonnut Seed
（马钱子，Maqianzi）
Wheat Fruit
（小麦，Xiaomai）
Blighted Wheat
（浮小麦，Fuxiaomai）
Feather Cockscomb Seed
（青葙子，Qingxiangzi）
Ginkgo Seed
（白果，Baiguo）
Gordon Euryale Seed
（芡实，Qianshi）
Areca Seed
（槟榔，Binlang）

Fruit Herbs

Cape Jasmine Fruit
（栀子，Zhizi）
Weeping Forsythia Capsule
（连翘，Lianqiao）
Medicinal Evodia Root
（吴茱萸，Wuzhuyu）
Fennel Fruit
（小茴香，Xiaohuixiang）
Long Pepper Fruit
（荜茇，Biba）
Mountain Spicy Tree Fruit
（荜澄茄，Bichengqie）
Shrub Chastetree Fruit
（蔓荆子，Manjingzi）
Chinese Date
（大枣，Dazao）
Sharpleaf Galangal Fruit
（益智仁，Yizhiren）
Longan Aril
（龙眼肉，Longyanrou）
Barbary Wolfberry Fruit
（枸杞子，Gouqizi）
Mulberry Solomonseal
（桑椹，Sangshen）
Chinese Magnoliavine
（五味子，Wuweizi）
Smoked Plum
（乌梅，Wumei）
Medicine Terminalia Fruit
（诃子，Hezi）

Immature Bitter Orange
（枳实，Zhishi）
Finger Citron Fruit
（佛手，Foshou）
Common Floweringquince Fruit
（木瓜，Mugua）
Villous Amomum Fruit
（砂仁，Sharen）
White Amomum Fruit
（白豆蔻，Baidoukou）
Caoguo
（草果，Caoguo）
Snakegourd Fruit
（瓜蒌，Gualou）
Dutchmanspipe Fruit
（马兜铃，Madouling）
Puncturevine Caltrop Fruit
（刺蒺藜，Cijili）
Hawthorn Fruit
（山楂，Shanzha）
Towel Gourd Vegetable Sponge
（丝瓜络，Sigualuo）
Hindu Lotus Receptacle
（莲房，Lianfang）
Pomegranate Rind Peel
（石榴皮，Shiliupi）
Tangerine Peel
（橘皮，Jupi）
Green Tangerine Peel
（青皮，Qingpi）
Chinese Honeylocust Fruit
（皂荚，Zaojia）
Asiatic Cornelian Cherry Fruit
（山茱萸，Shanzhuyu）
Szechwan chinaberry Fruit
（川楝子，Chuanlianzi）
Chinese Waxgourd Exocarp
（冬瓜皮，Dongguapi）

The Whole Herbs

Common Selfheal Spike
（夏枯草，Xiakucao）
Dandelion
（蒲公英，Pugongying）
Tokyo Violet Herb
（紫花地丁，Zihuadiding）
Heartlaef Houttuynia Herb
（鱼腥草，Yuxingcao）
Purslane Herb
（马齿苋，Machixian）
Whiteflower Patrinia Herb
（败酱草，Baijiangcao）
Barbed Skullcap Herb
（半枝莲，Banzhilian）
Spreading Hedyotis Herb
（白花蛇舌草，Baihuasheshecao）
Sweet Wormwood
（青蒿，Qinghao）
Common Ducksmeat Herb
（浮萍，Fuping）
Haichow Elsholtzia Herb
（香薷，Xiangru）
Yerbadetajo Herb
（墨旱莲，Mohanlian）
Motherwort Herb
（益母草，Yimucao）
Hirsute Shiny Bugleweed Herb
（泽兰，Zelan）
Diverse Wormwood Herb
（刘寄奴，Liujinu）
Japanese Thistle Herb or Root
（大蓟，Daji）
Common Cephalanoplos Herb
（小蓟，Xiaoji）
Hairvein Agrimonia Herb
（仙鹤草，Xianhecao）
Tamariskoid Spikemoss Herb
（卷柏，Juanbai）
Common St. Paulswort Herb
（豨莶草，Xixiancao）
Common Clubmoss Herb

(伸筋草, Shenjincao)
Wild Mint
(薄荷, Bohe)
Wrinkled Gianthyssop Herb
(藿香, Huoxiang)
Foutune Eupatorium Herb
(佩兰, Peilan)
Christina Loosetrife Herb
(金钱草, Jinqiancao)
Common Knotgrass Herb
(萹蓄, Bianxu)
Lilac Pink Herb
(瞿麦, Qumai)
Shorthorned Epimedium Herb
(淫羊藿, Yinyanghuo)
Capillary Wormwood Herb
(茵陈蒿, Yinchenhao)
Manchurian Wildginger Herb
(细辛, Xixin)

Mineral Drugs

Gypsum
(石膏, Shigao)
Actinolite
(阳起石, Yangqishi)
Red Halloysite
(赤石脂, Chishizhi)
Limonite
(禹余粮, Yuyuliang)
Talc
(滑石, Huashi)
Cinnabar
(朱砂, Zhusha)
Magnetite
(磁石, Cishi)
Hematite
(代赭石, Daizheshi)
Sulfur
(硫黄, Liuhuang)
Calamine
(炉甘石, Luganshi)
Borax
(硼砂, Pengsha)
Alumen
(明矾, Mingfan)
Mirabilite
(芒硝, Mangxiao)

Worm Drugs

Cicada Slough
(蝉蜕, Chantui)
Chinese Gall
(五倍子, Wubeizi)
Mantis Egg-case
(桑螵蛸, Sangpiaoxiao)
Ground Beetle
(䗪虫, Zhechong)
Leech
(水蛭, Shuizhi)
Gadfly
(虻虫, Mengchong)
Scorpion
(全蝎, Quanxie)
Centipede
(蜈蚣, Wugong)
Silkworm with Batrytis Larva
(白僵蚕, Baijiangcan)
Earth Worm
(地龙, Dilong)
Vasps Nest
(露蜂房, Lufengfang)

Animal Drugs

Buffalo Horn
(水牛角, Shuiniujiao)
Hairy Antler
(鹿茸, Lurong)
Pangolin Scales
(穿山甲, Chuanshanjia)
Ass-hide Glue

（阿胶，Ejiao）
Antelope Horn
（羚羊角，Lingyangjiao）
Musk
（麝香，Shexiang）
Chicken Gizzard Membrane
（鸡内金，Jineijin）
Tortoise's Shell and Plastron
（龟版，Guiban）
Cow-bezoar
（牛黄，Niuhuang）
Turtle Carapace
（鳖甲，Biejia）
Giant Gecko
（蛤蚧，Gejie）
Agkistrodon Acutus
（白花蛇，Baihuashe）

Sea Drugs

Cuttle Bone
（乌贼骨，Wuzeigu）
Clam Shell
（海蛤壳，Haigeqiao）
Seaweed
（海藻，Haizao）
Kelp
（昆布，Kunbu）
Oyster Shell
（牡蛎，Muli）
Pearl
（珍珠，Zhenzhu）
Ark Shell
（瓦楞子，Walengzi）
Abalone Shell
（石决明，Shijueming）

Edible Fungus Drugs

Tuckahoe
（茯苓，Fuling）
Umbellate Pore Fungus
（猪苓，Zhuling）
Lucid Ganoderma
（灵芝，Lingzhi）
Chinese Caterpillar Fungus
（冬虫夏草，Dongchongxiacao）
Puff-ball
（马勃，Mabo）

Other Kinds of Drugs

Malt Sugar
（饴糖，Yitang）
Honey
（蜂蜜，Fengmi）
Medicated Leaven
（神曲，Shenqu）
Camphor
（樟脑，Zhangnao）
Bamboo Juice
（竹沥，Zhuli）
Dried Human Placenta
（紫河车，Ziheche）
Charred Human Hair
（血余炭，Xueyutan）
Chinese Honeylocust Spine
（皂角，Zaojiao）
Tabasheer
（天竹黄，Tianzhuhuang）
Trogopterus Dung
（五灵脂，Wulingzhi）
Amber
（琥珀，Hupo）
Dragon's Bone
（龙骨，Longgu）
Borneol
（冰片，Bingpian）
Cattail Pollen
（蒲黄，Puhuang）
Aloes
（芦荟，Luhui）

Reference Ⅱ Clinical Application of Chinese Drugs Based on Pharmacological Research

Antivirotic Herbs

1. Anti-influenza virus: Indigowoad Leaf (大青叶, Daqingye) Indigwoad Root (板蓝根, Banlangen) Natural Indigo (青黛, Qingdai) Honeysuckle Flower (金银花, Jinyinhua) Weeping Forsythia Capsule (连翘, Lianqiao) Blackberrylily Rhizome (射干, Shegan) Baikal Skullcap Root (黄芩, Huangqin) Coptis Rhizome (黄连, Huanglian) Chinese Corktree Bark (黄柏, Huangbai) Rhubarb (大黄, Dahuang) Giant Knotweed Rhizome (虎杖, Huzhang) Sessile Stemona Root (百部, Baibu) Heartlaef Houttuynia Herb (鱼腥草, Yuxingcao) Fistular Onion (葱, Cong) Garlic Bulb (大蒜, Dasuan) Indian Chrysanthemum Flower (野菊花, Yejuhua) Chinese Thorowax Root (柴胡, Chaihu) Great Burdock Achene (牛蒡子, Niubangzi) Divaricate Saposhnikovia Root (防风, Fangfeng) Perilla Leaf (紫苏, Zisu) Male Fern Rhizome (贯众, Guanzhong) Root of Sinkiang Arnebia (紫草, Zicao) Red Peony Root (赤芍药, Chishaoyao) Tree Peony Bark (牡丹皮, Mudanpi) Capillary Wormwood Herb (茵陈蒿, Yinchenhao) Ephedra (麻黄, Mahuang) Cassia Twig (桂枝, Guizhi) Haichow Elsholtzia Herb (香薷, Xiangru) Foutune Eupatorium Herb (佩兰, Peilan) Small Centipeda Herb (鹅不食草, Ebushicao) Argy Wormwood Leaf (艾叶, Aiye) Tatarian Aster Root (紫苑, Ziyuan) Chinese Arborvitae Leafy Twig (侧柏叶, Cebaiye) Medicine Terminalia Fruit (诃子, Hezi) Siberian Solomonseal Rhizome (黄精, Huangjing) Chinese Magnoliavine (五味子, Wuweizi) Areca Seed (槟榔, Binlang) Olive (橄榄, Ganlan) Licorice Root (甘草, Shenggancao) Common Selfheal Spike (夏枯草, Xiakucao) Seaweed (海藻, Haizao) Common Dayflower Herb (鸭跖草, Yazhicao) Cherokee Rose Fruit (金樱子, Jinyingzi) Japanese Felt Fern Leaf (石韦, Shiwei) Lilac Daphne Flowerbud (芫花, Yuanhua)

2. Anti-parainfluenza virus: Great Burdock Achene (牛蒡子, Niubangzi)

3. Anti-rhinovirus: Male Fern Rhizome (贯众, Guanzhong) Apricot Seed (杏仁, Xingren) Tangerine Peel (橘皮, Jupi) Dried Human Placenta (紫河车, Ziheche) Centipede (蜈蚣, Wugong)

4. Anti-adenovirus: Blackberrylily Rhizome (射干, Shegan)

5. Anti-measles virus: Fineleaf Schizomepeta Herb (荆芥, Jingjie) Common Andrographis Herb (穿心莲, Chuanxinlian) Root of Sinkiang Arnebia (紫草, Zicao) Garter Snake (乌梢蛇, Wushaoshe)

6. Anti-herpesvirus: Honeysuckle Flower (金银花, Jinyinhua) Blackberrylily Rhizome (射干, Shegan) Giant Knotweed Rhizome (虎杖, Huzhang) Purslane Herb (马齿苋, Machixian) Red Peony Root (赤芍药, Chishaoyao) Siberian Solomonseal Rhizome (黄精, Huangjing) Chinese Arborvitae Leafy Twig (侧柏叶, Cebaiye)

7. Anti-poliovirus: Chinese Taxillus Twig

(桑寄生, Sangjisheng) Shorthorned Epimedium Herb (淫羊藿, Yinyanghuo) Root of Sinkiang Arnebia (紫草, Zicao) Chinese Thorowax Root (柴胡, Chaihu) Ephedra (麻黄, Mahuang) Cassia Twig (桂枝, Guizhi) Chinese Corktree Bark (黄柏, Huangbai) Giant Knotweed Rhizome (虎杖, Huzhang) Oyster Shell (牡蛎, Muli)

8. Anti-coxackievirus: Giant Knotweed Rhizome (虎杖, Huzhang) Blackberrylily Rhizome (射干, Shegan) Indigowoad Leaf (大青叶, Daqingye) Male Fern Rhizome (贯众, Guanzhong) Chinese Taxillus Twig (桑寄生, Sangjisheng)

9. Anti-ECHO virus: Blackberrylily Rhizome (射干, Shegan) Indigowoad Leaf (大青叶, Daqingye) Male Fern Rhizome (贯众, Guanzhong) Honeysuckle Flower (金银花, Jinyinhua) Common Andrographis Herb (穿心莲, Chuanxinlian) Heartlaef Houttuynia Herb (鱼腥草, Yuxingcao) Giant Knotweed Rhizome (虎杖, Huzhang) Indian Chrysanthemum Flower (野菊花, Yejuhua) Dandelion (蒲公英, Pugongying) Bunge Corydalis Herb (苦地丁, Kudiding) Sweet Wormwood (青蒿, Qinghao) Wild Mint (薄荷, Bohe) Common Ducksmeat Herb (浮萍, Fuping) Shrub Chastetree Fruit (蔓荆子, Manjingzi) Capillary Wormwood Herb (茵陈蒿, Yinchenhao) Common Selfheal Spike (夏枯草, Xiakucao) Cape Jasmine Fruit (栀子, Zhizi) Ephedra (麻黄, Mahuang) Cassia Twig (桂枝, Guizhi) Perilla Leaf (紫苏, Zisu) Haichow Elsholtzia Herb (香薷, Xiangru) Uniflower Swisscentaury Root (漏芦, Loulu) Dutchmanspipe Fruit (马兜铃, Madouling) Chinese Taxillus Twig (桑寄生, Sangjisheng)

10. Anti-arbovirus: Indigowoad Leaf (大青叶, Daqingye) Indigwoad Root (板蓝根, Banlangen) Natural Indigo (青黛, Qingdai) Common Dayflower Herb (鸭跖草, Yazhicao) Male Fern Rhizome (贯众, Guanzhong) Giant Knotweed Rhizome (虎杖, Huzhang) Snake Slough (蛇蜕, Shetui)

11. Anti-mumps virus: Indigowood Leaf (大青叶, Daqingye) Indigwoad Root (板蓝根, Banlangen) Honeysuckle Flower (金银花, Jinyinhua) Natural Indigo (青黛, Qingdai) Common Dayflower Herb (鸭跖草, Yazhicao) Snake Slough (蛇蜕, Shetui)

Antibacterial Herbs

1. Broad-spectrum antibiosis (including staphylococcus, a hemolytic streptococcus, beta hemolytic streptocooccus, Diplococcus pneumoniae, Diplococcus meningitidis, Bacillus enteritidis, Bacillus dysenteriae, typhoid bacillus, Bacillus paratyphosus, etc.): Honeysuckle Flower (金银花, Jinyinhua) Weeping Forsythia Capsule (连翘, Lianqiao) Indigowoad Leaf (大青叶, Daqingye) Indigwoad Root (板蓝根, Banlangen) Natural Indigo (青黛, Qingdai) Coptis Rhizome (黄连, Huanglian) Baikal Skullcap Root (黄芩, Huangqin) Chinese Corktree Bark (黄柏, Huangbai) Manyleaf Meadowrue Rhizome and Root (马尾莲, Maweilian) Tokyo Violet Herb (紫花地丁, Zihuadiding) Dandelion (蒲公英, Pugongying) Whiteflower Patrinia Herb (败酱草, Baijiangcao) Common Andrographis Herb (穿心莲, Chuanxinlian) Manyleaf Paris Rhizome (蚤休, Zaoxiu) Chinese Gentian Root (龙胆草, Longdancao) Tonkin Sophora Root (山豆根, Shandougen) Common Anemarrhea Rhizome (知母, Zhimu) Cape Jasmine Fruit (栀子, Zhizi) Officinal Magnolia Bark (厚朴, Houpo) Tree Peony Bark (牡丹皮, Mudanpi) White Peony

Root (白芍药, Baishaoyao) Common Selfheal Spike (夏枯草, Xiakucao) Snakegourd Fruit (瓜蒌, Gualou) Cow-bezoar (牛黄, Niuhuang) Largeleaf Gentian Root (秦艽, Qinjiao) Garlic Bulb (大蒜, Dasuan) Medicine Terminalia Fruit (诃子, Hezi) Leatherleaf Mahonia Leaf (十大功劳, Shidagonglao)

2. Anti-staphylococcus: Besides the above broad-spectrum antibiosis herbs, there are Heartlaef Houttuynia Herb (鱼腥草, Yuxingcao) Indian Chrysanthemum Flower (野菊花, Yejuhua) Balloonflower Root (桔梗, Jiegeng) Chinese Pulsatilla Root (白头翁, Baitouweng) Purslane Herb (马齿苋, Machixian) Giant Knotweed Rhizome (虎杖, Huzhang) Hairvein Agrimonia Herb (仙鹤草, Xianhecao) Yerbadetajo Herb (墨旱莲, Mohanlian) India Madder Root (茜草, Qiancao) Rhubarb (大黄, Dahuang) Lilac Pink Herb (瞿麦, Qumai) Common Knotgrass Herb (萹蓄, Bianxu) Great Burdock Achene (牛蒡子, Niubangzi) Common Perilla Leaf (苏叶, Suye) Fistular Onion Stalk (葱白, Congbai) Officinal Magnolia Bark (厚朴, Houpo) European Verbena Herb (马鞭草, Mabiancao) Common Dayflower Herb (鸭跖草, Yazhicao) Christina Loosetrife Herb (金钱草, Jinqiancao) Japanese Climbing Fern Spores (海金沙, Haijinsha) Male Fern Rhizome (贯众, Guanzhong) Siberian Cocklebur Fruit (苍耳子, Cangerzi) Clove Flower-bud (丁香, Dingxiang) Japanese Thistle Herb or Root (大蓟, Daji) Common Cephalanoplos Herb (小蓟, Xiaoji) Chinese Arborvitae Leafy Twig (侧柏叶, Cebaiye) Taiwan Beautybetter Leaf (紫珠, Zizhu) Pubescent Holly Root (毛冬青, Maodongqing) Borneol (冰片, Bingpian) Chinese Gall (五倍子, Wubeizi) Smoked Plum (乌梅, Wumei) Asiatic Cornelian Cherry Fruit (山茱萸, Shanzhuyu) Cherokee Rose Fruit (金樱子, Jinyingzi) Figwort Root (玄参, Xuanshen) Musk (麝香, Shexiang) Knoxia Root (红大戟, Hongdaji) Franchet Groundcherry Calyx or Fruit (锦灯笼, Jindenglong) Rhizome of Wild Buckwheat (野荞麦, Yeqiaomai)

3. Anti-a-hemolytic streptococcus, anti-beta hemolytic streptocooccus: Besides the above broad-spectrum antibiosis herbs, there are Giant Knotweed Rhizome (虎杖, Huzhang) Indian Chrysanthemum Flower (野菊花, Yejuhua) Heartlaef Houttuynia Herb (鱼腥草, Yuxingcao) Siberian Cocklebur Fruit (苍耳子, Cangerzi) Argy Wormwood Leaf (艾叶, Aiye) Borneol (冰片, Bingpian)

4. Anti-Diplococcus pnecemoniae: Besides the above broad-spectrum antibiosis herbs, there are Balloonflower Root (桔梗, Jiegeng) Giant Knotweed Rhizome (虎杖, Huzhang) Great Burdock Achene (牛蒡子, Niubangzi) Chinese Arborvitae Leafy Twig (侧柏叶, Cebaiye) Officinal Magnolia Bark (厚朴, Houpo) Sappan Wood (苏木, Sumu) Borneol (冰片, Bingpian) Argy Wormwood Leaf (艾叶, Aiye)

5. Anti-Diplococcus meningitidis: Besides the above broad-spectrum antibiosis herbs, there are Garlic Bulb (大蒜, Dasuan) Giant Knotweed Rhizome (虎杖, Huzhang) Japanese Thistle Herb or Root (大蓟, Daji)

6. Anti-catarrh: Indigowoad Leaf (大青叶, Daqingye) Tree Peony Bark (牡丹皮, Mudanpi) Giant Knotweed Rhizome (虎杖, Huzhang)

7. Anti-Hemophilus influenzae: Indigwoad Root (板蓝根, Banlangen) Blackberrylily Rhizome (射干, Shegan) Balloonflower Root (桔梗, Jiegeng) Dahurian Angelica Root (白芷, Baizhi) Whiteflower Patrinia Herb (败酱草, Baijiangcao) Snakegourd Fruit (瓜蒌,

Gualou) Lesser Galangal Rhizome (高良姜, Gaoliangjiang) Long Pepper Fruit (荜茇, Biba) Sappan Wood (苏木, Sumu) Chinese Magnoliavine (五味子, Wuweizi)

8. Anti-Mycobacterium tuberculosis: Sessile Stemona Root (百部, Baibu) Coptis Rhizome (黄连, Huanglian) Chinese Corktree Bark (黄柏, Huangbai) Common Selfheal Spike (夏枯草, Xiakucao) Lightyellow Sophora Root (苦参, Kushen) Honeysuckle Flower (金银花, Jinyinhua) Weeping Forsythia Capsule (连翘, Lianqiao) Tokyo Violet Herb (紫花地丁, Zihuadiding) Chinese Wolfberry Root-bark (地骨皮, Digupi) Siberian Solomonseal Rhizome (黄精, Huangjing) Fragrant Solomonseal Rhizome (玉竹, Yuzhu) Bletilla Rhizome (白及, Baiji) Thinleaf Milkwort Root (远志, Yuanzhi) Tatarian Aster Root (紫苑, Ziyuan) Common Coltsfoot Flower (款冬花, Kuandonghua) Scorpion (全蝎, Quanxie) Centipede (蜈蚣, Wugong) Pumice (海浮石, Haifushi) Clove Flower-bud (丁香, Dingxiang) Garden Burnet Root (地榆, Diyu) Musk (麝香, Shexiang) Dahurian Angelica Root (白芷, Baizhi) Chinese Thorowax Root (柴胡, Chaihu) Shunk Bugbane Rhizome (升麻, Shengma) Immature Bitter Orange (枳实, Zhishi) Capillary Wormwood Herb (茵陈蒿, Yinchenhao) Chinese Caterpillar Fungus (冬虫夏草, Dongchongxiacao) Dan-shen Root (丹参, Danshen) Ginkgo Seed (白果, Baiguo)

9. Anti-Bordetella pertussis: Baikal Skullcap Root (黄芩, Huangqin) Sessile Stemona Root (百部, Baibu) Hunifuse Euphorbia Herb (地锦草, Dijincao) Common Andrographis Herb (穿心莲, Chuanxinlian) Airpotato Yam Tuber (黄药子, Huangyaozi) Clove Flower-bud (丁香, Dingxiang) Bletilla Rhizome (白及, Baiji) Officinal Magnolia Bark (厚朴, Houpo) White Peony Root (白芍药, Baishaoyao) Common Cephalanoplos Herb (小蓟, Xiaoji)

10. Anti-Bacillus diphtheriae: Twotooth Achyranthes Root (土牛膝, Tuniuxi) European Verbena Herb (马鞭草, Mabiancao) Rehmannia Dried Root (生地黄, Shengdihuang) Figwort Root (玄参, Xuanshen) White Peony Root (白芍药, Baishaoyao) Tree Peony Bark (牡丹皮, Mudanpi) Hunifuse Euphorbia Herb (地锦草, Dijincao) Omoto Nipponlily (万年青, Wannianqing) Honeysuckle Flower (金银花, Jinyinhua) Weeping Forsythia Capsule (连翘, Lianqiao) Heartlaef Houttuynia Herb (鱼腥草, Yuxingcao) Indian Chrysanthemum Flower (野菊花, Yejuhua) Manyleaf Paris Rhizome (蚤休, Zaoxiu) Baikal Skullcap Root (黄芩, Huangqin) Common Anemarrhea Rhizome (知母, Zhimu) Tendrilleaf Fritillary Bulb (贝母, Beimu), Giant Knotweed Rhizome (虎杖, Huzhang) Fineleaf Schizomepeta Herb (荆芥, Jingjie) Dwarf Lilyturf Root (麦门冬, Maimendong) Cochinchinese Asparagus Root (天门冬, Tianmendong) Glossy Privet Fruit (女贞子, Nuzhenzi) Japanese Thistle Herb or Root (大蓟, Daji) Hairvein Agrimonia Herb (仙鹤草, Xianhecao) Yerbadetajo Herb (墨旱莲, Mohanlian) Chinese Angelica Root (当归, Danggui) Medicine Terminalia Fruit (诃子, Hezi) Garlic Bulb (大蒜, Dasuan) Common Aucklandia Root (木香, Muxiang) Japanese Felt Fern Leaf (石韦, Shiwei) Licorice Root (甘草, Gancao)

11. Anti-Bacillus enteritidis: Besides the above broad-spectrum antibiosis herbs, there are Hunifuse Euphorbia Herb (地锦草, Dijincao) Purslane Herb (马齿苋, Machixian) Largeleaf Chinese Ash Bark (秦皮, Qinpi) Yerbadetajo Herb (墨旱莲, Mohanlian)

Hairvein Agrimonia Herb (仙鹤草, Xianhecao) Heartlaef Houttuynia Herb (鱼腥草, Yuxingcao) Red Peony Root (赤芍药, Chishaoyao) Chinese Gall (五倍子, Wubeizi) Fineleaf Schizomepeta Herb (荆芥, Jingjie) Sweet Wormwood (青蒿, Qinghao) Chinese Wolfberry Root-bark (地骨皮, Digupi), Garden Burnet Root (地榆, Diyu)

12. Anti-Bacillus dysenteriae: Besides the above broad-spectrum antibiosis herbs, there are Purslane Herb (马齿苋, Machixian) Chinese Pulsatilla Root (白头翁, Baitouweng) Largeleaf Chinese Ash Bark (秦皮, Qinpi) Lightyellow Sophora Root (苦参, Kushen) Heartlaef Houttuynia Herb (鱼腥草, Yuxingcao) Common Aucklandia Root (木香, Muxiang) Giant Knotweed Rhizome (虎杖, Huzhang) Hairvein Agrimonia Herb (仙鹤草, Xianhecao) Common Heron's Bill Herb or Wilford Cranesbill Herb (老鹳草, Laoguancao) Japanese Thistle Herb or Root (大蓟, Daji)Common Perilla Leaf (苏叶, Suye) Divaricate Saposhnikovia Root (防风, Fangfeng) Fistular Onion Stalk (葱白, Congbai) Indian Chrysanthemum Flower (野菊花, Yejuhua) Japanese Climbing Fern Spores (海金沙, Haijinsha) Clove Flower-bud (丁香, Dingxiang) Garden Burnet Root (地榆, Diyu) Chinese Arborvitae Leafy Twig (侧柏叶, Cebaiye) Hawthorn Fruit (山楂, Shanzha) Chinese Gall (五倍子, Wubeizi) Smoked Plum (乌梅, Wumei) Pomegranate Rind Peel (石榴皮, Shiliupi) Tea Leaf-bud (茶叶, Chaye) Chinese Angelica Root (当归, Danggui) Common Knotgrass Herb (萹蓄, Bianxu) Chinese Magnoliavine (五味子, Wuweizi)

13. Anti-typhorid bacillus, anti-Bacillus paratyphosus: Besides the above broad-spectrum antibiosis herbs, there are Common Aucklandia Root (木香, Muxiang) Purslane Herb (马齿苋, Machixian) Officinal Magnolia Bark (厚朴, Houpo) Giant Knotweed Rhizome (虎杖, Huzhang) Japanese Climbing Fern Spores (海金沙, Haijinsha) Cassia Twig (桂枝, Guizhi) Clove Flower-bud (丁香, Dingxiang) Hairvein Agrimonia Herb (仙鹤草, Xianhecao) Japanese Thistle Herb or Root (大蓟, Daji) Common Cephalanoplos Herb (小蓟, Xiaoji) Garden Burnet Root (地榆, Diyu) Chinese Gall (五倍子, Wubeizi) Siberian Solomonseal Rhizome (黄精, Huangjing) Dwarf Lilyturf Root (麦门冬, Maimendong) Common Aucklandia Root (木香, Muxiang)

14. Anti-colibacillus: Indian Chrysanthemum Flower (野菊花, Yejuhua) Purslane Herb (马齿苋, Machixian) Hunifuse Euphorbia Herb (地锦草, Dijincao) Dandelion (蒲公英, Pugongying) Whiteflower Patrinia Herb (败酱草, Baijiangcao) European Verbena Herb (马鞭草, Mabiancao) Common Heron's Bill Herb or Wilford Cranesbill Herb (老鹳草, Laoguancao) Ciliate Bugle Herb (筋骨草, Jingucao) Baikal Skullcap Root (黄芩, Huangqin) Rhubarb (大黄, Dahuang) Snakegourd Fruit (瓜蒌, Gualou) Lightyellow Sophora Root (苦参, Kushen) Common Knotgrass Herb (萹蓄, Bianxu) Common Aucklandia Root (木香, Muxiang) Hairvein Agrimonia Herb (仙鹤草, Xianhecao) Japanese Thistle Herb or Root (大蓟, Daji) Common Cephalanoplos Herb (小蓟, Xiaoji) Dan-shen Root (丹参, Danshen) White Peony Root (白芍药, Baishaoyao) Musk (麝香, Shexiang) Garlic Bulb (大蒜, Dasuan) Smoked Plum (乌梅, Wumei) Dwarf Lilyturf Root (麦门冬, Maimendong) Barbed Skullcap Herb (半枝莲, Banzhilian) Common Carpesium Fruit (鹤虱, Heshi)

15. Anti-pseudomonas aeruginosa: Chinese Gall (五倍子, Wubeizi) Medicine Terminalia Fruit (诃子, Hezi) Manyleaf Paris Rhizome (蚤休, Zaoxiu) Common Selfheal Spike (夏枯草, Xiakucao) Honeysuckle Flower (金银花, Jinyinhua) Dandelion (蒲公英, Pugongying) Tokyo Violet Herb (紫花地丁, Zihuadiding) Tree Peony Bark (牡丹皮, Mudanpi) White Peony Root (白芍药, Baishaoyao) Chinese Pulsatilla Root (白头翁, Baitouweng) Baikal Skullcap Root (黄芩, Huangqin) Rhubarb (大黄, Dahuang) Giant Knotweed Rhizome (虎杖, Huzhang) Japanese Climbing Fern Spores (海金沙, Haijinsha) Chinese Lobelia Herb (半边莲, Banbianlian) Common Knotgrass Herb (萹蓄, Bianxu) Lilac Pink Herb (瞿麦, Qumai) Japanese Thistle Herb or Root (大蓟, Daji) Figwort Root (玄参, Xuanshen) Smoked Plum (乌梅, Wumei) Chinese Magnoliavine (五味子, Wuweizi) Common Heron's Bill Herb or Wilford Cranesbill Herb (老鹳草, Laoguancao) Cherokee Rose Fruit (金樱子, Jinyingzi) Knoxia Root (红大戟, Hongdaji) Waternut Corm (荸荠, Biqi)

16. Anti-brucellosis: Honeysuckle Flower (金银花, Jinyinhua) Medicine Terminalia Fruit (诃子, Hezi) Clove Flower-bud (丁香, Dingxiang) Barbed Skullcap Herb (半枝莲, Banzhilian) Lilac Pink Herb (瞿麦, Qumai) Bunge Pricklyash (花椒, Huajiao) Dan-shen Root (丹参, Danshen) White Peony Root (白芍药, Baishaoyao) Pubescent Holly Root (毛冬青, Maodongqing) Dwarf Lilyturf Root (麦门冬, Maimendong)

17. Anti-bacillus proteus: Coptis Rhizome (黄连, Huanglian) Manyleaf Meadowrue Rhizome and Root (马尾莲, Maweilian) Sargen Barberry Bark (三颗针, Sankezhen) Incised Notopterygium Rhizome and Root (羌活, Qianghuo)

18. Anti-bacillus leprae: European Hop Female-flower (啤酒花, Pijiuhua) Japanese Hop Herb (律草, Lvcao) Common Andrographis Herb (穿心莲, Chuanxinlian) Siberian Cocklebur Fruit (苍耳子, Cangerzi) Chinese Honeylocust Spine (皂角刺, Zaojiaoci) Garter Snake (乌梢蛇, Wushaoshe) Turmeric Root-tuber (郁金, Yujin) Rhubarb (大黄, Dahuang) Mirabilite (朴硝, Piaoxiao)

19. Anti-bacillus anthracis: Heartlaef Houttuynia Herb (鱼腥草, Yuxingcao) Indian Chrysanthemum Flower (野菊花, Yejuhua) Leatherleaf Mahonia Leaf (十大功劳, Shidagonglao) Shunk Bugbane Rhizome (升麻, Shengma) Wild Mint (薄荷, Bohe) Barbed Skullcap Herb (半枝莲, Banzhilian) Giant Knotweed Rhizome (虎杖, Huzhang) Largeleaf Gentian Root (秦艽, Qinjiao) Tuber Fleeceflower Root (何首乌, Heshouwu) Eucommia Bark (杜仲, Duzhong) Glossy Privet Fruit (女贞子, Nuzhenzi) Fortune's Drynaria Rhizome, Baron's Drynaria Rhizome (骨碎补, Gusuibu) Japanese Thistle Herb or Root (大蓟, Daji) India Madder Root (茜草, Qiancao) Hairvein Agrimonia Herb (仙鹤草, Xianhecao) Hirsute Shiny Bugleweed Herb (泽兰, Zelan) Argy Wormwood Leaf (艾叶, Aiye) Combined Spicebush Root (乌药, Wuyao) Bunge Pricklyash (花椒, Huajiao) Long Pepper Fruit (荜茇, Biba) Lesser Galangal Rhizome (高良姜, Gaoliangjiang), Clove Flower-bud (丁香, Dingxiang)

20. Anti-bacillus subtilis: Divaricate Saposhnikovia Root (防风, Fangfeng) Lesser Galangal Rhizome (高良姜, Gaoliangjiang), Long Pepper Fruit (荜茇, Biba) Common Aucklandia Root (木香, Muxiang) Garlic Bulb (大蒜, Dasuan) Dwarf Lilyturf Root (麦门冬, Maimendong) Cochinchinese As-

paragus Root (天门冬, Tianmendong) Membranous Milkvetch Root (黄芪, Huangqi)

21. Anti-epidermophyton rubrum (pathogenic dermatomycosis): Sulfur (硫黄, Liuhuang) Bark of Golden Larch (土槿皮, Tujinpi) Lightyellow Sophora Root (苦参, Kushen) Siberian Solomonseal Rhizome (黄精, Huangjing) Densefruit Pittany Root-bark (白鲜皮, Baixianpi) Blackberrylily Rhizome (射干, Shegan) Aloes (芦荟, Luhui) Rhubarb (大黄, Dahuang) Chinese Pulsatilla Root (白头翁, Baitouweng) Balloonflower Root (桔梗, Jiegeng) Heartlaef Houttuynia Herb (鱼腥草, Yuxingcao) Chinese Ligusticum Rhizome (藁本, Gaoben) Common Knotgrass Herb (萹蓄, Bianxu) Clove Flower-bud (丁香, Dingxiang) Szechwan chinaberry Fruit (川楝子, Chuanlianzi) Pomegranate Rind Peel (石榴皮, Shiliupi) Uniflower Swisscentaury Root (漏芦, Loulu) Tonkin Sophora Root (山豆根, Shandougen) Irkutsk Anemone Rhizome (九节菖蒲, Jiujiechangpu) Chaulmoogratree Seed (大风子, Dafengzi) Belvedere Fruit (地肤子, Difuzi) Capillary Wormwood Herb (茵陈蒿, Yinchenhao)

22. Anti-candida albicans: Chinese Corktree Bark (黄柏, Huangbai) Baikal Skullcap Root (黄芩, Huangqin) Tonkin Sophora Root (山豆根, Shandougen) Alumen (白矾, Baifan) Szechwan chinaberry Fruit (川楝子, Chuanlianzi) Bark of Golden Larch (土槿皮, Tujinpi)

23. Anti-bacillus tetani: Cherokee Rose Fruit (金樱子, Jinyingzi) Divaricate Saposhnikovia Root (防风, Fangfeng) Cicada Slough (蝉蜕, Chantui) Scorpion (全蝎, Quanxie)

Anti-spirochete Herbs

1. Anti-Leptospia: Indigowoad Leaf (大青叶, Daqingye) Indigwoad Root (板蓝根, Banlangen) Common Andrographis Herb (穿心莲, Chuanxinlian) Glabrous Greenbrier Rhizome (土茯苓, Tufuling) Coptis Rhizome (黄连, Huanglian) Baikal Skullcap Root (黄芩, Huangqin) Chinese Corktree Bark (黄柏, Huangbai) Weeping Forsythia Capsule (连翘, Lianqiao) Cape Jasmine Fruit (栀子, Zhizi) Garden Burnet Root (地榆, Diyu) Giant Knotweed Rhizome (虎杖, Huzhang) Cherokee Rose Fruit (金樱子, Jinyingzi)

2. Anti-treponema pallidum: Glabrous Greenbrier Rhizome (土茯苓, Tufuling)

Anti-protozoom Herbs

1. Anti-plasmodium: Sweet Wormwood (青蒿, Qinghao) Chinese Thorowax Root (柴胡, Chaihu) Antifebrile Dichroa Root (常山, Changshan) Caoguo (草果, Caoguo) Java Brucea Fruit (鸦胆子, Yadanzi) European Verbena Herb (马鞭草, Mabiancao) Common St. Paulswort Herb (豨莶草, Xixiancao) Baikal Skullcap Root (黄芩, Huangqin) Coptis Rhizome (黄连, Huanglian) Chinese Corktree Bark (黄柏, Huangbai) Chinese Gentian Root (龙胆草, Longdancao) Swordlike Atractylodes Rhizome (苍术, Cangzhu) Shunk Bugbane Rhizome (升麻, Shengma) Garden Burnet Root (地榆, Diyu) Smoked Plum (乌梅, Wumei) Turtle Carapace (鳖甲, Biejia) Hairvein Agrimonia Herb (仙鹤草, Xianhecao) Fourstamen Stephania Root

(防己，Fangji) Borax (硼砂，Pengsha)

2. Anti-ameba: Chinese Pulsatilla Root (白头翁，Baitouweng) Coptis Rhizome (黄连，Huanglian) Baikal Skullcap Root (黄芩，Huangqin) Lightyellow Sophora Root (苦参，Kushen) Largeleaf Chinese Ash Bark (秦皮，Qinpi) Sessile Stemona Root (百部，Baibu) Fourstamen Stephania Root (汉防已，Hanfangji) Java Brucea Fruit (鸦胆子，Yadanzi) Yerbadetajo Herb (墨旱莲，Mohanlian) Purslane Herb (马齿苋，Machixian) Chinese Clematis Root (威灵仙，Weilingxian) Mountain Spicy Tree Fruit (荜澄茄，Bichengqie)

3. Anti-trichomonas vaginatis: Common Cnidium Fruit (蛇床子，Shechuangzi) Lightyellow Sophora Root (苦参，Kushen) Chinese Pulsatilla Root (白头翁，Baitouweng) Chinaberry-tree Bark (苦楝根皮，Kuliangenpi) Wild Mint (薄荷，Bohe) Fistular Onion Stalk (葱白，Congbai) Garlic Bulb (大蒜，Dasuan) Radish Seed (莱菔子，Laifuzi) Frankincense (乳香，Ruxiang) Chinese Honeylocust Spine (皂角，Zaojiao)

Antiparasite Herbs

1. Anti-ascaris lumbricoides: Szechwan Chinaberry Bark (苦楝皮，Kulianpi) Szechwan chinaberry Fruit (川楝子，Chuanlianzi) Rangooncreeper Fruit (使君子，Shijunzi) Bigfruit Elm Fruit (芜荑，Wuyi) Cushaw Seed (南瓜子，Nanguazi) Grand Torreya Seed (榧子，Feizi) Male Fern Rhizome (贯众，Guanzhong) Pomegranate Rind Peel (石榴皮，Shiliupi) Smoked Plum (乌梅，Wumei) Bunge Pricklyash (花椒，Huajiao) Medicinal Evodia Root (吴茱萸，Wuzhuyu) Clove Flower-bud (丁香，Dingxiang) Officinal Magnolia Bark (厚朴，Houpo) Pharbitis Seed (牵牛子，Qianniuzi) Luffa Seed (丝瓜子，Siguazi) Common Knotgrass Herb (萹蓄，Bianxu) Areca Seed (槟榔，Binlang)

2. Anti-Enterobius vermicularis: Sessile Stemona Root (百部，Baibu) Szechwan Chinaberry Bark (苦楝皮，Kulianpi) Rangooncreeper Fruit (使君子，Shijunzi) Male Fern Rhizome (贯众，Guanzhong) Common Carpesium Fruit (鹤虱，Heshi) Garlic Bulb (大蒜，Dasuan) Grand Torreya Seed (榧子，Feizi) Pomegranate Rind Peel (石榴皮，Shiliupi) Medicinal Evodia Root (吴茱萸，Wuzhuyu) Java Brucea Fruit (鸦胆子，Yadanzi)

3. Anti-ancylostomum: Areca Seed (槟榔，Binlang) Stone-like Omphalia (fungus) (雷丸，Leiwan) Grand Torreya Seed (榧子，Feizi) Szechwan Chinaberry Bark (苦楝皮，Kulianpi) Pomegranate Rind Peel (石榴皮，Shiliupi)

4. Schistosomicide: Cushaw Seed (南瓜子，Nanguazi) Fennel Fruit (小茴香，Xiaohuixiang) Dan-shen Root (丹参，Danshen) Cape Jasmine Fruit (栀子，Zhizi) Lilac Pink Herb (瞿麦，Qumai) Toad Skin Secretion Cake (蟾酥，Chansu)

5. Filaricide: Chinese Clematis Root (威灵仙，Weilingxian) Stone-like Omphalia (fungus，雷丸，Leiwan) Sweet Wormwood (青蒿，Qinghao) Slenderstyle Acanthopanax Root-bark (北五加皮，Beiwujiapi) Glutinous Rice Rhizome and Root (糯稻根，Nuodaogen) Mulberry Leaf (桑叶，Sangye) Chinese Honeylocust Spine (猪牙皂，Zhuyazhao)

6. Anti-tenia: Areca Seed (槟榔，Binlang) Cushaw Seed (南瓜子，Nanguazi) Stone-like Omphalia (fungus) (雷丸，Leiwan) Male Fern Rhizome (贯众，Guanzhong) Grand Torreya Seed (榧子，Feizi) Common Carpesium Fruit (鹤虱，Heshi)

7. Anti-mastigote: Lightyellow Sophora Root (苦参，Kushen)

8. Anti-fasciolopsis: Ccocnut (椰子, Yezi) and Coconut Juice (椰子汁, Yezizhi)

Anticancer Herbs

Appendiculate Cremastra Pseudobulb (丽江山慈姑, Lijiangshancigu) Spreading Hedyotis Herb (白花蛇舌草, Baihuasheshecao) Zedoray (莪术, Ezhu) Manyleaf Paris Rhizome (蚤休, Zaoxiu) Snakegroud Root (天花粉, Tianhuafen) Coix Seed (薏苡仁, Yiyiren) Tuckahoe (茯苓, Fuling) Umbellate Pore Fungus (猪苓, Zhuling) Fig Receptacle (无花果, Wuhuaguo) Snakegourd Fruit (瓜蒌, Gualou) Tonkin Sophora Root (广豆根, Guangdougen) Blackberrylily Rhizome (射干, Shegan) Fourstamen Stephania Root (粉防己, Fenfangji) Black Nightshade Herb (龙葵, Longkui) Airpotato Yam Tuber (黄药子, Huangyaozi) Common Selfheal Spike (夏枯草, Xiakucao) Large Blister Beetle (斑蝥, Banmao) Ground Beetle (土鳖虫, Tubiechong) Scorpion (全蝎, Quanxie) Gecko (壁虎, Bihu) Centipede (蜈蚣, Wugong) Toad Skin Secretion Cake (蟾酥, Chansu) Leech (水蛭, Shuizhi) Barbed Skullcap Herb (半枝莲, Banzhilian) Chinese Lobelia Herb (半边莲, Banbianlian) Herb of Bittesweet (白英, Baiying) Dandelion (蒲公英, Pugongying) Heartlaef Houttuynia Herb (鱼腥草, Yuxingcao) Dan-shen Root (丹参, Danshen) Red Peony Root (赤芍药, Chishaoyao) Sanchi Root (三七, Sanqi) Japanese Thistle Herb or Root (大蓟, Daji) Common Cephalanoplos Herb (小蓟, Xiaoji) Java Brucea Fruit (鸦胆子, Yadanzi) Grassleaf Sweetflag Rhizome (石菖蒲, Shichangpu) Catechu (儿茶, Ercha) Root of Sinkiang Arnebia (紫草, Zicao) Jackinthep-ulpit Tuber (天南星, Tiannanxing) Chinese Clematis Root (威灵仙, Weilingxian) Garden Balsam Seed (急性子, Jixingzi) Malaytea Scurfpea Fruit (补骨脂, Buguzhi) Realgar (雄黄, Xionghuang) Arsenolite Ore (砒霜, Pishuang) Sal-ammoniac (硇砂, Naosha) Glossy Privet Fruit (女贞子, Nuzhenzi) Asiatic Cornelian Cherry Fruit (山茱萸, Shanzhuyu) Shorthorned Epimedium Herb (淫羊藿, Yinyanghuo) Pinellia Rhizome (半夏, Banxia) Kelp (海带, Haidai) Seaweed (海藻, Haizao) Kelp (昆布, Kunbu), Musk (麝香, Shexiang) Pubescent Holly Root (毛冬青, Maodongqing) Shorttube Lycoris Bulb (石蒜, Shisuan) Fig Receptacle (无花果, Wuhuaguo) Smoked Plum (乌梅, Wumei) Lilac Pink Herb (瞿麦, Qumai)

Anti-leukemia Herbs

Dried Toad (干蟾皮, Ganchanpi) Large Blister Beetle (斑蝥, Banmao) Diversifolious Patrinia Root (墓头回, Mutouhui) Nut-vomitive Poisonnut Seed (马钱子, Maqianzi) Figwortflower Picrorhiza Rhizome (胡黄连, Huhuanglian) Java Brucea Fruit (鸦胆子, Yadanzi) Chinese Pulsatilla Root (白头翁, Baitouweng) Puff-ball (马勃, Mabo) Sword-like Iris Root (马兰根, Malangen) Safflower (红花, Honghua) Oriental Stephania Root (白药子, Baiyaozi) Chinese Stellera Root (狼毒, Langdu) Tonkin Sophora Root (广豆根, Guangdougen) Centipede (蜈蚣, Wugong) Scorpion (全蝎, Quanxie)

Antipytetic Herbs

1. Anti-pyretic by regulating heat centre: Chinese Thorowax Root (柴胡, Chaihu) Baikal Skullcap Root (黄芩, Huangqin) Common Anemarrhea Rhizome (知母, Zhimu)

Gypsum（石膏，Shigao）Sweet Wormwood（青蒿，Qinghao）Common Dayflower Herb（鸭跖草，Yazhicao）Chinese Wolfberry Root-bark（地骨皮，Digupi），Capillary Wormwood Herb（茵陈蒿，Yinchenhao）Cape Jasmine Fruit（栀子，Zhizi）Tree Peony Bark（牡丹皮，Mudanpi）Coptis Rhizome（黄连，Huanglian）Manchurian Wildginger Herb（细辛，Xixin）Chrysanthemum Flower（菊花，Juhua）Divaricate Saposhnikovia Root（防风，Fangfeng）Fourstamen Stephania Root（汉防己，Hanfangji）Chinese Tamarish Twig（西河柳，Xiheliu）Shrub Chastetree Fruit（蔓荆子，Manjingzi）European Verbena Herb（马鞭草，Mabiancao）Starwort Root（银柴胡，Yinchaihu）Whiteflower hogfenel Root（前胡，Qianhu），Antelope Horn（羚羊角，Lingyangjiao）Asiatic Rhinoceros Horn（犀角，Xijiao）Buffalo Horn（水牛角，Shuiniujiao）Earth Worm（地龙，Dilong）Borneol（冰片，Bingpian）Dendrobium Herb（石斛，Shihu）Root of Sinkiang Arnebia（紫草，Zicao）Chinese Clematis Root（威灵仙，Weilingxian）Common Lophatherum Herb（淡竹叶，Danzhuye）

2. Antipyretic by exciting sudoriferous gland to sweat：Ephedra（麻黄，Mahuang）Cassia Twig（桂枝，Guizhi）Haichow Elsholtzia Herb（香薷，Xiangru）Common Perilla Leaf（苏叶，Suye）Fineleaf Schizomepeta Herb（荆芥，Jingjie）Divaricate Saposhnikovia Root（防风，Fangfeng）Largeleaf Gentian Root（秦艽，Qinjiao）Wild Mint（薄荷，Bohe）Great Burdock Achene（牛蒡子，Niubangzi）Chinese Thorowax Root（柴胡，Chaihu）Shunk Bugbane Rhizome（升麻，Shengma）Lobed Kudzuvine Root（葛根，Gegen）Fistular Onion Stalk（葱白，Congbai）Common Ducksmeat Herb（浮萍，Fuping）Densefruit Pittany Root-bark（白鲜皮，Baixianpi）

Herbs producing effect on nervous system

1. Sedation and hypnotism：Spine Date Seed（酸枣仁，Suanzaoren）Chinese Magnoliavine（五味子，Wuweizi）Yanhusuo（延胡索，Yanhusuo）Dan-shen Root（丹参，Danshen）Lucid Ganoderma（灵芝，Lingzhi）Chinese Angelica Root（当归，Danggui）Szechwan Lovage Rhizome（川芎，Chuanxiong）Sappan Wood（苏木，Sumu）Indian Bread with Hostwood（茯神，Fushen）Tall Gastrodia Rhizome（天麻，Tianma）Gambirplant Hooked Stem and Branch（钩藤，Gouteng）Puncturevine Caltrap Fruit（白蒺藜，Baijili）Shrub Chastetree Fruit（蔓荆子，Manjingzi）Chinese Ligusticum Rhizome（藁本，Gaoben）Cape Jasmine Fruit（栀子，Zhizi）Hindu Lotus Plumule（莲子心，Lianzixin）Scorpion（全蝎，Quanxie）Earth Worm（地龙，Dilong）Cicada Slough（蝉蜕，Chantui）Jackinthepulpit Tuber（天南星，Tiannanxing）Amber（琥珀，Hupo）Pearl（珍珠，Zhenzhu）Cinnabar（朱砂，Zhusha）Cow-bezoar（牛黄，Niuhuang）Magnetite Ore（磁石，Cishi）Dragon's Bone（龙骨，Longgu）Tuber Fleeceflower Stem and Leaf（夜交藤，Yejiaoteng）Chinese Arborvitae Seed（柏子仁，Baiziren）Silktree Albiziae Bark（合欢皮，Hehuanpi）Chinese Caterpillar Fungus（冬虫夏草，Dongchongxiacao）Chinese Thorowax Root（柴胡，Chaihu）Baikal Skullcap Root（黄芩，Huangqin）Gypsum（石膏，Shigao）Common Anemarrhea Rhizome（知母，Zhimu）Doubleteeth Pulbescent Angelica Root（独活，Duhuo）Nutgrass Galingale Rhizome（香附，Xiangfu）Harleguin Glorybower Leaf（臭梧桐，Chouwutong）Common St. Paulswort Herb（豨莶草，Xixiancao）Large-

leaf Chinese Ash Bark (秦皮, Qinpi) Largeleaf Gentian Root (秦艽, Qinjiao) Eucommia Bark (杜仲, Duzhong) Medicinal Indian-mulberry Root (巴戟天, Bajitian) Barbary Wolfberry Fruit (枸杞子, Gouqizi) Blighted Wheat (浮小麦, Fuxiaomai) Longan Aril (龙眼肉, Longyanrou) Tabasheer (天竹黄, Tianzhuhuang) Mongolian Gazelle Horn (黄羊角, Huangyangjiao) Heterophylla Falsestarwort Root (太子参, Taizishen) Dogbame Herb (罗布麻, Luobuma) Grassleaf Sweetflag Rhizome (石菖蒲, Shichangpu) Common Carpesium Fruit (鹤虱, Heshi) Paniculate Swallowwort Root (徐长卿, Xuchangqing) Manyleaf Paris Rhizome (七叶一枝花, Qiyeyizhihua) Spreading Hedyotis Herb (白花蛇舌草, Baihuasheshecao)

2. Anticonvulsion: Antelope Horn (羚羊角, Lingyangjiao) Scorpion (全蝎, Quanxie) Centipede (蜈蚣, Wugong) Earth Worm (地龙, Dilong) Silkworm with Batrytis Larva (白僵蚕, Baijiangcan) Jackinthepulpit Tuber (天南星, Tiannanxing) Gambirplant Hooked Stem and Branch (钩藤, Gouteng) Lucid Ganoderma (灵芝, Lingzhi) Tall Gastrodia Rhizome (天麻, Tianma) Snake Slough (蛇蜕, Shetui) Chinese Thorowax Root (柴胡, Chaihu) White Peony Root (白芍药, Baishaoyao) Tree Peony Bark (牡丹皮, Mudanpi) Biond Magnolia Flower-bud (辛夷, Xinyi) Largeleaf Chinese Ash Bark (秦皮, Qinpi) Mongolian Gazelle Horn (黄羊角, Huangyangjiao) Grassleaf Sweetflag Rhizome (石菖蒲, Shichangpu) Nacre (珍珠母, Zhenzhumu) Tabasheer (天竹黄, Tianzhuhuang)

3. Analgesia: Datura Flower (洋金花, Yangjinhua) Yanhusuo (延胡索, Yanhusuo) Opium Poppy Pericarp (罂粟壳, Yingsuqiao) Common Monksood (乌头, Wutou) Prepared Daughter Root of Common Monkshood (附子, Fuzi) Manchurian Wildginger Herb (细辛, Xixin) Cassia Twig (桂枝, Guizhi) Fourstamen Stephania Root (汉防己, Hanfangji) Toad Skin Secretion Cake (蟾酥, Chansu) Szechwan Lovage Rhizome (川芎, Chuanxiong) Dan-shen Root (丹参, Danshen) Chinese Angelica Root (当归, Danggui) White Peony Root (白芍药, Baishaoyao) Divaricate Saposhnikovia Root (防风, Fangfeng) Dahurian Angelica Root (白芷, Baizhi) Medicinal Evodia Root (吴茱萸, Wuzhuyu) Paniculate Swallowwort Root (徐长卿, Xuchangqing) Shrub Chastetree Fruit (蔓荆子, Manjingzi) Chinese Ligusticum Rhizome (藁本, Gaoben) Wild Mint (薄荷, Bohe) Largeleaf Gentian Root (秦艽, Qinjiao) Common St. Paulswort Herb (豨莶草, Xixiancao) Harleguin Glorybower Leaf (臭梧桐, Chouwutong) Cortex Acanthopanacis Radicis (五加皮, Wujiapi) Chinese Nardostachys Root and Rhizome or Spoonleaf Nardostachys Root and Rhizome (甘松, Gansong) Frankincense (乳香, Ruxiang) Myrrh (没药, Moyao) Orientvine Stem or Hair Orientvine Stem (青风藤, Qingfengteng) Twotooth Achyranthes Root (牛膝, Niuxi) Doubleteeth Pulbescent Angelica Root (独活, Duhuo) Chinese Clematis Root (威灵仙, Weilingxian) Cowherb Seed (王不留行, Wangbuliuxing) Nutgrass Galingale Rhizome (香附, Xiangfu) Turmeric Root-tuber (郁金, Yujin) Largeleaf Chinese Ash Bark (秦皮, Qinpi) Spreading Hedyotis Herb (白花蛇舌草, Baihuasheshecao) Manyleaf Paris Rhizome (蚤休, Zaoxiu) Sandalwood (檀香, Tanxiang) Obscured Homalamena Rhizome (千年健, Qiannianjian) Suberect Spatholobus Stem (鸡血藤, Jixueteng) Common Clubmoss Herb (伸筋草, Shenjincao) Nippon

Yam Rhizome (穿山龙, Chuanshanlong) Decumbent Corydalis Rhizome (夏天无, Xiatianwu) Chinese Starjasmine Stem (络石藤, Luoshiteng) Yangtao Actinidia Fruit (猕猴桃根, Mihoutaogen) Williams Elder (接骨木, Jiegumu) Small Centipeda Herb (鹅不食草, Ebushicao) Garter Snake (乌梢蛇, Wushaoshe) Aspongopus (九香虫, Jiuxiangchong) Stem of Chinese Photinial (石楠藤, Shinanteng) Towel Gourd Vegetable Sponge (丝瓜络, Sigualuo) Colored Mistletoe Herb (槲寄生, Hujisheng)

4. Anesthesia

(1) Local anesthesia: Common Monksood (乌头, Wutou) Manchurian Wildginger Herb (细辛, Xixin) Common Jasminorange Branchlet and Leaf (九里香, Jiulixiang) Arabian Jasmine Root (茉莉花根, Molihuagen) Bunge Pricklyash (花椒, Huajiao)

(2) General anesthesia: Datura Flower (洋金花, Yangjinhua)

5. Herbs for exciting nervous system: Ginseng (人参, Renshen) Chinese Magnoliavine (五味子, Wuweizi) Tea Leaf-bud (茶叶, Chaye) Membranous Milkvetch Root (黄芪, Huangqi) Tangshen Root (党参, Dangshen) Heterophylla Falsestarwort Root (太子参, Taizishen) Musk (麝香, Shexiang) Borneol (冰片, Bingpian) Storesin (苏合香, Suhexiang) Benzoin (安息香, Anxixiang) Camphor (樟脑, Zhangnao) Dahurian Angelica Root (白芷, Baizhi) Nut-vomitive Poisonnut Seed (马钱子, Maqianzi) Wild Mint (薄荷, Bohe) Weeping Forsythia Capsule (连翘, Lianqiao)

Herbs acting on cardiovascular system

1. Heart

(1) Cardiac: Toad Skin Secretion Cake (蟾酥, Chansu) Sweetscented Oleander Leaf or Bark (夹竹桃, Jiazhutao) Root of Dogbame (罗布麻根, Luobumagen) Chinese Starjasmine Stem (络石藤, Luoshiteng) Omoto Nipponlily (万年青, Wannianqing) Manyprickle Acanthopanax Root (刺五加, Ciwujia) Slenderstyle Acanthopanax Rootbark (北五加皮, Beiwujiapi), Chinese Pulsatilla Root (白头翁, Baitouweng) Musk (麝香, Shexiang) Hairy Antler (鹿茸, Lurong) Membranous Milkvetch Root (黄芪, Huangqi) Pepperweed Seed or Flixweed Tansymustard Seed (葶苈子, Tinglizi) Akebia Stem (木通, Mutong) Chinese Magnoliavine (五味子, Wuweizi) Tuber Fleeceflower Root (何首乌, Heshouwu) Prepared Daughter Root of Common Monkshood (附子, Fuzi) Lucid Ganoderma (灵芝, Lingzhi) Malaytea Scurfpea Fruit (补骨脂, Buguzhi) Common Cruculigo (仙茅, Xianmao) Sharpleaf Galangal Fruit (益智仁, Yizhiren) Fragrant Solomonseal Rhizome (玉竹, Yuzhu) Rehmannia Dried Root (生地黄, Shengdihuang) Prepared Rhizome of Adhesive Rehmannia (熟地黄, Shoudihuang) Figwort Root (玄参, Xuanshen) Dwarf Lilyturf Root (麦门冬, Maimendong) Glossy Privet Fruit (女贞子, Nuzhenzi) Sanchi Root (三七, Sanqi) Cassia Twig (桂枝, Guizhi) Hawthorn Fruit (山楂, Shanzha) Sappan Wood (苏木, Sumu) Hindu Lotus Plumule (莲子心, Lianzixin) Cow-bezoar (牛黄, Niuhuang) Asiatic Rhinoceros Horn (犀角, Xijiao) Common Selfheal Spike (夏枯草, Xiakucao) Root of Sinkiang Arnebia (紫草, Zicao) Hairvein Agrimonia Herb (仙鹤草, Xianhecao) Weeping Forsythia Capsule (连翘, Lianqiao) Common Ducksmeat Herb (浮萍, Fuping) Licorice Root (甘草, Gancao) Chinese Pyrola Herb (鹿衔草, Luxiancao) Im-

mature Bitter Orange (枳实, Zhishi) Tangerine Peel (橘皮, Jupi) Green Tangerine Peel (青皮, Qingpi) Combined Spicebush Root (乌药, Wuyao)

(2) Acceleration of heart rate: Ephedra (麻黄, Mahuang) Musk (麝香, Shexiang) Hairy Antler (鹿茸, Lurong) Datura Flower (洋金花, Yangjinhua) Tea Leaf-bud (茶叶, Chaye)

(3) Deceleration of heart rate: Chinese Azalea (羊踯躅, Yangzhizhu) Chinese Arborvitae Seed (柏子仁, Baiziren) Prepared Daughter Root of Common Monkshood (附子, Fuzi) Chinese Angelica Root (当归, Danggui) Lucid Ganoderma (灵芝, Lingzhi) Fragrant Solomonseal Rhizome (玉竹, Yuzhu) Dahurian Rhododendron Leaf (满山红, Manshanhong) Dodder Seed (菟丝子, Tusizi) Dendrobium Herb (石斛, Shihu) Paniculate Swallowwort Root (徐长卿, Xuchangqing) Common Jasminorange Branchlet and Leaf (九里香, Jiulixiang) Lilac Pink Herb (瞿麦, Qumai) Root of Dogbame (罗布麻根, Luobumagen) Phoenix Tree Leaf (梧桐叶, Wutongye)

(4) Antiarrhythmia: Licorice Root (甘草, Gancao) Ginseng (人参, Renshen) Rehmannia Dried Root (生地黄, Shengdihuang) Dwarf Lilyturf Root (麦门冬, Maimendong) Lightyellow Sophora Root (苦参, Kushen) Yanhusuo (延胡索, Yanhusuo) Red Peony Root (赤芍药, Chishaoyao) Chinese Thorowax Root (柴胡, Chaihu) Cassia Twig (桂枝, Guizhi) Capillary Wormwood Herb (茵陈蒿, Yinchenhao)

2. Blood vessel

(1) Dilating coronary artery and increaing coronary blood flow: Mongolian Snakeground Pericarp (瓜蒌皮, Gualoupi) Lobed Kudzuvine Root (葛根, Gegen) Pubescent Holly Root (毛冬青, Maodongqing) Szechwan Lovage Rhizome (川芎, Chuanxiong) Dan-shen Root (丹参, Danshen) Sanchi Root (三七, Sanqi) Tall Oplopanax Root (刺人参, Cirenshen) Safflower (红花, Honghua) Red Peony Root (赤芍药, Chishaoyao) Prepared Daughter Root of Common Monkshood (附子, Fuzi) Malaytea Scurfpea Fruit (补骨脂, Buguzhi) Common Cruculigo (仙茅, Xianmao) Chinese Taxillus Twig (桑寄生, Sangjisheng) Dodder Seed (菟丝子, Tusizi) Sharpleaf Galangal Fruit (益智仁, Yizhiren) Siberian Solomonseal Rhizome (黄精, Huangjing) Fragrant Solomonseal Rhizome (玉竹, Yuzhu) Whiteflower hogfenel Root (前胡, Qianhu) Apricot Seed (杏仁, Xingren) Fourstamen Stephania Root (汉防已, Hanfangji) Broadleaf Holly Leaf (苦丁茶, Kudingcha) Yunnan Madder Root (小红参, Xiaohongshen) Capillary Wormwood Herb (茵陈蒿, Yinchenhao) Honeysuckle Flower (金银花, Jinyinhua) Omoto Nipponlily (万年青, Wannianqing) Ginkgo Leaf (银杏叶, Yinxingye) Paniculate Swallowwort Root (徐长卿, Xuchangqing)

(2) Dilating cerebral arteries and increasing cerebral blood flow: Lobed Kudzuvine Root (葛根, Gegen) Ginkgo Leaf (银杏叶, Yinxingye) Incised Notopterygium Rhizome and Root (羌活, Qianghuo)

(3) Dilating renal artery and increaing renal blood flow: Membranous Milkvetch Root (黄芪, Huangqi) Eucommia Bark (杜仲, Duzhong) Dogbame Herb (罗布麻, Luobuma) Immature Bitter Orange (枳实, Zhishi)

(4) Reducing blood pressure: Fourstamen Stephania Root (汉防已, Hanfangji) Lobed Kudzuvine Root (葛根, Gegen) Common Devilpepper Root (萝芙木, Luofumu) Decumbent Corydalis Rhizome (夏天无, Xia-

tianwu) Harleguin Glorybower Leaf (臭梧桐, Chouwutong) Common St. Paulswort Herb (豨莶草, Xixiancao) Tall Gastrodia Rhizome (天麻, Tianma) Gambirplant Hooked Stem and Branch (钩藤, Gouteng) Puncturevine Caltrap Fruit (白蒺藜, Baijili) Abalone Shell (石决明, Shijueming) Scorpion (全蝎, Quanxie) Earth Worm (地龙, Dilong) Baikal Skullcap Root (黄芩, Huangqin) Leaf of Dogbame (罗布麻叶, Luobumaye) Pubescent Holly Root (毛冬青, Maodongqing) Hawthorn Fruit (山楂, Shanzha) Thickleaf Vladimiria Root (青木香, Qingmuxiang) Common Aucklandia Root (木香, Muxiang) Indian Chrysanthemum Flower (野菊花, Yejuhua) Weeping Forsythia Capsule (连翘, Lianqiao) Common Selfheal Spike (夏枯草, Xiakucao) Garden Burnet Root (地榆, Diyu) Japanese Pagodatree Flower (槐花, Huaihua) Japanese Thistle Herb or Root (大蓟, Daji) Figwort Root (玄参, Xuanshen) Coptis Rhizome (黄连, Huanglian) Tree Peony Bark (牡丹皮, Mudanpi) Cape Jasmine Fruit (栀子, Zhizi) Hindu Lotus Plumule (莲子心, Lianzixin) Shrub Chastetree Fruit (蔓荆子, Manjingzi) Chinese Ligusticum Rhizome (藁本, Gaoben) Feather Cockscomb Seed (青葙子, Qingxiangzi) Wormwoodlike Motherwort Seed (茺蔚子, Chongweizi) Motherwort Herb (益母草, Yimucao) Umbellate Pore Fungus (猪苓, Zhuling) Tuckahoe (茯苓, Fuling) Oriental Waterplantain Rhizome (泽泻, Zexie) Asiatic Plantain Herb (车前草, Cheqiancao) Asiatic Plantain Seed (车前子, Cheqianzi) White Mulberry Root-bark (桑白皮, Sangbaipi) Mazie Style (玉米须, Yumixu) Common Knotgrass Herb (萹蓄, Bianxu) Lilac Pink Herb (瞿麦, Qumai) Membranous Milkvetch Root (黄芪, Huangqi) Tangshen Root (党参, Dangshen) Siberian Solomonseal Rhizome (黄精, Huangjing) Dan-shen Root (丹参, Danshen) Szechwan Lovage Rhizome (川芎, Chuanxiong) Spine Date Seed (酸枣仁, Suanzaoren) Tuber Fleeceflower Root (何首乌, Heshouwu) Asiatic Cornelian Cherry Fruit (山茱萸, Shanzhuyu) Barbary Wolfberry Fruit (枸杞子, Gouqizi) Chinese Taxillus Twig (桑寄生, Sangjisheng) Eucommia Bark (杜仲, Duzhong) Twotooth Achyranthes Root (牛膝, Niuxi) Doubleteeth Pulbescent Angelica Root (独活, Duhuo) Medicinal Indian-mulberry Root (巴戟天, Bajitian) Chinese Pyrola Herb (鹿衔草, Luxiancao) Phoenix Tree Leaf (梧桐叶, Wutongye) Colored Mistletoe Herb (槲寄生, Hujisheng) Franchet Groundcherry Calyx or Fruit (锦灯笼, Jindenglong) Dahurian Rhododendron Leaf (满山红, Manshanhong) Shorthorned Epimedium Herb (淫羊藿, Yinyanghuo) Persimmon Leaf (柿树叶, Shishuye) Fig Receptacle (无花果, Wuhuaguo) Fortune Paulownia (泡桐, Paotong)

(5) Reducing blood-lipid and resisting atheroscleorsis: Cassia Seed (决明子, Juemingzi) Giant Knotweed Rhizome (虎杖, Huzhang) Rhubarb (大黄, Dahuang) Capillary Wormwood Herb (茵陈蒿, Yinchenhao) Asiatic Plantain Herb (车前草, Cheqiancao) Oriental Waterplantain Rhizome (泽泻, Zexie) Paniculate Swallowwort Root (徐长卿, Xuchangqing) Hawthorn Fruit (山楂, Shanzha) Tangerine Peel (橘皮, Jupi) Ginkgo Leaf (银杏叶, Yinxingye) Lucid Ganoderma (灵芝, Lingzhi) Tuber Fleeceflower Root (何首乌, Heshouwu) Eucommia Bark (杜仲, Duzhong) Phoenix Tree Leaf (梧桐叶, Wutongye) Chinese Taxillus Twig (桑寄生, Sangjisheng) Barbary Wolfberry Fruit (枸杞子, Gouqizi) Chrysanthemum Flower (菊花, Juhua) Siberian Solomonseal Rhizome (黄精,

Huangjing) Fragrant Solomonseal Rhizome (玉竹, Yuzhu) Gordon Euryale Seed (芡实, Qianshi) Cherokee Rose Fruit (金樱子, Jinyingzi) Membranous Milkvetch Root (黄芪, Huangqi) Chinese Angelica Root (当归, Danggui) Amber (琥珀, Hupo) Cluster Mallow Seed (冬葵子, Dongkuizi) Sanchi Root (三七, Sanqi) Common Cephalanoplos Herb (小蓟, Xiaoji) Flower Bud of Japanese Pagodatree (槐米, Huaimi) Bunge Pricklyash (花椒, Huajiao) Puncturevine Caltrap Fruit (白蒺藜, Baijili) Kelp (昆布, Kunbu), Turmeric Rhizome (姜黄, Jianghuang) Turmeric Root-tuber (郁金, Yujin) Grassleaf Sweetflag Rhizome (石菖蒲, Shichangpu) Buffalo Horn (水牛角, Shuiniujiao) Persimmon Leaf (柿树叶, Shishuye) Tea Root (茶树根, Chashugen) Hindu Lotus Leaf (荷叶, Heye) Honeysuckle Flower (金银花, Jinyinhua)

(6) Regulating blood pressure: Cortex Acanthopanacis Radicis (五加皮, Wujiapi) Chinese Magnoliavine (五味子, Wuweizi)

(7) Elevating blood pressure (improve hypotension): Ephedra (麻黄, Mahuang) Musk (麝香, Shexiang) Toad Skin Secretion Cake (蟾酥, Chansu) Immature Bitter Orange (枳实, Zhishi) Dahurian Angelica Root (白芷, Baizhi) Argy Wormwood Leaf (艾叶, Aiye) Malaytea Scurfpea Fruit (补骨脂, Buguzhi) Lucid Ganoderma (灵芝, Lingzhi) Common Cephalanoplos Herb (小蓟, Xiaoji) Purslane Herb (马齿苋, Machixian) Safflower (红花, Honghua) Manchurian Wildginger Herb (细辛, Xixin) Funneled Physochlaine Root (华山参, Huashanshen)

(8) Diastolizating peripheral capillary and improving blood circulation in skin: Membranous Milkvetch Root (黄芪, Huangqi) Danshen Root (丹参, Danshen) Cassia Bark (肉桂, Rougui) Cassia Twig (桂枝, Guizhi) Fresh Ginger (生姜, Shengjiang) Fistular Onion Stalk (葱白, Congbai) Cariander Herb (胡荽, Husui) Common Perilla Leaf (苏叶, Suye) Fineleaf Schizomepeta Herb (荆芥, Jingjie) Wild Mint (薄荷, Bohe) Great Burdock Achene (牛蒡子, Niubangzi) Chinese Tamarish Twig (西河柳, Xiheliu) Scorpion (全蝎, Quanxie)

(9) Systoling nasal mucosa blood vessels: Ephedra (麻黄, Mahuang) Biond Magnolia Flower-bud (辛夷, Xinyi) Siberian Cocklebur Fruit (苍耳子, Cangerzi) Manchurian Wildginger Herb (细辛, Xixin)

(10) Reducing capillary permeability: Flower Bud of Japanese Pagodatree (槐米, Huaimi) Japanese Pagodatree Flower (槐花, Huaihua) Weeping Forsythia Capsule (连翘, Lianqiao) Lalang Grass Rhizome (白茅根, Baimaogen) Membranous Milkvetch Root (黄芪, Huangqi) Sargentoglory Vine Stem (红藤, Hongteng) Baikal Skullcap Root (黄芩, Huangqin) Buffalo Horn (水牛角, Shuiniujiao) Largeleaf Gentian Root (秦艽, Qinjiao) Cortex Acanthopanacis Radicis (五加皮, Wujiapi) Green Tangerine Peel (青皮, Qingpi) Tangerine Peel (橘皮, Jupi)

Herbs Acting on Respiratory System

1. Exiting respiration center: Camphor (樟脑, Zhangnao) Musk (麝香, Shexiang) Toad Skin Secretion Cake (蟾酥, Chansu) Ephedra (麻黄, Mahuang) Datura Flower (洋金花, Yangjinhua) Argy Wormwood Leaf (艾叶, Aiye) Fresh Ginger (生姜, Shengjiang) Dahurian Angelica Root (白芷, Baizhi) Motherwort Herb (益母草, Yimucao) Safflower (红花, Honghua) Tall Gastrodia Rhi-

zome（天麻，Tianma）Doubleteeth Pulbescent Angelica Root（独活，Duhuo）Chinese Lobelia Herb（半边莲，Banbianlian）

2. Calming respiration center: Bitter Apricot Seed（苦杏仁，Kuxingren）Apricot Seed（甜杏仁，Tianxingren）Peach Seed（桃仁，Taoren）Ginkgo Seed（白果，Baiguo）Loquat Leaf（枇杷叶，Pipaye）Common Coltsfoot Flower（款冬花，Kuandonghua）Sessile Stemona Root（百部，Baibu）Scorpion（全蝎，Quanxie）Muskmelon Fruit Pedicel（瓜蒂，Guadi）Black Falsehellebore Root and Rhizome（藜芦，Lilu）

3. Diastolizating smooth muscle of bronchus: Ephedra（麻黄，Mahuang）Datura Flower（洋金花，Yangjinhua）Apricot Seed（杏仁，Xingren）Ginkgo Seed（白果，Baiguo）Ginkgo Leaf（银杏叶，Yinxingye）Earth Worm（地龙，Dilong）Pepperweed Seed or Flixweed Tansymustard Seed（葶苈子，Tinglizi）Common Perilla Leaf（苏叶，Suye）Perilla Seed（苏子，Suzi）Thunberg Fritillary Bulb（浙贝母，Zhebeimu）Pinellia Rhizome（半夏，Banxia）Japanese Felt Fern Leaf（石韦，Shiwei）Inula Flower（旋覆花，Xuanfuhua）Heartlaef Houttuynia Herb（鱼腥草，Yuxingcao）Chinese Arborvitae Leafy Twig（侧柏叶，Cebaiye）Capillary Wormwood Herb（茵陈蒿，Yinchenhao）Common Aucklandia Root（木香，Muxiang）Thickleaf Vladimiria Root（青木香，Qingmuxiang）Officinal Magnolia Bark（厚朴，Houpo）Chinese Magnoliavine（五味子，Wuweizi）Chinese Caterpillar Fungus（冬虫夏草，Dongchongxiacao）English Walnut Seed（胡桃肉，Hutaorou）Chinese Eaglewood Wood（沉香，Chenxiang）Tangerine Peel（橘皮，Jupi）Levant Cotton Root-bark（棉花根，Mianhuagen）Kelp（昆布，Kunbu），Manyleaf Paris Rhizome（蚤休，Zaoxiu）

4. Relieving cough: Bitter Apricot Seed（苦杏仁，Kuxingren）Common Coltsfoot Flower（款冬花，Kuandonghua）Remote Lemongrass Herb（芸香草，Yunxiangcao）Argy Wormwood Leaf（艾叶，Aiye）Giant Knotweed Rhizome（虎杖，Huzhang）Sessile Stemona Root（百部，Baibu）Tendrilleaf Fritillary Bulb（贝母，Beimu）Loquat Leaf（枇杷叶，Pipaye）Lilac Daphne Flower-bud（芫花，Yuanhua）Licorice Root（甘草，Gancao）Pinellia Rhizome（半夏，Banxia）Inula Flower（旋覆花，Xuanfuhua）Tatarian Aster Root（紫苑，Ziyuan）Whiteflower hogfenel Root（前胡，Qianhu）White Mulberry Root-bark（桑白皮，Sangbaipi）Dutchmanspipe Fruit（马兜铃，Madouling）Common Anemarrhea Rhizome（知母，Zhimu）Plantain Seed（车前子，Cheqianzi）Sensitiveplant Herb（含羞草，Hanxiucao）Cudweed Herb（鼠曲草，Shuqucao）Levant Cotton Root-bark（棉花根，Mianhuagen）Coastal Glehnia Root（北沙参，Beishashen）Lily Bulb（百合，Baihe）Cochinchinese Asparagus Root（天门冬，Tianmendong）Dwarf Lilyturf Root（麦门冬，Maimendong）Shorthorned Epimedium Herb（淫羊藿，Yinyanghuo）Perilla Seed（苏子，Suzi）Snakegourd Fruit（瓜蒌，Gualou）Thunberg Fritillary Bulb（浙贝母，Zhebeimu）Grosvenor Momordica Fruit（罗汉果，Luohanguo）

5. Removing the phlegm: Balloonflower Root（桔梗，Jiegeng）Thinleaf Milkwort Root（远志，Yuanzhi）Argy Wormwood Leaf（艾叶，Aiye）Tatarian Aster Root（紫苑，Ziyuan）Pinellia Rhizome（半夏，Banxia）Jackinthepulpit Tuber（天南星，Tiannanxing）Whiteflower hogfenel Root（前胡，Qianhu）Fourleaf Ladybell Root（南沙参，Nanshashen）Mongolian Snakeground Pericarp（瓜蒌皮，Gualoupi）Hempleaf Negundo

Chastetree (牡荆, Mujing) Licorice Root (甘草, Shenggancao) Chinese Honeylocust Fruit (皂荚, Zaojia) Manchurian Rhododendron Branchlet Leaf or Flower (照山白, Zhaoshanbai) Seniavin Rhododendron Root (满山白, Manshanbai) Ciliate Bugle Herb (筋骨草, Jingucao) Levant Cotton Root-bark (棉花根, Mianhuagen) Japanese Ardisia Herb (矮地茶, Aidicha) Honey (蜂蜜, Fengmi) Funneled Physochlaine Root (华山参, Huashanshen) Luffa Stem (丝瓜藤, Siguateng)

Herbs Acting on Digestive System

1. Herbs acting on salivary gland

(1) Stimulating salivary gland to secrete: Fresh Ginger (生姜, Shengjiang) Medicine Terminalia Fruit (诃子, Hezi) Chinese White Olive (青果, Qingguo) Smoked Plum (乌梅, Wumei) Chinese Magnoliavine (五味子, Wuweizi) Bunge Pricklyash (花椒, Huajiao) Dendrobium Herb (石斛, Shihu) Figwort Root (玄参, Xuanshen) Blackberrylily Rhizome (射干, Shegan) Cassia Twig (桂枝, Guizhi) Lobed Kudzuvine Root (葛根, Gegen) Areca Seed (槟榔, Binlang) Desertliving Cistanche (肉苁蓉, Roucongrong)

(2) Controlling secretion of salivary gland: Datura Flower (洋金花, Yangjinhua) Thunberg Fritillary Bulb (浙贝母, Zhebeimu) Tonkin Sophora Root (山豆根, Shandougen) Safflower (红花, Honghua) Sharpleaf Galangal Fruit (益智仁, Yizhiren)

2. Herbs acting on gastrointestinal digestive glands

(1) Increasing secretion of digestive juice: Chicken Gizzard Membrane (鸡内金, Jineijin) Hawthorn Fruit (山楂, Shanzha) Medicated Leaven (神曲, Shenqu) Rice Germinating Fruit (sprout) (谷芽, Guya) Malt (麦芽, Maiya) Chinese Gentian Root (龙胆草, Longdancao) Rhubarb (大黄, Dahuang) Coptis Rhizome (黄连, Huanglian) Villous Amomum Fruit (砂仁, Sharen) Fresh Ginger (生姜, Shengjiang) Tangerine Peel (橘皮, Jupi) Common Aucklandia Root (木香, Muxiang) Lesser Galangal Rhizome (高良姜, Gaoliangjiang), Wrinkled Gianthyssop Herb (藿香, Huoxiang) Fistular Onion Stalk (葱白, Congbai) Bunge Pricklyash (花椒, Huajiao) Clove Flower-bud (丁香, Dingxiang) Medicinal Evodia Root (吴茱萸, Wuzhuyu) Black Pepper Fruit (胡椒, Hujiao) Long Pepper Fruit (荜茇, Biba) Nutmeg Seed (肉豆蔻, Roudoukou) Cassia Bark (肉桂, Rougui) Tangshen Root (党参, Dangshen) Heterophylla Falsestarwort Root (太子参, Taizishen) Largehead Atractylodes Rhizome (白术, Baizhu) Dendrobium Herb (石斛, Shihu) Chinese Magnoliavine (五味子, Wuweizi) Cherokee Rose Fruit (金樱子, Jinyingzi) Desertliving Cistanche (肉苁蓉, Roucongrong) Combined Spicebush Root (乌药, Wuyao) Officinal Magnolia Bark (厚朴, Houpo) Areca Peel (大腹皮, Dafupi) Areca Seed (槟榔, Binlang) Grassleaf Sweetflag Rhizome (石菖蒲, Shichangpu) Turmeric Root-tuber (郁金, Yujin) Heterophylla Falsestarwort Root (太子参, Taizishen)

(2) Controlling secretion of digestive juice: Datura Flower (洋金花, Yangjinhua) Opium Poppy Pericarp (罂粟壳, Yingsuqiao) Nutmeg Seed (肉豆蔻, Roudoukou) White Peony Root (白芍药, Baishaoyao) Yanhusuo (延胡索, Yanhusuo)

3. Relieving Vomiting: Pinellia Rhizome (半夏, Banxia) Fresh Ginger (生姜, Shengjiang) Inula Flower (旋覆花, Xuanfuhua) Chinese Eaglewood Wood (沉香,

Chenxiang) Wrinkled Gianthyssop Herb (藿香, Huoxiang) Medicinal Evodia Root (吴茱萸, Wuzhuyu) Reed Rhizome (芦根, Lugen) Bamboo Shavings (竹茹, Zhuru) Bamboo leaf (竹叶, Zhuye) Clove Flower-bud (丁香, Dingxiang) Persimmon Calyx and Receptacle (柿蒂, Shidi) Sword Jackbean Seed (刀豆子, Daodouzi) Cooking Stove Earth (伏龙肝, Fulonggan) Yanhusuo (延胡索, Yanhusuo)

4. Emetic action: Muskmelon Fruit Pedicel (瓜蒂, Guadi) Black Falsehellebore Root and Rhizome (藜芦, Lilu) Chalcanthnium (胆矾, Danfan) Antifebrile Dichroa Root (常山, Changshan) Pinellia Rhizome (半夏, Banxia) Shorttube Lycoris Bulb (石蒜, Shisuan)

5. Controlling gastrointestinal smooth muscle: Datura Flower (洋金花, Yangjinhua) Opium Poppy Pericarp (罂粟壳, Yingsuqiao) Cassia Bark (肉桂, Rougui) Chinese Eaglewood Wood (沉香, Chenxiang) Medicinal Evodia Root (吴茱萸, Wuzhuyu) Wrinkled Gianthyssop Herb (藿香, Huoxiang) Combined Spicebush Root (乌药, Wuyao) Thunberg Fritillary Bulb (浙贝母, Zhebeimu) Baikal Skullcap Root (黄芩, Huangqin) Thickleaf Vladimiria Root (青木香, Qingmuxiang) Fennel Fruit (小茴香, Xiaohuixiang) Common Fenugreek Seed (胡芦巴, Huluba) Nutmeg Seed (肉豆蔻, Roudoukou) Tangerine Peel (橘皮, Jupi) Lesser Galangal Rhizome (高良姜, Gaoliangjiang), Katsumada Galangal Seed (草豆蔻, Caodoukou) Red Peony Root (赤芍药, Chishaoyao) White Peony Root (白芍药, Baishaoyao) Licorice Root (甘草, Gancao) Grassleaf Sweetflag Rhizome (石菖蒲, Shichangpu) Sanchi Root (三七, Sanqi) Scandent Schefflera Root (七叶莲, Qiyelian) Trogopterus Dung (五灵脂, Wulingzhi) Chinese Pulsatilla Root (白头翁, Baitouweng) Ephedra (麻黄, Mahuang) Twotooth Achyranthes Root (牛膝, Niuxi) Common Heron's Bill Herb or Wilford Cranesbill Herb (老鹳草, Laoguancao) Paniculate Swallowwort Root (徐长卿, Xuchangqing) Catechu (儿茶, Ercha) Smoked Plum (乌梅, Wumei) Siberian Solomonseal Rhizome (黄精, Huangjing) Chinese Caterpillar Fungus (冬虫夏草, Dongchongxiacao) Black Henbane Seed (天仙子, Tianxianzi) White Peony Root (白芍药, Baishaoyao) Red Peony Root (赤芍药, Chishaoyao)

6. Exciting gastrointestinal smooth muscle: Rhubarb (大黄, Dahuang) Immature Bitter Orange (枳实, Zhishi) Bitter Orange (枳壳, Zhiqiao) Mirabilite (芒硝, Mangxiao) Areca Seed (槟榔, Binlang) Radish Seed (莱菔子, Laifuzi) Common Aucklandia Root (木香, Muxiang) Villous Amomum Fruit (砂仁, Sharen) Clove Flower-bud (丁香, Dingxiang) Katsumada Galangal Seed (草豆蔻, Caodoukou) Caoguo (草果, Caoguo) Fresh Ginger (生姜, Shengjiang) Common Perilla Leaf (苏叶, Suye) Tuber Fleeceflower Root (何首乌, Heshouwu) Cassia Twig (桂枝, Guizhi) Cariander Herb (胡荽, Husui) Shunk Bugbane Rhizome (升麻, Shengma) Areca Peel (大腹皮, Dafupi) Akebia Stem (木通, Mutong) Dendrobium Herb (石斛, Shihu) Officinal Magnolia Bark (厚朴, Houpo) Combined Spicebush Root (乌药, Wuyao)

7. Antiacid: Cuttle Bone (乌贼骨, Wuzeigu) Calcined Concha Arcae (煅瓦楞子, Duanwalengzi) Oyster Shell (牡蛎, Muli) Nacre (珍珠母, Zhenzhumu) Egg-shell (鸡蛋壳, Jidanke) Stalactite (钟乳石, Zhongrushi)

8. Protecting and astringing gastrointestinal mucosa: Chinese Gall (五倍子, Wubeizi) Medicine Terminalia Fruit (诃子, Hezi) Talc (滑石, Huashi) Red Halloysite (赤石脂,

Chishizhi) Licorice Root (甘草, Gancao)

9. Enhancing secretion of bile: Christina Loosetrife Herb (金钱草, Jinqiancao) Capillary Wormwood Herb (茵陈蒿, Yinchenhao) Turmeric Root-tuber (郁金, Yujin) Turmeric Rhizome (姜黄, Jianghuang) Coptis Rhizome (黄连, Huanglian) Baikal Skullcap Root (黄芩, Huangqin) Chinese Corktree Bark (黄柏, Huangbai) Leatherleaf Mahonia Leaf (十大功劳, Shidagonglao) Cape Jasmine Fruit (栀子, Zhizi) Rhubarb (大黄, Dahuang) Chinese Thorowax Root (柴胡, Chaihu) Immature Bitter Orange (枳实, Zhishi) Smoked Plum (乌梅, Wumei) Chinese Magnoliavine (五味子, Wuweizi) Rugose Rose Flower (玫瑰花, Meiguihua) Common Cephalanoplos Herb (小蓟, Xiaoji) Purslane Herb (马齿苋, Machixian) Tall Gastrodia Rhizome (天麻, Tianma)

10. Relaxing sphincter muscle of biliary tract: Christina Loosetrife Herb (金钱草, Jinqiancao) Common Aucklandia Root (木香, Muxiang) Chinese Thorowax Root (柴胡, Chaihu) Turmeric Root-tuber (郁金, Yujin) Nutgrass Galingale Rhizome (香附, Xiangfu) Smoked Plum (乌梅, Wumei) Fourstamen Stephania Root (汉防己, Hanfangji) Officinal Magnolia Bark (厚朴, Houpo) Oriental Variegated Coralbean Bark (海桐皮, Haitongpi) Star Anise (八角茴香, Bajiaohuixiang)

11. Reducing transaminase: Holy Thistle Fruit (水飞蓟, Shuifeiji) Chinese Magnoliavine (五味子, Wuweizi) Herb of False Chinese Swertia (当药, Dangyao) Lucid Ganoderma (灵芝, Lingzhi) Chinese Gentian Root (龙胆草, Longdancao) Dan-shen Root (丹参, Danshen) Chinese Thorowax Root (柴胡, Chaihu) Stringy Stonecrop Herb (垂盆草, Chuipencao) Weeping Forsythia Capsule (连翘, Lianqiao) Licorice Root (甘草, Gancao) Chicken Gizzard Membrane (鸡内金, Jineijin) Indigowoad Leaf (大青叶, Daqingye) Buffalo Horn (水牛角, Shuiniujiao) Whiteflower Patrinia Herb (败酱草, Baijiangcao) Indian Chrysanthemum Flower (野菊花, Yejuhua) 豨 Common St. Paulswort Herb (豨莶草, Xixiancao)

12. Reducing thymol flocculation test, cephalin-cholesterol flocculation: Chinese Angelica Root (当归, Danggui) Dan-shen Root (丹参, Danshen) Peach Seed (桃仁, Taoren) Turmeric Root-tuber (郁金, Yujin)

13. Protecting liver and enhancing reproduction of liver cells: Chinese Angelica Root (当归, Danggui) Rehmannia Dried Root (生地黄, Shengdihuang) Membranous Milkvetch Root (黄芪, Huangqi) Largehead Atractylodes Rhizome (白术, Baizhu) Lucid Ganoderma (灵芝, Lingzhi) Chinese Thorowax Root (柴胡, Chaihu) Licorice Root (甘草, Gancao) Weeping Forsythia Capsule (连翘, Lianqiao) Buffalo Horn (水牛角, Shuiniujiao) Barbary Wolfberry Fruit (枸杞子, Gouqizi) Oriental Waterplantain Rhizome (泽泻, Zexie) Dan-shen Root (丹参, Danshen) Giant Knotweed Rhizome (虎杖, Huzhang) Ciliate Bugle Herb (筋骨草, Jingucao)

14. Reducing serum bilirubin: Capillary Wormwood Herb (茵陈蒿, Yinchenhao) Cape Jasmine Fruit (栀子, Zhizi) Indigowoad Leaf (大青叶, Daqingye)

15. Increacing serum albumin: Chinese Date (大枣, Dazao) Turmeric Root-tuber (郁金, Yujin) Tangshen Root (党参, Dangshen) Largehead Atractylodes Rhizome (白术, Baizhu) Cassia Bark (肉桂, Rougui)

16. Softening and contracting liver and spleen: Dan-shen Root (丹参, Danshen) Hirsute Shiny Bugleweed Herb (泽兰, Zelan) Cowherb Seed (王不留行, Wangbuliuxing) Chicken Gizzard Membrane (鸡内金, Jinei-

jin) Earth Worm (地龙, Dilong) Common Burreed Rhizome (三棱, Sanleng) Zedoray (莪术, Ezhu)

17. Arresting diarrhea: Chinese Gall (五倍子, Wubeizi) Medicine Terminalia Fruit (诃子, Hezi) Nutmeg Seed (肉豆蔻, Roudoukou) Opium Poppy Pericarp (罂粟壳, Yingsuqiao) Common Heron's Bill Herb or Wilford Cranesbill Herb (老鹳草, Laoguancao) Cherokee Rose Fruit (金樱子, Jinyingzi) Red Halloysite (赤石脂, Chishizhi) Alumen (明矾, Mingfan) Garden Burnet Root (地榆, Diyu)

18. Purgative herbs

(1) Irritanl purgative: Rhubarb (大黄, Dahuang) Aloes (芦荟, Luhui) Senna Leaf (番泻叶, Fanxieye) Giant Knotweed Rhizome (虎杖, Huzhang) Cassia Seed (决明子, Juemingzi) Tuber Fleeceflower Root (何首乌, Heshouwu) Sensitiveplant - like Senna Herb (山扁豆, Shanbiandou) Croton Seed (巴豆, Badou) Lilac Daphne Flower-bud (芫花, Yuanhua) Kansui Root (甘遂, Gansui) Peking Euphorbia Root (大戟, Daji) Pokeberry Root (商陆, Shanglu) Pharbitis Seed (牵牛子, Qianniuzi) Caper Euphorbia (续随子, Xusuizi)

(2) Bulk cathartic: Mirabilite (芒硝, Mangxiao)

(3) Caccagogue: Mongolian Snakegourd Seed (瓜蒌仁, Gualouren) Apricot Seed (杏仁, Xingren) Peach Seed (桃仁, Taoren) Hemp Seed (火麻仁, Huomaren) Bushcherry Seed (郁李仁, Yuliren) Oriental Sesame Seed (黑芝麻, Heizhima) Honey (蜂蜜, Fengmi) English Walnut (核桃肉, Hetaorou) Grosvenor Momordica Fruit (罗汉果, Luohanguo) Fig Receptacle (无花果, Wuhuaguo) Common Knotgrass Herb (萹蓄, Bianxu)

Herbs acting on urinary system

1. Diuretic herbs: Umbellate Pore Fungus (猪苓, Zhuling) Tuckahoe (茯苓, Fuling) Oriental Waterplantain Rhizome (泽泻, Zexie) Swordlike Atractylodes Rhizome (苍术, Cangzhu) Largehead Atractylodes Rhizome (白术, Baizhu) Asiatic Plantain Herb (车前草, Cheqiancao) Asiatic Plantain Seed (车前子, Cheqianzi) Akebia Stem (木通, Mutong) Common Lophatherum Herb (淡竹叶, Danzhuye) Amber (琥珀, Hupo) Common Knotgrass Herb (萹蓄, Bianxu) Lilac Pink Herb (瞿麦, Qumai) Chinese Lobelia Herb (半边莲, Banbianlian) Barbed Skullcap Herb (半枝莲, Banzhilian) Black Nightshade Herb (龙葵, Longkui) Japanese Climbing Fern Spores (海金沙, Haijinsha) Sevenlobed Yam Rhizome (萆薢, Bixie), Japanese Felt Fern Leaf (石韦, Shiwei) Talc (滑石, Huashi) Mazie Style (玉米须, Yumixu) Lalang Grass Rhizome (白茅根, Baimaogen) Reed Rhizome (芦根, Lugen) Chinese Waxgourd Exocarp (冬瓜皮, Dongguapi) Common Selfheal Spike (夏枯草, Xiakucao) Ephedra (麻黄, Mahuang) Haichow Elsholtzia Herb (香薷, Xiangru) Common Ducksmeat Herb (浮萍, Fuping) Common Dayflower Herb (鸭跖草, Yazhicao) Capillary Wormwood Herb (茵陈蒿, Yinchenhao) Lightyellow Sophora Root (苦参, Kushen) Baikal Skullcap Root (黄芩, Huangqin) Belvedere Fruit (地肤子, Difuzi) Motherwort Herb (益母草, Yimucao) Areca Peel (大腹皮, Dafupi) Fourstamen Stephania Root (防己, Fangji) Pepperweed Seed or Flixweed Tansymustard Seed (葶苈子, Tinglizi) Sweetscented Oleander Leaf or Bark (夹竹桃, Jiazhutao) Omoto Nipponlily (万年

青，Wannianqing）Slenderstyle Acanthopanax Root-bark（北五加皮，Beiwujiapi）Tea Leaf-bud（茶叶，Chaye）Membranous Milkvetch Root（黄芪，Huangqi）Chinese Taxillus Twig（桑寄生，Sangjisheng）Asiatic Cornelian Cherry Fruit（山茱萸，Shanzhuyu）Kansui Root（甘遂，Gansui）Peking Euphorbia Root（大戟，Daji）Lilac Daphne Flower-bud（芫花，Yuanhua）Pokeberry Root（商陆，Shanglu）Pharbitis Seed（牵牛子，Qianniuzi）Toothleaf Goldenray Root and Rhizome（葫芦，Hulu）Indian Stringbush Root（了哥王根，Liaogewanggen）Sensitiveplant-like Senna Herb（山扁豆，Shanbiandou）Inula Flower（旋覆花，Xuanfuhua）Crab Fossil（石蟹，Shixie）Ciliate Bugle Herb（筋骨草，Jingucao）Common Goldenrod Herb（一枝黄花，Yizhihuanghua）Chinese Lobelia Herb（半边莲，Banbianlian）

2. Increasing to excrete urate（treating for the gout）：Largeleaf Chinese Ash Bark（秦皮，Qinpi）Chinese Clematis Root（威灵仙，Weilingxian）Largeleaf Gentian Root（秦艽，Qinjiao）豨 Common St. Paulswort Herb（豨莶草，Xixiancao）Glabrous Greenbrier Rhizome（土茯苓，Tufuling）Plantain Seed（车前子，Cheqianzi）

3. Expelling away or dispelling lithangiuria：Snowbelleaf Tickclover Herb（金钱草，Jinqiancao）Christina Loosetrife Herb（金钱草，Jinqiancao）Japanese Climbing Fern Spores（海金沙，Haijinsha）Japanese Felt Fern Leaf（石韦，Shiwei）Amber（琥珀，Hupo）Common Knotgrass Herb（萹蓄，Bianxu）Lilac Pink Herb（瞿麦，Qumai）Gambirplant Hooked Stem and Branch（钩藤，Gouteng）Mazie Style（玉米须，Yumixu）Cluster Mallow Seed（冬葵子，Dongkuizi）Ground Ivy Herb（连钱草，Lianqiancao）

4. Chispelling chyluria：Sevenlobed Yam Rhizome（萆薢，Bixie）薢，Lilac Pink Herb（瞿麦，Qumai）Shepherdspurse Herb with Root（荠菜，Jicai）Mazie Style（玉米须，Yumixu）

5. Resuming renal function and dispelling proteinuria：Membranous Milkvetch Root（黄芪，Huangqi）Ginseng（人参，Renshen）Tangshen Root（党参，Dangshen）Largehead Atractylodes Rhizome（白术，Baizhu）Tuckahoe（茯苓，Fuling）Turtle Carapace Glue（鳖甲胶，Biejiajiao）Common Yam Rhizome（山药，Shanyao）Chinese Angelica Root（当归，Danggui）Barbary Wolfberry Fruit（枸杞子，Gouqizi）Cherokee Rose Fruit（金樱子，Jinyingzi）Mantis Egg-case（桑螵蛸，Sangpiaoxiao）Hindu Lotus Stamen（莲须，Lianxu）Twotooth Achyranthes Root（牛膝，Niuxi）Eucommia Bark（杜仲，Duzhong）Rehmannia Dried Root（生地黄，Shengdihuang）Figwort Root（玄参，Xuanshen）Dwarf Lilyturf Root（麦门冬，Maimendong）Dodder Seed（菟丝子，Tusizi）Glabrous Greenbrier Rhizome（土茯苓，Tufuling）Cicada Slough（蝉蜕，Chantui）Common Perilla Leaf（苏叶，Suye）Motherwort Herb（益母草，Yimucao）

6. Resisting diuresis：Chinese Clematis Root（威灵仙，Weilingxian）Datura Flower（洋金花，Yangjinhua）Ginseng（人参，Renshen）Cortex Acanthopanacis Radicis（五加皮，Wujiapi）Mantis Egg-case（桑螵蛸，Sangpiaoxiao）Flatstem Milkvetch Seed（沙苑子，Shayuanzi）Dodder Seed（菟丝子，Tusizi）Palmleaf Raspberry Fruit（覆盆子，Fupenzi）Malaytea Scurfpea Fruit（补骨脂，Buguzhi）Sharpleaf Galangal Fruit（益智仁，Yizhiren）Licorice Root（甘草，Gancao）Tangerine Peel（橘皮，Jupi）Safflower（红花，Honghua）Shorthorned Epimedium Herb（淫羊藿，Yinyanghuo）Chicken Gizzard Membrane（鸡内金，Jineijin）

Herbs acting on reproductive system

1. Exciting uterine contraction: Bitter Orange (枳壳, Zhiqiao) Immature Bitter Orange (枳实, Zhishi) Male Fern Rhizome (贯众, Guanzhong) Motherwort Herb (益母草, Yimucao) Wormwoodlike Motherwort Seed (茺蔚子, Chongweizi) Purslane Herb (马齿苋, Machixian) Cowherb Seed (王不留行, Wangbuliuxing) Cattail Pollen (蒲黄, Puhuang) Hawthorn Fruit (山楂, Shanzha) Coix Seed (薏苡仁, Yiyiren) Chinese Magnoliavine (五味子, Wuweizi) Garden Balsam Seed (急性子, Jixingzi) Safflower (红花, Honghua) Rhubarb (大黄, Dahuang) Musk (麝香, Shexiang) Chinese Honeylocust Spine (Chinese Honeylocust Spine (皂角, Zaojiao) 刺, Zaojiaoci) Antifebrile Dichroa Root (常山, Changshan) Levant Cotton Root-bark (棉花根, Mianhuagen) Franchet Groundcherry Calyx or Fruit (锦灯笼, Jindenglong)

2. Controlling uterine contraction: Chinese Angelica Root (当归, Danggui) Szechwan Lovage Rhizome (川芎, Chuanxiong) Nutgrass Galingale Rhizome (香附, Xiangfu) Eucommia Bark (杜仲, Duzhong) Largehead Atractylodes Rhizome (白术, Baizhu) Baikal Skullcap Root (黄芩, Huangqin) Largeleaf Gentian Root (秦艽, Qinjiao) Tangerine Peel (橘皮, Jupi) Common Perilla Stem (苏梗, Sugeng) Common Aucklandia Root (木香, Muxiang)

3. Impelling endometria to congest: Tree Peony Bark (牡丹皮, Mudanpi) Rhubarb (大黄, Dahuang) Dried Human Placenta (紫河车, Ziheche) Licorice Root (甘草, Gancao)

Herbs acting on endocrine glands

1. Pituitary gland-adrenocortical system: Prepared Daughter Root of Common Monkshood (附子, Fuzi) Common Monksood (乌头, Wutou) Ginseng (人参, Renshen) Ginseng Leaf (人参叶, Renshenye) Largeleaf Gentian Root (秦艽, Qinjiao) Fourstamen Stephania Root (汉防己, Hanfangji) Hairystalk Tinospora Root (金果榄, Jinguolan) Levant Cotton Root-bark (棉花根, Mianhuagen) Licorice Root (甘草, Gancao) Chinese Magnoliavine (五味子, Wuweizi) Silkworm with Batrytis Larva (白僵蚕, Baijiangcan) Aspisin (蜂毒, Fengdu) Royal Jelly (蜂乳, Fengru) Orientvine Stem or Hair Orientvine Stem (青风藤, Qingfengteng) Nippon Yam Rhizome (穿山龙, Chuanshanlong) Shorttube Lycoris Bulb (石蒜, Shisuan) Buffalo Horn (水牛角, Shuiniujiao)

2. Similar adrenocorticoids: Licorice Root (甘草, Gancao) Nippon Yam Rhizome (穿山龙, Chuanshanlong) Royal Jelly (蜂乳, Fengru) Membranous Milkvetch Root (黄芪, Huangqi) Tuber Fleeceflower Root (何首乌, Heshouwu) Fragrant Solomonseal Rhizome (玉竹, Yuzhu) Manyprickle Acanthopanax Root (刺五加, Ciwujia)

3. Promoting sexual gland: Hairy Antler (鹿茸, Lurong) Dried Human Placenta (紫河车, Ziheche) Prepared Daughter Root of Common Monkshood (附子, Fuzi) Shorthorned Epimedium Herb (淫羊藿, Yinyanghuo) Common Cruculigo (仙茅, Xianmao) Common Cnidium Fruit (蛇床子, Shechuangzi) Giant Gecko (蛤蚧, Gejie) De-

sertliving Cistanche（肉苁蓉，Roucongrong）Eucommia Bark（杜仲，Duzhong）Medicinal Indian - mulberry Root（巴戟天，Bajitian）Songaria Cynomorium Herb（锁阳，Suoyang）Royal Jelly（蜂乳，Fengru）Ginseng（人参，Renshen）Membranous Milkvetch Root（黄芪，Huangqi）Toad Skin Secretion Cake（蟾酥，Chansu）European Hop Female - flower（啤酒花，Pijiuhua）Dodder Seed（菟丝子，Tusizi）

4. Improving gonopoiesis and gonopoiesis: Hairy Antler（鹿茸，Lurong）Dried Human Placenta（紫河车，Ziheche）Shorthorned Epimedium Herb（淫羊藿，Yinyanghuo）

5. Improving the growth of mammary gland and woman genital organ: Dried Human Placenta（紫河车，Ziheche）Himalayan Teasel Root（续断，Xuduan）

6. Improving galacthidrosis: Root of Lance Asiabell（四叶参，Siyeshen）Cowherb Seed（王不留行，Wangbuliuxing）Dried Human Placenta（紫河车，Ziheche）Himalayan Teasel Root（续断，Xuduan）Tuckahoe（茯苓，Fuling）Ricepaperplant Pith（通草，Tongcao）Cushaw Seed（南瓜子，Nanguazi）Licorice Root（甘草，Gancao）Akebia Stem（木通，Mutong）Pangolin Scales（穿山甲，Chuanshanjia）Beautiful Sweetgum Fruit（路路通，Lulutong）Uniflower Swisscentaury Root（漏芦，Loulu）

7. Controlling milk-secretion: Charred Malt（焦麦芽，Jiaomaiya）Bunge Pricklyash（花椒，Huajiao）Mirabilite（芒硝，Mangxiao）

8. Resisting pituitary gonadotropic hormone and chronic gonadotropin: Snakegroud Root（天花粉，Tianhuafen）Root of Sinkiang Arnebia（紫草，Zicao）Musk（麝香，Shexiang）

9. Resisting atrophy of ovary: Garden Balsam Seed（急性子，Jixingzi）

10. Herbs acting on thyroid

(1) Containing iodine, used for goiter due to iodine deficiency: Kelp（昆布，Kunbu），Kelp（海带，Haidai）Seaweed（海藻，Haizao）Laver（紫菜，Zicai）

11. Promoting basic metabolism: Ginseng（人参，Renshen）Ephedra（麻黄，Mahuang）Tea Leaf - bud（茶叶，Chaye）Centipede（蜈蚣，Wugong）Great Burdock Achene（牛蒡子，Niubangzi）

12. Herbs for temperarily reducing basic metabolism: Kelp（昆布，Kunbu），Seaweed（海藻，Haizao）

13. Herbs for enhancing resistance and immunity: Ginseng（人参，Renshen）Membranous Milkvetch Root（黄芪，Huangqi）Dried Human Placenta（紫河车，Ziheche）Cortex Acanthopanacis Radicis（五加皮，Wujiapi）Shorthorned Epimedium Herb（淫羊藿，Yinyanghuo）Heartlaef Houttuynia Herb（鱼腥草，Yuxingcao）Mulberry Twig（桑枝，Sangzhi）

Herbs acting on blood system

1. Herbs stimulating hematopoietic system and increasing RBC and Hgb: Hairy Antler（鹿茸，Lurong）Antler（鹿角，Lujiao）Dried Human Placenta（紫河车，Ziheche）Ass-hide Glue（阿胶，Ejiao）Suberect Spatholobus Stem（鸡血藤，Jixueteng）Ginseng（人参，Renshen）Membranous Milkvetch Root（黄芪，Huangqi）Tangshen Root（党参，Dangshen）Tuber Fleeceflower Root（何首乌，Heshouwu）Root of Lance Asiabell（四叶参，Siyeshen）Chinese Angelica Root（当归，Danggui）Prepared Rhizome of Adhesive Rehmannia（熟地黄，Shoudihuang）Barbary Wolfberry Fruit（枸杞子，Gouqizi）Large-

head Atractylodes Rhizome (白术, Baizhu) Tuckahoe (茯苓, Fuling) Tuber Fleeceflower Stem and Leaf (夜交藤, Yejiaoteng) Longan Aril (龙眼肉, Longyanrou) Malaytea Scurfpea Fruit (补骨脂, Buguzhi) Songaria Cynomorium Herb (锁阳, Suoyang) Medicinal Indian-mulberry Root (巴戟天, Bajitian) Tangerine Peel (橘皮, Jupi) Dan-shen Root (丹参, Danshen)

2. Herbs increasing reticulated corpuscles: Hairy Antler (鹿茸, Lurong) Suberect Spatholobus Stem (鸡血藤, Jixueteng) Chinese Fevervine Herb and Root (鸡矢藤, Jishiteng) Spreading Hedyotis Herb (白花蛇舌草, Baihuasheshecao)

3. Herbs increasing white blood cells: Ginseng (人参, Renshen) Ciliate Bugle Herb (筋骨草, Jingucao) Suberect Spatholobus Stem (鸡血藤, Jixueteng) Dan-shen Root (丹参, Danshen) Musk (麝香, Shexiang) Pangolin Scales (穿山甲, Chuanshanjia) Toad Skin Secretion Cake (蟾酥, Chansu) Giant Knotweed Rhizome (虎杖, Huzhang) Japanese Felt Fern Leaf (石韦, Shiwei) Frankincense (乳香, Ruxiang) Myrrh (没药, Moyao) Trogopterus Dung (五灵脂, Wulingzhi)

4. Herbs reducing white blood cells: Asiatic Rhinoceros Horn (犀角, Xijiao) Tangshen Root (党参, Dangshen) Root of Lance Asiabell (四叶参, Siyeshen) Ground Beetle (土鳖虫, Tubiechong) Giant Knotweed Rhizome (虎杖, Huzhang)

5. Herbs exciting reticuloendothelial system: Honeysuckle Flower (金银花, Jinyinhua) Coptis Rhizome (黄连, Huanglian) Chinese Corktree Bark (黄柏, Huangbai) Indigowoad Leaf (大青叶, Daqingye) Indigwoad Root (板蓝根, Banlangen) Spreading Hedyotis Herb (白花蛇舌草, Baihuasheshecao) Common Andrographis Herb (穿心莲, Chuanxinlian) Tonkin Sophora Root (山豆根, Shandougen) Heartlaef Houttuynia Herb (鱼腥草, Yuxingcao) Common Goldenrod Herb (一枝黄花, Yizhihuanghua) Membranous Milkvetch Root (黄芪, Huangqi)

6. Herbs elevating the number of blood platelet: Chinese Angelica Root (当归, Danggui) White Peony Root (白芍药, Baishaoyao) Rehmannia Dried Root (生地黄, Shengdihuang) Prepared Rhizome of Adhesive Rehmannia (熟地黄, Shoudihuang) Asiatic Cornelian Cherry Fruit (山茱萸, Shanzhuyu) Dried Human Placenta (紫河车, Ziheche) Longan Aril (龙眼肉, Longyanrou) Chinese Date (大枣, Dazao) Rice Bean (赤小豆, Chixiaodou) Rhubarb (大黄, Dahuang) Patience Dock Root (牛西西, Niuxixi) Japanese Dock Root (羊蹄, Yangti) Sanchi Root (三七, Sanqi) Bletilla Rhizome (白及, Baiji) Hindu Lotus Rhizome-node (藕节, Oujie) Hairvein Agrimonia Herb (仙鹤草, Xianhecao) Desertliving Cistanche (肉苁蓉, Roucongrong) East Asian Tree Fern Rhizome (狗脊, Gouji) Buffalo Horn (水牛角, Shuiniujiao) Chinese Corktree Bark (黄柏, Huangbai) Weeping Forsythia Capsule (连翘, Lianqiao)

7. Herbs functioning as treating the reduction of white blood cells and blood platelet due to chemotherapy and radiotherapy

(1)Herbs functioning as treating the reduction of white blood celles and blood platelet: Membranous Milkvetch Root (黄芪, Huangqi) Heterophylla Falsestarwort Root (太子参, Taizishen) Largehead Atractylodes Rhizome (白术, Baizhu) Chinese Angelica Root (当归, Danggui) Ass-hide Glue (阿胶, Ejiao) Toad Skin Secretion Cake (蟾酥, Chansu) Pangolin Scales (穿山甲, Chuanshanjia) Tortoise's Shell and Plastron Glue

(龟版胶, Guibanjiao) Dan-shen Root (丹参, Danshen) Suberect Spatholobus Stem (鸡血藤, Jixueteng) Chinese Fevervine Herb and Root (鸡矢藤, Jishiteng) Rehmannia Dried Root (生地黄, Shengdihuang) Prepared Rhizome of Adhesive Rehmannia (熟地黄, Shoudihuang) Chinese Caterpillar Fungus (冬虫夏草, Dongchongxiacao) Barbary Wolfberry Fruit (枸杞子, Gouqizi) Chinese Magnoliavine (五味子, Wuweizi) Asiatic Cornelian Cherry Fruit (山茱萸, Shanzhuyu) Malaytea Scurfpea Fruit (补骨脂, Buguzhi) Glossy Privet Fruit (女贞子, Nuzhenzi) Japanese Felt Fern Leaf (石韦, Shiwei) Lucid Ganoderma (灵芝, Lingzhi) Figwort Root (玄参, Xuanshen) Dendrobium Herb (石斛, Shihu) Sharpleaf Galangal Fruit (益智仁, Yizhiren) Common Cnidium Fruit (蛇床子, Shechuangzi) Mushroom (蘑菇, Mogu)

(2)Herbs functioning as treating the reduction of blood platelet: Heterophylla Falsestarwort Root(太子参, Taizishen) Glossy Privet Fruit (女贞子, Nuzhenzi) Chinese Magnoliavine (五味子, Wuweizi) Chinese Date (大枣, Dazao)

8. Herbs functioning as stopping bleeding: Sanchi Root (三七, Sanqi) Dragon's Blood (血竭, Xuejie) Yerbadetajo Herb (墨旱莲, Mohanlian) Hairvein Agrimonia Herb (仙鹤草, Xianhecao) Bletilla Rhizome (白及, Baiji) Tree Peony Bark (牡丹皮, Mudanpi) Cape Jasmine Fruit (栀子, Zhizi) Ciliate Bugle Herb (筋骨草, Jingucao) Chinese Arborvitae Leafy Twig (侧柏叶, Cebaiye) Lalang Grass Rhizome (白茅根, Baimaogen) Ass-hide Glue (阿胶, Ejiao) Heartlaef Houttuynia Herb (鱼腥草, Yuxingcao) Ovateleaf Holly Bark (救必应, Jiubiying) Patience Dock Root (牛西西, Niuxixi) Japanese Dock Root (羊蹄, Yangti) India Madder Root (茜草, Qiancao) Hunifuse Euphorbia Herb (地锦草, Dijincao) Garden Burnet Root (地榆, Diyu) Japanese Pagodatree Flower (槐花, Huaihua) Japanese Pagodatree Fruit (槐角, Huaijiao) Cattail Pollen (蒲黄, Puhuang) Argy Wormwood Leaf (艾叶, Aiye) Male Fern Rhizome (贯众, Guanzhong) Charred Human Hair (血余炭, Xueyutan) Purslane Herb (马齿苋, Machixian) Chinese Gall (五倍子, Wubeizi) Puff-ball (马勃, Mabo) East Asian Tree Fern Rhizome (狗脊, Gouji) Cuttle Bone (乌贼骨, Wuzeigu) Ophicalcite (花蕊石, Huaruishi) Japanese Thistle Herb or Root (大蓟, Daji) Common Cephalanoplos Herb (小蓟, Xiaoji) Shepherdspurse Herb with Root (荠菜, Jicai) Eucommia Bark (杜仲, Duzhong) Malaytea Scurfpea Fruit (补骨脂, Buguzhi) Desertliving Cistanche (肉苁蓉, Roucongrong) Jew's Ear (木耳, Muer) Taiwan Beautybetter Leaf (紫珠, Zizhu) Hindu Lotus Rhizome-node (藕节, Oujie) Baked Rhizome (炮姜, Paojiang) Baikal Skullcap Root (黄芩, Huangqin) Fineleaf Schizomepeta Herb (荆芥, Jingjie) Coptis Rhizome (黄连, Huanglian) Smoked Plum (乌梅, Wumei) Ass-hide Glue (阿胶, Ejiao)

9. Herbs resisting blood coagulation: Leech (水蛭, Shuizhi) Seaweed (海藻, Haizao)

10. Herbs containing saponin with the function of hemolysis: Chinese Honeylocust Fruit (皂荚, Zaojia) Chinese Honeylocust Spine (皂角刺, Zaojiaoci) Balloonflower Root (桔梗, Jiegeng) Pinellia Rhizome (半夏, Banxia) Jackinthepulpit Tuber (天南星, Tiannanxing) Thinleaf Milkwort Root (远志, Yuanzhi) Tatarian Aster Root (紫苑, Ziyuan) Willowleaf Swallowwort Rhizome (白前, Baiqian) Whiteflower hogfenel Root (前胡, Qianhu) Sevenlobed Yam Rhizome (萆薢, Bixie)薢, Twotooth Achyranthes Root

(牛膝，Niuxi).

Herbs acting on striated muscle

1. Herbs with the function of relaxing striated muscle: Fourstamen Stephania Root (汉防己，Hanfangji) Yanhusuo (延胡索，Yanhusuo) Biond Magnolia Flower-bud (辛夷，Xinyi) Thickleaf Vladimiria Root (青木香，Qingmuxiang) Motherwort Herb (益母草，Yimucao) Common Carpesium Fruit (鹤虱，Heshi) Cicada Slough (蝉蜕，Chantui) Coix Seed (薏苡仁，Yiyiren) Common Floweringquince Fruit (木瓜，Mugua) Lucid Ganoderma (灵芝，Lingzhi) Amber (琥珀，Hupo)

2. Herbs with the function of convulting striated muscle: Nut-vomitive Poisonnut Seed (马钱子，Maqianzi) Dahurian Angelica Root (白芷，Baizhi)

Herbs with the function of antianaphylaxis

Smoked Plum (乌梅，Wumei) Earth Worm (地龙，Dilong) Dried Human Placenta (紫河车，Ziheche) Membranous Milkvetch Root (黄芪，Huangqi) Fourstamen Stephania Root (汉防已，Hanfangji) Luffa Stem (丝瓜藤，Siguateng) Pearl (珍珠，Zhenzhu) Tree Peony Bark (牡丹皮，Mudanpi) Japanese Felt Fern Leaf (石韦，Shiwei) Licorice Root (甘草，Gancao) Ephedra (麻黄，Mahuang) Largeleaf Gentian Root (秦艽，Qinjiao) Chinese Thorowax Root (柴胡，Chaihu) Snake Slough (蛇蜕，Shetui) Swordlike Atractylodes Rhizome (苍术，Cangzhu) Japanese Felt Fern Leaf (石韦，Shiwei) Pearl (珍珠，Zhenzhu) Tuber Fleeceflower Stem and Leaf (夜交藤，Yejiaoteng) Puncturevine Caltrap Fruit (白蒺藜，Baijili) Ginseng (人参，Renshen) Common Ducksmeat Herb (浮萍，Fuping) Paniculate Swallowwort Root (徐长卿，Xuchangqing) Cicada Slough (蝉蜕，Chantui) Wild Mint (薄荷，Bohe) Fineleaf Schizomepeta Herb (荆芥，Jingjie) Honeysuckle Stem (忍冬藤，Rendongteng) Incised Notopterygium Rhizome and Root (羌活，Qianghuo) Chinese Tamarish Twig (西河柳，Xiheliu) Belvedere Fruit (地肤子，Difuzi) Cape Jasmine Fruit (栀子，Zhizi) Silkworm Feculae (蚕砂，Cansha) Densefruit Pittany Root-bark (白鲜皮，Baixianpi)

Herbs resisting rheumatic arthritis

1. Herbs acting on analogous adrenocortical hormone: Fourstamen Stephania Root (汉防己，Hanfangji) Licorice Root (甘草，Gancao) Largeleaf Gentian Root (秦艽，Qinjiao) Orientvine Stem or Hair Orientvine Stem (青风藤，Qingfengteng) Aspisin (蜂毒，Fengdu) Nippon Yam Rhizome (穿山龙，Chuanshanlong) Ginseng Leaf (人参叶，Renshenye) Shorttube Lycoris Bulb (石蒜，Shisuan) Sanchi Root (三七，Sanqi) Prepared Daughter Root of Common Monkshood (附子，Fuzi) Common Monksood (乌头，Wutou) Kusnezoff Monkhood Root (草乌，Caowu) Musk (麝香，Shexiang) Silkworm with Batrytis Larva (白僵蚕，Baijiangcan) Paniculate Swallowwort Root (徐长卿，Xuchangqing) Largeleaf Chinese Ash Bark (秦皮，Qinpi) Oriental Variegated Coralbean Bark (海桐皮，Haitongpi) Kadsura Pepper Stem (海风藤，Haifengteng) Chinese Starjasmine Stem (络石藤，Luoshiteng)

2. Others: Rehmannia Dried Root (生地黄，Shengdihuang), Cortex Acanthopanacis Radicis (五加皮，Wujiapi), Manchurian Wildginger Herb (细辛，Xixin), Divaricate

Saposhnikovia Root (防风, Fangfeng), Dragon's Bone (龙骨, Longgu), Himalayan Teasel Root (续断, Xuduan), Eucommia Bark (杜仲, Duzhong), Twotooth Achyranthes Root (牛膝, Niuxi), Medicininal Cyathula Root (川牛膝, Chuanniuxi), Doubleteeth Pulbescent Angelica Root (独活, Duhuo), Incised Notopterygium Rhizome and Root (羌活, Qianghuo), Common Heron's Bill Herb or Wilford Cranesbill Herb (老鹳草, Laoguancao), Tuberculate Speranskia Herb (透骨草, Tougucao), Swordlike Atractylodes Rhizome (苍术, Cangzhu), Tall Gastrodia Rhizome (天麻, Tianma), Beautiful Sweetgum Fruit (路路通, Lulutong), Agkistrodon Acutus (白花蛇, Baihuashe), Garter Snake (乌梢蛇, Wushaoshe), Obscured Homalamena Rhizome (千年健, Qiannianjian), Stem of Chinese Photinial (石楠藤, Shinanteng), Chinese Pyrola Herb (鹿衔草, Luxiancao), Common Clubmoss Herb (伸筋草, Shenjincao), Common Threewingnut Root Leaf or Flower (雷公藤, Leigongteng), Chinese Clematis Root (威灵仙, Weilingxian).

Herbs with the function of glycometabolism

1. Herbs with the function of reducing blood sugar concentration: Ginseng (人参, Renshen) Membranous Milkvetch Root (黄芪, Huangqi) Tuckahoe (茯苓, Fuling) Largehead Atractylodes Rhizome (白术, Baizhu) Swordlike Atractylodes Rhizome (苍术, Cangzhu) Common Yam Rhizome (山药, Shanyao) Siberian Solomonseal Rhizome (黄精, Huangjing) Rehmannia Dried Root (生地黄, Shengdihuang) Prepared Rhizome of Adhesive Rehmannia (熟地黄, Shoudihuang) Figwort Root (玄参, Xuanshen) Dwarf Lilyturf Root (麦门冬, Maimendong) Common Anemarrhea Rhizome (知母, Zhimu) Snakegroud Root (天花粉, Tianhuafen) Fragrant Solomonseal Rhizome (玉竹, Yuzhu) Barbary Wolfberry Fruit (枸杞子, Gouqizi) Tuber Fleeceflower Root (何首乌, Heshouw u) Chinese Magnoliavine (五味子, Wuweizi) Shorthorned Epimedium Herb (淫羊藿, Yinyanghuo) Royal Jelly (蜂乳, Fengru) Lobed Kudzuvine Root (葛根, Gegen) Oriental Waterplantain Rhizome (泽泻, Zexie) Mazie Style (玉米须, Yumixu) Chinese Wolfberry Root-bark (地骨皮, Digupi), Giant Knotweed Rhizome (虎杖, Huzhang) Hairvein Agrimonia Herb (仙鹤草, Xianhecao) Cortex Acanthopanacis Radicis (五加皮, Wujiapi) Siberian Cocklebur Fruit (苍耳子, Cangerzi) Mulberry Leaf (桑叶, Sangye) Chinese Gall (五倍子, Wubeizi) Cochinchinese Asparagus Root (天门冬, Tianmendong)

2. Herbs with the function of increasing blood sugar concentration: Tangshen Root (党参, Dangshen) Root of Lance Asiabell (四叶参, Siyeshen) Dendrobium Herb (石斛, Shihu) Baikal Skullcap Root (黄芩, Huangqin) Largeleaf Gentian Root (秦艽, Qinjiao) Bamboo leaf (竹叶, Zhuye) Fresh Ginger (生姜, Shengjiang) Japanese Pagodatree Flower (槐花, Huaihua)

Reference Ⅲ Clinical Application of Chinese Drugs Based on the Syndromes

Fever

1. Fever affter invasion of exogenous pathogens

(1) Being invaded by wind-cold: Fineleaf Schizomepeta Herb (荆芥, Jingjie) Divaricate Saposhnikovia Root (防风, Fangfeng) Perilla Leaf (紫苏, Zisu) Incised Notopterygium Rhizome and Root (羌活, Qianghuo) Ephedra (麻黄, Mahuang) Cassia Twig (桂枝, Guizhi) Manchurian Wildginger Herb (细辛, Xixin) Dahurian Angelica Root (白芷, Baizhi) Cariander Herb (胡荽, Husui) Chinese Ligusticum Rhizome (藁本, Gaoben) Fresh Ginger (生姜, Shengjiang) Fistular Onion Stalk (葱白, Congbai)

(2) Being invaded by wind-heat: Honeysuckle Flower (金银花, Jinyinhua) Weeping Forsythia Capsule (连翘, Lianqiao) Wild Mint (薄荷, Bohe) Mulberry Leaf (桑叶, Sangye) Chrysanthemum Flower (菊花, Juhua) Great Burdock Achene (牛蒡子, Niubangzi) Reed Rhizome (芦根, Lugen) Chinese Thorowax Root (柴胡, Chaihu) Lobed Kudzuvine Root (葛根, Gegen) Bamboo leaf (竹叶, Zhuye) Common Ducksmeat Herb (浮萍, Fuping) Cicada Slough (蝉蜕, Chantui) Prepared Soybean (淡豆豉, Dandouchi)

(3) Being invaded by summer-wetness: Wrinkled Gianthyssop Herb (藿香, Huoxiang) Foutune Eupatorium Herb (佩兰, Peilan) Haichow Elsholtzia Herb (香薷, Xiangru) Sweet Wormwood (青蒿, Qinghao) Coptis Rhizome (黄连, Huanglian) Balsampear Fruit (苦瓜, Kugua) Hindu Lotus Leaf (荷叶, Heye) Hindu Lotus Petiole (荷梗, Hegeng) Watermelon Pericarp (西瓜皮, Xiguapi) Green Gram Seed (绿豆, Lvdou) Hyacinth Dolichos Flower (扁豆花, Biandouhua)

2. Fever caused by internal damage

(1) Interior heat caused by deficiency of yin: Starwort Root (银柴胡, Yinchaihu) Chinese Wolfberry Root-bark (地骨皮, Digupi), Sweet Wormwood (青蒿, Qinghao) Common Anemarrhea Rhizome (知母, Zhimu) Largeleaf Gentian Root (秦艽, Qinjiao) Turtle Carapace (鳖甲, Biejia) Blackend Swallowwort Root (白薇, Baiwei) Rice Germinating Fruit (sprout) (谷芽, Guya) Rehmannia Dried Root (生地黄, Shengdihuang) Tree Peony Bark (牡丹皮, Mudanpi) Figwortflower Picrorhiza Rhizome (胡黄连, Huhuanglian)

(2) Fever caused by deficiency of qi: Membranous Milkvetch Root (黄芪, Huangqi) Tangshen Root (党参, Dangshen) Largehead Atractylodes Rhizome (白术, Baizhu) Tuckahoe (茯苓, Fuling) Siberian Solomonseal Rhizome (黄精, Huangjing)

(3) Interior heat caused by deficiency of blood: Chinese Angelica Root (当归, Danggui) Prepared Rhizome of Adhesive Rehmannia (熟地黄, Shoudihuang) Red Peony Root (赤芍药, Chishaoyao) Tree Peony Bark (牡丹皮, Mudanpi) Dan-shen Root (丹参, Danshen) Root of Sinkiang Arnebia (紫草, Zicao) Blackend Swallowwort Root (白薇, Bai-

wei) Barbary Wolfberry Fruit (枸杞子, Gouqizi) Membranous Milkvetch Root (黄芪, Huangqi)

Headache

1. Invasion of exogenous pathogens

(1) Headache due to wind-cold: Fineleaf Schizomepeta Herb (荆芥, Jingjie) Divaricate Saposhnikovia Root (防风, Fangfeng) Dahurian Angelica Root (白芷, Baizhi) Chinese Ligusticum Rhizome (藁本, Gaoben) Manchurian Wildginger Herb (细辛, Xixin) Incised Notopterygium Rhizome and Root (羌活, Qianghuo) Szechwan Lovage Rhizome (川芎, Chuanxiong) Ephedra (麻黄, Mahuang) Cassia Twig (桂枝, Guizhi) Haichow Elsholtzia Herb (香薷, Xiangru) Doubleteeth Pulbescent Angelica Root (独活, Duhuo) Biond Magnolia Flower-bud (辛夷, Xinyi) Siberian Cocklebur Fruit (苍耳子, Cangerzi)

(2) Headache due to wind-heat: Mulberry Leaf (桑叶, Sangye) Chrysanthemum Flower (菊花, Juhua) Wild Mint (薄荷, Bohe) Gypsum (石膏, Shigao) Shrub Chastetree Fruit (蔓荆子, Manjingzi) Lobed Kudzuvine Root (葛根, Gegen) Fineleaf Schizomepeta Herb (荆芥, Jingjie) Great Burdock Achene (牛蒡子, Niubangzi) Silkworm with Batrytis Larva (白僵蚕, Baijiangcan) Common Lophatherum Herb (淡竹叶, Danzhuye) Cicada Slough (蝉蜕, Chantui) Common Scouring Rush Herb (木贼, Muzei) Honeysuckle Flower (金银花, Jinyinhua) Weeping Forsythia Capsule (连翘, Lianqiao) Shunk Bugbane Rhizome (升麻, Shengma)

(3) Headache due to wind-dampness: Incised Notopterygium Rhizome and Root (羌活, Qianghuo) Divaricate Saposhnikovia Root (防风, Fangfeng) Dahurian Angelica Root (白芷, Baizhi) Szechwan Lovage Rhizome (川芎, Chuanxiong) Siberian Cocklebur Fruit (苍耳子, Cangerzi) Doubleteeth Pulbescent Angelica Root (独活, Duhuo) Chinese Ligusticum Rhizome (藁本, Gaoben)

2. Internal damage

(1) Headache due to hyperactivity of liver-yang: ① Suppress the hyperactive liver: Tall Gastrodia Rhizome (天麻, Tianma) Gambirplant Hooked Stem and Branch (钩藤, Gouteng) Puncturevine Caltrap Fruit (白蒺藜, Baijili) White Peony Root (白芍药, Baishaoyao) Chrysanthemum Flower (菊花, Juhua) Common St. Paulswort Herb (豨莶草, Xixiancao) Cassia Seed (决明子, Juemingzi) Wormwoodlike Motherwort Seed (茺蔚子, Chongweizi) Feather Cockscomb Seed (青葙子, Qingxiangzi) Antelope Horn (羚羊角, Lingyangjiao) ② Subside yang: Abalone Shell (石决明, Shijueming) Nacre (珍珠母, Zhenzhumu) Dragon's Bone (龙骨, Longgu) Oyster Shell (牡蛎, Muli) Magnetite (磁石, Cishi) Hematite (代赭石, Daizheshi) Antelope Horn (羚羊角, Lingyangjiao) ③ Nourish the liver and kidney: Twotooth Achyranthes Root (牛膝, Niuxi) Chinese Taxillus Twig (桑寄生, Sangjisheng) Eucommia Bark (杜仲, Duzhong) Glossy Privet Fruit (女贞子, Nuzhenzi) Yerbadetajo Herb (墨旱莲, Mohanlian) Flatstem Milkvetch Seed (沙苑子, Shayuanzi) Mulberry Solomonseal (桑椹, Sangshen) ④ Clear away liver-fire: Chinese Gentian Root (龙胆草, Longdancao) Cape Jasmine Fruit (栀子, Zhizi) Baikal Skullcap Root (黄芩, Huangqin) Common Selfheal Spike (夏枯草, Xiakucao) Antelope Horn (羚羊角, Lingyangjiao)

(2) Headache caused by turbid phlegm: Pinellia Rhizome (半夏, Banxia) Largehead Atractylodes Rhizome (白术, Baizhu) Tall

Gastrodia Rhizome（天麻，Tianma）Puncturevine Caltrop Fruit（白蒺藜，Baijili）Medicinal Evodia Root（吴茱萸，Wuzhuyu）Jackinthepulpit Tuber（天南星，Tiannanxing）Giant Typhonium Rhizome（白附子，Baifuzi）Oyster Shell（牡蛎，Muli）

（3）Headache caused by blood stasis：Peach Seed（桃仁，Taoren）Safflower（红花，Honghua）Chinese Angelica Root（当归，Danggui）Szechwan Lovage Rhizome（川芎，Chuanxiong）Red Peony Root（赤芍药，Chishaoyao）Rehmannia Dried Root（生地黄，Shengdihuang）Twotooth Achyranthes Root（牛膝，Niuxi）Yanhusuo（延胡索，Yanhusuo）Musk（麝香，Shexiang）

（4）Headache caused by deficiency of kidney：① Deficiency of kidney-yin：Prepared Rhizome of Adhesive Rehmannia（熟地黄，Shoudihuang）Common Yam Rhizome（山药，Shanyao）Asiatic Cornelian Cherry Fruit（山茱萸，Shanzhuyu）Barbary Wolfberry Fruit（枸杞子，Gouqizi）Chrysanthemum Flower（菊花，Juhua）Glossy Privet Fruit（女贞子，Nuzhenzi）Yerbadetajo Herb（墨旱莲，Mohanlian）②Deficiency of kidney-yang：Eucommia Bark（杜仲，Duzhong）Common Curculigo（仙茅，Xianmao）Shorthorned Epimedium Herb（淫羊藿，Yinyanghuo）Malaytea Scurfpea Fruit（补骨脂，Buguzhi）Prepared Daughter Root of Common Monkshood（附子，Fuzi）Cassia Bark（肉桂，Rougui）

（5）Headache due to deficiency of both qi and blood：Tangshen Root（党参，Dangshen）Largehead Atractylodes Rhizome（白术，Baizhu）Tuckahoe（茯苓，Fuling）Licorice Root（甘草，Gancao）Chinese Angelica Root（当归，Danggui）Szechwan Lovage Rhizome（川芎，Chuanxiong）White Peony Root（白芍药，Baishaoyao）Prepared Rhizome of Adhesive Rehmannia（熟地黄，Shoudihuang）Siberian Solomonseal Rhizome（黄精，Huangjing）Tuber Fleeceflower Root（何首乌，Heshouwu）Mulberry Solomonseal（桑椹，Sangshen）Dried Human Placenta（紫河车，Ziheche）Ass-hide Glue（阿胶，Ejiao）

（6）Obstinate headache：Giant Typhonium Rhizome（白附子，Baifuzi）Manchurian Wildginger Herb（细辛，Xixin）Scorpion（全蝎，Quanxie）Centipede（蜈蚣，Wugong）

Dizziness

1. Hyperactivity of Liver-yang

（1）Suppress the hyperactive liver：Tall Gastrodia Rhizome（天麻，Tianma）Gambirplant Hooked Stem and Branch（钩藤，Gouteng）Chrysanthemum Flower（菊花，Juhua）Mulberry Leaf（桑叶，Sangye）Hindu Lotus Leaf（荷叶，Heye）Wild Mint（薄荷，Bohe）Common St. Paulswort Herb（豨莶草，Xixiancao）Cassia Seed（决明子，Juemingzi）Tortoise's Shell and Plastron（龟版，Guiban）White Peony Root（白芍药，Baishaoyao）Puncturevine Caltrop Fruit（刺蒺藜，Cijili）Feather Cockscomb Seed（青葙子，Qingxiangzi）Dogbame Herb（罗布麻，Luobuma）

（2）Subside yang：Nacre（珍珠母，Zhenzhumu）Abalone Shell（石决明，Shijueming）Oyster Shell（牡蛎，Muli）Hematite（代赭石，Daizheshi）Magnetite Ore（磁石，Cishi）Dragon's Bone（龙骨，Longgu）Arabic Cowry Shell（紫贝齿，Zibeichi），Antelope Horn（羚羊角，Lingyangjiao）

（3）Clear away liver-fire：Chinese Gentian Root（龙胆草，Longdancao）Common Selfheal Spike（夏枯草，Xiakucao）Baikal Skullcap Root（黄芩，Huangqin）Cape Jasmine Fruit（栀子，Zhizi）Cassia Seed（决明子，Juemingzi）Aloes（芦荟，Luhui）Feather Cockscomb Seed（青葙子，Qingxiangzi）Antelope Horn（羚羊角，Lingyangjiao）Dogbame Herb (罗布麻, Luobuma) Chrysanthemum Flower (菊花, Juhua) Japanese Pagodatree Flower (槐花, Huaihua)

(4) Nourish the liver and kidney: Eucommia Bark (杜仲, Duzhong) Twotooth Achyranthes Root (牛膝, Niuxi) Chinese Taxillus Twig (桑寄生, Sangjisheng) Prepared Rhizome of Adhesive Rehmannia (熟地黄, Shoudihuang) Asiatic Cornelian Cherry Fruit (山茱萸, Shanzhuyu) Barbary Wolfberry Fruit (枸杞子, Gouqizi) Chinese Magnoliavine (五味子, Wuweizi) Glossy Privet Fruit (女贞子, Nuzhenzi) Yerbadetajo Herb (墨旱莲, Mohanlian)

2. Deficiency of both qi and blood: Membranous Milkvetch Root (黄芪, Huangqi) Tangshen Root (党参, Dangshen) Largehead Atractylodes Rhizome (白术, Baizhu) Tuckahoe (茯苓, Fuling) Licorice Root (甘草, Gancao) Tuber Fleeceflower Root (何首乌, Heshouwu) Dan-shen Root (丹参, Danshen) Chinese Angelica Root (当归, Danggui) Prepared Rhizome of Adhesive Rehmannia (熟地黄, Shoudihuang) Longan Aril (龙眼肉, Longyanrou) Chinese Date (大枣, Dazao)

3. Deficiency of kidney-essence: Hairy Antler (鹿茸, Lurong) Antler Glue (鹿角胶, Lujiaojiao) Tortoise's Shell and Plastron Glue (龟版胶, Guibanjiao) Prepared Daughter Root of Common Monkshood (附子, Fuzi) Cassia Bark (肉桂, Rougui) Prepared Rhizome of Adhesive Rehmannia (熟地黄, Shoudihuang) Asiatic Cornelian Cherry Fruit (山茱萸, Shanzhuyu) Barbary Wolfberry Fruit (枸杞子, Gouqizi) Desertliving Cistanche (肉苁蓉, Roucongrong) Dodder Seed (菟丝子, Tusizi) Glossy Privet Fruit (女贞子, Nuzhenzi) Yerbadetajo Herb (墨旱莲, Mohanlian) Eucommia Bark (杜仲, Duzhong) English Walnut (核桃肉, Hetaorou)

4. Stagnation of turbid phlegm in middle-Jiao: Pinellia Rhizome (半夏, Banxia) Tangerine Peel (橘皮, Jupi) Tuckahoe (茯苓, Fuling) Largehead Atractylodes Rhizome (白术, Baizhu) Swordlike Atractylodes Rhizome (苍术, Cangzhu) Jackinthepulpit Tuber (天南星, Tiannanxing) Bamboo Shavings (竹茹, Zhuru) Silkworm with Batrytis Larva (白僵蚕, Baijiangcan) Oriental Waterplantain Rhizome (泽泻, Zexie)

Tinnitus Deafness

1. Excessive Fire in the liver and gallbladder: Chinese Gentian Root (龙胆草, Longdancao) Baikal Skullcap Root (黄芩, Huangqin) Cape Jasmine Fruit (栀子, Zhizi) Chinese Thorowax Root (柴胡, Chaihu) Chinese Angelica Root (当归, Danggui) Akebia Stem (木通, Mutong) Oriental Waterplantain Rhizome (泽泻, Zexie) Plantain Seed (车前子, Cheqianzi)

2. Stagnation of phlegm-fire: Tangerine Peel (橘皮, Jupi) Pinellia Rhizome (半夏, Banxia) Tuckahoe (茯苓, Fuling) Thinleaf Milkwort Root (远志, Yuanzhi) Grassleaf Sweetflag Rhizome (石菖蒲, Shichangpu) Chlorite-schist (礞石, Mengshi) Baikal Skullcap Root (黄芩, Huangqin) Coptis Rhizome (黄连, Huanglian) Rhubarb (大黄, Dahuang) Turmeric Root-tuber (郁金, Yujin) Chinese Eaglewood Wood (沉香, Chenxiang)

3. Comsumption of kidney-essence: Prepared Rhizome of Adhesive Rehmannia (熟地黄, Shoudihuang) Common Yam Rhizome (山药, Shanyao) Asiatic Cornelian Cherry Fruit (山茱萸, Shanzhuyu) Tuckahoe (茯苓, Fuling) Oriental Waterplantain Rhizome (泽泻, Zexie) Tree Peony Bark (牡丹皮,

Mudanpi) Chinese Magnoliavine (五味子, Wuweizi) Dodder Seed (菟丝子, Tusizi) Malaytea Scurfpea Fruit (补骨脂, Buguzhi) Magnetite Ore (磁石, Cishi)

4. Deficiency of spleen-qi and stomach-qi: Ginseng (人参, Renshen) Membranous Milkvetch Root (黄芪, Huangqi) Largehead Atractylodes Rhizome (白术, Baizhu) Tuckahoe (茯苓, Fuling) Shunk Bugbane Rhizome (升麻, Shengma) Lobed Kudzuvine Root (葛根, Gegen) Grassleaf Sweetflag Rhizome (石菖蒲, Shichangpu) Chinese Angelica Root (当归, Danggui) White Peony Root (白芍药, Baishaoyao) Licorice Root (甘草, Gancao)

Coma

1. Heat attacking the pericardium: Cowbezoar (牛黄, Niuhuang) Artificial Ox-gallstone (人工牛黄, Rengongniuhuang) Buffalo Horn (水牛角, Shuiniujiao) Antelope Horn (羚羊角, Lingyangjiao) Goat Horn (山羊角, Shanyangjiao) Borneol (冰片, Bingpian) Gypsum (石膏, Shigao) Mirabilite Crystal (寒水石, Hanshuishi) Shunk Bugbane Rhizome (升麻, Shengma) Coptis Rhizome (黄连, Huanglian) Cape Jasmine Fruit (栀子, Zhizi) Turmeric Root-tuber (郁金, Yujin) Baikal Skullcap Root (黄芩, Huangqin)

2. Mental Confusion due to phlegm: Storesin (苏合香, Suhexiang) Musk (麝香, Shexiang) Benzoin (安息香, Anxixiang) Borneol (冰片, Bingpian) Clove Flower-bud (丁香, Dingxiang) Frankincense (乳香, Ruxiang) Chinese Honeylocust Fruit (皂荚, Zaojia) Manchurian Wildginger Herb (细辛, Xixin) Grassleaf Sweetflag Rhizome (石菖蒲, Shichangpu) Thinleaf Milkwort Root (远志, Yuanzhi) Arisaema with Bile (胆南星, Dannanxing) Bamboo Juice (竹沥, Zhuli) Tabasheer (天竹黄, Tianzhuhuang) Alumen (白矾, Baifan) Turmeric Root-tuber (郁金, Yujin) Snake bile (蛇胆, Shedan)

Insomnia

1. Blood deficiency of both the heart and spleen: Tangshen Root (党参, Dangshen) Membranous Milkvetch Root (黄芪, Huangqi) Largehead Atractylodes Rhizome (白术, Baizhu) Indian Bread with Hostwood (茯神, Fushen) Spine Date Seed (酸枣仁, Suanzaoren) Thinleaf Milkwort Root (远志, Yuanzhi) Chinese Magnoliavine (五味子, Wuweizi) Chinese Arborvitae Seed (柏子仁, Baiziren) Tuber Fleeceflower Root (何首乌, Heshouwu) Tuber Fleeceflower Stem and Leaf (夜交藤, Yejiaoteng) Lucid Ganoderma (灵芝, Lingzhi) Prepared Rhizome of Adhesive Rehmannia (熟地黄, Shoudihuang) White Peony Root (白芍药, Baishaoyao) Chinese Angelica Root (当归, Danggui)

2. Hyperactivity of fire caused by deficiency of yin: Coptis Rhizome (黄连, Huanglian) Ass-hide Glue (阿胶, Ejiao) Dwarf Lilyturf Root (麦门冬, Maimendong) Rehmannia Dried Root (生地黄, Shengdihuang) Figwort Root (玄参, Xuanshen) Dan-shen Root (丹参, Danshen) Lily Bulb (百合, Baihe) Hindu Lotus Plumule (莲子心, Lianzixin) Glossy Privet Fruit (女贞子, Nuzhenzi) Yerbadetajo Herb (墨旱莲, Mohanlian) Bamboo leaf (竹叶, Zhuye) Cape Jasmine Fruit (栀子, Zhizi)

3. Timidness due to deficiency of the heart: Tangshen Root (党参, Dangshen) Indian Bread with Hostwood (茯神, Fushen) Tuber Fleeceflower Root (何首乌, Heshouwu) Tuber Fleeceflower Stem and Leaf (夜交藤, Yejiaoteng) Chinese Magnoliavine (五味子, Wuweizi) Spine Date Seed (酸枣仁, Suanzaoren) Dragon's Teeth (龙齿, Longchi) Thin-

leaf Milkwort Root (远志, Yuanzhi) Arabic Cowry Shell (紫贝齿, Zibeichi)

4. Disorder of the stomach: Charred Hawthorn Fruit (焦山楂, Jiaoshanzha) Charred Malt (焦麦芽, Jiaomaiya) Charred Medicated Leaven (焦神曲, Jiaoshenqu) Pinellia Rhizome (半夏, Banxia) Tangerine Peel (橘皮, Jupi) Tuckahoe (茯苓, Fuling) Bitter Orange (枳壳, Zhiqiao) Villous Amomum Fruit (砂仁, Sharen) Common Aucklandia Root (木香, Muxiang)

Swelling and Pain in the Throat

1. Excess Syndromes

(1) Affection of exogenous wind-heat: Wild Mint (薄荷, Bohe) Great Burdock Achene (牛蒡子, Niubangzi) Balloonflower Root (桔梗, Jiegeng) Puff-ball (马勃, Mabo) Honeysuckle Flower (金银花, Jinyinhua) Weeping Forsythia Capsule (连翘, Lianqiao) Franchet Groundcherry Calyx or Fruit (锦灯笼, Jindenglong) Cicada Slough (蝉蜕, Chantui) Olive (橄榄, Ganlan) Chrysanthemum Flower (菊花, Juhua) Common Dayflower Herb (鸭跖草, Yazhicao) Giant Knotweed Rhizome (虎杖, Huzhang) Heartlaef Houttuynia Herb (鱼腥草, Yuxingcao) Chinese Lobelia Herb (半边莲, Banbianlian) Spreading Hedyotis Herb (白花蛇舌草, Baihuasheshecao) Borneol (冰片, Bingpian) Shunk Bugbane Rhizome (升麻, Shengma) Silkworm with Batrytis Larva (白僵蚕, Baijiangcan) Mulberry Leaf (桑叶, Sangye)

(2) Overabundance of toxic heat: Honeysuckle Flower (金银花, Jinyinhua) Weeping Forsythia Capsule (连翘, Lianqiao) Coptis Rhizome (黄连, Huanglian) Baikal Skullcap Root (黄芩, Huangqin) Cape Jasmine Fruit (栀子, Zhizi) Blackberrylily Rhizome (射干, Shegan) Tonkin Sophora Root (山豆根, Shandougen) Hairystalk Tinospora Root (金果榄, Jinguolan) Indigowoad Leaf (大青叶, Daqingye) Common Andrographis Herb (穿心莲, Chuanxinlian) Twotooth Achyranthes Root (土牛膝, Tuniuxi) Franchet Groundcherry Calyx or Fruit (锦灯笼, Jindenglong) Shunk Bugbane Rhizome (升麻, Shengma) Cow-bezoar (牛黄, Niuhuang) Artificial Oxgallstone (人工牛黄, Rengongniuhuang) Toad Skin Secretion Cake (蟾酥, Chansu) Common Dayflower Herb (鸭跖草, Yazhicao) Boat-fruited Sterculia Seed (胖大海, Pangdahai) Dandelion (蒲公英, Pugongying) Mulberry Leaf (桑叶, Sangye) Thunberg Fritillary Bulb (浙贝母, Zhebeimu) Airpotato Yam Tuber (黄药子, Huangyaozi) Indigwoad Root (板蓝根, Banlangen) Puff-ball (马勃, Mabo) Great Burdock Achene (牛蒡子, Niubangzi) Balloonflower Root (桔梗, Jiegeng) Licorice Root (甘草, Gancao) Figwort Root (玄参, Xuanshen)

2. Deficiency Syndromes

(1) Insufficiency of lung-yin: Coastal Glehnia Root (北沙参, Beishashen) Dwarf Lilyturf Root (麦门冬, Maimendong) Snakegroud Root (天花粉, Tianhuafen) Lily Bulb (百合, Baihe) Fragrant Solomonseal Rhizome (玉竹, Yuzhu) Ass-hide Glue (阿胶, Ejiao) Rehmannia Dried Root (生地黄, Shengdihuang) Reed Rhizome (芦根, Lugen) Chinese White Olive (青果, Qingguo) Indian Trumpetflower Seed (木蝴蝶, Muhudie) Fig Receptacle (无花果, Wuhuaguo) Honey (蜂蜜, Fengmi) Dendrobium Herb (石斛, Shihu) Siberian Solomonseal Rhizome (黄精, Huangjing)

Hoarse voice: Boat-fruited Sterculia Seed (胖大海, Pangdahai) Medicine Terminalia Fruit (诃子, Hezi) Medicine Terminalia Immature Fruit (藏青果, Zangqingguo) Charred

Human Hair (血余炭, Xueyutan) Cicada Slough (蝉蜕, Chantui)

(2) Insufficiency of kidney-yin: Figwort Root (玄参, Xuanshen) Cochinchinese Asparagus Root (天门冬, Tianmendong) Prepared Rhizome of Adhesive Rehmannia (熟地黄, Shoudihuang) Asiatic Cornelian Cherry Fruit (山茱萸, Shanzhuyu) Chinese Magnoliavine (五味子, Wuweizi) Dendrobium Herb (石斛, Shihu) Common Anemarrhea Rhizome (知母, Zhimu) Chinese Corktree Bark (黄柏, Huangbai)

Cough

1. Exopathogen Affection

(1) Affection of exogenous wind-cold: Ephedra (麻黄, Mahuang) Apricot Seed (杏仁, Xingren) Tatarian Aster Root (紫苑, Ziyuan) Common Perilla Leaf (苏叶, Suye) Manchurian Wildginger Herb (细辛, Xixin) Balloonflower Root (桔梗, Jiegeng) Willowleaf Swallowwort Rhizome (白前, Baiqian) Tatarian Aster Root (紫苑, Ziyuan) Common Coltsfoot Flower (款冬花, Kuandonghua) Tangerine Peel (橘皮, Jupi) Whiteflower hogfenel Root (前胡, Qianhu), Fineleaf Schizomepeta Herb (荆芥, Jingjie) Divaricate Saposhnikovia Root (防风, Fangfeng)

(2) Affection of exogenous wind-heat: Mulberry Leaf (桑叶, Sangye) Chrysanthemum Flower (菊花, Juhua) Wild Mint (薄荷, Bohe) Great Burdock Achene (牛蒡子, Niubangzi) Thunberg Fritillary Bulb (浙贝母, Zhebeimu) Whiteflower hogfenel Root (前胡, Qianhu), Mongolian Snakeground Pericarp (瓜蒌皮, Gualoupi) White Mulberry Root-bark (桑白皮, Sangbaipi) Tonkin Sophora Root (山豆根, Shandougen) Honeysuckle Flower (金银花, Jinyinhua) Weeping Forsythia Capsule (连翘, Lianqiao)

2. Internal damage

(1) Cough due to Lung-heat: Baikal Skullcap Root (黄芩, Huangqin) Common Anemarrhea Rhizome (知母, Zhimu) Blackberrylily Rhizome (射干, Shegan) Arisaema with Bile (胆南星, Dannanxing) Mulberry Leaf (桑叶, Sangye) White Mulberry Root-bark (桑白皮, Sangbaipi) Cape Jasmine Fruit (栀子, Zhizi) Mongolian Snakeground Pericarp (瓜蒌皮, Gualoupi) Chinese Wolfberry Root-bark (地骨皮, Digupi), Plantain Seed (车前子, Cheqianzi) Reed Rhizome (芦根, Lugen) Lalang Grass Rhizome (白茅根, Baimaogen) Gypsum (石膏, Shigao) Mirabilite Crystal (寒水石, Hanshuishi) Baikal Skullcap Root (黄芩, Huangqin) Indigowoad Leaf (大青叶, Daqingye) Dyers Woad Root (板蓝根, Banlangen)

(2) Cough due to Lung-cold: Ephedra (麻黄, Mahuang) Manchurian Wildginger Herb (细辛, Xixin) Dried Ginger (干姜, Ganjiang) Tatarian Aster Root (紫苑, Ziyuan) Common Coltsfoot Flower (款冬花, Kuandonghua) Common Perilla Leaf (苏叶, Suye) Sessile Stemona Root (百部, Baibu)

(3) Excessive cold-phlegm: Tangerine Peel (橘皮, Jupi) Pinellia Rhizome (半夏, Banxia) Thinleaf Milkwort Root (远志, Yuanzhi) Balloonflower Root (桔梗, Jiegeng) Jackinthepulpit Tuber (天南星, Tiannanxing) Willowleaf Swallowwort Rhizome (白前, Baiqian) Perilla Seed (苏子, Suzi) White Mustard Seed (白芥子, Baijiezi) Radish Seed (莱菔子, Laifuzi) Chinese Honeylocust Fruit (皂荚, Zaojia) Inula Flower (旋覆花, Xuanfuhua) Manchurian Wildginger Herb (细辛, Xixin) Chinese Magnoliavine (五味子, Wuweizi) Dried Ginger (干姜, Ganjiang)

(4) Excessive heat-phlegm: Baikal Skullcap

Root（黄芩，Huangqin）Snakegourd Fruit（瓜蒌，Gualou）Thunberg Fritillary Bulb（浙贝母，Zhebeimu）Arisaema with Bile（胆南星，Dannanxing）Tabasheer（天竹黄，Tianzhuhuang）Heartlaef Houttuynia Herb（鱼腥草，Yuxingcao）Chinese Waxgourd Seed（冬瓜子，Dongguazi）Clam Shell（海蛤壳，Haigeqiao）Pumice（海浮石，Haifushi）Whiteflower hogfenel Root（前胡，Qianhu），Dutchmanspipe Fruit（马兜铃，Madouling）Bamboo Juice（竹沥，Zhuli）Bamboo Shavings（竹茹，Zhuru）

（5）Cough due to lung deficiency：①Moisten the lung and arrest cough：Coastal Glehnia Root（北沙参，Beishashen）Dwarf Lilyturf Root（麦门冬，Maimendong）Cochinchinese Asparagus Root（天门冬，Tianmendong）Lily Bulb（百合，Baihe）Fragrant Solomonseal Rhizome（玉竹，Yuzhu）Tendrilleaf Fritillary Bulb（贝母，Beimu）Apricot Seed（甜杏仁，Tianxingren）Ass-hide Glue（阿胶，Ejiao）Honey（蜂蜜，Fengmi）Tatarian Aster Root（紫苑，Ziyuan）Common Coltsfoot Flower（款冬花，Kuandonghua）Sessile Stemona Root（百部，Baibu）Fig Receptacle（无花果，Wuhuaguo）Dried Chinese Woodfrog（哈士蟆油，Hashimayou）Licorice Root（甘草，Gancao）② Astringe Lung-qi and relieve cough：Chinese Magnoliavine（五味子，Wuweizi）Medicine Terminalia Fruit（诃子，Hezi）Smoked Plum（乌梅，Wumei）Chinese Caterpillar Fungus（冬虫夏草，Dongchongxiacao）Chinese Gall（五倍子，Wubeizi）Ginkgo Seed（白果，Baiguo）Opium Poppy Pericarp（罂粟壳，Yingsuqiao）

Asthma（Dyspnea）

1．Excess Syndromes

（1）Dyspnea caused by adversed flow of qi：Ephedra（麻黄，Mahuang）Perilla Seed（苏子，Suzi）Pepperweed Seed or Flixweed Tansymustard Seed（葶苈子，Tinglizi）Inula Flower（旋覆花，Xuanfuhua）Apricot Seed（杏仁，Xingren）Earth Worm（地龙，Dilong）Officinal Magnolia Bark（厚朴，Houpo）Chinese Eaglewood Wood（沉香，Chenxiang）Datura Flower（洋金花，Yangjinhua）

（2）Dyspnea caused by water-retention：Pepperweed Seed or Flixweed Tansymustard Seed（葶苈子，Tinglizi）Radish Seed（莱菔子，Laifuzi）White Mustard Seed（白芥子，Baijiezi）Inula Flower（旋覆花，Xuanfuhua）Pinellia Rhizome（半夏，Banxia）Dried Ginger（干姜，Ganjiang）Manchurian Wildginger Herb（细辛，Xixin）White Mulberry Root-bark（桑白皮，Sangbaipi）Japanese Felt Fern Leaf（石韦，Shiwei）

2．Deficiency Syndromes

（1）Dysfunction of Lung-qi：Chinese Magnoliavine（五味子，Wuweizi）Medicine Terminalia Fruit（诃子，Hezi）Opium Poppy Pericarp（罂粟壳，Yingsuqiao）Smoked Plum（乌梅，Wumei）Ginkgo Seed（白果，Baiguo）

（2）Dyspnea due to deficiency of the lung：Ginseng（人参，Renshen）Tangshen Root（党参，Dangshen）Membranous Milkvetch Root（黄芪，Huangqi）Chinese Magnoliavine（五味子，Wuweizi）Dried Human Placenta（紫河车，Ziheche）Ass-hide Glue（阿胶，Ejiao）Chinese Caterpillar Fungus（冬虫夏草，Dongchongxiacao）

（3）Failure of the kidney in receiving qi：Prepared Daughter Root of Common Monkshood（附子，Fuzi）Cassia Bark（肉桂，Rougui）Prepared Rhizome of Adhesive Rehmannia（熟地黄，Shoudihuang）Siberian Solomonseal Rhizome（黄精，Huangjing）Chinese Magnoliavine（五味子，Wuweizi）Barbary Wolfberry Fruit（枸杞子，Gouqizi）Malaytea Scurfpea Fruit（补骨脂，Buguzhi）

Chinese Eaglewood Wood (沉香, Chenxiang) Giant Gecko (蛤蚧, Gejie) English Walnut (核桃肉, Hetaorou) Magnetite (磁石, Cishi) Levant Cotton Root-bark (棉花根, Mianhuagen)

Fluid-retention Syndrome

1. Food retention in the (epigastric) stomach and intestine (e.g. disturbane of gastrointestinal function): Tuckahoe (茯苓, Fuling) Cassia Twig (桂枝, Guizhi) Largehead Atractylodes Rhizome (白术, Baizhu) Pinellia Rhizome (半夏, Banxia) Fresh Ginger (生姜, Shengjiang) Bunge Pricklyash Seed (椒目, Jiaomu) Pepperweed Seed or Flixweed Tansymustard Seed (葶苈子, Tinglizi) Tangerine Peel (橘皮, Jupi)

2. Fluid-retention in the chest and hypochondrium (e.g. exudative pleurisy): Perilla Seed (苏子, Suzi) White Mustard Seed (白芥子, Baijiezi) Radish Seed (莱菔子, Laifuzi) Pepperweed Seed or Flixweed Tansymustard Seed (葶苈子, Tinglizi) Peking Euphorbia Root (大戟, Daji) Kansui Root (甘遂, Gansui) Lilac Daphne Flower-bud (芫花, Yuanhua) Chinese Thorowax Root (柴胡, Chaihu) Snakegourd Fruit (瓜蒌, Gualou)

3. Stagnation of the lung by fluid-retention (e.g. chonic bronchitis, bronchial asthma): Ephedra (麻黄, Mahuang) Cassia Twig (桂枝, Guizhi) Dried Ginger (干姜, Ganjiang) Manchurian Wildginger Herb (细辛, Xixin) Pinellia Rhizome (半夏, Banxia) Chinese Magnoliavine (五味子, Wuweizi) Apricot Seed (杏仁, Xingren) Tatarian Aster Root (紫苑, Ziyuan) Common Coltsfoot Flower (款冬花, Kuandonghua) Inula Flower (旋覆花, Xuanfuhua) Licorice Root (甘草, Gancao) Tuckahoe (茯苓, Fuling)

Palpitation

1. Restlessness of heart-mind: Magnetite (磁石, Cishi) Cinnabar (朱砂, Zhusha) Amber (琥珀, Hupo) Dragon's Teeth (龙齿, Longchi) Dragon's Bone (龙骨, Longgu) Oyster Shell (牡蛎, Muli) Thinleaf Milkwort Root (远志, Yuanzhi) Poria Cum Ligno Hospite (茯神, Fushen) Silktree Albizia Immature Flower (合欢花, Hehuanhua) Tuber Fleeceflower Stem and Leaf (夜交藤, Yejiaoteng)

2. Insufficiency of heart and spleen: Membranous Milkvetch Root (黄芪, Huangqi) Tangshen Root (党参, Dangshen) Largehead Atractylodes Rhizome (白术, Baizhu) Licorice Root (甘草, Gancao) Chinese Angelica Root (当归, Danggui) Prepared Rhizome of Adhesive Rehmannia (熟地黄, Shoudihuang) Spine Date Seed (酸枣仁, Suanzaore n) Thinleaf Milkwort Root (远志, Yuanzhi) Chinese Arborvitae Seed (柏子仁, Baiziren) Dan-shen Root (丹参, Danshen) Tuber Fleeceflower Root (何首乌, Heshouwu) Longan Aril (龙眼肉, Longyanrou) Chinese Date (大枣, Dazao)

3. Hyperactivity of fire due to yin deficiency: Rehmannia Dried Root (生地黄, Shengdihuang) Figwort Root (玄参, Xuanshen) Cochinchinese Asparagus Root (天门冬, Tianmendong) Dwarf Lilyturf Root (麦门冬, Maimendong) Fragrant Solomonseal Rhizome (玉竹, Yuzhu) Chinese Angelica Root (当归, Danggui) Dan-shen Root (丹参, Danshen) Chinese Magnoliavine (五味子, Wuweizi) Lily Bulb (百合, Baihe) Glossy Privet Fruit (女贞子, Nuzhenzi) Hindu Lotus Plumule (莲子心, Lianzixin) Common Anemarrhea Rhizome (知母, Zhimu)

4. Deficiency of heart-yang: Cassia Twig (桂枝, Guizhi) Dragon's Bone (龙骨, Long-

gu) Oyster Shell (牡蛎, Muli) Prepared Daughter Root of Common Monkshood (附子, Fuzi) Cassia Bark (肉桂, Rougui) Longstament Onion Bulb (薤白, Xiebai) Chinese Magnoliavine (五味子, Wuweizi) Dried Ginger (干姜, Ganjiang) Licorice Root (甘草, Gancao) Thinleaf Milkwort Root (远志, Yuanzhi)

5. Heat evil attacking the heart meridian: Bamboo leaf (竹叶, Zhuye) Cape Jasmine Fruit (栀子, Zhizi) Coptis Rhizome (黄连, Huanglian) Hindu Lotus Plumule (莲子心, Lianzixin) Akebia Stem (木通, Mutong) Cicada Slough (蝉蜕, Chantui) Rehmannia Dried Root (生地黄, Shengdihuang) Turmeric Root-tuber (郁金, Yujin) Dan－shen Root (丹参, Danshen)

Bleeding

1. Heat in the blood: Buffalo Horn (水牛角, Shuiniujiao) Rehmannia Dried Root (生地黄, Shengdihuang) Tree Peony Bark (牡丹皮, Mudanpi) Red Peony Root (赤芍药, Chishaoyao) Yerbadetajo Herb (墨旱莲, Mohanlian) Bletilla Rhizome (白及, Baiji) Hairvein Agrimonia Herb (仙鹤草, Xianhecao) Lalang Grass Rhizome (白茅根, Baimaogen) Hindu Lotus Rhizome-node (藕节, Oujie) Chinese Arborvitae Leafy Twig (侧柏叶, Cebaiye) Ophicalcite (花蕊石, Huaruishi) Japanese Thistle Herb or Root (大蓟, Daji) Common Cephalanoplos Herb (小蓟, Xiaoji) Cape Jasmine Fruit (栀子, Zhizi) Root of Sinkiang Arnebia (紫草, Zicao) India Madder Root (茜草, Qiancao) Garden Burnet Root (地榆, Diyu) Japanese Pagodatree Flower (槐花, Huaihua) Ramie Root (苎麻根, Zhumagen) Charred Human Hair (血余炭, Xueyutan)

2. Blood stasis: Sanchi Root (三七, Sanqi) Frankincense (乳香, Ruxiang) Myrrh (没药, Moyao) Dragon's Blood (血竭, Xuejie) Cattail Pollen (蒲黄, Puhuang) Giant Knotweed Rhizome (虎杖, Huzhang) Charred Human Hair (血余炭, Xueyutan) India Madder Root (茜草, Qiancao) Ophicalcite (花蕊石, Huaruishi) Rhubarb (大黄, Dahuang)

3. Qi failing to control blood: Ginseng (人参, Renshen) Membranous Milkvetch Root (黄芪, Huangqi) Tangshen Root (党参, Dangshen) Largehead Atractylodes Rhizome (白术, Baizhu) Tuckahoe (茯苓, Fuling) Antler Glue (鹿角胶, Lujiaojiao) Longan Aril (龙眼肉, Longyanrou) Argy Wormwood Leaf (艾叶, Aiye) Baked Rhizome (炮姜, Paojiang) Burnt Clay-lining of Kitchen Range (灶心土, Zaoxintu)

4. Traumatic bleeding: Sanchi Root (三七, Sanqi) Puff-ball (马勃, Mabo) Bletilla Rhizome (白及, Baiji) Catechu (儿茶, Ercha) Cuttle Bone (乌贼骨, Wuzeigu) East Asian Tree Fern Rhizome (狗脊, Gouji) Cattail Pollen (蒲黄, Puhuang) Yerbadetajo Herb (墨旱莲, Mohanlian) Densefruit Pittany Root-bark (白鲜皮, Baixianpi) Frankincense (乳香, Ruxiang) Myrrh (没药, Moyao)

Hypochondriac Pain

1. Stagnation of qi: Chinese Thorowax Root (柴胡, Chaihu) Nutgrass Galingale Rhizome (香附, Xiangfu) Bitter Orange (枳壳, Zhiqiao) Immature Bitter Orange (枳实, Zhishi) Green Tangerine Peel (青皮, Qingpi) Tangerine Peel (橘皮, Jupi) Turmeric Root-tuber (郁金, Yujin) Thickleaf Vladimiria Root (青木香, Qingmuxiang) Chinese Eaglewood Wood (沉香, Chenxiang) Sandalwood (檀香, Tanxiang) Combined Spicebush Root

(乌药, Wuyao) Finger Citron Fruit (佛手, Foshou) Wild Mint (薄荷, Bohe) Fiveleaf Akebia Fruit (八月札, Bayuezha) Rugose Rose Flower (玫瑰花, Meiguihua) Plum Flower Bud (绿萼梅, Lvemei) Chinese Buckeye Seed (娑罗子, Suoluozi) Aspongopus (九香虫, Jiuxiangchong) Lychee Seed (荔枝核, Lizhihe) Yanhusuo (延胡索, Yanhusuo) Szechwan chinaberry Fruit (川楝子, Chuanlianzi)

2. Blood stasis: Chinese Angelica Root (当归, Danggui) Red Peony Root (赤芍药, Chishaoyao) Szechwan Lovage Rhizome (川芎, Chuanxiong) Peach Seed (桃仁, Taoren) Safflower (红花, Honghua) Sanchi Root (三七, Sanqi) Dragon's Blood (血竭, Xuejie) Frankincense (乳香, Ruxiang) Myrrh (没药, Moyao) Dan-shen Root (丹参, Danshen) Common Burreed Rhizome (三棱, Sanleng) Zedoray (莪术, Ezhu) Ground Beetle (土鳖虫, Tubiechong) Cattail Pollen (蒲黄, Puhuang) Trogopterus Dung (五灵脂, Wulingzhi) Chinese Thorowax Root (柴胡, Chaihu) Bitter Orange (枳壳, Zhiqiao) Turmeric Rhizome (姜黄, Jianghuang) Turmeric Roottuber (郁金, Yujin) Chinese Honeylocust Spine (皂角刺, Zaojiaoci) Puncturevine Caltrap Fruit (白蒺藜, Baijili) Yanhusuo (延胡索, Yanhusuo) Rosewood (降香, Jiangxiang) Pubescent Holly Root (毛冬青, Maodongqing) Hawthorn Fruit (山楂, Shanzha) Chinese Rose Flower (月季花, Yuejihua) Turtle Carapace (鳖甲, Biejia) Pangolin Scales (穿山甲, Chuanshanjia) Silktree Albiziae Bark (合欢皮, Hehuanpi)

3. Damp-heat in the liver and gallbladder: Chinese Gentian Root (龙胆草, Longdancao) Baikal Skullcap Root (黄芩, Huangqin) Cape Jasmine Fruit (栀子, Zhizi) Common Selfheal Spike (夏枯草, Xiakucao) Capillary Wormwood Herb (茵陈蒿, Yinchenhao) Akebia Stem (木通, Mutong) Oriental Waterplantain Rhizome (泽泻, Zexie) Plantain Seed (车前子, Cheqianzi) Chinese Thorowax Root (柴胡, Chaihu) Szechwan Chinaberry Fruit (川楝子, Chuanlianzi) hepatolith: Christina Loosetrife Herb (金钱草, Jinqiancao) Japanese Climbing Fern Spores (海金沙, Haijinsha) Chicken Gizzard Membrane (鸡内金, Jineijin)

4. Chest pain syndrome: Mongolian Snakeground Pericarp (瓜蒌皮, Gualoupi) Longstament Onion Bulb (薤白, Xiebai) Pinellia Rhizome (半夏, Banxia) Cassia Twig (桂枝, Guizhi) Immature Bitter Orange (枳实, Zhishi) Long Pepper Fruit (荜茇, Biba) Sandalwood (檀香, Tanxiang) Lesser Galangal Rhizome (高良姜, Gaoliangjiang), Musk (麝香, Shexiang) Rosewood (降香, Jiangxiang) Chinese Eaglewood Wood (沉香, Chenxiang) Storesin (苏合香, Suhexiang) combining with blood stasis: Dan-shen Root (丹参, Danshen) Safflower (红花, Honghua) Pubescent Holly Root (毛冬青, Maodongqing) Szechwan Lovage Rhizome (川芎, Chuanxiong) Peach Seed (桃仁, Taoren)

5. Stagnation of toxic heat in the lung: Reed Rhizome (芦根, Lugen) Coix Seed (薏苡仁, Yiyiren) Chinese Waxgourd Seed (冬瓜子, Dongguazi) Peach Seed (桃仁, Taoren) Heartlaef Houttuynia Herb (鱼腥草, Yuxingcao) Baikal Skullcap Root (黄芩, Huangqin) Coptis Rhizome (黄连, Huanglian) Snakegourd Fruit (瓜蒌, Gualou) Honeysuckle Flower (金银花, Jinyinhua) Weeping Forsythia Capsule (连翘, Lianqiao) Cape Jasmine Fruit (栀子, Zhizi)

6. Stagnation of phlegm: Snakegourd Fruit (瓜蒌, Gualou) Pinellia Rhizome (半夏, Banxia) Officinal Magnolia Bark (厚朴,

Houpo) Tangerine Peel (橘皮, Jupi) Cassia Twig (桂枝, Guizhi) White Mustard Seed (白芥子, Baijiezi) Immature Bitter Orange (枳实, Zhishi) Longstament Onion Bulb (薤白, Xiebai)

7. Yang deficiency: Prepared Daughter Root of Common Monkshood (附子, Fuzi) Cassia Twig (桂枝, Guizhi) Longstament Onion Bulb (薤白, Xiebai) Shorthorned Epimedium Herb (淫羊藿, Yinyanghuo)

Vomiting

1. Excess Syndromes

(1) Invasion of exogenous wind, cold and summer wetness: Wrinkled Gianthyssop Herb (藿香, Huoxiang) Perilla Leaf (紫苏, Zisu) Fresh Ginger (生姜, Shengjiang) Pinellia Rhizome (半夏, Banxia) Officinal Magnolia Bark (厚朴, Houpo) Tangerine Peel (橘皮, Jupi) Tuckahoe (茯苓, Fuling) Foutune Eupatorium Herb (佩兰, Peilan) Round Cardamom Seed (白豆蔻, Baidoukou) Villous Amomum Fruit (砂仁, Sharen) Haichow Elsholtzia Herb (香薷, Xiangru)

(2) Retention of food and drink: Medicated Leaven (神曲, Shenqu) Charred Hawthorn Fruit (焦山楂, Jiaoshanzha) Charred Malt (焦麦芽, Jiaomaiya) Rice Germinating Fruit (sprout) (谷芽, Guya) Radish Seed (莱菔子, Laifuzi) Tuckahoe (茯苓, Fuling) Tangerine Peel (橘皮, Jupi) Pinellia Rhizome (半夏, Banxia) Immature Bitter Orange (枳实, Zhishi) Weeping Forsythia Capsule (连翘, Lianqiao)

(3) Accumulation of fluid-retention in the body: Pinellia Rhizome (半夏, Banxia) Fresh Ginger (生姜, Shengjiang) Tuckahoe (茯苓, Fuling) Cassia Twig (桂枝, Guizhi) Large-head Atractylodes Rhizome (白术, Baizhu) Officinal Magnolia Bark (厚朴, Houpo) Tangerine Peel (橘皮, Jupi) Inula Flower (旋覆花, Xuanfuhua)

(4) Adverse rising of stomach-qi: Inula Flower (旋覆花, Xuanfuhua) Hematite (代赭石, Daizheshi) Clove Flower-bud (丁香, Dingxiang) Pinellia Rhizome (半夏, Banxia) Common Perilla Stem (苏梗, Sugeng) Chinese Eaglewood Wood (沉香, Chenxiang) Round Cardamom Seed (白豆蔻, Baidoukou)

(5) Vomiting due to stomach-heat: Coptis Rhizome (黄连, Huanglian) Gypsum (石膏, Shigao) Tangerine Peel (橘皮, Jupi) Pinellia Rhizome (半夏, Banxia) Tuckahoe (茯苓, Fuling) Immature Bitter Orange (枳实, Zhishi) Bamboo Shavings (竹茹, Zhuru) Reed Rhizome (芦根, Lugen) Loquat Leaf (枇杷叶, Pipaye) Lalang Grass Rhizome (白茅根, Baimaogen)

(6) Vomiting due to Qi stagnation: Tangerine Peel (橘皮, Jupi) Perilla Leaf (紫苏, Zisu) Villous Amomum Fruit (砂仁, Sharen) Persimmon Calyx and Receptacle (柿蒂, Shidi) Sandalwood (檀香, Tanxiang) Sword Jackbean Seed (刀豆子, Daodouzi) Chinese Eaglewood Wood (沉香, Chenxiang) Finger Citron Fruit (佛手, Foshou) Medicinal Citron Fruit (香橼, Xiangyuan) Inula Flower (旋覆花, Xuanfuhua) Round Cardamom Seed (白豆蔻, Baidoukou) Katsumada Galangal Seed (草豆蔻, Caodoukou) Common Aucklandia Root (木香, Muxiang)

(7) Vomiting due to cold evil attacking the stomach: Medicinal Evodia Root (吴茱萸, Wuzhuyu) Lesser Galangal Rhizome (高良姜, Gaoliangjiang), Round Cardamom Seed (白豆蔻, Baidoukou) Mountain Spicy Tree Fruit (荜澄茄, Bichengqie) Fennel Fruit (小茴香, Xiaohuixiang) Pinellia Rhizome (半夏, Banxia) Dried Ginger (干姜, Ganjiang) Fresh Ginger (生姜, Shengjiang) Clove Flower-bud (丁香, Dingxiang) Villous Amo-

mum Fruit（砂仁，Sharen）Sandalwood（檀香，Tanxiang）Caoguo（草果，Caoguo）Bunge Pricklyash（花椒，Huajiao）Black Pepper Fruit（胡椒，Hujiao）Chinese Eaglewood Wood（沉香，Chenxiang）Sword Jackbean Seed（刀豆子，Daodouzi）Burnt Clay-lining of Kitchen Range（灶心土，Zaoxintu）

2. Deficiency Syndrome

(1) Vomiting caused by deficiency cold of the stomach: Tangshen Root（党参，Dangshen）Largehead Atractylodes Rhizome（白术，Baizhu）Dried Ginger（干姜，Ganjiang）Pinellia Rhizome（半夏，Banxia）Medicinal Evodia Root（吴茱萸，Wuzhuyu）Round Cardamom Seed（白豆蔻，Baidoukou）Villous Amomum Fruit（砂仁，Sharen）Clove Flower-bud（丁香，Dingxiang）Burnt Clay-lining of Kitchen Range（灶心土，Zaoxintu）

(2) Insufficiency of stomach-yin: Coastal Glehnia Root（北沙参，Beishashen）Dwarf Lilyturf Root（麦门冬，Maimendong）Reed Rhizome（芦根，Lugen）Snakegroud Root（天花粉，Tianhuafen）Dendrobium Herb（石斛，Shihu）Common Anemarrhea Rhizome（知母，Zhimu）Twotooth Achyranthes Root（牛膝，Niuxi）Rice Fruit（粳米，Jingmi）Licorice Root（甘草，Gancao）

Stomachache (Epigastralgia)

1. Stagnation of qi: Szechwan chinaberry Fruit（川楝子，Chuanlianzi）Yanhusuo（延胡索，Yanhusuo）Chinese Thorowax Root（柴胡，Chaihu）Nutgrass Galingale Rhizome（香附，Xiangfu）Common Aucklandia Root（木香，Muxiang）Villous Amomum Fruit（砂仁，Sharen）Green Tangerine Peel（青皮，Qingpi）Tangerine Peel（橘皮，Jupi）Bitter Orange（枳壳，Zhiqiao）Combined Spicebush Root（乌药，Wuyao）Thickleaf Vladimiria Root（青木香，Qingmuxiang）Chinese Nardostachys Root and Rhizome or Spoonleaf Nardostachys Root and Rhizome（甘松，Gansong）Lychee Seed（荔枝核，Lizhihe）Sandalwood（檀香，Tanxiang）Rugose Rose Flower（玫瑰花，Meiguihua）Aspongopus（九香虫，Jiuxiangchong）Plum Flower Bud（绿萼梅，Lvemei）Chinese Buckeye Seed（娑罗子，Suoluozi）Finger Citron Fruit（佛手，Foshou）Medicinal Citron Fruit（香橼，Xiangyuan）

With acid-eructation: Cuttle Bone（乌贼骨，Wuzeigu）Calcined Concha Arcae（煅瓦楞子，Duanwalengzi）Egg-shell（鸡蛋壳，Jidanke）

With indigestion: Chicken Gizzard Membrane（鸡内金，Jineijin）Medicated Leaven（神曲，Shenqu）Charred Hawthorn Fruit（焦山楂，Jiaoshanzha）Charred Malt（焦麦芽，Jiaomaiya）

2. Deficiency of the spleen and stomach: Tangshen Root（党参，Dangshen）Membranous Milkvetch Root（黄芪，Huangqi）Largehead Atractylodes Rhizome（白术，Baizhu）Tuckahoe（茯苓，Fuling）Licorice Root（甘草，Gancao）Chinese Date（大枣，Dazao）Tangerine Peel（橘皮，Jupi）Common Aucklandia Root（木香，Muxiang）Villous Amomum Fruit（砂仁，Sharen）Round Cardamom Seed（白豆蔻，Baidoukou）White Peony Root（白芍药，Baishaoyao）Malt Sugar（饴糖，Yitang）

With deficiency of stomach yin: Coastal Glehnia Root（北沙参，Beishashen）Dwarf Lilyturf Root（麦门冬，Maimendong）Dendrobium Herb（石斛，Shihu）Smoked Plum（乌梅，Wumei）

3. Stomach cold: Lesser Galangal Rhizome（高良姜，Gaoliangjiang），Nutgrass Galingale Rhizome（香附，Xiangfu）Fresh Ginger（生姜，Shengjiang）Dried Ginger（干姜，Gan-

jiang) Medicinal Evodia Root (吴茱萸, Wuzhuyu) Bunge Pricklyash (花椒, Huajiao) Clove Flower-bud (丁香, Dingxiang) Cassia Bark (肉桂, Rougui) Prepared Daughter Root of Common Monkshood (附子, Fuzi) Mountain Spicy Tree Fruit (荜澄茄, Bichengqie) Aspongopus (九香虫, Jiuxiangchong) Round Cardamom Seed (白豆蔻, Baidoukou) Villous Amomum Fruit (砂仁, Sharen) Sandalwood (檀香, Tanxiang) Caoguo (草果, Caoguo) Chinese Nardostachys Root and Rhizome or Spoonleaf Nardostachys Root and Rhizome (甘松, Gansong)

4. Heat in the stomach: Coptis Rhizome (黄连, Huanglian) Gypsum (石膏, Shigao) Chinese Thorowax Root (柴胡, Chaihu) White Peony Root (白芍药, Baishaoyao) Szechwan chinaberry Fruit (川楝子, Chuanlianzi) Immature Bitter Orange (枳实, Zhishi) Cape Jasmine Fruit (栀子, Zhizi) Turmeric Root-tuber (郁金, Yujin) Rhubarb (大黄, Dahuang)

5. Blood stasis (stagnation of blood): Cattail Pollen (蒲黄, Puhuang) Trogopterus Dung (五灵脂, Wulingzhi) Sanchi Root (三七, Sanqi) Dan-shen Root (丹参, Danshen) Chinese Angelica Root (当归, Danggui) White Peony Root (白芍药, Baishaoyao) Frankincense (乳香, Ruxiang) Myrrh (没药, Moyao) Common Burreed Rhizome (三棱, Sanleng) Zedoray (莪术, Ezhu) Yanhusuo (延胡索, Yanhusuo) Szechwan chinaberry Fruit (川楝子, Chuanlianzi)

6. Indigestion: Green Tangerine Peel (青皮, Qingpi) Chicken Gizzard Membrane (鸡内金, Jineijin) Hawthorn Fruit (山楂, Shanzha) Medicated Leaven (神曲, Shenqu) Diverse Wormwood Herb (刘寄奴, Liujinu) Common Burreed Rhizome (三棱, Sanleng) Zedoray (莪术, Ezhu)

Abdominal Pain

1. Abdominal pain caused by stagnation of qi: Chinese Thorowax Root (柴胡, Chaihu) Immature Bitter Orange (枳实, Zhishi) Bitter Orange (枳壳, Zhiqiao) White Peony Root (白芍药, Baishaoyao) Common Aucklandia Root (木香, Muxiang) Areca Seed (槟榔, Binlang) Green Tangerine Peel (青皮, Qingpi) Tangerine Peel (橘皮, Jupi) Nutgrass Galingale Rhizome (香附, Xiangfu) Szechwan chinaberry Fruit (川楝子, Chuanlianzi) Yanhusuo (延胡索, Yanhusuo) Turmeric Root-tuber (郁金, Yujin) Officinal Magnolia Bark (厚朴, Houpo) Round Cardamom Seed (白豆蔻, Baidoukou) Villous Amomum Fruit (砂仁, Sharen) Thickleaf Vladimiria Root (青木香, Qingmuxiang) Combined Spicebush Root (乌药, Wuyao) Sandalwood (檀香, Tanxiang) Chinese Nardostachys Root and Rhizome or Spoonleaf Nardostachys Root and Rhizome (甘松, Gansong) Finger Citron Fruit (佛手, Foshou) Chinese Eaglewood Wood (沉香, Chenxiang)

2. Abdominal pain caused by blood stasis: Chinese Angelica Root (当归, Danggui) Szechwan Lovage Rhizome (川芎, Chuanxiong) Red Peony Root (赤芍药, Chishaoyao) Cattail Pollen (蒲黄, Puhuang) Trogopterus Dung (五灵脂, Wulingzhi) Frankincense (乳香, Ruxiang) Myrrh (没药, Moyao) Peach Seed (桃仁, Taoren) Safflower (红花, Honghua) Dan-shen Root (丹参, Danshen) Sanchi Root (三七, Sanqi) Common Burreed Rhizome (三棱, Sanleng) Zedoray (莪术, Ezhu) Nutgrass Galingale Rhizome (香附, Xiangfu) Hirsute Shiny Bugleweed Herb (泽兰, Zelan) Motherwort Herb (益母草, Yimucao) Rhubarb (大黄, Dahuang) Ground Beetle (土鳖虫, Tubiechong) Leech (水蛭,

Shuizhi) Ark Shell (瓦楞子, Walengzi) Garden Balsam Seed (急性子, Jixingzi) Sinkiang Giantfennal Resin (阿魏, Awei) Musk (麝香, Shexiang) Diverse Wormwood Herb (刘寄奴, Liujinu) Chinese Rose Flower (月季花, Yuejihua) Sappan Wood (苏木, Sumu) Whiteflower Patrinia Herb (败酱草, Baijiangcao) Hawthorn Fruit (山楂, Shanzha) Yanhusuo (延胡索, Yanhusuo)

3. Abdominal pain caused by dystentery due to damp-heat: Coptis Rhizome (黄连, Huanglian) Chinese Corktree Bark (黄柏, Huangbai) White Peony Root (白芍药, Baishaoyao) Chinese Pulsatilla Root (白头翁, Baitouweng) Largeleaf Chinese Ash Bark (秦皮, Qinpi) Common Aucklandia Root (木香, Muxiang) Areca Seed (槟榔, Binlang) Common Andrographis Herb (穿心莲, Chuanxinlian) Hunifuse Euphorbia Herb (地锦草, Dijincao) Copperleaf Herb (铁苋菜, Tiexiangcai) Garlic Bulb (大蒜, Dasuan)

4. Abdominal pain caused by acute appendicitis: Rhubarb (大黄, Dahuang) Mirabilite (芒硝, Mangxiao) Peach Seed (桃仁, Taoren) Chinese Waxgourd Seed (冬瓜子, Dongguazi) Tree Peony Bark (牡丹皮, Mudanpi) Red Peony Root (赤芍药, Chishaoyao) Spreading Hedyotis Herb (白花蛇舌草, Baihuasheshecao) Sargentoglory Vine Stem (红藤, Hongteng) Whiteflower Patrinia Herb (败酱草, Baijiangcao) Honeysuckle Flower (金银花, Jinyinhua) Weeping Forsythia Capsule (连翘, Lianqiao) Dandelion (蒲公英, Pugongying) Radish Seed (莱菔子, Laifuzi) Coix Seed (薏苡仁, Yiyiren)

5. Abdominal pain due to stagnation of food: Medicated Leaven (神曲, Shenqu) Charred Hawthorn Fruit (焦山楂, Jiaoshanzha) Charred Malt (焦麦芽, Jiaomaiya) Chicken Gizzard Membrane (鸡内金, Jineijin) Radish Seed (莱菔子, Laifuzi) Tuckahoe (茯苓, Fuling) Pinellia Rhizome (半夏, Banxia) Tangerine Peel (橘皮, Jupi) Immature Bitter Orange (枳实, Zhishi) Officinal Magnolia Bark (厚朴, Houpo)

6. Abdominal pain due to parasitic infestation: Rangooncreeper Fruit (使君子, Shijunzi) Szechwan Chinaberry Bark (苦楝皮, Kulianpi) Smoked Plum (乌梅, Wumei) Bunge Pricklyash (花椒, Huajiao) Clove Flower-bud (丁香, Dingxiang) Elecampane Inula Root (土木香, Tumuxiang) Luffa Seed (丝瓜子, Siguazi)

Diarrhea

1. Acute diarrhea

(1) Diarrhea caused by cold-damp: Wrinkled Gianthyssop Herb (藿香, Huoxiang) Perilla Leaf (紫苏, Zisu) Largehead Atractylodes Rhizome (白术, Baizhu) Swordlike Atractylodes Rhizome (苍术, Cangzhu) Tuckahoe (茯苓, Fuling) Officinal Magnolia Bark (厚朴, Houpo) Areca Peel (大腹皮, Dafupi) Tangerine Peel (橘皮, Jupi) Baked Rhizome (炮姜, Paojiang) Villous Amomum Fruit (砂仁, Sharen) Caoguo (草果, Caoguo) Katsumada Galangal Seed (草豆蔻, Caodoukou)

(2) Diarrhea caused by damp-heat: Coptis Rhizome (黄连, Huanglian) Baikal Skullcap Root (黄芩, Huangqin) Chinese Corktree Bark (黄柏, Huangbai) Lobed Kudzuvine Root (葛根, Gegen) Chinese Pulsatilla Root (白头翁, Baitouweng) Largeleaf Chinese Ash Bark (秦皮, Qinpi) Hunifuse Euphorbia Herb (地锦草, Dijincao) Copperleaf Herb (铁苋菜, Tiexiangcai) Purslane Herb (马齿苋, Machixian)

(3) Diarrhea caused by improper food: Charred Hawthorn Fruit (焦山楂, Jiaoshanzha) Charred Malt (焦麦芽, Jiao-

maiya) Medicated Leaven (神曲, Shenqu) Radish Seed (莱菔子, Laifuzi) Chicken Gizzard Membrane (鸡内金, Jineijin) Tangerine Peel (橘皮, Jupi) Areca Seed (槟榔, Binlang) Bitter Orange (枳壳, Zhiqiao) Officinal Magnolia Bark (厚朴, Houpo)

(4) Watery diarrhea: Umbellate Pore Fungus (猪苓, Zhuling) Tuckahoe (茯苓, Fuling) Oriental Waterplantain Rhizome (泽泻, Zexie) Largehead Atractylodes Rhizome (白术, Baizhu) Swordlike Atractylodes Rhizome (苍术, Cangzhu) Plantain Seed (车前子, Cheqianzi) Coix Seed (薏苡仁, Yiyiren) Talc (滑石, Huashi)

(5) Diarrhea due to Qi stagnation: Common Aucklandia Root (木香, Muxiang) Areca Seed (槟榔, Binlang)

(6) Diarrhea due to summer dampness: Plantain Seed (车前子, Cheqianzi) Talc (滑石, Huashi) Hyacinth Bean (扁豆, Biandou) Honeysuckle Flower (金银花, Jinyinhua)

(7) Diarrhea due to spleen cold: Medicinal Evodia Root (吴茱萸, Wuzhuyu) Prepared Daughter Root of Common Monkshood (附子, Fuzi) Villous Amomum Fruit (砂仁, Sharen) Dried Ginger (干姜, Ganjiang) Bunge Pricklyash (花椒, Huajiao) Long Pepper Fruit (荜茇, Biba) Lesser Galangal Rhizome (高良姜, Gaoliangjiang), Black Pepper Fruit (胡椒, Hujiao)

2. Chronic Diarrhea

(1) Diarrhea caused by deficiency of the spleen: ①Diarrhea due to deficiency of spleen-qi: Tangshen Root (党参, Dangshen) Membranous Milkvetch Root (黄芪, Huangqi) Largehead Atractylodes Rhizome (白术, Baizhu) Swordlike Atractylodes Rhizome (苍术, Cangzhu) Tuckahoe (茯苓, Fuling) Common Yam Rhizome (山药, Shanyao) Coix Seed (薏苡仁, Yiyiren) Hyacinth Bean (扁豆, Biandou) Hindu Lotus Seed (莲子, Lianzi), Lobed Kudzuvine Root (葛根, Gegen) Gordon Euryale Seed (芡实, Qianshi) Common Aucklandia Root (木香, Muxiang) Shunk Bugbane Rhizome (升麻, Shengma) Argy Wormwood Leaf (艾叶, Aiye) Hairvein Agrimonia Herb (仙鹤草, Xianhecao) ②Diarrhea due to deficiency of spleen - yang: Villous Amomum Fruit (砂仁, Sharen) Sharpleaf Galangal Fruit (益智仁, Yizhiren) Nutmeg Seed (肉豆蔻, Roudoukou) Prepared Daughter Root of Common Monkshood (附子, Fuzi) Cassia Bark (肉桂, Rougui) Dried Ginger (干姜, Ganjiang)

(2) Diarrhea caused by deficiency of both the spleen and kidney: Malaytea Scurfpea Fruit (补骨脂, Buguzhi) Chinese Magnoliavine (五味子, Wuweizi) Medicinal Evodia Root (吴茱萸, Wuzhuyu) Nutmeg Seed (肉豆蔻, Roudoukou) Gordon Euryale Seed (芡实, Qianshi) Sharpleaf Galangal Fruit (益智仁, Yizhiren) Prepared Daughter Root of Common Monkshood (附子, Fuzi) Cassia Bark (肉桂, Rougui)

(3) Diarrhea caused by deficiency of the intestine: Medicine Terminalia Fruit (诃子, Hezi) Nutmeg Seed (肉豆蔻, Roudoukou) Smoked Plum (乌梅, Wumei) Pomegranate Rind Peel (石榴皮, Shiliupi) Chinese Gall (五倍子, Wubeizi) Chinese Magnoliavine (五味子, Wuweizi) Red Halloysite (赤石脂, Chishizhi) Limonite(禹余粮, Yuyuliang)

Jaundice

1. Yang Jaundice: Capillary Wormwood Herb (茵陈蒿, Yinchenhao) Cape Jasmine Fruit (栀子, Zhizi) Rhubarb (大黄, Dahuang) Giant Knotweed Rhizome (虎杖, Huzhang) Chinese Gentian Root (龙胆草, Longdancao) Baikal Skullcap Root (黄芩,

Huangqin) Chinese Corktree Bark (黄柏, Huangbai) Christina Loosetrife Herb (金钱草, Jinqiancao) Indian Bread Pink Epidermis (赤茯苓, Chifuling) Oriental Waterplantain Rhizome (泽泻, Zexie) Asiatic Plantain Herb (车前草, Cheqiancao) Indigowoad Leaf (大青叶, Daqingye) Purslane Herb (马齿苋, Machixian) Common Cephalanoplos Herb (小蓟, Xiaoji) Glutinous Rice Rhizome and Root (糯稻根, Nuodaogen) Tonkin Sophora Root (山豆根, Shandougen) Lightyellow Sophora Root (苦参, Kushen) Manyleaf Meadowrue Rhizome and Root (马尾莲, Maweilian) Figwortflower Picrorhiza Rhizome (胡黄连, Huhuanglian) Turmeric Root-tuber (郁金, Yujin) Largeleaf Gentian Root (秦艽, Qinjiao) Japanese Ardisia Herb (矮地茶, Aidicha) Dandelion (蒲公英, Pugongying) Hunifuse Euphorbia Herb (地锦草, Dijincao) Densefruit Pittany Root-bark (白鲜皮, Baixianpi) Rice Bean (赤小豆, Chixiaodou) Lalang Grass Rhizome (白茅根, Baimaogen)

2. Yin Jaundice: Capillary Wormwood Herb (茵陈蒿, Yinchenhao) Prepared Daughter Root of Common Monkshood (附子, Fuzi) Largehead Atractylodes Rhizome (白术, Baizhu) Dried Ginger (干姜, Ganjiang) Tuckahoe (茯苓, Fuling) Turmeric Rhizome (姜黄, Jianghuang) Turmeric Root-tuber (郁金, Yujin) Mazie Style (玉米须, Yumixu) Cassia Bark (肉桂, Rougui)

Edema

1. Wind attacking the lung: Ephedra (麻黄, Mahuang) Gypsum (石膏, Shigao) Largehead Atractylodes Rhizome (白术, Baizhu) Weeping Forsythia Capsule (连翘, Lianqiao) Rice Bean (赤小豆, Chixiaodou) White Mulberry Root-bark (桑白皮, Sangbaipi) Apricot Seed (杏仁, Xingren) Fresh Ginger (生姜, Shengjiang) Common Ducksmeat Herb (浮萍, Fuping) Pepperweed Seed or Flixweed Tansymustard Seed (葶苈子, Tinglizi) Common Dayflower Herb (鸭跖草, Yazhicao) Fourstamen Stephania Root (汉防己, Hanfangji)

2. Retention of water-damp: Umbellate Pore Fungus (猪苓, Zhuling) Tuckahoe (茯苓, Fuling) Oriental Waterplantain Rhizome (泽泻, Zexie) Swordlike Atractylodes Rhizome (苍术, Cangzhu) Largehead Atractylodes Rhizome (白术, Baizhu) White Mulberry Root-bark (桑白皮, Sangbaipi) Tangerine Peel (橘皮, Jupi) Fresh Ginger Peel (生姜皮, Shengjiangpi) Areca Peel (大腹皮, Dafupi) Peel of Tuckahoe (茯苓皮, Fulingpi) Chinese Waxgourd Exocarp (冬瓜皮, Dongguapi) Fourstamen Stephania Root (汉防己, Hanfangji) Akebia Stem (木通, Mutong) Ricepaperplant Pith (通草, Tongcao) Plantain Seed (车前子, Cheqianzi) Japanese Felt Fern Leaf (石韦, Shiwei) Mazie Style (玉米须, Yumixu) Largehead Atractylodes Rhizome (白术, Baizhu) Chinese Lobelia Herb (半边莲, Banbianlian) Barbed Skullcap Herb (半枝莲, Banzhilian) Infected Foxtail Millet Spike's Bran (糠谷老, Kanggulao)

3. Deficiency of spleen-yang: Membranous Milkvetch Root (黄芪, Huangqi) Tangshen Root (党参, Dangshen) Dried Ginger (干姜, Ganjiang) Largehead Atractylodes Rhizome (白术, Baizhu) Tuckahoe (茯苓, Fuling) Coix Seed (薏苡仁, Yiyiren) Chinese Date (大枣, Dazao) Caoguo (草果, Caoguo) Officinal Magnolia Bark (厚朴, Houpo) Common Aucklandia Root (木香, Muxiang)

4. Deficiency of kidney-yang: Prepared Daughter Root of Common Monkshood (附子, Fuzi) Cassia Bark (肉桂, Rougui) Malaytea Scurfpea Fruit (补骨脂, Buguzhi)

Common Fenugreek Seed (胡芦巴, Huluba) Chinese Magnoliavine (五味子, Wuweizi) Umbellate Pore Fungus (猪苓, Zhuling) Tuckahoe (茯苓, Fuling) Largehead Atractylodes Rhizome (白术, Baizhu) Oriental Waterplantain Rhizome (泽泻, Zexie) Plantain Seed (车前子, Cheqianzi) Twotooth Achyranthes Root (牛膝, Niuxi) Sea Horse (海马, Haima) Pipefish (海龙, Hailong)

Constipation

1. Excess Syndromes

(1) Constipation of heat type: Rhubarb (大黄, Dahuang) Mirabilite (芒硝, Mangxiao) Anhydrous Sodium Sulfate (玄明粉, Xuanmingfen) Immature Bitter Orange (枳实, Zhishi) Senna Leaf (番泻叶, Fanxieye) Aloes (芦荟, Luhui) Cassia Seed (决明子, Juemingzi) Coffee Senna Stem and Leaf (望江南, Wangjiangnan) Japanese Dock Root (羊蹄, Yangti)

(2) Constipation due to disorder of qi: Common Aucklandia Root (木香, Muxiang) Areca Seed (槟榔, Binlang) Immature Bitter Orange (枳实, Zhishi) Officinal Magnolia Bark (厚朴, Houpo) Combined Spicebush Root (乌药, Wuyao) Chinese Eaglewood Wood (沉香, Chenxiang)

2. Deficiency syndromes

(1) Constipation caused by deficiency of qi: Membranous Milkvetch Root (黄芪, Huangqi) Tangshen Root (党参, Dangshen) Largehead Atractylodes Rhizome (白术, Baizhu) Tuckahoe (茯苓, Fuling) Honey (蜂蜜, Fengmi) Chinese Thorowax Root (柴胡, Chaihu)

(2) Constipation caused by dryness of the intestine due to blood deficiency: Chinese Angelica Root (当归, Danggui) Tuber Fleeceflower Root (何首乌, Heshouwu) Prepared Rhizome of Adhesive Rehmannia (熟地黄, Shoudihuang) Siberian Solomonseal Rhizome (黄精, Huangjing) Figwort Root (玄参, Xuanshen) Dwarf Lilyturf Root (麦门冬, Maimendong) Hemp Seed (火麻仁, Huomaren) Bushcherry Seed (郁李仁, Yuliren) Mulberry Solomonseal (桑椹, Sangshen) Oriental Sesame Seed (黑芝麻, Heizhima) Peach Seed (桃仁, Taoren) 松子仁, Chinese Arborvitae Seed (柏子仁, Baiziren) Mongolian Snakegourd Seed (瓜蒌仁, Gualouren) Fig Receptacle (无花果, Wuhuaguo) Honey (蜂蜜, Fengmi)

(3) Constipation due to deficiency of yang: Songaria Cynomorium Herb (锁阳, Suoyang) Desertliving Cistanche (肉苁蓉, Roucongrong) Twotooth Achyranthes Root (牛膝, Niuxi) English Walnut (核桃肉, Hetaorou)

Lumbago

1. Lumbago due to cold-damp: Dried Ginger (干姜, Ganjiang) Swordlike Atractylodes Rhizome (苍术, Cangzhu) Tuckahoe (茯苓, Fuling) Doubleteeth Pulbescent Angelica Root (独活, Duhuo) Manchurian Wildginger Herb (细辛, Xixin) Cassia Twig (桂枝, Guizhi) Common Monksood (乌头, Wutou) Eucommia Bark (杜仲, Duzhong) Twotooth Achyranthes Root (牛膝, Niuxi) Chinese Taxillus Twig (桑寄生, Sangjisheng) Himalayan Teasel Root (续断, Xuduan)

2. Lumbago due to damp-heat: Chinese Corktree Bark (黄柏, Huangbai) Swordlike Atractylodes Rhizome (苍术, Cangzhu) Twotooth Achyranthes Root (牛膝, Niuxi) Coix Seed (薏苡仁, Yiyiren) Fourstamen Stephania Root (防己, Fangji) Sevenlobed Yam Rhizome (萆薢, Bixie)

3. Lumbago due to deficiency of the kidney: Prepared Rhizome of Adhesive Rehman-

nia（熟地黄，Shoudihuang）Common Yam Rhizome（山药，Shanyao）Asiatic Cornelian Cherry Fruit（山茱萸，Shanzhuyu）Barbary Wolfberry Fruit（枸杞子，Gouqizi）Dodder Seed（菟丝子，Tusizi）Eucommia Bark（杜仲，Duzhong）Malaytea Scurfpea Fruit（补骨脂，Buguzhi）English Walnut（核桃肉，Hetaorou）Chinese Taxillus Twig（桑寄生，Sangjisheng）East Asian Tree Fern Rhizome（狗脊，Gouji）Himalayan Teasel Root（续断，Xuduan）Nutgrass Galingale Rhizome（香附，Xiangfu）Cassia Bark（肉桂，Rougui）Prepared Daughter Root of Common Monkshood（附子，Fuzi）Antler Glue（鹿角胶，Lujiaojiao）Tortoise's Shell and Plastron Glue（龟版胶，Guibanjiao）Tuber Onion Seed（韭子，Jiuzi）Twotooth Achyranthes Root（牛膝，Niuxi）

4．Lumbago due to blood stasis：Chinese Angelica Root（当归，Danggui）Szechwan Lovage Rhizome（川芎，Chuanxiong）Peach Seed（桃仁，Taoren）Safflower（红花，Honghua）Myrrh（没药，Moyao）Yanhusuo（延胡索，Yanhusuo）Trogopterus Dung（五灵脂，Wulingzhi）Ground Beetle（土鳖虫，Tubiechong）Nutgrass Galingale Rhizome（香附，Xiangfu）Largeleaf Gentian Root（秦艽，Qinjiao）Twotooth Achyranthes Root（牛膝，Niuxi）

Arthralgia Syndrome

1．Dominance of pathogenic wind（mignatory arthralgia）：Incised Notopterygium Rhizome and Root（羌活，Qianghuo）Doubleteeth Pulbescent Angelica Root（独活，Duhuo）Cassia Twig（桂枝，Guizhi）Ephedra（麻黄，Mahuang）Divaricate Saposhnikovia Root（防风，Fangfeng）Manchurian Wildginger Herb（细辛，Xixin）Dahurian Angelica Root（白芷，Baizhi）Chinese Clematis Root（威灵仙，Weilingxian）Chinese Arborvitae Leafy Twig（侧柏叶，Cebaiye）Giant Knotweed Rhizome（虎杖，Huzhang）Wooly Dutchmanspipe Leaf（寻骨风，Xungufeng）Silkworm with Batrytis Larva（白僵蚕，Baijiangcan）Kadsura Pepper Stem（海风藤，Haifengteng）

2．Dominance of pathogenic cold（arthralgia aggravated）：Common Monksood（乌头，Wutou）Prepared Daughter Root of Common Monkshood（附子，Fuzi）Nut-vomitive Poisonnut Seed（马钱子，Maqianzi）Cassia Bark（肉桂，Rougui）Ephedra（麻黄，Mahuang）Cassia Twig（桂枝，Guizhi）Manchurian Wildginger Herb（细辛，Xixin）Chinese Clematis Root（威灵仙，Weilingxian）Turmeric Rhizome（姜黄，Jianghuang）Obscured Homalamena Rhizome（千年健，Qiannianjian）Stem of Chinese Photinial（石楠藤，Shinanteng）

3．Dominance of pathogenic damp（arthralgra chrefly caused by damp）：Coix Seed（薏苡仁，Yiyiren）Swordlike Atractylodes Rhizome（苍术，Cangzhu）Common Floweringquince Fruit（木瓜，Mugua）Siberian Cocklebur Fruit（苍耳子，Cangerzi）Fourstamen Stephania Root（防己，Fangji）Doubleteeth Pulbescent Angelica Root（独活，Duhuo）Cortex Acanthopanacis Radicis（五加皮，Wujiapi）Harleguin Glorybower Leaf（臭梧桐，Chouwutong）Obscured Homalamena Rhizome（千年健，Qiannianjian）

4．Dominance of pathogenic heat（arthralgra chiefly cuased by heat）：Gypsum（石膏，Shigao）Common Anemarrhea Rhizome（知母，Zhimu）Fourstamen Stephania Root（防己，Fangji）Largeleaf Gentian Root（秦艽，Qinjiao）Common St. Paulswort Herb（豨莶草，Xixiancao）Chinese Starjasmine Stem（络石藤，Luoshiteng）Honeysuckle Stem（忍冬

藤, Rendongteng) Mulberry Twig (桑枝, Sangzhi) Dan-shen Root (丹参, Danshen)

5. Arthralgia due to insufficiency of kidney-yin: Chinese Taxillus Twig (桑寄生, Sangjisheng) Himalayan Teasel Root (续断, Xuduan) Eucommia Bark (杜仲, Duzhong) Suberect Spatholobus Stem (鸡血藤, Jixueteng) Twotooth Achyranthes Root (牛膝, Niuxi) Cortex Acanthopanacis Radicis (五加皮, Wujiapi) East Asian Tree Fern Rhizome (狗脊, Gouji) Chinese Angelica Root (当归, Danggui) White Peony Root (白芍药, Baishaoyao) Szechwan Lovage Rhizome (川芎, Chuanxiong) Prepared Rhizome of Adhesive Rehmannia (熟地黄, Shoudihuang) Tangshen Root (党参, Dangshen) Largehead Atractylodes Rhizome (白术, Baizhu) Tuckahoe (茯苓, Fuling) Siberian Solomonseal Rhizome (黄精, Huangjing) Tall Gastrodia Rhizome (天麻, Tianma) Chinese Photinia Leaf (石楠叶, Shinanye)

Eye-diseases

1. Wind-heat: Mulberry Leaf (桑叶, Sangye) Wild Mint (薄荷, Bohe) Chrysanthemum Flower (菊花, Juhua) Common Scouring Rush Herb (木贼, Muzei) Red Peony Root (赤芍药, Chishaoyao) Tokyo Violet Herb (紫花地丁, Zihuadiding) Largeleaf Chinese Ash Bark (秦皮, Qinpi) Cassia Seed (决明子, Juemingzi) Puncturevine Caltrop Fruit (刺蒺藜, Cijili) Abalone Shell (石决明, Shijueming) Shrub Chastetree Fruit (蔓荆子, Manjingzi) Cicada Slough (蝉蜕, Chantui)

2. Liver-heat: Chrysanthemum Flower (菊花, Juhua) Mulberry Leaf (桑叶, Sangye) Common Selfheal Spike (夏枯草, Xiakucao) Pale Butterflybush Flower (密蒙花, Mimenghua) Feather Cockscomb Seed (青葙子, Qingxiangzi) Red Peony Root (赤芍药, Chishaoyao) Tokyo Violet Herb (紫花地丁, Zihuadiding) Largeleaf Chinese Ash Bark (秦皮, Qinpi) Cassia Seed (决明子, Juemingzi) Antelope Horn (羚羊角, Lingyangjiao) Nacre (珍珠母, Zhenzhumu) Pearl (珍珠, Zhenzhu) Arabic Cowry Shell (紫贝齿, Zibeichi), Plantain Seed (车前子, Cheqianzi) Wormwoodlike Motherwort Seed (茺蔚子, Chongweizi) Chalcanthnium (胆矾, Danfan) Bear Gall (熊胆, Xiongdan) Rhubarb (大黄, Dahuang) Mirabilite (芒硝, Mangxiao) Silkworm with Batrytis Larva (白僵蚕, Baijiangcan)

3. Blurred vision due to Liver-yin deficiency: Flatstem Milkvetch Seed (沙苑子, Shayuanzi) Dodder Seed (菟丝子, Tusizi) Dendrobium Herb (石斛, Shihu) Barbary Wolfberry Fruit (枸杞子, Gouqizi) Mulberry Solomonseal (桑椹, Sangshen) Glossy Privet Fruit (女贞子, Nuzhenzi) Oriental Sesame Seed (黑芝麻, Heizhima)

4. Eye nebula: Cicada Slough (蝉蜕, Chantui) Snake Slough (蛇蜕, Shetui) Pearl (珍珠, Zhenzhu) Borax (硼砂, Pengsha) Calamine (炉甘石, Luganshi) Abalone Shell (石决明, Shijueming) Juice of Pig Bladder (猪胆汁, Zhudanzhi)

Thirsty

1. Wind-heat: Reed Rhizome (芦根, Lugen) Lobed Kudzuvine Root (葛根, Gegen)

2. Heat in the stomach: Gypsum (石膏, Shigao) Common Anemarrhea Rhizome (知母, Zhimu)

3. Impairment of body fluids: Dendrobium Herb (石斛, Shihu) Fragrant Solomonseal Rhizome (玉竹, Yuzhu) Snakegroud Root (天花粉, Tianhuafen) Rehmannia Dried Root (生地黄, Shengdihuang) Figwort Root (玄

参, Xuanshen) Dwarf Lilyturf Root (麦门冬, Maimendong) Coastal Glehnia Root, and Fourleaf Ladybell Root (沙参, Shashen) Reed Rhizome (芦根, Lugen)

4. Water retention: Pinellia Rhizome (半夏, Banxia) Tuckahoe (茯苓, Fuling)

Bitter taste in the mouth: Chinese Gentian Root (龙胆草, Longdancao) Capillary Wormwood Herb (茵陈蒿, Yinchenhao); Sweet taste in the mouth: Tuckahoe (茯苓, Fuling) Foutune Eupatorium Herb (佩兰, Peilan)

Toothache

1. Stomach-heat: Gypsum (石膏, Shigao) Shunk Bugbane Rhizome (升麻, Shengma) Coptis Rhizome (黄连, Huanglian) Rhubarb (大黄, Dahuang) Bamboo leaf (竹叶, Zhuye) Dahurian Angelica Root (白芷, Baizhi)

2. Kidney-deficiency: Fortune's Drynaria Rhizome, Baron's Drynaria Rhizome (骨碎补, Gusuibu) Manchurian Wildginger Herb (细辛, Xixin) Twotooth Achyranthes Root (牛膝, Niuxi)

3. Cold-wind: Dahurian Angelica Root (白芷, Baizhi) Chinese Ligusticum Rhizome (藁本, Gaoben) Manchurian Wildginger Herb (细辛, Xixin) Long Pepper Fruit (荜茇, Biba)

Pulmonary abscess

Reed Stem (苇茎, Weijing) Heartlaef Houttuynia Herb (鱼腥草, Yuxingcao) Common Selfheal Spike (夏枯草, Xiakucao) Balloonflower Root (桔梗, Jiegeng) Coix Seed (薏苡仁, Yiyiren) Chinese Waxgourd Seed (冬瓜子, Dongguazi) Dandelion (蒲公英, Pugongying) Common Andrographis Herb (穿心莲, Chuanxinlian) Common Buckwheat Seed (荞麦, Qiaomai) Whiteflower Patrinia Herb (败酱草, Baijiangcao) Peach Seed (桃仁, Taoren) Honeysuckle Flower (金银花, Jinyinhua)

Hernia pain

Combined Spicebush Root (乌药, Wuyao) Fennel Fruit (小茴香, Xiaohuixiang) Medicinal Evodia Root (吴茱萸, Wuzhuyu) Tangerine Seed (橘核, Juhe) Lychee Seed (荔枝核, Lizhihe) Green Tangerine Peel (青皮, Qingpi) Szechwan chinaberry Fruit (川楝子, Chuanlianzi) Cassia Bark (肉桂, Rougui) Chinese Eaglewood Wood (沉香, Chenxiang)

Hiccup

Persimmon Calyx and Receptacle (柿蒂, Shidi) Sword Jackbean Seed (刀豆子, Daodouzi) Clove Flower-bud (丁香, Dingxiang) Chinese Eaglewood Wood (沉香, Chenxiang) Hematite (代赭石, Daizheshi) Inula Flower (旋覆花, Xuanfuhua) Mountain Spicy Tree Fruit (荜澄茄, Bichengqie)

Dysentery

1. Dysentery of heat-dampness type: Chinese Corktree Bark (黄柏, Huangbai) Coptis Rhizome (黄连, Huanglian) Baikal Skullcap Root (黄芩, Huangqin) Lightyellow Sophora Root (苦参, Kushen) Largeleaf Chinese Ash Bark (秦皮, Qinpi) Purslane Herb (马齿苋, Machixian) Chinese Pulsatilla Root (白头翁, Baitouweng) Common Andrographis Herb (穿心莲, Chuanxinlian) Honeysuckle Flower (金银花, Jinyinhua) Rhubarb (大黄, Dahuang) Hairvein Agrimonia Herb (仙鹤草, Xianhecao)

2. Dysentery of cold-dampness type: Swordlike Atractylodes Rhizome (苍术, Cangzhu) Officinal Magnolia Bark (厚朴, Houpo) Common Aucklandia Root (木香,

Muxiang) Baked Rhizome (炮姜, Paojiang) Cassia Bark (肉桂, Rougui)

Prolapse of anus

Chinese Thorowax Root (柴胡, Chaihu) Shunk Bugbane Rhizome (升麻, Shengma) Membranous Milkvetch Root (黄芪, Huangqi) Immature Bitter Orange (枳实, Zhishi) Bitter Orange (枳壳, Zhiqiao) Balloonflower Root (桔梗, Jiegeng) Lobed Kudzuvine Root (葛根, Gegen) Alumen (白矾, Baifan) Chinese Gall (五倍子, Wubeizi)

Diabetes

1. Diabetes involving the upper-jiao: Snakegroud Root (天花粉, Tianhuafen) Chinese Magnoliavine (五味子, Wuweizi) Ginseng (人参, Renshen) Dwarf Lilyturf Root (麦门冬, Maimendong)

2. Diabetes involving the middle-jiao: Lobed Kudzuvine Root (葛根, Gegen) Dendrobium Herb (石斛, Shihu) Siberian Solomonseal Rhizome (黄精, Huangjing) Snakegroud Root (天花粉, Tianhuafen) Gypsum (石膏, Shigao) Common Anemarrhea Rhizome (知母, Zhimu)

3. Diabetes involving the lower-jiao: Prepared Rhizome of Adhesive Rehmannia (熟地黄, Shoudihuang) Asiatic Cornelian Cherry Fruit (山茱萸, Shanzhuyu) Chinese Magnoliavine (五味子, Wuweizi) Common Anemarrhea Rhizome (知母, Zhimu)

Malarial disease

Chinese Thorowax Root (柴胡, Chaihu) Antifebrile Dichroa Root (常山, Changshan) Sweet Wormwood (青蒿, Qinghao) Caoguo (草果, Caoguo) Areca Seed (槟榔, Binlang) European Verbena Herb (马鞭草, Mabiancao) Baikal Skullcap Root (黄芩, Huangqin) Tuber Fleeceflower Root (何首乌, Heshouwu) Cinnabar (朱砂, Zhusha) Hairvein Agrimonia Herb (仙鹤草, Xianhecao) Realgar (雄黄, Xionghuang) Arsenolite Ore (砒石, Pishi) Minium (铅丹, Qiandan) Japanese Buttercup Herb (毛茛, Maogen)

Rash

1. Rash due to heat in the blood: Rehmannia Dried Root (生地黄, Shengdihuang) Asiatic Rhinoceros Horn (犀角, Xijiao) Figwort Root (玄参, Xuanshen) Red Peony Root (赤芍药, Chishaoyao) Tree Peony Bark (牡丹皮, Mudanpi) Indigowoad Leaf (大青叶, Daqingye) Saffron Crocus Stigma (藏红花, Zanghonghua) Root of Sinkiang Arnebia (紫草, Zicao) Natural Indigo (青黛, Qingdai)

2. Measles: Lobed Kudzuvine Root (葛根, Gegen) Shunk Bugbane Rhizome (升麻, Shengma) Wild Mint (薄荷, Bohe) Great Burdock Achene (牛蒡子, Niubangzi) Fineleaf Schizomepeta Herb (荆芥, Jingjie) Root of Sinkiang Arnebia (紫草, Zicao) Chinese Tamarish Twig (西河柳, Xiheliu) Cicada Slough (蝉蜕, Chantui) Common Ducksmeat Herb (浮萍, Fuping) Haichow Elsholtzia Herb (香薷, Xiangru)

3. Rubella: Divaricate Saposhnikovia Root (防风, Fangfeng) Lightyellow Sophora Root (苦参, Kushen) Fineleaf Schizomepeta Herb (荆芥, Jingjie) Cicada Slough (蝉蜕, Chantui) Belvedere Fruit (地肤子, Difuzi) Common Cnidium Fruit (蛇床子, Shechuangzi) Chinese Trumpetcreeper Flower (凌霄花, Lingxiaohua) Dahurian Angelica Root (白芷, Baizhi) Puncturevine Caltrop Fruit (刺蒺藜, Cijili)

4. Eczema: Baikal Skullcap Root (黄芩, Huangqin) Common Andrographis Herb (穿心莲, Chuanxinlian) Densefruit Pittany Root-

bark（白鲜皮，Baixianpi）Paniculate Swallowwort Root（徐长卿，Xuchangqing）Oriental Variegated Coralbean Bark（海桐皮，Haitongpi）Silkworm Feculae（蚕砂，Cansha）Wrinkled Gianthyssop Herb（藿香，Huoxiang）Ricepaperplant Pith（通草，Tongcao）Garden Burnet Root（地榆，Diyu）Dragon's Bone（龙骨，Longgu）Cuttle Bone（乌贼骨，Wuzeigu）Nacre（珍珠母，Zhenzhumu）Sulfur（硫黄，Liuhuang）Alumen（明矾，Mingfan）Common Cnidium Fruit（蛇床子，Shechuangzi）Colophony（松香，Songxiang）Calamine（炉甘石，Luganshi）Lightyellow Sophora Root（苦参，Kushen）

Scabies and tinea

Croton Seed（巴豆，Badou）Lilac Daphne Flower-bud（芫花，Yuanhua）Fortune Euphorbin Seed（千金子，Qianjinzi）Oriental Variegated Coralbean Bark（海桐皮，Haitongpi）Japanese Dock Root（羊蹄，Yangti）Bigfruit Elm Fruit（芜荑，Wuyi）Chinese Trumpetcreeper Flower（凌霄花，Lingxiaohua）Common Cnidium Fruit（蛇床子，Shechuangzi）Colophony（松香，Songxiang）Garlic Bulb（大蒜，Dasuan）Melanterite（皂矾，Zaofan）Alumen（明矾，Mingfan）Magnetite（磁石，Cishi）Realgar（雄黄，Xionghuang）Sulfur（硫黄，Liuhuang）Szechwan chinaberry Fruit（川楝子，Chuanlianzi）Paniculate Swallowwort Root（徐长卿，Xuchangqing）Arsenolite Ore（砒石，Pishi）Large Blister Beetle（斑蝥，Banmao）Aloes（芦荟，Luhui）Camphor（樟脑，Zhangnao）

Scrofula and goiter

Pangolin Scales（穿山甲，Chuanshanjia）Common Selfheal Spike（夏枯草，Xiakucao）Chinese Rose Flower（月季花，Yuejihua）Chinese Trumpetcreeper Flower（凌霄花，Lingxiaohua）Giant Typhonium Rhizome（白附子，Baifuzi）Pumice（海浮石，Haifushi）Clam Shell（海蛤壳，Haigeqiao）Airpotato Yam Tuber（黄药子，Huangyaozi）Silkworm with Batrytis Larva（白僵蚕，Baijiangcan）Vasps Nest（露蜂房，Lufengfang）Ark Shell（瓦楞子，Walengzi）Musk（麝香，Shexiang）Large Blister Beetle（斑蝥，Banmao）Arsenolite Ore（砒石，Pishi）Thunberg Fritillary Bulb（浙贝母，Zhebeimu）Pinellia Rhizome（半夏，Banxia）Peking Euphorbia Root（大戟，Daji）Weeping Forsythia Capsule（连翘，Lianqiao）Figwort Root（玄参，Xuanshen）Realgar（雄黄，Xionghuang）Sulfur（硫黄，Liuhuang）Oyster Shell（牡蛎，Muli）Kelp（昆布，Kunbu），Seaweed（海藻，Haizao）Gecko（守宫，Shougong）Scorpion（全蝎，Quanxie）Centipede（蜈蚣，Wugong）Catclaw Buttercup Root（猫爪草，Maozhuacao）

Traumatic injury

Tree Peony Bark（牡丹皮，Mudanpi）Red Peony Root（赤芍药，Chishaoyao）Sargentoglory Vine Stem（红藤，Hongteng）Rhubarb（大黄，Dahuang）Chinese Pine Node（松节，Songjie）Sanchi Root（三七，Sanqi）Szechwan Lovage Rhizome（川芎，Chuanxiong）Frankincense（乳香，Ruxiang）Myrrh（没药，Moyao）Giant Knotweed Rhizome（虎杖，Huzhang）Peach Seed（桃仁，Taoren）Safflower（红花，Honghua）Twotooth Achyranthes Root（牛膝，Niuxi）Ground Beetle（䗪虫，Zhechong）Leech（水蛭，Shuizhi）Gadfly（虻虫，Mengchong）Rosewood（降香，Jiangxiang）Hirsute Shiny Bugleweed Herb（泽兰，Zelan）Sappan Wood（苏木，Sumu）Musk（麝香，Shexiang）Himalayan Teasel Root（续断，Xuduan）Chinese Angelica Root（当归，Danggui）Dragon's Blood（血竭，Xuejie）Camphor（樟脑，

Zhangnao) Nut-vomitive Poisonnut Seed (马钱子, Maqianzi) Silktree Albiziae Bark (合欢皮, Hehuanpi) Datura Flower (洋金花, Yangjinhua) Japanese Ardisia Herb (矮地茶, Aidicha) Diverse Wormwood Herb (刘寄奴, Liujinu) Pyrite (自然铜, Zirantong) Motherwort Herb (益母草, Yimucao) Kadsura Pepper Stem (海风藤, Haifengteng) Wooly Dutchmanspipe Leaf (寻骨风, Xungufeng) Paniculate Swallowwort Root (徐长卿, Xuchangqing) Cottonrose Hibiscus Leaf (木芙蓉叶, Mufurongye)

Dysmenorrhea

1. Qi-stagnation: Chinese Thorowax Root (柴胡, Chaihu) Nutgrass Galingale Rhizome (香附, Xiangfu) Combined Spicebush Root (乌药, Wuyao) Wild Mint (薄荷, Bohe) Szechwan chinaberry Fruit (川楝子, Chuanlianzi) Turmeric Root-tuber (郁金, Yujin) Lychee Seed (荔枝核, Lizhihe)

2. Blood-stagnation: Szechwan Lovage Rhizome (川芎, Chuanxiong) Dan-shen Root (丹参, Danshen) Motherwort Herb (益母草, Yimucao) Peach Seed (桃仁, Taoren) Safflower (红花, Honghua) Chinese Angelica Root (当归, Danggui) Trogopterus Dung (五灵脂, Wulingzhi) Cattail Pollen (蒲黄, Puhuang) Frankincense (乳香, Ruxiang) Myrrh (没药, Moyao) Cowherb Seed (王不留行, Wangbuliuxing) Sappan Wood (苏木, Sumu) Chinese Rose Flower (月季花, Yuejihua) Hirsute Shiny Bugleweed Herb (泽兰, Zelan) Red Peony Root (赤芍药, Chishaoyao) Twotooth Achyranthes Root (牛膝, Niuxi) Common Burreed Rhizome (三棱, Sanleng) Zedoray (莪术, Ezhu) Cassia Twig (桂枝, Guizhi) Hawthorn Fruit (山楂, Shanzha) Lilac Pink Herb (瞿麦, Qumai) Yanhusuo (延胡索, Yanhusuo) Turmeric Root-tuber (郁金, Yujin) Turmeric Rhizome (姜黄, Jianghuang) Giant Knotweed Rhizome (虎杖, Huzhang) Suberect Spatholobus Stem (鸡血藤, Jixueteng) Pangolin Scales (穿山甲, Chuanshanjia) 䗪 Ground Beetle (䗪虫, Zhechong) Leech (水蛭, Shuizhi) India Madder Root (茜草, Qiancao) Agkistrodon Acutus (白花蛇, Baihuashe) Chinese Trumpetcreeper Flower (凌霄花, Lingxiaohua) Diverse Wormwood Herb (刘寄奴, Liujinu) Tree Peony Bark (牡丹皮, Mudanpi) Japanese Ardisia Herb (矮地茶, Aidicha) Amber (琥珀, Hupo) Musk (麝香, Shexiang) Dragon's Blood (血竭, Xuejie) Sargentoglory Vine Stem (红藤, Hongteng) Fortune Euphorbin Seed (千金子, Qianjinzi)

3. Cold-dampness: Cassia Bark (肉桂, Rougui) Cassia Twig (桂枝, Guizhi) Medicinal Evodia Root (吴茱萸, Wuzhuyu) Argy Wormwood Leaf (艾叶, Aiye) Baked Rhizome (炮姜, Paojiang) Combined Spicebush Root (乌药, Wuyao)

Threatened abortion

1. Qi-deficiency: Ginseng (人参, Renshen) Membranous Milkvetch Root (黄芪, Huangqi) Largehead Atractylodes Rhizome (白术, Baizhu)

2. Blood-deficiency: Chinese Angelica Root (当归, Danggui) White Peony Root (白芍药, Baishaoyao) Prepared Rhizome of Adhesive Rehmannia (熟地黄, Shoudihuang) Asshide Glue (阿胶, Ejiao)

3. Kidney-deficiency: Chinese Taxillus Twig (桑寄生, Sangjisheng) Himalayan Teasel Root (续断, Xuduan) Eucommia Bark (杜仲, Duzhong) Dodder Seed (菟丝子, Tusizi)

4. Heat in the blood: Baikal Skullcap Root (黄芩, Huangqin) Ramie Root (苎麻根, Zhumagen)

5. Qi stagnation: Villous Amomum Fruit

(砂仁, Sharen) Common Perilla Stem (苏梗, Sugeng)

Galactostasis

Pangolin Scales (穿山甲, Chuanshanjia) Cowherb Seed (王不留行, Wangbuliuxing) Uniflower Swisscentaury Root (漏芦, Loulu) Beautiful Sweetgum Fruit (路路通, Lulutong) Akebia Stem (木通, Mutong) Ricepaperplant Pith (通草, Tongcao) Cluster Mallow Seed (冬葵子, Dongkuizi) Towel Gourd Vegetable Sponge (丝瓜络, Sigualuo) Puncturevine Caltrop Fruit (刺蒺藜, Cijili) Pig Feet (猪蹄, Zhuti)

Leukorrhea

1. Heat-dampness: Chinese Corktree Bark (黄柏, Huangbai) Lightyellow Sophora Root (苦参, Kushen) Oriental Waterplantain Rhizome (泽泻, Zexie) Coptis Rhizome (黄连, Huanglian)

2. Cold of deficiency type: Ginkgo Seed (白果, Baiguo) Argy Wormwood Leaf (艾叶, Aiye) East Asian Tree Fern Rhizome (狗脊, Gouji) Hairy Antler (鹿茸, Lurong)

3. Cold-dampness: Dahurian Angelica Root (白芷, Baizhi) Swordlike Atractylodes Rhizome (苍术, Cangzhu) Largehead Atractylodes Rhizome (白术, Baizhu) Argy Wormwood Leaf (艾叶, Aiye) Cuttle Bone (乌贼骨, Wuzeigu)

4. Kidney deficiency: Dragon's Bone (龙骨, Longgu) Oyster Shell (牡蛎, Muli) Dodder Seed (菟丝子, Tusizi) Flatstem Milkvetch Seed (沙苑子, Shayuanzi) Tuber Onion Seed (韭子, Jiuzi) Pomegranate Rind Peel (石榴皮, Shiliupi) Lotus Seed (莲子, Lianzi) Gordon Euryale Seed (芡实, Qianshi) Cherokee Rose Fruit (金樱子, Jinyingzi) Mantis Egg - case (桑螵蛸, Sangpiaoxiao) Cuttle Bone (乌贼骨, Wuzeigu)

Reference Ⅳ Clinical Application of Chinese Drugs Based on Differentiation of Zangfu Organs

Heart

1. Insufficiency of Heart-qi: pale complexion, palpitation and short of breath, pale tongue, tiredness and lack of strength, corpalent and tender tongue, whitish tongue coating with deficient pulse. It is advisable to invigorate the Heart-qi.

Ginseng (人参, Renshen) Membranous Milkvetch Root (黄芪, Huangqi) Tangshen Root (党参, Dangshen) Tuckahoe (茯苓, Fuling) Chinese Magnoliavine (五味子, Wuweizi) Licorice Root (甘草, Gancao) Heterophylla Falsestarwort Root (太子参, Taizishen) Chinese Date (大枣, Dazao)

2. Deficiency of Heart-yang: coldness of the body with chills, pale complexion, suffocation in the chest, shortness of breath and palpitation, frequent spontaneous perspiration, pale or dark-purple tongue, thready and weak pulse or irregularly knotted intermittent pulse, dripping sweat in severe case, extreme cold of the four limbs, cyanotic lips, shallow breathing, faint pulse being about to disappear. It is advisable to warm the heart-yang.

Cassia Twig (桂枝, Guizhi) Cassia Bark

(肉桂, Rougui) Prepared Daughter Root of Common Monkshood (附子, Fuzi) Longstament Onion Bulb (薤白, Xiebai) Dried Ginger (干姜, Ganjiang) Chinese Date (大枣, Dazao)

3. Deficiency of Heart-blood: Lusterless complexion, dizziness and blurred vision, palpitation and being susceptible to fright. Forgetfulness and insomnia; pale tongue and lips, thready and weak pulse. It is advisable to invigorate the heart-blood.

Chinese Angelica Root (当归, Danggui) Dan-shen Root (丹参, Danshen) White Peony Root (白芍药, Baishaoyao) Suberect Spatholobus Stem (鸡血藤, Jixueteng) Longan Aril (龙眼肉, Longyanrou) Dried Human Placenta (紫河车, Ziheche) Prepared Rhizome of Adhesive Rehmannia (熟地黄, Shoudihuang) Tuber Fleeceflower Root (何首乌, Heshouwu) Ass-hide Glue (阿胶, Ejiao)

4. Deficiency of heart-yin: palpitation and restlessness, dysphoria with feverish sensation in the chest, palms and soles, low fever and night sweating, dry mouth, forgetfulness and insomnia, thready and rapid pulse. It is advisable to tonify the heart-yin.

Rehmannia Dried Root (生地黄, Shengdihuang) Dwarf Lilyturf Root (麦门冬, Maimendong) Fragrant Solomonseal Rhizome (玉竹, Yuzhu) Ass-hide Glue (阿胶, Ejiao) Lily Bulb (百合, Baihe) Chinese Magnoliavine (五味子, Wuweizi) Spine Date Seed (酸枣仁, Suanzaoren) American Ginseng Root (西洋参, Xiyangshen) Tortoise's Shell and Plastron (龟版, Guiban)

5. Restlessness of heart-mind: Deficiency of both heart-blood and heart-yin may lead to loss of nourishment of heart-mind, it may be manifested as insomnia, forgetfulness, easily awaking etc. Besides the drugs (used) for reinforcing heart blood and heart-yin, those used for nourishing the heart and tranquilizing the mind can also be prescribed in the treatment.

Nourishing the heart and tranquilizing: Spine Date Seed (酸枣仁, Suanzaoren) Tuber Fleeceflower Stem (何首乌藤, Heshouwuteng) Thinleaf Milkwort Root (远志, Yuanzhi) Silktree Albiziae Bark (合欢皮, Hehuanpi) Silktree Albizia Immature Flower (合欢花, Hehuanhua) Dwarf Lilyturf Root (麦门冬, Maimendong)

Calming the heart and tranquilizing: Amber (琥珀, Hupo) Cinnabar (朱砂, Zhusha) Dragon's Bone (龙骨, Longgu) Dragon's Teeth (龙齿, Longchi) Nacre (珍珠母, Zhenzhumu), Magnetite (磁石, Cishi) Iron Scales (生铁落, Shengtieluo) Oyster Shell (牡蛎, Muli)

6. Excessive fire in the heart: restless and hot feeling in the epigastrium, irritability and insomnia, thirst, erosion of mucous membrane of the oral cavity and the tongue, red tip of the tongue or reddish tongue, rapid pulse. It is advisable to clear away the heart-fire.

Buffalo Horn (水牛角, Shuiniujiao) Cowbezoar (牛黄, Niuhuang) Coptis Rhizome (黄连, Huanglian) Manyleaf Meadowrue Rhizome and Root (马尾莲, Maweilian) Cape Jasmine Fruit (栀子, Zhizi) Hindu Lotus Plumule (莲子心, Lianzixin) Lily Bulb (百合, Baihe) Bamboo leaf (竹叶, Zhuye) Akebia Stem (木通, Mutong) Weeping Forsythia Capsule (连翘, Lianqiao) Rehmannia Dried Root (生地黄, Shengdihuang) Tree Peony Bark (牡丹皮, Mudanpi)

7. Phlegm blocking the orifice of the heart: mental derangement, unconsciousness or dull looking and expression, talking to oneself, ab-

normal behavior, deep, stringy and slippery pulse, white and greasy tongue coating, sudden fall with loss of consciousness in severe case, wheezing due to retention of sputum in the throat. It is advisable to induce resuscitation and resolve phlegm.

Musk (麝香, Shexiang) Artificial Musk (人工麝香, Shexiang) Storesin (苏合香, Suhexiang) Cow-bezoar (牛黄, Niuhuang) Borneol (冰片, Bingpian) Toad Skin Secretion Cake (蟾酥, Chansu) Grassleaf Sweetflag Rhizome (石菖蒲, Shichangpu) Thinleaf Milkwort Root (远志, Yuanzhi) Turmeric Root-tuber (郁金, Yujin) Manchurian Wildginger Herb (细辛, Xixin) Chinese Honeylocust Spine (猪牙皂, Zhuyazhao) Bamboo Juice (竹沥, Zhuli) Chlorite-schist (礞石, Mengshi)

8. Stagnation of heart-blood: palpitation, stabbing and suffocating pain in the pericardial region, radiating to the medial part of the left arm, in the way of coming and going. In the severe case, there may appear cyamotic face, lips and fingers, extreme cold of the limbs, dark red of the tongue, or with purple colored spot, thin tongue coating, faint, thready or hesitant pulse. It is advisable to promote blood circulation to remove blood stasis, and regulate qi to relieve pain.

Dan-shen Root (丹参, Danshen) Peach Seed (桃仁, Taoren) Safflower (红花, Honghua) Szechwan Lovage Rhizome (川芎, Chuanxiong) Sanchi Root (三七, Sanqi) Red Peony Root (赤芍药, Chishaoyao) Turmeric Root-tuber (郁金, Yujin) Pubescent Holly Root (毛冬青, Maodongqing) Ginkgo Seed (白果, Baiguo) Long Pepper Fruit (荜茇, Biba) Sandalwood (檀香, Tanxiang) Rosewood (降香, Jiangxiang) Chinese Eaglewood Wood (沉香, Chenxiang) Clove Flower-bud (丁香, Dingxiang) Frankincense (乳香, Ruxiang) Artificial Musk (人工麝香, Shexiang) Storesin (苏合香, Suhexiang)

Small Intestine

1. Deficiency-cold of small intestine: Pain in the lower abdomen, distention and borborygums in the abdomen, relieved by pressure, or pain due to hernia, white tongue coating and weak pulse. It is advisable to warm the cold of small intestine.

Nutmeg Seed (肉豆蔻, Roudoukou) Combined Spicebush Root (乌药, Wuyao) Cassia Bark (肉桂, Rougui) Fennel Fruit (小茴香, Xiaohuixiang) Tangerine Seed (橘核, Juhe) Green Tangerine Peel (青皮, Qingpi) Medicinal Evodia Root (吴茱萸, Wuzhuyu)

2. Excess-heat of small intestine: excess-fire of the heart transferring heat to the small intestine, irritability and heat over the chest, frequent urine leading to pain, erosion and pain of the mouth and tongue. It is advisable to clear away heat of the small intestine.

Akebia Stem (木通, Mutong) Bamboo leaf (竹叶, Zhuye) Common Cephalanoplos Herb (小蓟, Xiaoji) Oriental Waterplantain Rhizome (泽泻, Zexie) Lalang Grass Rhizome (白茅根, Baimaogen) Rehmannia Dried Root (生地黄, Shengdihuang) Indian Bread Pink Epidermis (赤茯苓, Chifuling) Umbellate Pore Fungus (猪苓, Zhuling) Common Rush Stem Pith (灯芯, Dengxin) Talc (滑石, Huashi) Mazie Style (玉米须, Yumixu) Rice Bean (赤小豆, Chixiaodou) Lightyellow Sophora Root (苦参, Kushen) Japanese Thistle Herb or Root (大蓟, Daji)

Liver

1. Deficiency of Liver-yin: headache and dizziness, dull pain in the hypochrondrium,

tinnitus and insomnia, feverish sensation of the chest, palms and soles, dry mouth and throat, night sweating, reddish tongue with thin coating, stringy, thready or rapid pulse. It is advisable to nourish liver-yin.

Asiatic Cornelian Cherry Fruit (山茱萸, Shanzhuyu) Barbary Wolfberry Fruit (枸杞子, Gouqizi) Glossy Privet Fruit (女贞子, Nuzhenzi) Yerbadetajo Herb (墨旱莲, Mohanlian) White Peony Root (白芍药, Baishaoyao) Rehmannia Dried Root (生地黄, Shengdihuang) Prepared Rhizome of Adhesive Rehmannia (熟地黄, Shoudihuang) Flatstem Milkvetch Seed (沙苑子, Shayuanzi) Tortoise's Shell and Plastron (龟版, Guiban) Turtle Carapace (鳖甲, Biejia) Tuber Fleeceflower Root (何首乌, Heshouwu)

2. Deficiency of liver-blood: Dizziness and headache, numbness or trembling of the four limbs, insomnia, dryness and uneasy feeling of the eyes, small amount of menses of amenorrhea, yellow complexion, pale tongue and lips, deep and thready pulse. It is advisable to reinforce and tonify liver-blood.

Chinese Angelica Root (当归, Danggui) White Peony Root (白芍药, Baishaoyao) Tuber Fleeceflower Root (何首乌, Heshouwu) Ass-hide Glue (阿胶, Ejiao) Suberect Spatholobus Stem (鸡血藤, Jixueteng) Barbary Wolfberry Fruit (枸杞子, Gouqizi) Common Floweringquince Fruit (木瓜, Mugua) Twotooth Achyranthes Root (牛膝, Niuxi) Prepared Rhizome of Adhesive Rehmannia (熟地黄, Shoudihuang) Szechwan Lovage Rhizome (川芎, Chuanxiong) Mulberry Solomonseal (桑椹, Sangshen)

3. Stagnation of liver-qi: distending pain over the hypochondrium, oppressive feeling in the chest, mental depression, anorexia, dizziness and blurred vision, stringy pulse, white and slippery tongue coating, irregular menstruation, dysmenorrhea, or distending feeling of the breaths before the menses. It is advisable to disperse the stagnated liver-qi to relieve the stagnation of qi.

Chinese Thorowax Root (柴胡, Chaihu) Nutgrass Galingale Rhizome (香附, Xiangfu) Turmeric Root-tuber (郁金, Yujin) Szechwan chinaberry Fruit (川楝子, Chuanlianzi) Yanhusuo (延胡索, Yanhusuo) Common Aucklandia Root (木香, Muxiang) Green Tangerine Peel (青皮, Qingpi) Bitter Orange (枳壳, Zhiqiao) Tangerine Leaf (橘叶, Jvye) Finger Citron Fruit (佛手, Foshou), Plum Flower Bud (绿萼梅, Lvemei) Rugose Rose Flower (玫瑰花, Meiguihua) Puncturevine Caltrap Fruit (白蒺藜, Baijili) Wild Mint (薄荷, Bohe)

4. Hyperactivity of liver-yang: headache, distending feeling of the head, vertigo with intermittent mild and severe ease, tinnitus and deafness of the ear, dry mouth and throat, dryness and uneasy feeling of the eyes, insomnia and forgetfulness, numbness and trembling of the limbs, reddish tongue with scanty body fluid, stringy and strong pulse It is advisable to nourish yin, suppress the hyperactive liver and subside yang.

Drugs for nourishing yin: Rehmannia Dried Root (生地黄, Shengdihuang) Prepared Rhizome of Adhesive Rehmannia (熟地黄, Shoudihuang) Asiatic Cornelian Cherry Fruit (山茱萸, Shanzhuyu) Barbary Wolfberry Fruit (枸杞子, Gouqizi) Glossy Privet Fruit (女贞子, Nuzhenzi) Yerbadetajo Herb (墨旱莲, Mohanlian) Turtle Carapace (鳖甲, Biejia)

Drugs for suppressing the hyperactive liver: Tall Gastrodia Rhizome (天麻, Tianma) Gambirplant Hooked Stem and Branch (钩藤,

Gouteng) Chrysanthemum Flower (菊花, Juhua) Puncturevine Caltrap Fruit (白蒺藜, Baijili) Cassia Seed (决明子, Juemingzi)

Drugs for subsiding yang: Nacre (珍珠母, Zhenzhumu) Abalone Shell (石决明, Shijueming) Dragon's Bone (龙骨, Longgu) Oyster Shell (牡蛎, Muli) Magnetite (磁石, Cishi) Hematite (代赭石, Daizheshi) Twotooth Achyranthes Root (牛膝, Niuxi)

5. Flaming up of liver-fire: headache and dizziness, tinnitus and deafness of the ear, flushed face with red ears, bitter taste in the mouth, yellowish urine, red tongue with yellowish coating, stringy and rapid pulse, hemoptysis hematemesis and epistaxis in severe case. It is advisable to clear away liver-fire.

Mulberry Leaf (桑叶, Sangye) Chrysanthemum Flower (菊花, Juhua) Cassia Seed (决明子, Juemingzi) Chinese Gentian Root (龙胆草, Longdancao) Cape Jasmine Fruit (栀子, Zhizi) Tree Peony Bark (牡丹皮, Mudanpi) Common Selfheal Spike (夏枯草, Xiakucao) Natural Indigo (青黛, Qingdai) Rhubarb (大黄, Dahuang) Capillary Wormwood Herb (茵陈蒿, Yinchenhao) Antelope Horn (羚羊角, Lingyangjiao)

6. Damp-heat in the liver and gallbladder: fullness and oppressive feeling in the hypochondrium, jaundice, scanty dark urine, or yellowish and turbid urine, or yellowish leukorrhea with fishy odour, itch of vulva, or swelling pain and redness of tastis, yellowish and greasy tongue coating, stringy and rapid pulse. It is advisable to clear away damp-heat from the liver and gallbladder.

Chinese Gentian Root (龙胆草, Longdancao) Baikal Skullcap Root (黄芩, Huangqin) Cape Jasmine Fruit (栀子, Zhizi) Capillary Wormwood Herb (茵陈蒿, Yinchenhao) Akebia Stem (木通, Mutong) Oriental Waterplantain Rhizome (泽泻, Zexie) Asiatic Plantain Herb (车前草, Cheqiancao) Chinese Thorowax Root (柴胡, Chaihu) Christina Loosetrife Herb (金钱草, Jinqiancao)

7. Liver-wind stirring-up internally: dizziness, numbness, spasm, and trembling of the limbs trembling of the tongue, red tongue without coating, stringy pulse. Liver-yang changing into liver-mind may lead to sudden fall with loss of consciousness, stiff tongue, difficult speech, and hemiplegia. Extreme heat causing wind syndrome may lead to convulsion due to high fever and unconsciousness. Wind syndrome due to blood deficiency may lead to yellowish complexion, blurred vision, and spasm of hands and feet. It is advisable to suppress the hyperactive-liver to relieve the wind syndrome, reinforce and tonify liver blood.

Drugs for suppressing the hyperactive liver to relieve the wind syndrome: Tall Gastrodia Rhizome (天麻, Tianma) Gambirplant Hooked Stem and Branch (钩藤, Gouteng) White Peony Root (白芍药, Baishaoyao) Antelope Horn (羚羊角, Lingyangjiao) Goat Horn (山羊角, Shanyangjiao) Centipede (蜈蚣, Wugong) Scorpion (全蝎, Quanxie) Earth Worm (地龙, Dilong) Silkworm with Batrytis Larva (白僵蚕, Baijiangcan) Cicada Slough (蝉蜕, Chantui) Jackinthepulpit Tuber (天南星, Tiannanxing) Puncturevine Caltrap Fruit (白蒺藜, Baijili)

补养肝血: Chinese Angelica Root (当归, Danggui) Tuber Fleeceflower Root (何首乌, Heshouwu) White Peony Root (白芍药, Baishaoyao) Prepared Rhizome of Adhesive Rehmannia (熟地黄, Shoudihuang) Ass-hide Glue (阿胶, Ejiao) Suberect Spatholobus Stem (鸡血藤, Jixueteng) Barbary Wolfberry

Fruit (枸杞子, Gouqizi) Oriental Sesame Seed (黑芝麻, Heizhima)

8. Cold stagnating the liver meridian: distending pain in the lower abdomen radiating to the testis, or distension of teitis, or contraction of scratum, moist tongue with white coating, deep and stringy pulse It is advisable to warm the liver to disperse cold.

Medicinal Evodia Root (吴茱萸, Wuzhuyu) Cassia Bark (肉桂, Rougui) Fennel Fruit (小茴香, Xiaohuixiang) Combined Spicebush Root (乌药, Wuyao) Shorthorned Epimedium Herb (淫羊藿, Yinyanghuo) Desertliving Cistanche (肉苁蓉, Roucongrong) Bunge Pricklyash (花椒, Huajiao) Tangerine Seed (橘核, Juhe) Lychee Seed (荔枝核, Lizhihe) Asiatic Cornelian Cherry Fruit (山茱萸, Shanzhuyu) Medicinal Indian-mulberry Root (巴戟天, Bajitian) Flatstem Milkvetch Seed (潼蒺藜, Tongjili)

Gallbladder

The liver and gallbladder are interiorly and exteriorly related. Similar symptoms can be found if liver and gallbladder diseases occur. However, these symptoms are mainly caused by liver disorder, which should be treated at first in the treatment. Liver disorder is mainly manifested as jaundice, hypochondriac pain, intermittent cold and heat, bitter taste in the mouth, vomiting bitter fluid, etc.

Chinese Thorowax Root (柴胡, Chaihu) Baikal Skullcap Root (黄芩, Huangqin) White Peony Root (白芍药, Baishaoyao) Weeping Forsythia Capsule (连翘, Lianqiao) Chinese Gentian Root (龙胆草, Longdancao) Capillary Wormwood Herb (茵陈蒿, Yinchenhao) Cape Jasmine Fruit (栀子, Zhizi) Christina Loosetrife Herb (金钱草, Jinqiancao) Common Selfheal Spike (夏枯草, Xiakucao) Rhubarb (大黄, Dahuang) Szechwan chinaberry Fruit (川楝子, Chuanlianzi)

Spleen

1. Deficiency of spleen-qi: Deficiency of spleen-qi refers to dyfunction of the spleen, sinking due to spleen deficiency and failure of spleen to control circulating blood.

(1) Dysfunction of the spleen: decreased amount of food taken distending feel after meal, watery stool, or edema of the limbs, difficulty in urination, accompanied with fatigue and weakness, short ness of breath and unwillingness of speech, yellowish complexion. Pale and tender tongue with white coating, moderate and weak pulse. It is advisable to invigorate the spleen and benefit qi and promote digestion.

Tangshen Root (党参, Dangshen) Largehead Atractylodes Rhizome (白术, Baizhu) Tuckahoe (茯苓, Fuling) Common Yam Rhizome (山药, Shanyao) Coix Seed (薏苡仁, Yiyiren) Hyacinth Bean (扁豆, Biandou) Common Aucklandia Root (木香, Muxiang) Villous Amomum Fruit (砂仁, Sharen) Pinellia Rhizome (半夏, Banxia) Tangerine Peel (橘皮, Jupi) Chicken Gizzard Membrane (鸡内金, Jineijin) Charred Medicated Leaven (焦神曲, Jiaoshenqu) Charred Hawthorn Fruit (焦山楂, Jiaoshanzha) Charred Malt (焦麦芽, Jiaomaiya)

(2) Sinking of qi due to spleen deficiency: Prolapse of uterus, prolapse of the rectum, gastroptosia, chronic diarrhea, decreased amount of food taken, distending feeling after meal, falling sensation in the lower abdomen, lassitude, shortness of breath and unwillingness of speech, yellowish complesion, pale tongue with white coating, faint pulse. It is advisable to invigorate the spleen and benefit

qi，reinforce qi and ascend spleen-qi.

Membranous Milkvetch Root（黄芪，Huangqi）Tangshen Root（党参，Dangshen）Heterophylla Falsestarwort Root（太子参，Taizishen）Largehead Atractylodes Rhizome（白术，Baizhu）Tangerine Peel（橘皮，Jupi）Shunk Bugbane Rhizome（升麻，Shengma）Chinese Thorowax Root（柴胡，Chaihu）Lobed Kudzuvine Root（葛根，Gegen）Immature Bitter Orange（枳实，Zhishi）

（3）Failure of spleen to control circulating blood：pale or yellowish complexion，decreased amount of food taken，lassitude，shortness of breath，bleeding of skin bloody stoot，profuse menstruation in women or metrorrhagia and metrostaxis，pale tongue，thready and weak pulse. It is advisable to arrest bleeding by invigorateing the spleen and conduct blood to the meridian(s).

Chinese Date（大枣，Dazao）Common Aucklandia Root（木香，Muxiang）Cuttle Bone（乌贼骨，Wuzeigu）Hairvein Agrimonia Herb（仙鹤草，Xianhecao）Yerbadetajo Herb（墨旱莲，Mohanlian）Burnt Clay-lining of Kitchen Range（灶心土，Zaoxintu）Argy Wormwood Leaf（艾叶，Aiye）Hindu Lotus Rhizome-node（藕节，Oujie）Baked Rhizome（炮姜，Paojiang）

2. Deficiency of spleen-yang：decreased amount of food taken，shortness of breath and unwillingness of speech，coldness of the body with chills，lassitude，pale complexion，cold pain in the abdomen，fallness of the abdomen，relieved by warmth，diarrhea or diarrhea with undigested food. It is advisable to warm the spleen-yang.

Prepared Daughter Root of Common Monkshood（附子，Fuzi）Dried Ginger（干姜，Ganjiang）Medicinal Evodia Root（吴茱萸，Wuzhuyu）Nutmeg Seed（肉豆蔻，Roudoukou）Villous Amomum Fruit（砂仁，Sharen）Round Cardamom Seed（白豆蔻，Baidoukou）Sharpleaf Galangal Fruit（益智仁，Yizhiren）

3. Cold-damp disturbing the spleen：distension and fullness in the abdomen，heaviness sensation over the head and body，decreased amount of food taken，nausea and Vomiting，without thirst，loose stool，difficulty in urination，leukorrhea，white and greasy or thick tongue coating，slow，moderate and soft pulse. It is advisable to warm the spleen and remove dampness.

Wrinkled Gianthyssop Herb（藿香，Huoxiang）Foutune Eupatorium Herb（佩兰，Peilan）Swordlike Atractylodes Rhizome（苍术，Cangzhu）Officinal Magnolia Bark（厚朴，Houpo）Pinellia Rhizome（半夏，Banxia）Coix Seed（薏苡仁，Yiyiren）Tuckahoe（茯苓，Fuling）Katsumada Galangal Seed（草豆蔻，Caodoukou）Largehead Atractylodes Rhizome（白术，Baizhu）Dried Ginger（干姜，Ganjiang）

4. Damp-heat in the spleen and stomach：sallow complexion like an orange，distension and fullness in the abdomen，anorexia，aversion to oily food，nausea and Vomiting，fatigue and heaviness sensation of the body，fever，bitter taste in the mouth，scanty and yellowish urine，yellow and greasy tongue coating，soft and rapid pulse It is advisable to dear away and remove damp-heat.

Capillary Wormwood Herb（茵陈蒿，Yinchenhao）Chinese Thorowax Root（柴胡，Chaihu）Chinese Gentian Root（龙胆草，Longdancao）Chinese Corktree Bark（黄柏，Huangbai）Cape Jasmine Fruit（栀子，Zhizi）Rhubarb（大黄，Dahuang）Umbellate Pore Fungus（猪苓，Zhuling）Indian Bread Pink Epidermis（赤茯苓，Chifuling）Oriental Waterplantain Rhizome（泽泻，Zexie）Coix Seed（薏苡仁，Yiyiren）Asiatic Plantain Herb（车前草，Cheqiancao）Ricepaperplant Pith（通草，Tongcao）

Stomach

1. Cold in the stomach: Stomachache，(epigastralgia) lingering pain in mild case and bad pain in severe case，with intermittent onset，aggravated by cold and relieved by warmth，Vomiting，watery fluid，white and slippery tongue coating，deep and slow or deep and stringy pulse. It is advisable to warm the stomach and remove cold.

Lesser Galangal Rhizome（高良姜，Gaoliangjiang），Long Pepper Fruit（荜茇，Biba）Spiked Gingerlily Rhizome（土良姜，Tuliangjiang）Fresh Ginger（生姜，Shengjiang）Medicinal Evodia Root（吴茱萸，Wuzhuyu）Round Cardamom Seed（白豆蔻，Baidoukou）Clove Flower-bud（丁香，Dingxiang）Cassia Bark（肉桂，Rougui）Dried Ginger（干姜，Ganjiang）Malt Sugar（饴糖，Yitang）Cassia Twig（桂枝，Guizhi）

2. Heat in the stomach: burning heat and pain in the stomach，thirsty with excessive drinks or thirsty with cold drink，rapid digestion of food and polyorexia，swelling and pain in the gams foul breath，acid regurgitation，red tongue with yellow coating，slippery and rapid pulse. It is advisable to clear away stomach-fire.

Gypsum（石膏，Shigao）Common Anemarrhea Rhizome（知母，Zhimu）Coptis Rhizome（黄连，Huanglian）Baikal Skullcap Root（黄芩，Huangqin）Cape Jasmine Fruit（栀子，Zhizi）Reed Rhizome（芦根，Lugen）Indigowoad Leaf（大青叶，Daqingye）Snakegroud Root（天花粉，Tianhuafen）Lalang Grass Rhizome（白茅根，Baimaogen）Loquat Leaf（枇杷叶，Pipaye）

3. Retention of food in the stomach: distension and fullness in the stomach，Vomiting indigested food with sour and fetid odour，eructation and acid regurgitation，anorexia，diarrhea or constipation，thick and greasy tongue coating，slippery pulse. It is advisable to promote digestion and remove stagnated food.

Charred Medicated Leaven（焦神曲，Jiaoshenqu）Charred Hawthorn Fruit（焦山楂，Jiaoshanzha）Charred Malt（焦麦芽，Jiaomaiya）Chicken Gizzard Membrane（鸡内金，Jineijin）Radish Seed（莱菔子，Laifuzi）Areca Seed（槟榔，Binlang）Tea Leaf-bud（茶叶，Chaye）Rhubarb（大黄，Dahuang）Officinal Magnolia Bark（厚朴，Houpo）Papaya Fruit（番木瓜，Fanmugua）

4. Adverse rising of the stomach-qi: nausea and Vomiting，hiccup and belching，poor appetite，distention and oppressed feeling in the stomach and abdomen，or Vomiting after meal: Inula Flower（旋覆花，Xuanfuhua）Hematite（代赭石，Daizheshi）Common Perilla Stem（苏梗，Sugeng）Tangerine Peel（橘皮，Jupi）Pinellia Rhizome（半夏，Banxia）Fresh Ginger（生姜，Shengjiang）Loquat Leaf（枇杷叶，Pipaye）Bamboo Shavings（竹茹，Zhuru）Clove Flower-bud（丁香，Dingxiang）Persimmon Calyx and Receptacle（柿蒂，Shidi）Chinese Eaglewood Wood（沉香，Chenxiang）Officinal Magnolia Bark（厚朴，Houpo）

5. Deficiency of stomach-yin: dry mouth and throat，aggravated after sleep，anorexia，irritability，low fever，difficulty in passing stool，nausea without Vomiting，red tongue with little or without coating，thready and rapid pulse. It is advisable to nourish stomach-yin.

Dendrobium Herb（石斛，Shihu）

Snakegroud Root（天花粉，Tianhuafen）Coastal Glehnia Root（北沙参，Beishashen）Dwarf Lilyturf Root（麦门冬，Maimendong）White Peony Root（白芍药，Baishaoyao）Reed Rhizome（芦根，Lugen）Siberian Solomonseal Rhizome（黄精，Huangjing）Fragrant Solomonseal Rhizome（玉竹，Yuzhu）Smoked Plum（乌梅，Wumei）

Lung

1. Deficiency of lung-qi: faint cough with dyspnea, shortness of breath and unwillingness of speech, feeble voice, dyspnea aggravated by strength, lassitude, spontaneous perspiration, pale complexion, pale and tender tongue, faint pulse. It is advisable to reinforce lung-qi.

Ginseng（人参，Renshen）Tangshen Root（党参，Dangshen）Membranous Milkvetch Root（黄芪，Huangqi）Common Yam Rhizome（山药，Shanyao）Licorice Root（甘草，Gancao）Largehead Atractylodes Rhizome（白术，Baizhu）Chinese Caterpillar Fungus（冬虫夏草，Dongchongxiacao）

For failure of lung-qi to astring: Ginkgo Seed（白果，Baiguo）Chinese Magnoliavine（五味子，Wuweizi）English Walnut（核桃肉，Hetaorou）Medicine Terminalia Fruit（诃子，Hezi）Smoked Plum（乌梅，Wumei）Opium Poppy Pericarp（罂粟壳，Yingsuqiao）

2. Deficiency of lung-yin: severe cough, dry cough with phlegm or sticky sputum, dry and itch feeling of the throat, hoarse, emaciated physique, red tongue with little body fluid, thready and weak plse. In case of hyperactivity of fire caused by deficiency of yin: cough with bloody sputum, dry thirst with willingness for drinks, low fever in the afternoon, night sweating, flushed checks, red tongue, thready and rapid pulse. It is advisable to nourish lung-yin or adding drugs for arresting bleeding.

Drugs for nourishing lung-yin: Coastal Glehnia Root（北沙参，Beishashen）Dwarf Lilyturf Root（麦门冬，Maimendong）Cochinchinese Asparagus Root（天门冬，Tianmendong）Ass-hide Glue（阿胶，Ejiao）Dendrobium Herb（石斛，Shihu）Snakegroud Root（天花粉，Tianhuafen）Lily Bulb（百合，Baihe）Sessile Stemona Root（百部，Baibu）Fragrant Solomonseal Rhizome（玉竹，Yuzhu）Siberian Solomonseal Rhizome（黄精，Huangjing）

To stop bleeding in the lung: Bletilla Rhizome（白及，Baiji）Sanchi Root（三七，Sanqi）Ass-hide Glue（阿胶，Ejiao）Hairvein Agrimonia Herb（仙鹤草，Xianhecao）Taiwan Beautybetter Leaf（紫珠，Zizhu）Hindu Lotus Rhizome-node（藕节，Oujie）Tatarian Aster Root（紫苑，Ziyuan）Baikal Skullcap Root（黄芩，Huangqin）

3. Wind-cold tightening the lung: cough or dyspnea, whitish and clear sputum with foam, without desire for drinks, accompanied by watery nasal, discharge or fever and aveision to cold, headache, general acheass, white and thin tongue coating, floating or stringy and tense pulse. It is advisable to disperse lung-qi and dredge athe nasal passage, dispel cold and resolve phlegm.

Drugs for dispersing lung-qi: Apricot Seed（杏仁，Xingren）Balloonflower Root（桔梗，Jiegeng）Whiteflower hogfenel Root（前胡，Qianhu），Sessile Stemona Root（百部，Baibu）Ephedra（麻黄，Mahuang）

Drugs for dredging the nasal passage: Siberian Cocklebur Fruit（苍耳子，Cangerzi）Biond Magnolia Flower-bud（辛夷，Xinyi）Dahurian Angelica Root（白芷，Baizhi）Small Centipeda Herb（鹅不食草，Ebushicao）

Manchurian Wildginger Herb (细辛, Xixin)

Drugs for dispelling cold: Ephedra (麻黄, Mahuang) Manchurian Wildginger Herb (细辛, Xixin) Fresh Ginger (生姜, Shengjiang) Common Perilla Leaf (苏叶, Suye) Cassia Twig (桂枝, Guizhi)

Drugs for resolving phlegm and arresting cough: Pinellia Rhizome (半夏, Banxia) Inula Flower (旋覆花, Xuanfuhua) Radish Seed (莱菔子, Laifuzi) White Mustard Seed (白芥子, Baijiezi) Jackinthepulpit Tuber (天南星, Tiannanxing) Giant Typhonium Rhizome (白附子, Baifuzi) Tatarian Aster Root (紫苑, Ziyuan) Common Coltsfoot Flower (款冬花, Kuandonghua)

4. Wind-heat invading the lung: Cough with yellowish and thick sputum, difficulty in spitting, sputum with blood and pus in severe case, usually accompanied by sorethroat, turbid nasal discharge, thirst with desie for drinks, red tip of the tongue, floating and rapid pulse. It is advisable to clear away Lung-heat and resolve phlegm-heat.

Drugs for clearing away lung-heat: Baikal Skullcap Root (黄芩, Huangqin) Blackberrylily Rhizome (射干, Shegan) Common Anemarrhea Rhizome (知母, Zhimu) Cape Jasmine Fruit (栀子, Zhizi) Mongolian Snakeground Pericarp (瓜蒌皮, Gualoupi) Chinese Wolfberry Root-bark (地骨皮, Digupi) White Mulberry Root-bark (桑白皮, Sangbaipi) Reed Rhizome (芦根, Lugen) Lalang Grass Rhizome (白茅根, Baimaogen)

Drugs for clear away phlegm-heat: Thunberg Fritillary Bulb (浙贝母, Zhebeimu) Arisaema with Bile (胆南星, Dannanxing) Bamboo Juice (竹沥, Zhuli) Clam Shell (海蛤壳, Haigeqiao) Pumice (海浮石, Haifushi) Snakegourd Fruit (瓜蒌, Gualou) Loquat Leaf (枇杷叶, Pipaye) Tabasheer (天竺黄, Tianzhuhuang)

Dispelling wind and removing heat: Mulberry Leaf (桑叶, Sangye) Wild Mint (薄荷, Bohe) Reed Rhizome (芦根, Lugen) Cicada Slough (蝉蜕, Chantui) Fineleaf Schizomepeta Herb (荆芥, Jingjie) Divaricate Saposhnikovia Root (防风, Fangfeng) Honeysuckle Flower (金银花, Jinyinhua) Weeping Forsythia Capsule (连翘, Lianqiao) White-flower hogfenel Root (前胡, Qianhu)

5. Turbid phlegm obstructing in the lung: Cough with profuse sputum, whitish and sticky, easy to spit, dyspnea leading to oppressive feeling in the chest, nausea, white and greasy tongue coating, slippery pulse. It is advisable to remove dampness and resolve phlegm.

Pinellia Rhizome (半夏, Banxia) Tangerine Peel (橘皮, Jupi) Tuckahoe (茯苓, Fuling) Swordlike Atractylodes Rhizome (苍术, Cangzhu) Largehead Atractylodes Rhizome (白术, Baizhu) Caoguo (草果, Caoguo) White Mustard Seed (白芥子, Baijiezi) Perilla Seed (苏子, Suzi) Radish Seed (莱菔子, Laifuzi) Chinese Honeylocust Spine (皂角, Zaojiao) Chlorite-schist (礞石, Mengshi) Chinese Waxgourd Exocarp (冬瓜皮, Dongguapi) Pepperweed Seed or Flixweed Tansymustard Seed (葶苈子, Tinglizi)

Large Intestine

1. Damp-heat in the large intestine: abdominal pain with diarrhea, tenesmus, passing stool with blood and pus, burning heat in the anus, scanty dark urine, yellow and greasy tongue coating, slippery and rapid pulse. It is advisable to clear away damp-heat.

Coptis Rhizome (黄连, Huanglian) Baikal Skullcap Root (黄芩, Huangqin) Chinese Corktree Bark (黄柏, Huangbai) Rhubarb (大黄, Dahuang) Chinese Pulsatilla Root (白

头翁，Baitouweng）Largeleaf Chinese Ash Bark（秦皮，Qinpi）Lightyellow Sophora Root（苦参，Kushen）Purslane Herb（马齿苋，Machixian）Copperleaf Herb（铁苋菜，Tiexiangcai）Japanese Pagodatree Flower（槐花，Huaihua）Garden Burnet Root（地榆，Diyu）Whiteflower Patrinia Herb（败酱草，Baijiangcao）

2. Deficiency of fluid in the large intestine: dry stool or constipation, difficulty in passing stool, probably once for a few days, accompanied by dizziness, foul breath, thready pulse, red tongne with little body fluid. It is advisable to use lubricant drugs to relieve constipation.

Hemp Seed（火麻仁，Huomaren）Bushcherry Seed（郁李仁，Yuliren）Peach Seed（桃仁，Taoren）Apricot Seed（杏仁，Xingren）Mongolian Snakegourd Seed（瓜蒌仁，Gualouren）Chinese Arborvitae Seed（柏子仁，Baiziren）Tuber Fleeceflower Root（何首乌，Heshouwu）Desertliving Cistanche（肉苁蓉，Roucongrong）Chinese Angelica Root（当归，Danggui）Figwort Root（玄参，Xuanshen）Dwarf Lilyturf Root（麦门冬，Maimendong）Rehmannia Dried Root（生地黄，Shengdihuang）Mulberry Solomonseal（桑椹，Sangshen）Honey（蜂蜜，Fengmi）

Kidney

1. Deficiency of kidney-yin: dizziness and blurred vision, tinnitus and deafness of the ear, loose teeth, insomnia, seminal emission, dry mouth and throat, feverish sensation in the chest, palms and soles, night sweating, ache of the waist and knees, red tongue, thready and rapid pulse. It is advisable to nourish and reinforce kidney-yin.

Prepared Rhizome of Adhesive Rehmannia（熟地黄，Shoudihuang）Asiatic Cornelian Cherry Fruit（山茱萸，Shanzhuyu）Barbary Wolfberry Fruit（枸杞子，Gouqizi）Glossy Privet Fruit（女贞子，Nuzhenzi）Yerbadetajo Herb（墨旱莲，Mohanlian）Figwort Root（玄参，Xuanshen）Cochinchinese Asparagus Root（天门冬，Tianmendong）Siberian Solomonseal Rhizome（黄精，Huangjing）Tuber Fleeceflower Root（何首乌，Heshouwu）Common Anemarrhea Rhizome（知母，Zhimu）Ass-hide Glue（阿胶，Ejiao）Tortoise's Shell and Plastron（龟版，Guiban）Turtle Carapace（鳖甲，Biejia）

2. Deficiency of kidney-yang: Coldness of the body with chills, mental dapression, ache of the waist and knees or impotence, pale tongue with white coating, deep and slow pulse, weakness of chi pulse, It is advisable to warm the kidney yang.

Prepared Daughter Root of Common Monkshood（附子，Fuzi）Cassia Bark（肉桂，Rougui）Hairy Antler（鹿茸，Lurong）Antler Glue（鹿角胶，Lujiaojiao）Common Cruculigo（仙茅，Xianmao）Shorthorned Epimedium Herb（淫羊藿，Yinyanghuo）Malaytea Scurfpea Fruit（补骨脂，Buguzhi）Medicinal Indian-mulberry Root（巴戟天，Bajitian）Desertliving Cistanche（肉苁蓉，Roucongrong）Russian Boschniakia Herb（草苁蓉，Caocongrong）East Asian Tree Fern Rhizome（狗脊，Gouji）Himalayan Teasel Root（续断，Xuduan）Flatstem Milkvetch Seed（沙苑子，Shayuanzi）Songaria Cynomorium Herb（锁阳，Suoyang）

3. Instability of kidney-qi: Spermatorrhea, premature ejaculation, dribbling of urine, frequent and clear urine, incontinence of urine in severe case, soreness of the spinal column, pale complexion, decreased hearing ability. Pale tongue with white coating, thready and weak pulse. It is advisable to reinforce kidney-qi with astringents.

Chinese Magnoliavine (五味子, Wuweizi) Asiatic Cornelian Cherry Fruit (山茱萸, Shanzhuyu) Palmleaf Raspberry Fruit (覆盆子, Fupenzi) Gordon Euryale Seed (芡实, Qianshi) Cherokee Rose Fruit (金樱子, Jinyingzi) Hindu Lotus Stamen (莲须, Lianxu) Sharpleaf Galangal Fruit (益智仁, Yizhiren) Mantis Egg-case (桑螵蛸, Sangpiaoxiao) Dragon's Bone (龙骨, Longgu) Oyster Shell (牡蛎, Muli) Dodder Seed (菟丝子, Tusizi)

4. Failure of the kidney in receiving qi: dyspnea due to qi deficiency, dyspnea while acting, being liable to sweating, coldness of the limbs, aversion to wind-cold, edema of the face, faint and floating pulse, pale tongue. It is advisable to reinforce the kidney and receive qi.

Chinese Magnoliavine (五味子, Wuweizi) Ginkgo Seed (白果, Baiguo) Chinese Eaglewood Wood (沉香, Chenxiang) Giant Gecko (蛤蚧, Gejie) Sulfur (硫黄, Liuhuang) Magnetite (磁石, Cishi) Chinese Caterpillar Fungus (冬虫夏草, Dongchongxiacao) English Walnut Seed (核桃仁, Hetaoren)

5. Edema due to deficiency of the kidney: edema all over the body, severe case in the lower limbs, fingers are depressed white pressing, ache of the waist, distension and fullness in the abdomen, scanty urine accompanied by dyspnea, dyspnea and cough with rele, pale and enlarged tongue white tongue coating, deep and thready pulse It is advisable to warm kidney yang and promote diuresis.

Prepared Daughter Root of Common Monkshood (附子, Fuzi) Cassia Bark (肉桂, Rougui) Umbellate Pore Fungus (猪苓, Zhuling) Tuckahoe (茯苓, Fuling) Oriental Waterplantain Rhizome (泽泻, Zexie) Large-head Atractylodes Rhizome (白术, Baizhu) Malaytea Scurfpea Fruit (补骨脂, Buguzhi) Common Fenugreek Seed (胡芦巴, Huluba) Chinese Magnoliavine (五味子, Wuweizi) Plantain Seed (车前子, Cheqianzi) Twotooth Achyranthes Root (牛膝, Niuxi)

6. Softness of bones due to kidney deficiency: soreness of the waist and knees, weakness of the muscle and joints. It is advisable to reinforce the liver and kidney, strengthen the muscle and bones.

Eucommia Bark (杜仲, Duzhong) Himalayan Teasel Root (续断, Xuduan) Chinese Taxillus Twig (桑寄生, Sangjisheng) Twotooth Achyranthes Root (牛膝, Niuxi) East Asian Tree Fern Rhizome (狗脊, Gouji) Cortex Acanthopanacis Radicis (五加皮, Wujiapi) Common Heron's Bill Herb or Wilford Cranesbill Herb (老鹳草, Laoguancao)

7. Hyperactivity of kidney-fire: deficiency of kidney-yin make deficient-fire possible, restlessness in sleep, dizziness and palpitation, excessive sexual desire. It is advisable to nourish yin and dispel fire

Common Anemarrhea Rhizome (知母, Zhimu) Chinese Corktree Bark (黄柏, Huangbai) Figwort Root (玄参, Xuanshen) Prepared Rhizome of Adhesive Rehmannia (熟地黄, Shoudihuang) Asiatic Cornelian Cherry Fruit (山茱萸, Shanzhuyu) Oriental Waterplantain Rhizome (泽泻, Zexie) Hindu Lotus Plumule (莲子心, Lianzixin) Tree Peony Bark (牡丹皮, Mudanpi)

Urinary Bladder

1. Damp-heat in the urinary bladder: difficulty in urination, frequent urine, urgency of micturition, urodynia, yellow and turbid urine with pus and blood. It is advisable to clear away damp-heat.

Plantain Seed (车前子, Cheqianzi) Asiatic Plantain Herb (车前草, Cheqiancao) Akebia

Stem（木通，Mutong）Capillary Wormwood Herb（茵陈蒿，Yinchenhao）Common Knotgrass Herb（萹蓄，Bianxu）Lilac Pink Herb（瞿麦，Qumai）Indian Bread Pink Epidermis（赤茯苓，Chifuling）Sevenlobed Yam Rhizome（萆薢，Bixie），Oriental Waterplantain Rhizome（泽泻，Zexie）Fourstamen Stephania Root（防己，Fangji）Talc（滑石，Huashi）Belvedere Fruit（地肤子，Difuzi）Common Dayflower Herb（鸭跖草，Yazhicao）Mazie Style（玉米须，Yumixu）

2. Stones in the urinary bladder: dribbling urine with stones, contraction of the urinary bladder, urinary bladder pain radiating to the lower abdomen. It is advisable to remove dampness and dissolve stones.

Christina Loosetrife Herb（金钱草，Jinqiancao）Japanese Climbing Fern Spores（海金沙，Haijinsha）Japanese Felt Fern Leaf（石韦，Shiwei）Akebia Stem（木通，Mutong）Cluster Mallow Seed（冬葵子，Dongkuizi）Talc（滑石，Huashi）Ural Licorice Root Tip（甘草梢，Gancaoshao）Sevenlobed Yam Rhizome（萆薢，Bixie），Gambirplant Hooked Stem and Branch（钩藤，Gouteng）Japanese Thistle Herb or Root（大蓟，Daji）Common Cephalanoplos Herb（小蓟，Xiaoji）Chicken Gizzard Membrane（鸡内金，Jineijin）

Major Drugs of the Six Meridians

1. Taiyang Meridian
2. Shaoyang Meridian
3. Yangming Meridian
4. Taiyin Meridian
5. Shaoyin Meridian
6. Jueyin Meridian

Reference Ⅴ Clinical Application of Chinese Drugs Based on Diseases

Infectious diseases and Parasitosis

Influenza: Black Nightshade Herb（龙葵，Longkui）Sweet Wormwood（青蒿，Qinghao）Haichow Elsholtzia Herb（香薷，Xiangru）Indian Chrysanthemum Flower（野菊花，Yejuhua）Capillary Wormwood Herb（茵陈蒿，Yinchenhao）Indigowoad Leaf（大青叶，Daqingye）Vinegar（醋，Cu）Gypsum（石膏，Shigao）European Verbena Herb（马鞭草，Mabiancao）Chinese Thorowax Root（柴胡，Chaihu）Male Fern Rhizome（贯众，Guanzhong）Cottonrose Hibiscus Leaf（木芙蓉叶，Mufurongye）Garlic Bulb（蒜，Suan）Honeysuckle Flower（金银花，Jinyinhua）Weeping Forsythia Capsule（连翘，Lianqiao）Dyers Woad Root（板蓝根，Banlangen）Natural Indigo（青黛，Qingdai）Blackberrylily Rhizome（射干，Shegan）Baikal Skullcap Root（黄芩，Huangqin）Coptis Rhizome（黄连，Huanglian）Chinese Corktree Bark（黄柏，Huangbai）Argy Wormwood Leaf（艾叶，Aiye）Tatarian Aster Root（紫菀，Ziyuan）Chinese Arborvitae Leafy Twig（侧柏叶，Cebaiye）Medicine Terminalia Fruit（诃子，Hezi）Siberian Solomonseal Rhizome（黄精，Huangjing）Chinese Magnoliavine（五味子，Wuweizi）Rhubarb（大黄，Dahuang）Giant

Knotweed Rhizome (虎杖, Huzhang) Sessile Stemona Root (百部, Baibu) Heartlaef Houttuynia Herb (鱼腥草, Yuxingcao) Great Burdock Achene (牛蒡子, Niubangzi) Divaricate Saposhnikovia Root (防风, Fangfeng) Perilla Leaf (紫苏, Zisu) Root of Sinkiang Arnebia (紫草, Zicao) Red Peony Root (赤芍药, Chishaoyao) Tree Peony Bark (牡丹皮, Mudanpi) Ephedra (麻黄, Mahuang) Cassia Twig (桂枝, Guizhi) Foutune Eupatorium Herb (佩兰, Peilan) Areca Seed (槟榔, Binlang) Olive (橄榄, Ganlan) Licorice Root (甘草, Shenggancao) Common Selfheal Fruit-spike (Common Selfheal Spike (夏枯草, Xiakucao) Xiakucao) Seaweed (海藻, Haizao) Common Dayflower Herb (鸭跖草, Yazhicao) Cherokee Rose Fruit (金樱子, Jinyingzi) Japanese Felt Fern Leaf (石韦, Shiwei)

Measles: Wild Mint (薄荷, Bohe) Coptis Rhizome (黄连, Huanglian) Root of Sinkiang Arnebia (紫草根, Zicaogen) Combined Spice-bush Root (乌药, Wuyao) Cariander Herb (胡荽, Husui) Carrot Root (胡萝卜, Huluobo) Shepherdspurse Herb with Root (荠菜, Jicai) Divaricate Saposhnikovia Root (防风, Fangfeng) Fineleaf Schizomepeta Herb (荆芥, Jingjie) Cicada Slough (蝉蜕, Chantui) Great Burdock Achene (牛蒡子, Niubangzi) Reed Rhizome (芦根, Lugen)

Measles associated laryngopharyngitis: Twotooth Achyranthes Root (牛膝, Niuxi)

Measles associated pneumonia: Rhubarb (大黄, Dahuang) Shunk Bugbane Rhizome (升麻, Shengma) Alumen (明矾, Mingfan)

Chickenpox: Common Dayflower Herb (鸭跖草, Yazhicao) Talc (滑石, Huashi)

Parotitis: Asiatic Plantain Herb (车前草, Cheqiancao) Whiteflower Patrinia Herb (败酱草, Baijiangcao) Indian Chrysanthemum Flower (野菊花, Yejuhua) Mirabilite (朴硝, Piaoxiao) Manyleaf Paris Rhizome (蚤休, Zaoxiu) Indian Mockstrawberry Herb (蛇莓, Shemei) Jackinthepulpit Tuber (天南星, Tiannanxing) Japanese Climbing Fern Spores (海金沙, Haijinsha) Common Knotgrass Herb (萹蓄, Bianxu) Natural Indigo (青黛, Qingdai) Chinese Thorowax Root (柴胡, Chaihu) Alumen (明矾, Mingfan) Vasps Nest (露蜂房, Lufengfang) Centipede (蜈蚣, Wugong) Earthworm (蚯蚓, Qiuyin) Chinese Gall (五倍子, Wubeizi) Chinese Corktree Bark (黄柏, Huangbai) Todpole (蝌蚪, Kedou) Medicinal Evodia Root (吴茱萸, Wuzhuyu) Rice Bean (赤小豆, Chixiaodou) Dandelion (蒲公英, Pugongying) Chinese Arborvitae Leafy Twig (侧柏叶, Cebaiye) Green Gram Seed (绿豆, Lvdou) Chinese Clematis Root (威灵仙, Weilingxian) Realgar (雄黄, Xionghuang) Male Fern Rhizome (贯众, Guanzhong)

Encephalitis: Indigowoad Leaf (大青叶, Daqingye) Common Anemarrhea Rhizome (知母, Zhimu) Chinese Gentian Root (龙胆草, Longdancao) Earthworm (蚯蚓, Qiuyin) Sweet Wormwood (青蒿, Qinghao) Cow-bezoar (牛黄, Niuhuang) Asiatic Rhinoceros Horn (犀角, Xijiao) Garlic Bulb (大蒜, Dasuan) Gypsum (石膏, Shigao)

Virus hepatiis: Common Aucklandia Root (木香, Muxiang) Dwarf Lilyturf Root (麦门冬, Maimendong) Asiatic Plantain Herb (车前草, Cheqiancao) Common Dayflower Herb (鸭跖草, Yazhicao) Whiteflower Patrinia Herb (败酱草, Baijiangcao) Sweet Wormwood (青蒿, Qinghao) Capillary Wormwood Herb (茵陈蒿, Yinchenhao) Common Scouring Rush Herb (木贼, Muzei) Common St. Paulswort Herb (豨莶草, Xixiancao) Rehmannia Dried Root (生地黄, Shengdihuang) Malt (麦芽, Maiya) Hindu Datura

Flower (曼陀罗花, Mantuoluohua) Chinese Magnoliavine (五味子, Wuweizi) Turmeric Root-tuber (郁金, Yujin) Rhubarb (大黄, Dahuang) White Peony Root (白芍药, Baishaoyao) Giant Knotweed Rhizome (虎杖, Huzhang) Soyben (黄大豆, Huangdadou) Weeping Forsythia Capsule (连翘, Lianqiao) Natural Indigo (青黛, Qingdai) European Verbena Herb (马鞭草, Mabiancao) Danshen Root (丹参, Danshen) Root of Sinkiang Arnebia (紫草根, Zicaogen) Sanchi Root (三七, Sanqi) Cassia Twig (桂枝, Guizhi) Doubleteeth Pulbescent Angelica Root (独活, Duhuo) Baikal Skullcap Root (黄芩, Huangqin) Licorice Root (甘草, Gancao) Chinese Angelica Root (当归, Danggui) Lalang Grass Rhizome (白茅根, Baimaogen) Chinese Gentian Root (龙胆草, Longdancao) Appendiculate Cremastra Pseudobulb (山慈姑, Shancigu) Creeping Woodsorred Herb (酢浆草, Zuojiangcao) Wrinkled Gianthyssop Herb (藿香, Huoxiang) Hirsute Shiny Bugleweed Herb (泽兰, Zelan) Magnetite (磁石, Cishi) Lightyellow Sophora Root (苦参, Kushen) Common Selfheal Fruit-spike (Common Selfheal Spike (夏枯草, Xiakucao) Xiakucao) Ginseng (人参, Renshen) Alumen (明矾, Mingfan) Tuckahoe (茯苓, Fuling) Centipede (蜈蚣, Wugong) Olive (橄榄, Ganlan) Umbellate Pore Fungus (猪苓, Zhuling) Ground Beetle (䗪虫, Zhechong) Large Blister Beetle (斑蝥, Banmao) Honeysuckle Stem(忍冬藤, Rendongteng) Chinese Corktree Bark (黄柏, Huangbai) Officinal Magnolia Bark (厚朴, Houpo) Beardie (泥鳅鱼, Niqiuyu) Babylon Weeping Willow Branchlet (柳枝, Liuzhi) Common Floweringquince Fruit (木瓜, Mugua) Carrot Root (胡萝卜, Huluobo) Cow-bezoar (牛黄, Niuhuang) Dandelion (蒲公英, Pugongying) Bittersweet Herb (白毛藤, Baimaoteng) Tonkin Sophora Root (山豆根, Shandougen) Lilac Daphne Flower-bud (芫花, Yuanhua) Japanese Buttercup Herb (毛茛, Maogen) Hawthorn Fruit (山楂, Shanzha) Chinese Clematis Root (威灵仙, Weilingxian) Garlic Bulb (大蒜, Dasuan) Japanese Ardisia Herb (矮地茶, Aidicha) Inula Flower (旋覆花, Xuanfuhua) Membranous Milkvetch Root (黄芪, Huangqi) Male Fern Rhizome (贯众, Guanzhong) Buffalo Horn (水牛角, Shuiniujiao) Chinese Thorowax Root (柴胡, Chaihu)

Jaundice: Benzoin (安息香, Anxixiang) Hawthorn Fruit (山楂, Shanzha) Clove Flower-bud (丁香, Dingxiang) Capillary Wormwood Herb (茵陈蒿, Yinchenhao) Christina Loosetrife Herb (金钱草, Jinqiancao) Baikal Skullcap Root (黄芩, Huangqin) Coptis Rhizome (黄连, Huanglian) Chinese Corktree Bark (黄柏, Huangbai) Cape Jasmine Fruit (栀子, Zhizi) Chinese Gentian Root (龙胆草, Longdancao) Chinese Thorowax Root (柴胡, Chaihu)

Epidemic hemorrhagic fever: Dan-shen Root (丹参, Danshen) Membranous Milkvetch Root (黄芪, Huangqi) Common Anemarrhea Rhizome (知母, Zhimu) Lalang Grass Rhizome (白茅根, Baimaogen) Hirsute Shiny Bugleweed Herb (泽兰, Zelan) Siberian Solomonseal Rhizome (黄精, Huangjing) Umbellate Pore Fungus (猪苓, Zhuling) Common Yam Rhizome (山药, Shanyao)

Scarlet fever: Coptis Rhizome (黄连, Huanglian) Baikal Skullcap Root (黄芩, Huangqin)

Epidemic cerebrospinal meningitis: Largeleaf Gentian Root (秦艽, Qinjiao) Coptis Rhizome (黄连, Huanglian) Baikal Skullcap Root (黄芩, Huangqin) Male Fern Rhizome (贯众, Guanzhong) Chinese Corktree Bark

(黄柏, Huangbai) Scorpion (全蝎, Quanxie) Climbing Groundsel Herb (千里光, Qianliguang) Tuber Fleeceflower Root (何首乌, Heshouwu) Garlic Bulb (蒜, Suan)

Virus mentingitis: Cow-bezoar (牛黄, Niuhuang) Garlic Bulb (大蒜, Dasuan)

Diphtheria: Chalcanthnium (胆矾, Danfan) Nut-vomitive Poisonnut Seed (马钱子, Maqianzi) Indian Mockstrawberry Herb (蛇莓, Shemei) Cinnabar (朱砂, Zhusha) Yerbadetajo Herb (墨旱莲, Mohanlian) European Verbena Herb (马鞭草, Mabiancao) Coptis Rhizome (黄连, Huanglian) Common Selfheal Fruit-spike (Common Selfheal Spike (夏枯草, Xiakucao) Xiakucao) Alumen (明矾, Mingfan) Chinese Gall (五倍子, Wubeizi) Croton Seed (巴豆, Badou) Slug (蛞蝓, Kuoyu) Garlic Bulb (大蒜, Dasuan)

Chin cough: Plantain Seed (车前子, Cheqianzi) Pepperweed Seed or Flixweed Tansymustard Seed (葶苈子, Tinglizi) Ephedra (麻黄, Mahuang) Tatarian Aster Root (紫菀, Ziyuan) Indigowoad Leaf (大青叶, Daqingye) Inula Flower (旋覆花, Xuanfuhua) Talc (滑石, Huashi) Kansui Root (甘遂, Gansui) Natural Indigo (青黛, Qingdai) European Verbena Herb (马鞭草, Mabiancao) Coptis Rhizome (黄连, Huanglian) Bletilla Rhizome (白及, Baiji) Chlorite-schist (礞石, Mengshi) Tendrilleaf Fritillary Bulb (贝母, Beimu) Borax (硼砂, Pengsha) Siberian Solomonseal Rhizome (黄精, Huangjing) Centipede (蜈蚣, Wugong) Small Centipeda Herb (鹅不食草, Ebushicao) Scorpion (全蝎, Quanxie) Aloes (芦荟, Luhui) Largeleaf Chinese Ash Bark (秦皮, Qinpi) Loquat Flower (枇杷花, Pipahua) Hyacinth Bean (扁豆, Biandou) Radish Seed (莱菔子, Laifuzi) Purslane Herb (马齿苋, Machixian) Chinese Arborvitae Leafy Twig (侧柏叶, Cebaiye) Bear Gall (熊胆, Xiongdan) Gambirplant Hooked Stem and Branch (钩藤, Gouteng) Airpotato Yam Tuber (黄药子, Huangyaozi) Heartlaef Houttuynia Herb (鱼腥草, Yuxingcao) Tuber Fleeceflower Root (何首乌, Heshouwu) Sessile Stemona Root (百部, Baibu) Garlic Bulb (大蒜, Dasuan)

Ileotyphus: Coptis Rhizome (黄连, Huanglian) Thinleaf Adina Stem and Leaf (水杨梅, Shuiyangmei) Garlic Bulb (大蒜, Dasuan) Herb of Siberian Cocklebur (苍耳草, Cangercao) Garden Burnet Root (地榆, Diyu)

Bacillary dysentery: Common Floweringquince Fruit (木瓜, Mugua) Black Nightshade Herb (龙葵, Longkui) Plantain Seed (车前子, Cheqianzi) Siberian Cocklebur Fruit (苍耳子, Cangerzi) Common Carpesium Fruit (鹤虱, Heshi) Diverse Wormwood Herb (刘寄奴, Liujinu) Common Cephalanoplos Herb (小蓟, Xiaoji) Talc (滑石, Huashi) Vinegar (醋, Cu) Indian Mockstrawberry Herb (蛇莓, Shemei) Chinese Magnoliavine (五味子, Wuweizi) Rhubarb (大黄, Dahuang) Japanese Climbing Fern Spores (海金沙, Haijinsha) Common Knotgrass Herb (萹蓄, Bianxu) Yerbadetajo Herb (墨旱莲, Mohanlian) Chinese Elder Flower (陆英, Luting) Whiteflower hogfenel Root (前胡, Qianhu) Coptis Rhizome (黄连, Huanglian) Chinese Pulsatilla Root (白头翁, Baitouweng) Chinese Sage Herb (紫参, Zishen) Baikal Skullcap Root (黄芩, Huangqin) Shunk Bugbane Rhizome (升麻, Shengma) Bistort Rhizome (拳参, Quanshen) Creeping Woodsorred Herb (酢浆草, Zuojiangcao) Honeysuckle Flower (金银花, Jinyinhua) Thinleaf Adina Stem and Leaf (水杨梅, Shuiyangmei) Flowery Woodrust Herb or Fruit (地杨梅, Diyangmei) Flaccid Knotweed Herb (辣蓼草, Laliaocao)

Lightyellow Sophora Root（苦参，Kushen）Swordlike Atractylodes Rhizome（苍术，Cangzhu）Vasps Nest（露蜂房，Lufengfang）Purpleflower Holly Leaf（冬青叶，Dongqingye）Shrubalthea Bark（木槿皮，Mujinpi）Ass-hide Glue（阿胶，Ejiao）Chinese Gall（五倍子，Wubeizi）Honeysuckle Stem（忍冬藤，Rendongteng）Chinese Corktree Bark（黄柏，Huangbai）Officinal Magnolia Bark（厚朴，Houpo）Largeleaf Chinese Ash Bark（秦皮，Qinpi）Chinese White Olive（青果，Qingguo）Broadbean Seed（蚕豆，Candou）Luffa Fruit（丝瓜，Sigua）Opium Poppy Pericarp（罂粟壳，Yingsuqiao）Fresh Ginger（生姜，Shengjiang）Purslane Herb（马齿苋，Machixian）Common Jasminorange Branchlet and Leaf（九里香，Jiulixiang）Lobed Kudzuvine Root（葛根，Gegen）Hawthorn Fruit（山楂，Shanzha）Japanese Ampelopsis Root（白蔹，Bailian）Honey（蜂蜜，Fengmi）Humifuse Euphorbia Herb（地锦草，Dijincao）Glabrous Greenbrier Rhizome（土茯苓，Tufuling）Garlic Bulb（大蒜，Dasuan）

Malaria: Sweet Wormwood（青蒿，Qinghao）Talc（滑石，Huashi）Arsenolite Ore（砒石，Pishi）Lithargyrum（密陀僧，Mituoseng）Soot（百草霜，Baicaoshuang）Pinellia Rhizome（半夏，Banxia）Yerbadetajo Herb（墨旱莲，Mohanlian）European Verbena Herb（马鞭草，Mabiancao）Paniculate Swallowwort Root（徐长卿，Xuchangqing）Flaccid Knotweed Herb（辣蓼草，Laliaocao）Cuttle Bone（乌贼骨，Wuzeigu）Great-ventral Garden Spider（蜘蛛，Zhizhu）Chinese Wolfberry Root-bark（地骨皮，Digupi）Small Centipeda Herb（鹅不食草，Ebushicao）Cicada Slough（蝉蜕，Chantui）Croton Seed（巴豆，Badou）Large Blister Beetle（斑蝥，Banmao）Black Pepper Fruit（胡椒，Hujiao）Sinkiang Giantfennal Resin（阿魏，Awei）Common Floweringquince Fruit（木瓜，Mugua）Cassia Twig（桂枝，Guizhi）Lilac Daphne Flowerbud（芫花，Yuanhua）Japanese Buttercup Herb（毛茛，Maogen）Realgar（雄黄，Xionghuang）Tuber Fleeceflower Root（何首乌，Heshouwu）Honey（蜂蜜，Fengmi）Chinese Thorowax Root（柴胡，Chaihu）

Schistosomiasis: Sweet Wormwood（青蒿，Qinghao）Chinese Lobelia Herb（半边莲，Banbianlian）European Verbena Herb（马鞭草，Mabiancao）Silkworm with Batrytis Larva（白僵蚕，Baijiangcan）Bunge Pricklyash（花椒，Huajiao）Babylon Weeping Willow Leaf（柳叶，Liuye）Mountain Spicy Tree Fruit（荜澄茄，Bichengqie）Japanese Buttercup Herb（毛茛，Maogen）Areca Seed（槟榔，Binlang）Sessile Stemona Root（百部，Baibu）Garlic Bulb（大蒜，Dasuan）

Amebic dysentery: Chinese Pulsatilla Root（白头翁，Baitouweng）Mountain Spicy Tree Fruit（荜澄茄，Bichengqie）Szechwan chinaberry Fruit（川楝子，Chuanlianzi）Fourstamen Stephania Root（防已，Fangji）Garlic Bulb（蒜，Suan）

Pulmonary tuberculosis: Dwarf Lilyturf Root（麦门冬，Maimendong）Japanese Thistle Herb or Root（大蓟，Daji）Indian Chrysanthemum Flower（野菊花，Yejuhua）Chinese Stellera Root（狼毒，Langdu）Yerbadetajo Herb（墨旱莲，Mohanlian）Weeping Forsythia Capsule（连翘，Lianqiao）Coptis Rhizome（黄连，Huanglian）Chinese Sage Herb（石见穿，Shijianchuan）Bletilla Rhizome（白及，Baiji）Membranous Milkvetch Root（黄芪，Huangqi）Licorice Root（甘草，Gancao）Bistort Rhizome（拳参，Quanshen）Tendrilleaf Fritillary Bulb（贝母，Beimu）Acacia Catechu（孩儿茶，Haiercha）Stalactite（钟乳石，Zhongrushi）Common Selfheal Spike（夏枯草，Xiakucao）Siberian Solomonseal Rhizome (黄精, Huangjing) Alumen (明矾, Mingfan) Centipede (蜈蚣, Wugong) Pangolin Scales (穿山甲, Chuanshanjia) Chinese Gall (五倍子, Wubeizi) Honeysuckle Flower (金银花, Jinyinhua) Chinese Corktree Bark (黄柏, Huangbai) Long Usnae Filament (松萝, Songluo) Ginkgo Seed (白果, Baiguo) White Mustard Seed (白芥子, Baijiezi) Purslane Herb (马齿苋, Machixian) Ass-hide Glue (阿胶, Ejiao) Hunifuse Euphorbia Herb (地锦草, Dijincao) Sessile Stemona Root (百部, Baibu) Garlic Bulb (大蒜, Dasuan)

Infantile paralysis: Chinese Pyrola Herb (鹿衔草, Luxiancao) Shorthorned Epimedium Herb (淫羊藿, Yinyanghuo) Large Blister Beetle (斑蝥, Banmao) Eucommia Bark (杜仲, Duzhong) Fourstamen Stephania Root (防己, Fangji) Ginseng (人参, Renshen) Hairy Antler (鹿茸, Lurong) Tortoise's Shell and Plastron (龟版, Guiban) Turtle Carapace (鳖甲, Biejia)

Lymphoid tuberculosis: Rhubarb (大黄, Dahuang) Arsenolite Ore (砒石, Pishi) Gypsum (石膏, Shigao) Chinese Stellera Root (狼毒, Langdu) Kansui Root (甘遂, Gansui) Magnetite (磁石, Cishi) Tortoise's Shell and Plastron (龟版, Guiban) Centipede (蜈蚣, Wugong) Ground Beetle (䗪虫, Zhechong) Chinese Corktree Bark (黄柏, Huangbai) Scorpion (全蝎, Quanxie) Figwort Root (玄参, Xuanshen) Oyster Shell (牡蛎, Muli) Common Selfheal Spike (夏枯草, Xiakucao) Seaweed (海藻, Haizao) Kelp (昆布, Kunbu) Thunberg Fritillary Bulb (浙贝母, Zhebeimu) Croton Seed (巴豆, Badou) Dragon's Bone (龙骨, Longgu) Slug (蛞蝓, Kuoyu) Lizard (蜥蜴, Xiyi) Dragon's Blood (血竭, Xuejie) Discolor Cinquefoil Herb with Root (翻白草, Fanbaicao) Pharbitis Seed (牵牛子, Qianniuzi) Myrrh (没药, Moyao) Musk (麝香, Shexiang) Chinese Clematis Root (威灵仙, Weilingxian) Pig Gall (猪胆, Zhudan) Garlic Bulb (大蒜, Dasuan)

Leprosy: Herb of Siberian Cocklebur (苍耳草, Cangercao) Brevicaude Pit Viper (蝮蛇, Fushe) Chaulmoogratree Seed (大风子, Dafengzi) Realgar (雄黄, Xionghuang)

Leptospirosis: Coptis Rhizome (黄连, Huanglian) Baikal Skullcap Root (黄芩, Huangqin) Lightyellow Sophora Root (苦参, Kushen) Honeysuckle Flower (金银花, Jinyinhua) Tonkin Sophora Root (山豆根, Shandougen) Weeping Forsythia Capsule (连翘, Lianqiao) Heartlaef Houttuynia Herb (鱼腥草, Yuxingcao) Glabrous Greenbrier Rhizome (土茯苓, Tufuling)

Brucellosis: Coptis Rhizome (黄连, Huanglian) Garlic Bulb (蒜, Suan)

Ascariasis: Rangooncreeper Fruit (使君子, Shijunzi) Chinaberry-tree Bark (苦楝根皮, Kuliangenpi) Fistular Onion Stalk (葱白, Congbai) Areca Seed (槟榔, Binlang)

Filariasis: European Verbena Herb (马鞭草, Mabiancao) Mulberry Twig (桑枝, Sangzhi) Lilac Daphne Flower-bud (芫花, Yuanhua) Ture Lacquertree Dried Lacquer (干漆, Ganqi) Areca Seed (槟榔, Binlang) Chinese Clematis Root (威灵仙, Weilingxian)

Oxyuriasis: Vinegar (醋, Cu) Sulfur (硫黄, Liuhuang) Stone-like Omphalia (fungus) (雷丸, Leiwan) Bunge Pricklyash (花椒, Huajiao) Medicinal Evodia Root (吴茱萸, Wuzhuyu) Camphor (樟脑, Zhangnao) Apricot Seed (杏仁, Xingren) Fistular Onion Stalk (葱白, Congbai) Pharbitis Seed (牵牛子, Qianniuzi) Realgar (雄黄, Xionghuang) Sessile Stemona Root (百部, Baibu) Garlic Bulb (蒜, Suan)

Cestodiasis: Stone-like Omphalia (fungus)

(雷丸, Leiwan) Cushaw Seed (南瓜子, Nanguazi) Chinaberry-tree Bark (苦楝根皮, Kuliangenpi) Areca Seed (槟榔, Binlang)

Hypertrophic trematodiasis: Areca Seed (槟榔, Binlang)

Flagellosis: Lightyellow Sophora Root (苦参, Kushen) Areca Seed (槟榔, Binlang)

Ancylostomiasis (hookworm disease): Common Carpesium Fruit (鹤虱, Heshi) Stone-like Omphalia (fungus) (雷丸, Leiwan) Small Centipeda Herb (鹅不食草, Ebushicao) Szechwan Chinaberry Bark (苦楝皮, Kulianpi) Purslane Herb (马齿苋, Machixian) Areca Seed (槟榔, Binlang) Realgar (雄黄, Xionghuang) Hunifuse Euphorbia Herb (地锦草, Dijincao)

Respiratory disease

Upper respiratory tract infection: Common Dayflower Herb (鸭跖草, Yazhicao) Haichow Elsholtzia Herb (香薷, Xiangru) Cudweed Herb (鼠曲草, Shuqucao) Indigowoad Leaf (大青叶, Daqingye) Common Rush Stem Pith (灯芯, Dengxin) Chinese Thorowax Root (柴胡, Chaihu) Membranous Milkvetch Root (黄芪, Huangqi) Male Fern Rhizome (贯众, Guanzhong) Wrinkled Gianthyssop Herb (藿香, Huoxiang) Tendrilleaf Fritillary Bulb (贝母, Beimu) Szechwan Lovage Rhizome (川芎, Chuanxiong) Swordlike Atractylodes Rhizome (苍术, Cangzhu) Pubescent Holly Root (毛冬青, Maodongqing) Small Centipeda Herb (鹅不食草, Ebushicao) Loquat Leaf (枇杷叶, Pipaye) Cow-bezoar (牛黄, Niuhuang) Herb of Bittesweet (白英, Baiying) Heartlaef Houttuynia Herb (鱼腥草, Yuxingcao) Chinese Clematis Root (威灵仙, Weilingxian) Honeysuckle Flower (金银花, Jinyinhua) Weeping Forsythia Capsule (连翘, Lianqiao) Figwort Root (玄参, Xuanshen) Cicada Slough (蝉蜕, Chantui) Great Burdock Achene (牛蒡子, Niubangzi) Dyers Woad Root (板蓝根, Banlangen) Dwarf Lilyturf Root (麦门冬, Maimendong) Heartlaef Houttuynia Herb (鱼腥草, Yuxingcao)

Acute bronchitis: Loquat Leaf (枇杷叶, Pipaye) Ephedra (麻黄, Mahuang) Apricot Seed (杏仁, Xingren) Sessile Stemona Root (百部, Baibu) Tendrilleaf Fritillary Bulb (贝母, Beimu) Heartlaef Houttuynia Herb (鱼腥草, Yuxingcao)

Chronic bronchitis: Asiatic Plantain Herb (车前草, Cheqiancao) Tatarian Aster Root (紫苑, Ziyuan) Ephedra (麻黄, Mahuang) Sweet Wormwood (青蒿, Qinghao) Zedoray (莪术, Ezhu) Hindu Datura Flower (曼陀罗花, Mantuoluohua) Nut-vomitive Poisonnut Seed (马钱子, Maqianzi) Yunnan Manyleaf Pairs Rhizome (重楼, Chonglou) Pink Plumepoppy Herb with Root (博落回, Boluohui) Pinellia Rhizome (半夏, Banxia) Pokeberry Root (商陆, Shanglu) Giant Knotweed Rhizome (虎杖, Huzhang) Soyben (黄大豆, Huangdadou) Puncturevine Caltrap Fruit (白蒺藜, Baijili) Tree Peony Bark (牡丹皮, Mudanpi) Shorthorned Epimedium Herb (淫羊藿, Yinyanghuo) Chinese Sage Herb (石见穿, Shijianchuan) Baikal Skullcap Root (黄芩, Huangqin) Doubleteeth Pulbescent Angelica Root (独活, Duhuo) Membranous Milkvetch Root (黄芪, Huangqi) Chinese Angelica Root (当归, Danggui) Paniculate Swallowwort Root (徐长卿, Xuchangqing) Siberian Solomonseal Rhizome (黄精, Huangjing) Alumen (明矾, Mingfan) Earth Worm (地龙, Dilong) Pubescent Holly Root (毛冬青, Maodongqing) Manyprickle Acanthopanax Root (刺五加, Ciwujia) Grassleaf

Sweetflag Rhizome（石菖蒲，Shichangpu）Japanese Felt Fern Leaf（石韦，Shiwei）Loquat Leaf（枇杷叶，Pipaye）Ginkgo Seed（白果，Baiguo）Cochinchinese Asparagus Root（天门冬，Tianmendong）Largeleaf Chinese Ash Bark（秦皮，Qinpi）Long Usnae Filament（松萝，Songluo）Bunge Pricklyash（花椒，Huajiao）Luffa Fruit（丝瓜，Sigua）Babylon Weeping Willow Branchlet（柳枝，Liuzhi） Snakegourd Stem（瓜蒌藤，Gualouteng）Apricot Seed（杏仁，Xingren）Blackberrylily Rhizome（射干，Shegan）Chinese Arborvitae Leafy Twig（侧柏叶，Cebaiye）White Mustard Seed（白芥子，Baijiezi）India Madder Root（茜草，Qiancao）Tonkin Sophora Root（山豆根，Shandougen）Lilac Daphne Flower-bud（芫花，Yuanhua）Heartlaef Houttuynia Herb（鱼腥草，Yuxingcao）Myrrh（没药，Moyao）Chinese Clematis Root（威灵仙，Weilingxian）Sessile Stemona Root（百部，Baibu）Argy Wormwood Leaf（艾叶，Aiye）

Bronchial asthma: Common Coltsfoot Flower（款冬花，Kuandonghua）Ephedra（麻黄，Mahuang）Hindu Datura Flower（曼陀罗花，Mantuoluohua）Alumen（白矾，Baifan）Kansui Root（甘遂，Gansui）Pinellia Rhizome（半夏，Banxia）Prepared Daughter Root of Common Monkshood（附子，Fuzi）Soyben（黄大豆，Huangdadou）Membranous Milkvetch Root（黄芪，Huangqi）Licorice Root（甘草，Gancao）Common Cnidium Fruit（蛇床子，Shechuangzi）Yanhusuo（延胡索，Yanhusuo）Stalactite（钟乳石，Zhongrushi）Lightyellow Sophora Root（苦参，Kushen）Szechwan Lovage Rhizome（川芎，Chuanxiong）Ginseng（人参，Renshen）Malaytea Scurfpea Fruit（补骨脂，Buguzhi）Cuttle Bone（乌贼骨，Wuzeigu）Earth Worm（地龙，Dilong）Grassleaf Sweetflag Rhizome（石菖蒲，Shichangpu）Japanese Felt Fern Leaf（石韦，Shiwei）Giant Gecko（蛤蚧，Gejie）Toad（蟾蜍，Chanchu）Croton Seed（巴豆，Badou）Chinese Honeylocust Spine（皂角，Zaojiao）Bunge Pricklyash（花椒，Huajiao）Aspongopus（九香虫，Jiuxiangchong）Cassia Bark（肉桂，Rougui）White Mustard Seed（白芥子，Baijiezi）Gambirplant Hooked Stem and Branch（钩藤，Gouteng）Musk（麝香，Shexiang）

Bronchiectasis: Bletilla Rhizome（白及，Baiji）Ass-hide Glue（阿胶，Ejiao）Lily Bulb（百合，Baihe）Ramie Root（苎麻根，Zhumagen）

Pneumonia: Tatarian Aster Root（紫苑，Ziyuan）Ephedra（麻黄，Mahuang）Chinese Pyrola Herb（鹿衔草，Luxiancao）Rhubarb（大黄，Dahuang）Gypsum（石膏，Shigao）Giant Knotweed Rhizome（虎杖，Huzhang）Weeping Forsythia Capsule（连翘，Lianqiao）European Verbena Herb（马鞭草，Mabiancao）Coptis Rhizome（黄连，Huanglian）Pubescent Holly Root（毛冬青，Maodongqing）Chinese Corktree Bark（黄柏，Huangbai）Heartlaef Houttuynia Herb（鱼腥草，Yuxingcao）Garlic Bulb（大蒜，Dasuan）

Pulmonary abscess: Weeping Forsythia Capsule（连翘，Lianqiao）Coptis Rhizome（黄连，Huanglian）Balloonflower Root（桔梗，Jiegeng）Common Buckwheat Seed（荞麦，Qiaomai）Chinese Waxgourd Seed（冬瓜子，Dongguazi）Heartlaef Houttuynia Herb（鱼腥草，Yuxingcao）Dandelion（蒲公英，Pugongying）Reed Rhizome（芦根，Lugen）Coix Seed（薏苡仁，Yiyiren）Baikal Skullcap Root（黄芩，Huangqin）Peach Seed（桃仁，Taoren）

Pyothorax: Coptis Rhizome（黄连，Huanglian）Heartlaef Houttuynia Herb（鱼腥草，Yuxingcao）Pepperweed Seed or Flixweed

Tansymustard Seed (葶苈子, Tinglizi) White Mulberry Root-bark (桑白皮, Sangbaipi) Inula Flower (旋覆花, Xuanfuhua) Balloonflower Root (桔梗, Jiegeng)

Chronic pulmonary heart disease: Ephedra (麻黄, Mahuang) Membranous Milkvetch Root (黄芪, Huangqi) Szechwan Lovage Rhizome (川芎, Chuanxiong) Leech (水蛭, Shuizhi) Snakegourd Fruit (瓜蒌, Gualou) Heartlaef Houttuynia Herb (鱼腥草, Yuxingcao) Dan-shen Root (丹参, Danshen) Chinese Magnoliavine (五味子, Wuweizi)

Pleuritis: Pepperweed Seed or Flixweed Tansymustard Seed (葶苈子, Tinglizi) Nutgrass Galingale Rhizome (香附, Xiangfu) Inula Flower (旋覆花, Xuanfuhua) Kansui Root (甘遂, Gansui) Common Selfheal Spike (夏枯草, Xiakucao) White Mustard Seed (白芥子, Baijiezi) Longstament Onion Bulb (薤白, Xiebai) Snakegourd Fruit (瓜蒌, Gualou) Immature Bitter Orange (枳实, Zhishi) Coptis Rhizome (黄连, Huanglian)

Natural pneumatothorax: Pepperweed Seed or Flixweed Tansymustard Seed (葶苈子, Tinglizi)

Dry cough: Indian Chrysanthemum Flower (野菊花, Yejuhua) Dwarf Lilyturf Root (麦门冬, Maimendong) Common Anemarrhea Rhizome (知母, Zhimu) Coastal Glehnia Root, and Fourleaf Ladybell Root (沙参, Shashen) Tendrilleaf Fritillary Bulb (贝母, Beimu) Lily Bulb (百合, Baihe) Tatarian Aster Root (紫苑, Ziyuan) Common Coltsfoot Flower (款冬花, Kuandonghua) Ginkgo Seed (白果, Baiguo) Opium Poppy Pericarp (罂粟壳, Yingsuqiao)

Irritating dry cough: Dwarf Lilyturf Root (麦门冬, Maimendong) White Mulberry Root-bark (桑白皮, Sangbaipi) Honey (蜂蜜, Fengmi) Snakegroud Root (天花粉, Tianhuafen) Loquat Leaf (枇杷叶, Pipaye) Sessile Stemona Root (百部, Baibu) Lily Bulb (百合, Baihe) Fragrant Solomonseal Rhizome (玉竹, Yuzhu) Coastal Glehnia Root, and Fourleaf Ladybell Root (沙参, Shashen) Tendrilleaf Fritillary Bulb (贝母, Beimu)

Pulmonary encephalopathy: Grassleaf Sweetflag Rhizome (石菖蒲, Shichangpu) Thinleaf Milkwort Root (远志, Yuanzhi) Turmeric Root-tuber (郁金, Yujin)

Acute fever: Common Aucklandia Root (木香, Muxiang) Indian Chrysanthemum Flower (野菊花, Yejuhua) Pink Plumepoppy Herb with Root (博落回, Boluohui) Figwort Root (玄参, Xuanshen) Lightyellow Sophora Root (苦参, Kushen) Swordlike Atractylodes Rhizome (苍术, Cangzhu) Dan-shen Root (丹参, Danshen) Honeysuckle Flower (金银花, Jinyinhua) Chinese Corktree Bark (黄柏, Huangbai) Babylon Weeping Willow Leaf (柳叶, Liuye) Dutchmanspipe Fruit (马兜铃, Madouling) Common Fibraurea Stem (黄藤, Huangteng) Dandelion (蒲公英, Pugongying) Climbing Groundsel Herb (千里光, Qianliguang) Gypsum (石膏, Shigao) Cinnabar (朱砂, Zhusha) Indigowoad Leaf (大青叶, Daqingye) Chinese Thorowax Root (柴胡, Chaihu) Common Anemarrhea Rhizome (知母, Zhimu)

High fever: Sweet Wormwood (青蒿, Qinghao) Indian Mockstrawberry Herb (蛇莓, Shemei) Chlorite-schist (礞石, Mengshi) Chinese Waxgourd Exocarp (冬瓜皮, Dongguapi) Gypsum (石膏, Shigao) Common Anemarrhea Rhizome (知母, Zhimu) Indigowoad Leaf (大青叶, Daqingye) Cape Jasmine Fruit (栀子, Zhizi) Chinese Thorowax Root (柴胡, Chaihu)

Hemptysis: Inula Flower (旋覆花, Xuanfuhua) Rhubarb (大黄, Dahuang) Soot (百

草霜，Baicaoshuang）Baikal Skullcap Root（黄芩，Huangqin）Sanchi Root（三七，Sanqi）Heartlaef Houttuynia Herb（鱼腥草，Yuxingcao）Lalang Grass Rhizome（白茅根，Baimaogen）Bletilla Rhizome（白及，Baiji）Ramie Root（苎麻根，Zhumagen）Chinese Arborvitae Leafy Twig（侧柏叶，Cebaiye）

Pneumoconiosis: Pinellia Rhizome（半夏，Banxia）Bletilla Rhizome（白及，Baiji）Common Selfheal Spike（夏枯草，Xiakucao）Fourstamen Stephania Root（汉防己，Hanfangji）

Circulatory system diseases

Coronary heart disease: Twotooth Achyranthes Root（牛膝，Niuxi）Chinese Pyrola Herb（鹿衔草，Luxiancao）Safflower（红花，Honghua）Chrysanthemum Flower（菊花，Juhua）Zedoray（莪术，Ezhu）Hindu Datura Flower（曼陀罗花，Mantuoluohua）Turmeric Rhizome（姜黄，Jianghuang）Pinellia Rhizome（半夏，Banxia）Red Peony Root（赤芍药，Chishaoyao）Yerbadetajo Herb（墨旱莲，Mohanlian）Dan-shen Root（丹参，Danshen）Sanchi Root（三七，Sanqi）Membranous Milkvetch Root（黄芪，Huangqi）Common Burreed Rhizome（三棱，Sanleng）Yanhusuo（延胡索，Yanhusuo）Motherwort Herb（益母草，Yimucao）Szechwan Lovage Rhizome（川芎，Chuanxiong）Siberian Solomonseal Rhizome（黄精，Huangjing）Manyprickle Acanthopanax Root（刺五加，Ciwujia）Glossy Privet Leaf（女贞叶，Nvzhenye）Chinese Taxillus Twig（桑寄生，Sangjisheng）Ground Beetle（䗪虫，Zhechong）Ginkgo Seed（白果，Baiguo）Storesin（苏合香，Suhexiang）Leech（水蛭，Shuizhi）Sandalwood（檀香，Tanxiang）Babylon Weeping Willow Leaf（柳叶，Liuye）Snakegourd Fruit（瓜蒌，Gualou）Cow-bezoar（牛黄，Niuhuang）Hawthorn Fruit（山楂，Shanzha）Garlic Bulb（大蒜，Dasuan）

Angina pectoris: Manchurian Wildginger Herb（细辛，Xixin）Fourstamen Stephania Root（汉防己，Hanfangji）Lobed Kudzuvine Root（葛根，Gegen）Musk（麝香，Shexiang）Cattail Pollen（蒲黄，Puhuang）Honey（蜂蜜，Fengmi）Szechwan Lovage Rhizome（川芎，Chuanxiong）Sanchi Root（三七，Sanqi）Yanhusuo（延胡索，Yanhusuo）Trogopterus Dung（五灵脂，Wulingzhi）Dan-shen Root（丹参，Danshen）Cassia Twig（桂枝，Guizhi）

Acute myocardial infarction: Szechwan Lovage Rhizome（川芎，Chuanxiong）Lobed Kudzuvine Root（葛根，Gegen）Sanchi Root（三七，Sanqi）Dan-shen Root（丹参，Danshen）Musk（麝香，Shexiang）Storesin（苏合香，Suhexiang）Sandalwood（檀香，Tanxiang）

High blood pressure: Common Aucklandia Root（木香，Muxiang）Plantain Seed（车前子，Cheqianzi）Chinese Pyrola Herb（鹿衔草，Luxiancao）Black Nightshade Herb（龙葵，Longkui）Safflower（红花，Honghua）Feather Cockscomb Seed（青葙子，Qingxiangzi）Wild Mint（薄荷，Bohe）Indian Chrysanthemum Flower（野菊花，Yejuhua）Chrysanthemum Flower（菊花，Juhua）Rehmannia Dried Root（生地黄，Shengdihuang）Vinegar（醋，Cu）Turmeric Rhizome（姜黄，Jianghuang）Tree Peony Bark（牡丹皮，Mudanpi）Puncturevine Caltrap Fruit（白蒺藜，Baijili）Coptis Rhizome（黄连，Huanglian）Common Cruculigo（仙茅，Xianmao）Baikal Skullcap Root（黄芩，Huangqin）Sanchi Root（三七，Sanqi）Chinese Angelica Root（当归，Danggui）Chinese Gentian Root（龙胆草，Longdancao）Yanhusuo（延胡索，Yanhusuo）Magnetite（磁石，Cishi）Common Selfheal Fruit-spike（Common Selfheal Spike

(夏枯草，Xiakucao) Xiakucao) Ginseng (人参，Renshen) Acaleph (海蜇，Haizhe) Earthworm (蚯蚓，Qiuyin) Chinese Wolfberry Root-bark (地骨皮，Digupi) Eucommia Bark (杜仲，Duzhong) Medicinal Evodia Root (吴茱萸，Wuzhuyu) Common Buckwheat Seed (荞麦，Qiaomai) Dutchmanspipe Fruit (马兜铃，Madouling) Babylon Weeping Willow Leaf (柳叶，Liuye) Radish Seed (莱菔子，Laifuzi) Rice Bean (赤小豆，Chixiaodou) Gambirplant Hooked Stem and Branch (钩藤，Gouteng) Green Gram Seed (绿豆，Lvdou) Fourstamen Stephania Root (汉防己，Hanfangji) Oriental Waterplantain Rhizome (泽泻，Zexie) Lobed Kudzuvine Root (葛根，Gegen) Hawthorn Fruit (山楂，Shanzha) Honey (蜂蜜，Fengmi) Garlic Bulb (蒜，Suan) Tall Gastrodia Rhizome (天麻，Tianma) Cassia Seed (决明子，Juemingzi) Abalone Shell (石决明，Shijueming) Antelope Horn (羚羊角，Lingyangjiao) Twotooth Achyranthes Root (牛膝，Niuxi) Magnetite (磁石，Cishi) Hematite (代赭石，Daizheshi) Dan-shen Root (丹参，Danshen) Bear Gall (熊胆，Xiongdan)

Shock: Immature Bitter Orange (枳实，Zhishi) Green Tangerine Peel (青皮，Qingpi) Prepared Daughter Root of Common Monkshood (附子，Fuzi) Dried Ginger (干姜，Ganjiang) Ginseng (人参，Renshen)

Hypotension: Licorice Root (甘草，Gancao) Siberian Solomonseal Rhizome (黄精，Huangjing) Cassia Twig (桂枝，Guizhi) Ephedra (麻黄，Mahuang) Immature Bitter Orange (枳实，Zhishi) Prepared Daughter Root of Common Monkshood (附子，Fuzi)

Viral myocarclitis: Common Lophatherum Herb (淡竹叶，Danzhuye) Shorthorned Epimedium Herb (淫羊藿，Yinyanghuo) Motherwort Herb (益母草，Yimucao) Cassia Twig (桂枝，Guizhi)

Ke-shan disease: Whiteflower Patrinia Herb (败酱草，Baijiangcao) Camphortree Wood (樟木，Zhangmu) Hawthorn Fruit (山楂，Shanzha)

Congestive heart failure: Pepperweed Seed or Flixweed Tansymustard Seed (葶苈子，Tinglizi) Prepared Daughter Root of Common Monkshood (附子，Fuzi) Dan-shen Root (丹参，Danshen) Fragrant Solomonseal Rhizome (玉竹，Yuzhu) Ginseng (人参，Renshen) Immature Bitter Orange (枳实，Zhishi) Cortex Acanthopanacis Radicis (五加皮，Wujiap i) Szechwan Lovage Rhizome (川芎，Chuanxiong) Safflower (红花，Honghua)

Arrhythmia: Turmeric Root-tuber (郁金，Yujin) Prepared Daughter Root of Common Monkshood (附子，Fuzi) Dan-shen Root (丹参，Danshen) Chinese Angelica Root (当归，Danggui) Yanhusuo (延胡索，Yanhusuo) Lightyellow Sophora Root (苦参，Kushen) Chinese Taxillus Twig (桑寄生，Sangjisheng) Tonkin Sophora Root (山豆根，Shandougen) Lobed Kudzuvine Root (葛根，Gegen) Licorice Root (甘草，Gancao) Longan Aril (龙眼肉，Longyanrou) Chinese Date (大枣，Dazao) Blighted Wheat (浮小麦，Fuxiaomai) Lightyellow Sophora Root (苦参，Kushen)

Sinus tachycardia: Swordlike Atractylodes Rhizome (苍术，Cangzhu) Green Tangerine Peel (青皮，Qingpi) Fourstamen Stephania Root (防己，Fangji)

Extra systole: Safflower (红花，Honghua) Capillary Wormwood Herb (茵陈蒿，Yinchenhao) Membranous Milkvetch Root (黄芪，Huangqi) Licorice Root (甘草，Gancao) Yanhusuo (延胡索，Yanhusuo) Lightyellow Sophora Root (苦参，Kushen) Alumen (白矾，Baifan) Amur Barberry Root and Branchlet (小蘖, Xiaonie)

Atrioventricular block: Prepared Daughter Root of Common Monkshood (附子, Fuzi) Hairy Antler (鹿茸, Lurong)

Inadequacy of sinatrial node: Prepared Daughter Root of Common Monkshood (附子, Fuzi) Manchurian Wildginger Herb (细辛, Xixin) Siberian Solomonseal Rhizome (黄精, Huangjing) Malaytea Scurfpea Fruit (补骨脂, Buguzhi) Cassia Twig (桂枝, Guizhi)

Digestive system diseases

Inflammation of esophagus: Coastal Glehnia Root, and Fourleaf Ladybell Root (沙参, Shashen) Dwarf Lilyturf Root (麦门冬, Maimendong) Dendrobium Herb (石斛, Shihu) Fragrant Solomonseal Rhizome (玉竹, Yuzhu)

Acute gastroenteritis: Hyacinth Bean (扁豆, Biandou) Dried Ginger (干姜, Ganjiang) Clove Flower-bud (丁香, Dingxiang) Common Aucklandia Root (木香, Muxiang) Villous Amomum Fruit (砂仁, Sharen) Wrinkled Gianthyssop Herb (藿香, Huoxiang) Common Perilla Stem (苏梗, Sugeng) Bitter Orange (枳壳, Zhiqiao) Coptis Rhizome (黄连, Huanglian) Purslane Herb (马齿苋, Machixian)

Chronic gastritis: Talc (滑石, Huashi) Pinellia Rhizome (半夏, Banxia) Broadbean Seed (蚕豆, Candou) Opium Poppy Pericarp (罂粟壳, Yingsuqiao) Nutgrass Galingale Rhizome (香附, Xiangfu) Chinese Angelica Root (当归, Danggui) Dwarf Lilyturf Root (麦门冬, Maimendong) White Peony Root (白芍药, Baishaoyao) Membranous Milkvetch Root (黄芪, Huangqi) Barbary Wolfberry Fruit (枸杞子, Gouqizi) Sandalwood (檀香, Tanxiang) Fresh Ginger (生姜, Shengjiang) Garlic Bulb (蒜, Suan)

Vomiting: Hematite (代赭石, Daizheshi) Pinellia Rhizome (半夏, Banxia) Cooking Stove Earth (伏龙肝, Fulonggan) Inula Flower (旋覆花, Xuanfuhua) Fresh Ginger (生姜, Shengjiang) Loquat Leaf (枇杷叶, Pipaye) Reed Rhizome (芦根, Lugen) Wrinkled Gianthyssop Herb (藿香, Huoxiang) Finger Citron Fruit (佛手, Foshou)

Hiccup: Chinese Clematis Root (威灵仙, Weilingxian) Hawthorn Fruit (山楂, Shanzha) Iron Scales (生铁落, Shengtieluo) White Peony Root (白芍药, Baishaoyao) Rice Bean (赤小豆, Chixiaodou) Tuber Onion Seed (韭菜子, Jiucaozi) Persimmon Calyx and Receptacle (柿蒂, Shidi) Clove Flower-bud (丁香, Dingxiang) Sword Jackbean Seed (刀豆子, Daodouzi)

Hemorrhage of upper digestive tract: Hematite (代赭石, Daizheshi) Japanese Thistle Herb or Root (大蓟, Daji) Rehmannia Dried Root (生地黄, Shengdihuang) Rhubarb (大黄, Dahuang) Yerbadetajo Herb (墨旱莲, Mohanlian) Garden Burnet Root (地榆, Diyu) Sanchi Root (三七, Sanqi) Cuttle Bone (乌贼骨, Wuzeigu) Chinese Gall (五倍子, Wubeizi) Cooking Stove Earth (伏龙肝, Fulonggan) Pokeberry Root (商陆, Shanglu) Giant Knotweed Rhizome (虎杖, Huzhang) Chinese Angelica Root (当归, Danggui) Acacia Catechu (孩儿茶, Haiercha) Dragon's Blood (血竭, Xuejie) Cattail Pollen (蒲黄, Puhuang) Bletilla Rhizome (白及, Baiji) Copperleaf Root (苋菜根, Xiangcaigen) Chinese Arborvitae Leafy Twig (侧柏叶, Cebaiye) Oriental Stephania Root (白药子, Baiyaozi) Ramie Root (苎麻根, Zhumagen) Coptis Rhizome (黄连, Huanglian) Cape Jasmine Fruit (栀子, Zhizi)

Gastroptosia: Shunk Bugbane Rhizome (升

麻，Shengma）Swordlike Atractylodes Rhizome（苍术，Cangzhu）Immature Bitter Orange（枳实，Zhishi）Tangshen Root（党参，Dangshen）Membranous Milkvetch Root（黄芪，Huangqi）Chinese Thorowax Root（柴胡，Chaihu）

Stomachache：Lesser Galangal Rhizome（高良姜，Gaoliangjiang）Salt（食盐，Shiyan）Cooking Stove Earth（伏龙肝，Fulonggan）White Peony Root（白芍药，Baishaoyao）Dahurian Angelica Root（白芷，Baizhi）Ginseng（人参，Renshen）Black Pepper Fruit（胡椒，Hujiao）Chinese Eaglewood Wood（沉香，Chenxiang）Lily Bulb（百合，Baihe）Dried Ginger（干姜，Ganjiang）White Mustard Seed（白芥子，Baijiezi）Dandelion（蒲公英，Pugongying）Fennel Fruit（茴香，Huixiang）Japanese Buttercup Herb（毛茛，Maogen）Scabrous Doellingeria Herb（东风菜，Dongfengcai）Areca Seed（槟榔，Binlang）Common Aucklandia Root（木香，Muxiang）Nutgrass Galingale Rhizome（香附，Xiangfu）Officinal Magnolia Bark（厚朴，Houpo）Tangerine Peel（橘皮，Jupi）Szechwan chinaberry Fruit（川楝子，Chuanlianzi）

Gastroduodenal ulcer：Common Aucklandia Root（木香，Muxiang）Plantain Seed（车前子，Cheqianzi）Safflower（红花，Honghua）White Peony Root（白芍药，Baishaoyao）Garden Burnet Root（地榆，Diyu）Bletilla Rhizome（白及，Baiji）Membranous Milkvetch Root（黄芪，Huangqi）Songaria Cynomorium Herb（锁阳，Suoyang）Licorice Root（甘草，Gancao）Densefruit Pittany Root-bark（白鲜皮，Baixianpi）Tendrilleaf Fritillary Bulb（贝母，Beimu）Yanhusuo（延胡索，Yanhusuo）Acacia Catechu（孩儿茶，Haiercha）Alumen（白矾，Baifan）Cuttle Bone（乌贼骨，Wuzeigu）Earthworm（蚯蚓，Qiuyin）Pubescent Holly Root（毛冬青，Maodongqing）Clam Shell（海蛤壳，Haigeqiao）Oyster Shell（牡蛎，Muli）Large Blister Beetle（斑蝥，Banmao）Immature Bitter Orange（枳实，Zhishi）Malt Sugar（饴糖，Yitang）Jew's Ear（木耳，Muer）Myrrh（没药，Moyao）Honey（蜂蜜，Fengmi）Chinese Date（大枣，Dazao）Fresh Ginger（生姜，Shengjiang）Trogopterus Dung（五灵脂，Wulingzhi）Sanchi Root（三七，Sanqi）

Cirrhosis：Dan-shen Root（丹参，Danshen）Appendiculate Cremastra Pseudobulb（山慈姑，Shancigu）Largehead Atractylodes Rhizome（白术，Baizhu）Turtle Carapace（鳖甲，Biejia）Akebia Stem（木通，Mutong）Musk（麝香，Shexiang）Szechwan Lovage Rhizome（川芎，Chuanxiong）Zedoray（莪术，Ezhu）Green Tangerine Peel（青皮，Qingpi）Common Burreed Rhizome（三棱，Sanleng）

Chronic nonspecific ulcerative colitis：Rhubarb（大黄，Dahuang）Limonite（禹余粮，Yuyuliang）Pinellia Rhizome（半夏，Banxia）Natural Indigo（青黛，Qingdai）Acacia Catechu（孩儿茶，Haiercha）Chinese Corktree Bark（黄柏，Huangbai）Purslane Herb（马齿苋，Machixian）Diverse Wormwood Herb（刘寄奴，Liujinu）Coptis Rhizome（黄连，Huanglian）Alumen（明矾，Mingfan）Ass-hide Glue（阿胶，Ejiao）Cattail Pollen（蒲黄，Puhuang）

Acute hemorrhage necrotic enteritis：Rhubarb（大黄，Dahuang）Yerbadetajo Herb（墨旱莲，Mohanlian）Sanchi Root（三七，Sanqi）

Fungal enteritis：Acacia Catechu（孩儿茶，Haiercha）Chinese Corktree Bark（黄柏，Huangbai）Coix Seed（薏苡仁，Yiyiren）

Chronic dysentry：Sweet Wormwood（青蒿，Qinghao）Salt（食盐，Shiyan）Mirabilite Crystal（寒水石，Hanshuishi）Acacia Catechu

(孩儿茶, Haiercha) Longan Aril (龙眼肉, Longyanrou) Common Buckwheat Seed (荞麦, Qiaomai) India Madder Root (茜草, Qiancao) Wheat Fruit (小麦, Xiaomai) Hairy Antler (鹿茸, Lurong) Clove Flower-bud (丁香, Dingxiang) Garden Burnet Root (地榆, Diyu) Red Halloysite (赤石脂, Chishizhi) Limonite(禹余粮, Yuyuliang) Smoked Plum (乌梅, Wumei)

Bloody stool: Japanese Pagodatree Fruit (槐角, Huaijiao) Japanese Pagodatree Flower (槐花, Huaihua) Garden Burnet Root (地榆, Diyu) Bletilla Rhizome (白及, Baiji) Burnt Clay-lining of Kitchen Range (灶心土, Zaoxintu) Baked Rhizome (炮姜, Paojiang) Hindu Lotus Rhizome-node (藕节, Oujie) Smoked Plum (乌梅, Wumei)

Summer diarrhea: Wrinkled Gianthyssop Herb (藿香, Huoxiang) Talc (滑石, Huashi) Plantain Seed (车前子, Cheqianzi) Coptis Rhizome (黄连, Huanglian) Tuckahoe (茯苓, Fuling) Hyacinth Dolichos Flower (扁豆花, Biandouhua) Officinal Magnolia Immature Flower (厚朴花, Houpohua)

Constipation: Cassia Seed (决明子, Juemingzi) Hematite (代赭石, Daizheshi) Rhubarb (大黄, Dahuang) Chinese Angelica Root (当归, Danggui) Anhydrous Sodium Sulfate (玄明粉, Xuanmingfen) Bee Wax (蜂蜡, Fengla) Officinal Magnolia Bark (厚朴, Houpo) Mulberry Solomonseal (桑椹, Sangshen) Radish Seed (莱菔子, Laifuzi) Oriental Sesame Seed (黑芝麻, Heizhima) Tuber Fleeceflower Root (何首乌, Heshouwu) Honey (蜂蜜, Fengmi) Croton Seed (巴豆, Badou) Pharbitis Seed (牵牛子, Qianniuzi) Bushcherry Seed (郁李仁, Yuliren) Hemp Seed (火麻仁, Huomaren) Chinese Arborvitae Seed (柏子仁, Baiziren) Mongolian Snakegourd Seed (瓜蒌仁, Gualouren) Peach Seed (桃仁, Taoren)

Heat stroke: Talc (滑石, Huashi) Salt (食盐, Shiyan) Hyacinth Bean (扁豆, Biandou) Rice Bean (赤小豆, Chixiaodou) Green Gram Seed (绿豆, Lvdou)

Viral enteritis: Chinese Pyrola Herb (鹿衔草, Luxiancao) Chinese Gall (五倍子, Wubeizi) Camphortree Wood (樟木, Zhangmu)

Acute pancreatitis: Rhubarb (大黄, Dahuang) White Peony Root (白芍药, Baishaoyao) Cow-bezoar (牛黄, Niuhuang)

Ascites: Lilac Daphne Flower-bud (芫花, Yuanhua) Kansui Root (甘遂, Gansui) Oyster Shell (牡蛎, Muli) Carp (鲤鱼, Liyu) Chinese Corktree Bark (黄柏, Huangbai) Pepperweed Seed or Flixweed Tansymustard Seed (葶苈子, Tinglizi) Whiteflower Patrinia Herb (败酱草, Baijiangcao) Chinese Elder Flower (陆英, Luting) Areca Peel (大腹皮, Dafupi) Areca Seed (槟榔, Binlang) Pharbitis Seed (牵牛子, Qianniuzi)

Urinary system diseases

Acute glomerulonephritis: Asiatic Plantain Herb (车前草, Cheqiancao) Pepperweed Seed or Flixweed Tansymustard Seed (葶苈子, Tinglizi) Ephedra (麻黄, Mahuang) Common Rush Stem Pith (灯芯, Dengxin) Turmeric Root-tuber (郁金, Yujin) Chinese Lobelia Herb (半边莲, Banbianlian) Japanese Climbing Fern Spores (海金沙, Haijinsha) Weeping Forsythia Capsule (连翘, Lianqiao) European Verbena Herb (马鞭草, Mabiancao) Baikal Skullcap Root (黄芩, Huangqin) Membranous Milkvetch Root (黄芪, Huangqi) Lalang Grass Rhizome (白茅根, Baimaogen) Motherwort Herb (益母草, Yimucao) Flaccid Knotweed Herb (辣蓼草,

Laliaocao) Cicada Slough (蝉蜕, Chantui) Black Pepper Fruit (胡椒, Hujiao) Honeysuckle Flower (金银花, Jinyinhua) Human Milk (人乳汁, Renruzhi) Tuber Onion Leaf (韭菜, Jiucao) Garlic Bulb (大蒜, Dasuan) Japanese Felt Fern Leaf (石韦, Shiwei) Common Ducksmeat Herb (浮萍, Fuping)

Chronic nephritis: Motherwort Herb (益母草, Yimucao) Thinleaf Adina Stem and Leaf (水杨梅, Shuiyangmei) Szechwan Lovage Rhizome (川芎, Chuanxiong) Carp (鲤鱼, Liyu) Leech (水蛭, Shuizhi)

Urinaemia: Prepared Daughter Root of Common Monkshood (附子, Fuzi) Dandelion (蒲公英, Pugongying) Rhubarb (大黄, Dahuang)

Purpura nephritis: Motherwort Herb (益母草, Yimucao) Amber (琥珀, Hupo)

Chronic renal failure: Rhubarb (大黄, Dahuang) Prepared Daughter Root of Common Monkshood (附子, Fuzi)

Urinary infection: Plantain Seed (车前子, Cheqianzi) Talc (滑石, Huashi) Rhubarb (大黄, Dahuang) Dodder Seed (菟丝子, Tusizi) Japanese Pagodatree Fruit (槐角, Huaijiao) Purslane Herb (马齿苋, Machixian) Common Knotgrass Herb (萹蓄, Bianxu) Lilac Pink Herb (瞿麦, Qumai) Akebia Stem (木通, Mutong) Japanese Climbing Fern Spores (海金沙, Haijinsha) Japanese Felt Fern Leaf (石韦, Shiwei) Sevenlobed Yam Rhizome (萆薢, Bixie)

Acute pyelonephritis: Pubescent Holly Root (毛冬青, Maodongqing) Hawthorn Fruit (山楂, Shanzha) Christina Loosetrife Herb (金钱草, Jinqiancao) Japanese Climbing Fern Spores (海金沙, Haijinsha) Sevenlobed Yam Rhizome (萆薢, Bixie) Akebia Stem (木通, Mutong) Plantain Seed (车前子, Cheqianzi)

Cystitis: Talc (滑石, Huashi) Purslane Herb (马齿苋, Machixian) Ass-hide Glue (阿胶, Ejiao)

Anuresis: Tatarian Aster Root (紫苑, Ziyuan) Sweet Wormwood (青蒿, Qinghao) Diverse Wormwood Herb (刘寄奴, Liujinu) Salt (食盐, Shiyan) Kansui Root (甘遂, Gansui) Balloonflower Root (桔梗, Jiegeng) Licorice Root (甘草, Gancao) Chinese Angelica Root (当归, Danggui) Borax (硼砂, Pengsha) Alumen (白矾, Baifan) Dragon's Blood (血竭, Xuejie) Cochinchina Momordica Seed (木鳖子, Mubiezi) Fresh Ginger (生姜, Shengjiang) Shepherdspurse Herb with Root (荠菜, Jicai) Garlic Bulb (蒜, Suan) Earth Worm (地龙, Dilong) Christina Loosetrife Herb (金钱草, Jinqiancao) Akebia Stem (木通, Mutong) Japanese Climbing Fern Spores (海金沙, Haijinsha) Plantain Seed (车前子, Cheqianzi) Oriental Waterplantain Rhizome (泽泻, Zexie) Common Knotgrass Herb (萹蓄, Bianxu)

Hematuria: European Verbena Herb (马鞭草, Mabiancao) Sanchi Root (三七, Sanqi) Amber (琥珀, Hupo) India Madder Root (茜草, Qiancao) Lilac Pink Herb (瞿麦, Qumai) Common Cephalanoplos Herb (小蓟, Xiaoji) Japanese Thistle Herb or Root (大蓟, Daji) Japanese Felt Fern Leaf (石韦, Shiwei) Japanese Climbing Fern Spores (海金沙, Haijinsha) Lalang Grass Rhizome (白茅根, Baimaogen)

Chyluria: Thinleaf Milkwort Root (远志, Yuanzhi) Blackberrylily Rhizome (射干, Shegan) Shepherdspurse Herb with Root (荠菜, Jicai) Chinaroot Greenbrier Rhizome (菝葜, Baqia) Sevenlobed Yam Rhizome (萆薢, Bixie)

Hydrops: Chalcanthnium (胆矾, Danfan) Pokeberry Root (商陆, Shanglu) Lightyellow

Sophora Root (苦参, Kushen) Tuckahoe (茯苓, Fuling) Broadbean Seed (蚕豆, Candou) Watermelon Pericarp (西瓜皮, Xiguapi) White Mulberry Root-bark (桑白皮, Sangbaipi) Rice Bean (赤小豆, Chixiaodou) Umbellate Pore Fungus (猪苓, Zhuling) Oriental Waterplantain Rhizome (泽泻, Zexie) Plantain Seed (车前子, Cheqianzi) Areca Peel (大腹皮, Dafupi) Cortex Acanthopanacis Radicis (五加皮, Wujiapi) Fresh Ginger Peel (生姜皮, Shengjiangpi) Fourstamen Stephania Root (防己, Fangji)

Hematopathy

Iron-deficiency anemia: Ginseng (人参, Renshen) Ass-hide Glue (阿胶, Ejiao) Chinese Angelica Root (当归, Danggui) Mulberry Solomonseal (桑椹, Sangshen) Longan Aril (龙眼肉, Longyanrou) White Peony Root (白芍药, Baishaoyao) Dried Human Placenta (紫河车, Ziheche) Prepared Rhizome of Adhesive Rehmannia (熟地黄, Shoudihuang)

Aplastic anemia: Membranous Milkvetch Root (黄芪, Huangqi) Turtle (鳖, Bie) Hairy Antler (鹿茸, Lurong) Ginseng (人参, Renshen) Chinese Angelica Root (当归, Danggui) Prepared Rhizome of Adhesive Rehmannia (熟地黄, Shoudihuang)

Polycythemia vera: Motherwort Herb (益母草, Yimucao) Leech (水蛭, Shuizhi) Realgar (雄黄, Xionghuang) Dan-shen Root (丹参, Danshen)

Leukemia: Natural Indigo (青黛, Qingdai) Chinese Gentian Root (龙胆草, Longdancao) Cow-bezoar (牛黄, Niuhuang) Realgar (雄黄, Xionghuang)

Leukopenia: Suberect Spatholobus Stem (鸡血藤, Jixueteng) Giant Knotweed Rhizome (虎杖, Huzhang) Shorthorned Epimedium Herb (淫羊藿, Yinyanghuo) Membranous Milkvetch Root (黄芪, Huangqi) Largehead Atractylodes Rhizome (白术, Baizhu) Lightyellow Sophora Root (苦参, Kushen) Siberian Solomonseal Rhizome (黄精, Huangjing) Malaytea Scurfpea Fruit (补骨脂, Buguzhi) Manyprickle Acanthopanax Root (刺五加, Ciwujia) Glossy Privet Fruit (女贞子, Nuzhenzi) Walnut (胡桃仁, Hutaoren) India Madder Root (茜草, Qiancao)

Primary thrombocytopenic purpura: Chinese Pyrola Herb (鹿衔草, Luxiancao) Common Scouring Rush Herb (木贼, Muzei) Pokeberry Root (商陆, Shanglu) Weeping Forsythia Capsule (连翘, Lianqiao) Chinese Thorowax Root (柴胡, Chaihu) Root of Sinkiang Arnebia (紫草, Zicao) Songaria Cynomorium Herb (锁阳, Suoyang) Licorice Root (甘草, Gancao) Ass-hide Glue (阿胶, Ejiao) Buffalo Horn (水牛角, Shuiniujiao) Membranous Milkvetch Root (黄芪, Huangqi) Hairy Antler (鹿茸, Lurong)

Immune system diseases, collagen diseases

Rheumatic fever: Sweet Wormwood (青蒿, Qinghao) Membranous Milkvetch Root (黄芪, Huangqi) Fourstamen Stephania Root (防己, Fangji) Honeysuckle Stem(忍冬藤, Rendongteng) Largeleaf Gentian Root (秦艽, Qinjiao) Chinese Corktree Bark (黄柏, Huangbai) Akebia Stem (木通, Mutong) Scorpion (全蝎, Quanxie) Garter Snake (乌梢蛇, Wushaoshe)

Rheumatic arthritis: Nut-vomitive Poisonnut Seed (马钱子, Maqianzi) Chinese Magnoliavine (五味子, Wuweizi) Tall Gastrodia Rhizome (天麻, Tianma) Silkworm Feculae (蚕砂, Cansha) Manyprickle Acanthopanax

Root（刺五加，Ciwujia）Brevicaude Pit Viper（蝮蛇，Fushe）Dung Beetle（蜣螂，Qianglang）Scorpion（全蝎，Quanxie）Chinese Honeylocust Spine（皂角刺，Zaojiaoci）Solomonseal（桑椹，Sangshen）Dasheen Tuber（芋头，Yutou）India Madder Root（茜草，Qiancao）Lilac Daphne Flower-bud（芫花，Yuanhua）Chinaroot Greenbrier Rhizome（菝葜，Baqia）Japanese Buttercup Herb（毛茛，Maogen）Garter Snake（乌梢蛇，Wushaoshe）Doubleteeth Pulbescent Angelica Root（独活，Duhuo）Chinese Clematis Root（威灵仙，Weilingxian）Largeleaf Gentian Root（秦艽，Qinjiao）Common Floweringquince Fruit（木瓜，Mugua）Prepared Daughter Root of Common Monkshood（附子，Fuzi）Kadsura Pepper Stem（海风藤，Haifengteng）

Rheumatoid arthritis：Herb of Siberian Cocklebur（苍耳草，Cangercao)Common St. Paulswort Herb（豨莶草，Xixiancao）Rehmannia Dried Root（生地黄，Shengdihuang）Nut-vomitive Poisonnut Seed（马钱子，Maqianzi）Kansui Root（甘遂，Gansui）Giant Knotweed Rhizome（虎杖，Huzhang）Doubleteeth Pulbescent Angelica Root（独活，Duhuo）Chinese Angelica Root（当归，Danggui）Membranous Milkvetch Root（黄芪，Huangqi）Divaricate Saposhnikovia Root（防风，Fangfeng）Manchurian Wildginger Herb（细辛，Xixin）Ant（蚂蚁，Mayi）Dung Beetle（蜣螂，Qianglang）Brevicaude Pit Viper（蝮蛇，Fushe）Large Blister Beetle（斑蝥，Banmao）Iunate Peltate Sundew Herb（茅膏菜，Maogaocai）Chinese Clematis Root（威灵仙，Weilingxian）Garlic Bulb（蒜，Suan）

Ostecarthrosis deformans endemica：Gypsum（石膏，Shigao）Chinese Pine Node（松节，Songjie）

Metabolism endocrinopathy

Diabetes: Dwarf Lilyturf Root（麦门冬，Maimendong）Rehmannia Dried Root（生地黄，Shengdihuang）Gypsum（石膏，Shigao）White Peony Root（白芍药，Baishaoyao）Siberian Solomonseal Rhizome（黄精，Huangjing）Ginseng（人参，Renshen）Silkworm with Batrytis Larva（白僵蚕，Baijiangcan）Chinese Wolfberry Root-bark（地骨皮，Digupi）Manyprickle Acanthopanax Root（刺五加，Ciwujia）Chinese Gall（五倍子，Wubeizi）Lychee Fruit（荔枝，Lizhi）Radish Seed（莱菔子，Laifuzi）Rice Bean（赤小豆，Chixiaodou）Chinaroot Greenbrier Rhizome（菝葜，Baqia）Common Yam Rhizome（山药，Shanyao）Mazie Style（玉米须，Yumixu）

Adiposis：Plantain Seed（车前子，Cheqianzi）Uniflower Swisscentaury Root（漏芦，Loulu）Barbary Wolfberry Fruit（枸杞子，Gouqizi）White Mustard Seed（白芥子，Baijiezi）Senna Leaf（番泻叶，Fanxieye）

Hypertipoproteinemia：Cassia Seed（决明子，Juemingzi）Indian Chrysanthemum Flower（野菊花，Yejuhua）Capillary Wormwood Herb（茵陈蒿，Yinchenhao）Chrysanthemum Flower（菊花，Juhua）Turmeric Root-tuber（郁金，Yujin）Turmeric Rhizome（姜黄，Jianghuang）Giant Knotweed Rhizome（虎杖，Huzhang）Sanchi Root（三七，Sanqi）Fragrant Solomonseal Rhizome（玉竹，Yuzhu）Tall Gastrodia Rhizome（天麻，Tianma）Szechwan Lovage Rhizome（川芎，Chuanxiong）Siberian Solomonseal Rhizome（黄精，Huangjing）Alumen（白矾，Baifan）Pubescent Holly Root（毛冬青，Maodongqing）Silkworm with Batrytis Larva（白僵蚕，Baijiangcan）Manyprickle Acanthopanax Root (刺五加, Ciwujia) Honeysuckle Flower (金银花, Jinyinhua) Ginkgo Seed (白果, Baiguo) Sevenlobed Yam Rhizome (萆薢, Bixie) Leech (水蛭, Shuizhi) Coix Seed (薏苡仁, Yiyiren) Malt (麦芽, Maiya) Oriental Waterplantain Rhizome (泽泻, Zexie) Hawthorn Fruit (山楂, Shanzha) Cattail Pollen (蒲黄, Puhuang) Myrrh (没药, Moyao) Garlic Bulb (蒜, Suan) Tuber Fleeceflower Root (何首乌, Heshouwu)

Gout: Appendiculate Cremastra Pseudobulb (山慈姑, Shancigu) Garter Snake (乌蛇, Wushe) Prepared Daughter Root of Common Monkshood (附子, Fuzi) Kusnezoff Monkhood Root (草乌, Caowu) Scorpion (全蝎, Quanxie) Centipede (蜈蚣, Wugong) Manchurian Wildginger Herb (细辛, Xixin)

Nervous system diseases

Cerebral infarction: Twotooth Achyranthes Root (牛膝, Niuxi) Safflower (红花, Honghua) Chinese Angelica Root (当归, Danggui) Szechwan Lovage Rhizome (川芎, Chuanxiong) Manchurian Wildginger Herb (细辛, Xixin) Centipede (蜈蚣, Wugong) Earth Worm (地龙, Dilong) Manyprickle Acanthopanax Root (刺五加, Ciwujia) Brevicaude Pit Viper (蝮蛇, Fushe) Camphor (樟脑, Zhangnao) Leech (水蛭, Shuizhi) Snakegourd Fruit (瓜蒌, Gualou) Cow-bezoar (牛黄, Niuhuang) Gambirplant Hooked Stem and Branch (钩藤, Gouteng) Lobed Kudzuvine Root (葛根, Gegen) Blackend Swallowwort Root(白薇, Baiwei) Nut-vomitive Poisonnut Seed (马钱子, Maqianzi) Suberect Spatholobus Stem (鸡血藤, Jixueteng) Membranous Milkvetch Root (黄芪, Huangqi) Dan-shen Root (丹参, Danshen) Musk (麝香, Shexiang)

Cerebral arteriosclerosis: Safflower (红花, Honghua) Dan-shen Root (丹参, Danshen) Tall Gastrodia Rhizome (天麻, Tianma) Chinese Angelica Root (当归, Danggui) Lobed Kudzuvine Root (葛根, Gegen)

Epilepsy: Chalcanthnium (胆矾, Danfan) Hematite (代赭石, Daizheshi) Nut-vomitive Poisonnut Seed (马钱子, Maqianzi) Turmeric Root-tuber (郁金, Yujin) Iron Scales (生铁落, Shengtieluo) Cinnabar (朱砂, Zhusha) Kansui Root (甘遂, Gansui) Arisaema with Bile (胆南星, Dannanxing) Natural Indigo (青黛, Qingdai) Tall Gastrodia Rhizome (天麻, Tianma) Chlorite-schist (礞石, Mengshi) Borax (硼砂, Pengsha) Manchurian Wildginger Herb (细辛, Xixin) Silkworm with Batrytis Larva (白僵蚕, Baijiangcan) Centipede (蜈蚣, Wugong) Earthworm (蚯蚓, Qiuyin) Grassleaf Sweetflag Rhizome (石菖蒲, Shichangpu) Scorpion (全蝎, Quanxie) Lizard (蜥蝎, Xiyi) Black Pepper Fruit (胡椒, Hujiao) Olive (橄榄, Ganlan) Ginkgo Seed (白果, Baiguo) Medicated Leaven (神曲, Shenqu) Pharbitis Seed (牵牛子, Qianniuzi) Antelope Horn (羚羊角, Lingyangjiao)

Cysticercosis: Ture Lacquertree Dried Lacquer (干漆, Ganqi) Areca Seed (槟榔, Binlang)

Facial neuritis: Cinnabar (朱砂, Zhusha) Chinese Honeylocust Spine (皂角, Zaojiao) Dragon's Blood (血竭, Xuejie) Lobed Kudzuvine Root (葛根, Gegen) Chinese Clematis Root (威灵仙, Weilingxian) Centipede (蜈蚣, Wugong) Scorpion (全蝎, Quanxie)

Peripheral neuritis: Ass-hide Glue (阿胶, Ejiao) Common Cnidium Fruit (蛇床子, Shechuangzi)

Facial paralysis: Nut-vomitive Poisonnut Seed (马钱子, Maqianzi) Dahurian Angelica Root (白芷, Baizhi) Jackinthepulpit Tuber (天南星, Tiannanxing) Small Centipeda

Herb (鹅不食草, Ebushicao) Large Blister Beetle (斑蝥, Banmao) Scorpion (全蝎, Quanxie) Croton Seed (巴豆, Badou) Mud Eel (鳝鱼, Shanyu) Cochinchina Momordica Seed (木鳖子, Mubiezi) Cassia Twig (桂枝, Guizhi) Fistular Onion Stalk (葱白, Congbai) White Mustard Seed (白芥子, Baijiezi) Divaricate Saposhnikovia Root (防风, Fangfeng) Centipede (蜈蚣, Wugong)

Prosopalgia (trigeminal neuralgia): Nutvomitive Poisonnut Seed (马钱子, Maqianzi) White Peony Root (白芍药, Baishaoyao) Manchurian Wildginger Herb (细辛, Xixin) Silkworm with Batrytis Larva (白僵蚕, Baijiangcan) Earth Worm (地龙, Dilong) Spine Date Seed (酸枣仁, Suanzaoren) Paniculate Swallowwort Root (徐长卿, Xuchangqing) Yanhusuo (延胡索, Yanhusuo)

Neurosism: Manyprickle Acanthopanax Root (刺五加, Ciwujia) Ass-hide Glue (阿胶, Ejiao) Siberian Solomonseal Rhizome (黄精, Huangjing) Whiteflower Patrinia Herb (败酱草, Baijiangcao) Chrysanthemum Flower (菊花, Juhua) Inula Flower (旋覆花, Xuanfuhua) Iron Scales (生铁落, Shengtieluo) Chinese Magnoliavine (五味子, Wuweizi) Thinleaf Milkwort Root (远志, Yuanzhi) Shorthorned Epimedium Herb (淫羊藿, Yinyanghuo) Tall Gastrodia Rhizome (天麻, Tianma) Paniculate Swallowwort Root (徐长卿, Xuchangqing) Ginseng (人参, Renshen) Ant (蚂蚁, Mayi) Spine Date Seed (酸枣仁, Suanzaoren) Lily Bulb (百合, Baihe) Wheat Fruit (小麦, Xiaomai) Honey (蜂蜜, Fengmi) Chinese Angelica Root (当归, Danggui)

Insomnia: Yanhusuo (延胡索, Yanhusuo) Lightyellow Sophora Root (苦参, Kushen) Ass-hide Glue (阿胶, Ejiao) Silktree Albiziae Bark (合欢皮, Hehuanpi) Spine Date Seed (酸枣仁, Suanzaoren) Dragon's Teeth (龙齿, Longchi) Lily Bulb (百合, Baihe) Coptis Rhizome (黄连, Huanglian) Wheat Fruit (小麦, Xiaomai) Tuber Fleeceflower Root (何首乌, Heshouwu) Tuber Fleeceflower Stem and Leaf (夜交藤, Yejiaoteng) Cinnabar (朱砂, Zhusha) Amber (琥珀, Hupo) Dragon's Bone (龙骨, Longgu)

Vertigo: Inula Flower (旋覆花, Xuanfuhua) Tall Gastrodia Rhizome (天麻, Tianma) Medicinal Evodia Root (吴茱萸, Wuzhuyu) Babylon Weeping Willow Branchlet (柳枝, Liuzhi) Fresh Ginger (生姜, Shengjiang) Largehead Atractylodes Rhizome (白术, Baizhu) Pinellia Rhizome (半夏, Banxia) Hematite (代赭石, Daizheshi) Chrysanthemum Flower (菊花, Juhua) Abalone Shell (石决明, Shijueming) Oriental Waterplantain Rhizome (泽泻, Zexie) Tuckahoe (茯苓, Fuling)

Headache: Twotooth Achyranthes Root (牛膝, Niuxi) Tall Gastrodia Rhizome (天麻, Tianma) Chinese Angelica Root (当归, Danggui) Szechwan Lovage Rhizome (川芎, Chuanxiong) Manchurian Wildginger Herb (细辛, Xixin) Cicada Slough (蝉蜕, Chantui) Ginkgo Seed (白果, Baiguo) Medicinal Evodia Root (吴茱萸, Wuzhuyu) Scorpion (全蝎, Quanxie) Camphor (樟脑, Zhangnao) Common Buckwheat Seed (荞麦, Qiaomai) Lobed Kudzuvine Root (葛根, Gegen) Clove Flower-bud (丁香, Dingxiang) Salt (食盐, Shiyan) Dahurian Angelica Root (白芷, Baizhi) Divaricate Saposhnikovia Root (防风, Fangfeng) Gambirplant Hooked Stem and Branch (钩藤, Gouteng) Glabrous Greenbrier Rhizome (土茯苓, Tufuling) Mulberry Leaf (桑叶, Sangye) Chrysanthemum Flower (菊花, Juhua) Fineleaf Schizomepeta Herb (荆芥, Jingjie)

Psychosis

Schizophrenia: Safflower (红花, Honghua) Hematite (代赭石, Daizheshi) Hindu Datura Flower (曼陀罗花, Mantuoluohua) Iron Scales (生铁落, Shengtieluo) Cinnabar (朱砂, Zhusha) Pinellia Rhizome (半夏, Banxia) Prepared Daughter Root of Common Monkshood (附子, Fuzi) Chlorite-schist (礞石, Mengshi) Magnetite (磁石, Cishi) Lightyellow Sophora Root (苦参, Kushen) Tuckahoe (茯苓, Fuling) Earthworm (蚯蚓, Qiuyin) Grassleaf Sweetflag Rhizome (石菖蒲, Shichangpu) Chinese Eaglewood Wood (沉香, Chenxiang) Radish Seed (莱菔子, Laifuzi) Cow-bezoar (牛黄, Niuhuang) Tuber Fleeceflower Root (何首乌, Heshouwu) Turmeric Root-tuber (郁金, Yujin)

Reactive psychosis: Datura Flower (洋金花, Yangjinhua)

Hysteria: Wheat Fruit (小麦, Xiaomai) Licorice Root (甘草, Gancao) Chinese Date (大枣, Dazao) Lily Bulb (百合, Baihe)

Nosotoxicosis

Food poisoning: Chalcanthnium (胆矾, Danfan) Licorice Root (甘草, Gancao) Shunk Bugbane Rhizome (升麻, Shengma) Honeysuckle Flower (金银花, Jinyinhua) Hyacinth Bean (扁豆, Biandou) Cushaw Fruit Stem (南瓜藤, Nanguateng) Apricot Back (杏树皮, Xingshupi) Dasheen Tuber (芋头, Yutou) Green Gram Seed (绿豆, Lvdou) Fourstamen Stephania Root (防己, Fangji) Lobed Kudzuvine Root (葛根, Gegen) Honey (蜂蜜, Fengmi) Fresh Ginger (生姜, Shengjiang) Perilla Leaf (紫苏, Zisu)

White arsenic poisoning: Divaricate Saposhnikovia Root (防风, Fangfeng) Green Gram Seed (绿豆, Lvdou)

Lead poisoning: Male Fern Rhizome (贯众, Guanzhong) Garlic Bulb (大蒜, Dasuan)

Acute alcoholism: Lobed Kudzuvine Flower (葛花, Gehua)

Soft tissue diseases

Wound, scabies, cellulitis, carbuncle: Siberian Cocklebur Fruit (苍耳子, Cangerzi) Indian Chrysanthemum Flower (野菊花, Yejuhua) Vinegar (醋, Cu) Manyleaf Paris Rhizome (蚤休, Zaoxiu) Nut-vomitive Poisonnut Seed (马钱子, Maqianzi) Chinese Lobelia Herb (半边莲, Banbianlian) Soot (百草霜, Baicaoshuang) Giant Knotweed Rhizome (虎杖, Huzhang) Puncturevine Caltrap Fruit (白蒺藜, Baijili) European Verbena Herb (马鞭草, Mabiancao) Chinese Pulsatilla Root (白头翁, Baitouweng) Common Cruculigo (仙茅, Xianmao) Doubleteeth Pulbescent Angelica Root (独活, Duhuo) Membranous Milkvetch Root (黄芪, Huangqi) Sulfur (硫黄, Liuhuang) Figwortflower Picrorhiza Rhizome (胡黄连, Huhuanglian) Magnetite (磁石, Cishi) Vasps Nest (露蜂房, Lufengfang) Silkworm with Batrytis Larva (白僵蚕, Baijiangcan) Barbary Wolfberry Fruit (枸杞子, Gouqizi) Centipede (蜈蚣, Wugong) Toad (蟾蜍, Chanchu) Chinese Gall (五倍子, Wubeizi) Officinal Magnolia Bark (厚朴, Houpo) Slug (蛞蝓, Kuoyu) Common Buckwheat Seed (荞麦, Qiaomai) Human Milk (人乳汁, Renruzhi) Lily Bulb (百合, Baihe) Rice Bean (赤小豆, Chixiaodou) Dandelion (蒲公英, Pugongying) Wheat Fruit (小麦, Xiaomai) Green Gram Seed (绿豆, Lvdou) Weeping Forsythia Capsule (连翘, Lianqiao)

Honeysuckle Flower（金银花，Jinyinhua）Tokyo Violet Herb（紫花地丁，Zihuadiding）

Ersipelas：Common Dayflower Herb（鸭跖草，Yazhicao）Indian Chrysanthemum Flower（野菊花，Yejuhua）Mirabilite（朴硝，Piaoxiao）Nut－vomitive Poisonnut Seed（马钱子，Maqianzi）Earthworm（蚯蚓，Qiuyin）Scorpion（全蝎，Quanxie）Glabrous Greenbrier Rhizome（土茯苓，Tufuling）Indigowoad Leaf（大青叶，Daqingye）Dyers Woad Root（板蓝根，Banlangen）Tokyo Violet Herb（紫花地丁，Zihuadiding）

Acute phlegmon：Babylon Weeping Willow Leaf（柳叶，Liuye）Dandelion（蒲公英，Pugongying）Honeysuckle Flower（金银花，Jinyinhua）Indigowoad Leaf（大青叶，Daqingye）

Tetanus：Divaricate Saposhnikovia Root（防风，Fangfeng）Centipede（蜈蚣，Wugong）Cicada Slough（蝉蜕，Chantui）Scorpion（全蝎，Quanxie）Mulberry Twig（桑枝，Sangzhi）Common Floweringquince Fruit（木瓜，Mugua）Musk（麝香，Shexiang）Jackinthepulpit Tuber（天南星，Tiannanxing）Garter Snake（乌蛇，Wushe）

Cervical part diseases

Simple goiter：Chinese Gall（五倍子，Wubeizi）Airpotato Yam Tuber（黄药子，Huangyaozi）Common Selfheal Spike（夏枯草，Xiakucao）Babylon Weeping Willow Leaf（柳叶，Liuye）Seaweed（海藻，Haizao）Kelp（昆布，Kunbu）Figwort Root（玄参，Xuanshen）

Hyperthyroidism：Pinellia Rhizome（半夏，Banxia）Dandelion（蒲公英，Pugongying）Copperleaf Root（苋菜根，Xiancaigen）Airpotato Yam Tuber（黄药子，Huangyaozi）

Lymphadenectasis：Chinese Pulsatilla Root（白头翁，Baitouweng）Figwort Root（玄参，Xuanshen）Amber（琥珀，Hupo）Realgar（雄黄，Xionghuang）Oyster Shell（牡蛎，Muli）Thunberg Fritillary Bulb（浙贝母，Zhebeimu）Seaweed（海藻，Haizao）Common Selfheal Spike（夏枯草，Xiakucao）

Mastosis

Gynecogenic breast：Myrrh（没药，Moyao）

Chronic cystic mastitis：Uniflower Swisscentaury Root（漏芦，Loulu）Pokeberry Root（商陆，Shanglu）Szechwan Lovage Rhizome（川芎，Chuanxiong）Pangolin Scales（穿山甲，Chuanshanjia）Croton Seed（巴豆，Badou）Leech（水蛭，Shuizhi）Medicated Leaven（神曲，Shenqu）Frankincense（乳香，Ruxiang）Scorpion（全蝎，Quanxie）Snakegroud Root（天花粉，Tianhuafen）Chinese Angelica Root（当归，Danggui）Membranous Milkvetch Root（黄芪，Huangqi）White Mustard Seed（白芥子，Baijiezi）

Acute mastitis：Cowherb Seed（王不留行，Wangbuliuxing）Belvedere Fruit（地肤子，Difuzi）Cassia Seed（决明子，Juemingzi）Japanese Thistle Herb or Root（大蓟，Daji）Mirabilite（朴硝，Piaoxiao）Turmeric Roottuber（郁金，Yujin）Pinellia Rhizome（半夏，Banxia）Anhydrous Sodium Sulfate（玄明粉，Xuanmingfen）Red Peony Root（赤芍药，Chishaoyao）Thinleaf Milkwort Root（远志，Yuanzhi）Licorice Root（甘草，Gancao）Hirsute Shiny Bugleweed Herb（泽兰，Zelan）Alumen（明矾，Mingfan）Bee Wax（蜂蜡，Fengla）Vasps Nest（露蜂房，Lufengfang）Silkworm with Batrytis Larva（白僵蚕，Baijiangcan）Centipede（蜈蚣，Wugong）Scorpion（全蝎，Quanxie）Croton Seed（巴豆，Badou）Chinese Honeylocust Spine（皂角，Zaojiao）Beardie（泥鳅鱼，Niqiuyu）Tangerine Peel (橘皮, Jupi) Flower Bud of Japanese Pagodatree (槐米, Huaimi) Fistular Onion Stalk (葱白, Congbai) Dandelion (蒲公英, Pugongying) Antler (鹿角, Lujiao) Lilac Daphne Flower-bud (芫花, Yuanhua) Myrrh (没药, Moyao) Chinese Clematis Root (威灵仙, Weilingxian) Garlic Bulb (蒜, Suan) Honeysuckle Flower (金银花, Jinyinhua) Weeping Forsythia Capsule (连翘, Lianqiao) Snakegroud Root (天花粉, Tianhuafen) Thunberg Fritillary Bulb (浙贝母, Zhebeimu)

Abdominal diseases

Acute perforation of gastroduodenal ulcer: Bletilla Rhizome (白及, Baiji) Cuttle Bone (乌贼骨, Wuzeigu) Sanchi Root (三七, Sanqi)

Acute appendicitis: Whiteflower Patrinia Herb (败酱草, Baijiangcao) Mirabilite (朴消, Poxiao) Indian Mockstrawberry Herb (蛇莓, Shemei) Rhubarb (大黄, Dahuang) Spanishneedles Herb (鬼针草, Guizhengcao) Giant Knotweed Rhizome (虎杖, Huzhang) Chinese Gentian Root (龙胆草, Longdancao) Flaccid Knotweed Herb (辣蓼草, Laliaocao) Croton Seed (巴豆, Badou) Purslane Herb (马齿苋, Machixian) Garlic Bulb (蒜, Suan) Peach Seed (桃仁, Taoren) Coix Seed (薏苡仁, Yiyiren) Tree Peony Bark (牡丹皮, Mudanpi) Chinese Waxgourd Seed (冬瓜子, Dongguazi) Sargentoglory Vine Stem (红藤, Hongteng)

Periappendicular abscess: Common Burreed Rhizome (三棱, Sanleng) Peach Seed (桃仁, Taoren) Coix Seed (薏苡仁, Yiyiren)

Acute intestinal obstruction: Pepperweed Seed or Flixweed Tansymustard Seed (葶苈子, Tinglizi) Common arpesium Root and Leaf (天名精, Tianmingjing) Inula Flower (旋覆花, Xuanfuhua) Rhubarb (大黄, Dahuang) Salt (食盐, Shiyan) Anhydrous Sodium Sulfate (玄明粉, Xuanmingfen) Kansui Root (甘遂, Gansui) Chinese Angelica Root (当归, Danggui) Croton Seed (巴豆, Badou) Juice of Pig Bladder (猪胆汁, Zhudanzhi) Immature Bitter Orange (枳实, Zhishi) Chinese Honeylocust Spine (皂角刺, Zaojiaoci) Bunge Pricklyash (花椒, Huajiao) Combined Spicebush Root (乌药, Wuyao) Chinese Eaglewood Wood (沉香, Chenxiang) Dried Ginger (干姜, Ganjiang) Radish Seed (莱菔子, Laifuzi) Fresh Ginger (生姜, Shengjiang) Musk (麝香, Shexiang) Honey (蜂蜜, Fengmi) Common Floweringquince Fruit (木瓜, Mugua) Officinal Magnolia Bark (厚朴, Houpo) Areca Seed (槟榔, Binlang) Bitter Orange (枳壳, Zhiqiao)

Liver and gall bladder diseases

Cholelithiasis (cholecystolithiasis): Capillary Wormwood Herb (茵陈蒿, Yinchenhao) Turmeric Root-tuber (郁金, Yujin) Rhubarb (大黄, Dahuang) Chinese Clematis Root (威灵仙, Weilingxian) Christina Loosetrife Herb (金钱草, Jinqiancao) Cape Jasmine Fruit (栀子, Zhizi)

Biliary colic: Common Aucklandia Root (木香, Muxiang) Szechwan chinaberry Fruit (川楝子, Chuanlianzi) Nutgrass Galingale Rhizome (香附, Xiangfu) Yanhusuo (延胡索, Yanhusuo) Chinese Thorowax Root (柴胡, Chaihu) Turmeric Root-tuber (郁金, Yujin)

Ascariasis of biliary tract: Common Aucklandia Root (木香, Muxiang) Capillary Wormwood Herb (茵陈蒿, Yinchenhao)

Mirabilite（朴消，Piaoxiao）Common Knotgrass Herb（萹蓄，Bianxu）Male Fern Rhizome（贯众，Guanzhong）Bunge Pricklyash（花椒，Huajiao）Fresh Ginger（生姜，Shengjiang）Realgar（雄黄，Xionghuang）Smoked Plum（乌梅，Wumei）Coptis Rhizome（黄连，Huanglian）Chinese Corktree Bark（黄柏，Huangbai）

Chronic cholecystitis：Sweet Wormwood（青蒿，Qinghao）Rhubarb（大黄，Dahuang）Rice Bean（赤小豆，Chixiaodou）Bear Gall（熊胆，Xiongdan）Christina Loosetrife Herb（金钱草，Jinqiancao）Turmeric Root-tuber（郁金，Yujin）Chinese Thorowax Root（柴胡，Chaihu）

Bacterial gallbladder enlangement：Chinese Gentian Root（龙胆草，Longdancao）Silktree Albiziae Bark（合欢皮，Hehuanpi）Cape Jasmine Fruit（栀子，Zhizi）

Urogenital system diseases

Ureter stone：Twotooth Achyranthes Root（牛膝，Niuxi）Talc（滑石，Huashi）Zedoray（莪术，Ezhu）Turmeric Root-tuber（郁金，Yujin）Pokeberry Root（商陆，Shanglu）Japanese Climbing Fern Spores（海金沙，Haijinsha）Earthworm（蚯蚓，Qiuyin）Walnut（胡桃仁，Hutaoren）Ginkgo Seed（白果，Baiguo）Chinese Clematis Root（威灵仙，Weilingxian）Christina Loosetrife Herb（金钱草，Jinqiancao）Chicken Gizzard Membrane（鸡内金，Jineijin）Cattail Pollen（蒲黄，Puhuang）Japanese Felt Fern Leaf（石韦，Shiwei）Plantain Seed（车前子，Cheqianzi）

Chronic prostatitis：Indian Chrysanthemum Flower（野菊花，Yejuhua）Spanishneedles Herb（鬼针草，Guizhengcao）Membranous Milkvetch Root（黄芪，Huangqi）Amber（琥珀，Hupo）Gordon Euryale Seed（芡实，Qianshi）Leech（水蛭，Shuizhi）Garlic Bulb（大蒜，Dasuan）Chinese Corktree Bark（黄柏，Huangbai）

Prostatic hyperplasis：Twotooth Achyranthes Root（牛膝，Niuxi）Talc（滑石，Huashi）Fortune Windmillpalm（棕榈炭，Zonglutan）Combined Spicebush Root（乌药，Wuyao）

Male inferticity：Fresh Ginger（生姜，Shengjiang）Desertliving Cistanche（肉苁蓉，Roucongrong）Barbary Wolfberry Fruit（枸杞子，Gouqizi）Dodder Seed（菟丝子，Tusizi）Palmleaf Raspberry Fruit（覆盆子，Fupenzi）Shorthorned Epimedium Herb（淫羊藿，Yinyanghuo）Medicinal Indian-mulberry Root（巴戟天，Bajitian）

Hydrocele of tunica vaginalis：Alumen（白矾，Baifan）Common Knotgrass Herb（萹蓄，Bianxu）Hindu Lotus Rhizome-node（藕节，Oujie）Fennel Fruit（小茴香，Xiaohuixiang）Tangerine Seed（橘核，Juhe）

Orchitis：Chinese Gentian Root（龙胆草，Longdancao）Creeping Woodsorred Herb（酢浆草，Zuojiangcao）Szechwan chinaberry Fruit（川楝子，Chuanlianzi）

Impotence：Actinolite（阳起石，Yangqishi）Prepared Rhizome of Adhesive Rehmannia（熟地黄，Shoudihuang）Shorthorned Epimedium Herb（淫羊藿，Yinyanghuo）Common Cruculigo（仙茅，Xianmao）Magnetite（磁石，Cishi）Manchurian Wildginger Herb（细辛，Xixin）Ginseng（人参，Renshen）Ant（蚂蚁，Mayi）Silkworm with Batrytis Larva（白僵蚕，Baijiangcan）Centipede（蜈蚣，Wugong）Ass-hide Glue（阿胶，Ejiao）Leech（水蛭，Shuizhi）Aspongopus（九香虫，Jiuxiangchong）Hairy Antler（鹿茸，Lurong）Medicinal Indian-mulberry Root（巴戟天，Bajitian）

Seminal emission：Common Knotgrass

Herb (萹蓄, Bianxu) Tuber Onion Seed (韭菜子, Jiucaozi) Oriental Waterplantain Rhizome (泽泻, Zexie) Chicken Gizzard Membrane (鸡内金, Jineijin) Chinese Magnoliavine (五味子, Wuweizi) Smoked Plum (乌梅, Wumei) Combined Spicebush Root (乌药, Wuyao) Gordon Euryale Seed (芡实, Qianshi) Chinese Corktree Bark (黄柏, Huangbai)

Scald and burn

Scald: Gypsum (石膏, Shigao) Weeping Forsythia Capsule (连翘, Lianqiao) Garden Burnet Root (地榆, Diyu) Swordlike Atractylodes Rhizome (苍术, Cangzhu) Barbary Wolfberry Fruit (枸杞子, Gouqizi) Pond Forg (青蛙, Qingwa) Dragon's Bone (龙骨, Longgu) Phoenix Tree Leaf (梧桐叶, Wutongye) Camphor (樟脑, Zhangnao) Babylon Weeping Willow Branchlet (柳枝, Liuzhi) Opium Poppy Seed (罂粟, Yingsu) Fresh Ginger (生姜, Shengjiang) Chinaroot Greenbrier Rhizome (菝葜, Baqia) Honey (蜂蜜, Fengmi) Rhubarb (大黄, Dahuang)

Burn: Talc (滑石, Huashi) Zedoray (莪术, Ezhu) Rhubarb (大黄, Dahuang) Salt (食盐, Shiyan) Mirabilite Crystal (寒水石, Hanshuishi) Gypsum (石膏, Shigao) Giant Knotweed Rhizome (虎杖, Huzhang) Natural Indigo (青黛, Qingdai) Coptis Rhizome (黄连, Huanglian) Root of Sinkiang Arnebia (紫草, Zicao) Bletilla Rhizome (白及, Baiji) Licorice Root (甘草, Gancao) Calix (石灰, Shihui) Acacia Catechu (孩儿茶, Haiercha) Calamine (炉甘石, Luganshi) Tortoise's Shell and Plastron (龟版, Guiban) Earthworm (蚯蚓, Qiuyin) Pubescent Holly Root (毛冬青, Maodongqing) Glossy Privet Fruit (女贞子, Nuzhenzi) Chinese Gall (五倍子, Wubeizi) Chinese Corktree Bark (黄柏, Huangbai) Bunge Pricklyash (花椒, Huajiao) Chinese Fir Bark (杉树皮, Shanshupi) Dandelion (蒲公英, Pugongying) Green Gram Seed (绿豆, Lvdou) Myrrh (没药, Moyao) Frankincense (乳香, Ruxiang) Honey (蜂蜜, Fengmi) Garden Burnet Root (地榆, Diyu)

Capillary ending diseases

Thromboangiitis obliterans: Safflower (红花, Honghua) Prepared Daughter Root of Common Monkshood (附子, Fuzi) Hindu Datura Flower (曼陀罗花, Mantuoluohua) Manyleaf Paris Rhizome (蚤休, Zaoxiu) Danshen Root (丹参, Danshen) Root of Sinkiang Arnebia (紫草, Zicao) Pubescent Holly Root (毛冬青, Maodongqing) Chinese Angelica Root (当归, Danggui) Leech (水蛭, Shuizhi) Colophony (松香, Songxiang) Peach Seed (桃仁, Taoren) Suberect Spatholobus Stem (鸡血藤, Jixueteng) Szechwan Lovage Rhizome (川芎, Chuanxiong) Pangolin Scales (穿山甲, Chuanshanjia)

Thrombophlebitis: Licorice Root (甘草, Gancao) Wrinkled Gianthyssop Herb (藿香, Huoxiang) Motherwort Herb (益母草, Yimucao)

Skin diseases

Bed sore: Safflower (红花, Honghua) Alumen (明矾, Mingfan) Sal-ammoniac (硇砂, Naosha) Cuttle Bone (乌贼骨, Wuzeigu) Barbary Wolfberry Fruit (枸杞子, Gouqizi) Myrrh (没药, Moyao)

Pyogenic diseases: Honeysuckle Flower (金银花, Jinyinhua) Purslane Herb (马齿苋, Machixian) Chinaroot Greenbrier Rhizome (菝葜, Baqia) Japanese Ampelopsis Root (白

蔹, Bailian) Garlic Bulb (蒜, Suan) Calamine (炉甘石, Luganshi) Common Selfheal Spike (夏枯草, Xiakucao) Ginseng (人参, Renshen) Vasps Nest (露蜂房, Lufengfang) Ground Beetle (䗪虫, Zhechong) Chinese Honeylocust Spine (皂角刺, Zaojiaoci) Ass-hide Glue (阿胶, Ejiao) Clove Flower-bud (丁香, Dingxiang) Dragon's Bone (龙骨, Longgu) Cuttle Bone (乌贼骨, Wuzeigu) Chinese Wolfberry Root-bark (地骨皮, Digupi) Dragon's Blood (血竭, Xuejie) Cassia Bark (肉桂, Rougui) Radish Seed (莱菔子, Laifuzi) Climbing Groundsel Herb(千里光, Qianliguang) Heartlaef Houttuynia Herb (鱼腥草, Yuxingcao) Honey (蜂蜜, Fengmi) Bletilla Rhizome (白及, Baiji) Sea Horse (海马, Haima) Chinese Gall (五倍子, Wubeizi) Aquatic Malachium Herb (鹅肠菜, Echangcai) Weeping Forsythia Capsule (连翘, Lianqiao) Dandelion (蒲公英, Pugongying) Peach Seed (桃仁, Taoren)

Chronic ulcer in the lower limbs: Poisonous Buttercup Fruit (石龙芮, Shilongrui) Nut-vomitive Poisonnut Seed (马钱子, Maqianzi) Iron Scales (生铁落, Shengtieluo) Soyben (黄大豆, Huangdadou) Calamine (炉甘石, Luganshi) Alumen (白矾, Baifan) Cuttle Bone (乌贼骨, Wuzeigu) Pubescent Holly Root (毛冬青, Maodongqing) Slug (蛞蝓, Kuoyu) Lizard (蜥蜴, Xiyi) Camphor (樟脑, Zhangnao) Purslane Herb (马齿苋, Machixian) Myrrh (没药, Moyao) Garden Burnet Root (地榆, Diyu) Manchurian Catalpa Leaf (楸木皮, Qiumupi)

Traumatic hemorrhage: Asiatic Plantain Herb (车前草, Cheqiancao) Rhubarb (大黄, Dahuang) Yerbadetajo Herb (墨旱莲, Mohanlian) Cuttle Bone (乌贼骨, Wuzeigu) Aloes (芦荟, Luhui) Colophony (松香, Songxiang) India Madder Root (茜草, Qiancao) Sanchi Root (三七, Sanqi) Puff-ball (马勃, Mabo) Cattail Pollen (蒲黄, Puhuang)

Tragomaschalia: Talc (滑石, Huashi) Lithargyrum (密陀僧, Mituoseng) Alumen (白矾, Baifan) Wall Spider (壁钱, Biqian) Camphor (樟脑, Zhangnao) Dragon's Blood (血竭, Xuejie)

Pregnancy diseases

Habitual abortion: Sharpleaf Galangal Fruit (益智仁, Yizhiren) Ass-hide Glue (阿胶, Ejiao) Largehead Atractylodes Rhizome (白术, Baizhu) Perilla Leaf (紫苏, Zisu) Baikal Skullcap Root (黄芩, Huangqin) Eucommia Bark (杜仲, Duzhong) Chinese Taxillus Twig (桑寄生, Sangjisheng) Argy Wormwood Leaf (艾叶, Aiye) Himalayan Teasel Root (续断, Xuduan) Villous Amomum Fruit (砂仁, Sharen) Wrinkled Gianthyssop Herb (藿香, Huoxiang)

Vomiting of pregnancy: Inula Flower (旋覆花, Xuanfuhua) Hematite (代赭石, Daizheshi) Cooking Stove Earth (伏龙肝, Fulonggan) Pinellia Rhizome (半夏, Banxia) Largehead Atractylodes Rhizome (白术, Baizhu) Barbary Wolfberry Fruit (枸杞子, Gouqizi) Fresh Ginger (生姜, Shengjiang) Common Yam Rhizome (山药, Shanyao) Clove Flower-bud (丁香, Dingxiang) Common Perilla Stem (苏梗, Sugeng) Villous Amomum Fruit (砂仁, Sharen) Wrinkled Gianthyssop Herb (藿香, Huoxiang)

Hypertension of pregnancy: Soyben (黄大豆, Huangdadou) Hindu Datura Flower (曼陀罗花, Mantuoluohua)

Abnormal fetal position: Plantain Seed (车前子, Cheqianzi) Chinese Angelica Root (当归, Danggui) Szechwan Lovage Rhizome (川芎, Chuanxiong)

White lesions of vnlva and pruritus vulvae

White lesions of vulva: Nut-vomitive Poisonnut Seed（马钱子，Maqianzi）Chinese Gentian Root（龙胆草，Longdancao）Malaytea Scurfpea Fruit（补骨脂，Buguzhi）Dragon's Blood（血竭，Xuejie）Tuber Fleeceflower Root（何首乌，Heshouwu）Acacia Catechu（孩儿茶，Haiercha）

Pruritus of vulva: Natural Indigo（青黛，Qingdai）Common Cnidium Fruit（蛇床子，Shechuangzi）Chinese Corktree Bark（黄柏，Huangbai）Bunge Pricklyash（花椒，Huajiao）Lightyellow Sophora Root（苦参，Kushen）Alumen（明矾，Mingfan）

Inflammation of female reproductive system

Vaginitis: European Verbena Herb（马鞭草，Mabiancao）Root of Sinkiang Arnebia（紫草，Zicao）Common Cnidium Fruit（蛇床子，Shechuangzi）Pubescent Holly Root（毛冬青，Maodongqing）

Monilial vaginitis: Haichow Elsholtzia Herb（香薷，Xiangru）Zedoray（莪术，Ezhu）Giant Knotweed Rhizome（虎杖，Huzhang）Natural Indigo（青黛，Qingdai）Divaricate Saposhnikovia Root（防风，Fangfeng）Common Cnidium Fruit（蛇床子，Shechuangzi）Borax（硼砂，Pengsha）Calamine（炉甘石，Luganshi）

Trichomonal vaginitis: Vinegar（醋，Cu）Coptis Rhizome（黄连，Huanglian）Common Cnidium Fruit（蛇床子，Shechuangzi）Chinese Ligusticum Rhizome（藁本，Gaoben）Lightyellow Sophora Root（苦参，Kushen）Malaytea Scurfpea Fruit（补骨脂，Buguzhi）Hyacinth Bean（扁豆，Biandou）Cochinchina Momordica Seed（木鳖子，Mubiezi）Radish Seed（莱菔子，Laifuzi）Honey（蜂蜜，Fengmi）Sessile Stemona Root（百部，Baibu）Garlic Bulb（大蒜，Dasuan）Hairvein Agrimonia Herb（仙鹤草，Xianhecao）

Cervicitis: Black Nightshade Herb（龙葵，Longkui）Talc（滑石，Huashi）Zedoray（莪术，Ezhu）Nut-vomitive Poisonnut Seed（马钱子，Maqianzi）Giant Knotweed Rhizome（虎杖，Huzhang）Root of Sinkiang Arnebia（紫草，Zicao）Common Cnidium Fruit（蛇床子，Shechuangzi）Pinellia Rhizome（半夏，Banxia）Acacia Catechu（孩儿茶，Haiercha）Borax（硼砂，Pengsha）Lightyellow Sophora Root（苦参，Kushen）Ginseng（人参，Renshen）Alumen（白矾，Baifan）Chinese Gall（五倍子，Wubeizi）Honeysuckle Flower（金银花，Jinyinhua）Chinese Corktree Bark（黄柏，Huangbai）Camphor（樟脑，Zhangnao）Tonkin Sophora Root（山豆根，Shandougen）Airpotato Yam Tuber（黄药子，Huangyaozi）Heartlaef Houttuynia Herb（鱼腥草，Yuxingcao）Musk（麝香，Shexiang）

Inflammation of internal genitals: Chinese Angelica Root（当归，Danggui）Common Burreed Rhizome（三棱，Sanleng）Chinese Corktree Bark（黄柏，Huangbai）Chinese Honeylocust Spine（皂角刺，Zaojiaoci）

Ovariosalpingitis: Pangolin Scales（穿山甲，Chuanshanjia）Bock Greenbrier Rhizome（金刚藤，Jingangteng）

Profused leukorrhea: Black Nightshade Herb（龙葵，Longkui）Longan Aril（龙眼肉，Longyanrou）Ginkgo Seed（白果，Baiguo）Hyacinth Bean（扁豆，Biandou）Gordon Euryale Seed（芡实，Qianshi）Herb of Bittesweet（白英，Baiying）Common Yam Rhizome（山药，Shanyao）Swordlike Atractylodes Rhizome（苍术，Cangzhu）Chinese Corktree Bark (黄柏, Huangbai) Lightyellow Sophora Root (苦参, Kushen) Largehead Atractylodes Rhizome (白术, Baizhu)

Tumor in female genital organ

Hysteromyoma: Zedoray (莪术, Ezhu) Ass-hide Glue (阿胶, Ejiao) Medicated Leaven (神曲, Shenqu) Szechwan Lovage Rhizome (川芎, Chuanxiong)

Oophoritic cyst: Pangolin Scales (穿山甲, Chuanshanjia)

Menstrual disorder

Irregular menstruation: Manyleaf Paris Rhizome (蚤休, Zaoxiu) Chinese Angelica Root (当归, Danggui) Malaytea Scurfpea Fruit (补骨脂, Buguzhi) Argy Wormwood Leaf (艾叶, Aiye) Cochinchinese Asparagus Root (天门冬, Tianmendong) Fortune Windmillpalm (棕榈炭, Zonglütan) Radish Seed (莱菔子, Laifuzi) Akebia Stem (木通, Mutong) Ass-hide Glue (阿胶, Ejiao) Safflower (红花, Honghua) Szechwan Lovage Rhizome (川芎, Chuanxiong) Nutgrass Galingale Rhizome (香附, Xiangfu) Dan-shen Root (丹参, Danshen) Motherwort Herb (益母草, Yimucao)

Retrograde menstrution: Hematite (代赭石, Daizheshi) Twotooth Achyranthes Root (牛膝, Niuxi)

Massive metrorrhagia: Vinegar (醋, Cu) White Peony Root (白芍药, Baishaoyao) Garden Burnet Root (地榆, Diyu) Common Cruculigo (仙茅, Xianmao) Membranous Milkvetch Root (黄芪, Huangqi) Divaricate Saposhnikovia Root (防风, Fangfeng) Silkworm Feculae (蚕砂, Cansha) Loquat Root (枇杷根, Pipagen) Ginkgo Seed (白果, Baiguo) Radish Seed (莱菔子, Laifuzi) India Madder Root (茜草, Qiancao) Ass-hide Glue (阿胶, Ejiao) Deglued Antler Powder (鹿角霜, Lujiaoshuang) Sanchi Root (三七, Sanqi) Argy Wormwood Leaf (艾叶, Aiye) Burnt Clay-lining of Kitchen Range (灶心土, Zaoxintu) Hairvein Agrimonia Herb (仙鹤草, Xianhecao)

Amenorrhea: Rehmannia Dried Root (生地黄, Shengdihuang) Soot (百草霜, Baicaoshuang) Membranous Milkvetch Root (黄芪, Huangqi) Hawthorn Fruit (山楂, Shanzha) Szechwan Lovage Rhizome (川芎, Chuanxiong) Twotooth Achyranthes Root (牛膝, Niuxi) Safflower (红花, Honghua) Peach Seed (桃仁, Taoren) Ground Beetle (䗪虫, Zhechong) Rhubarb (大黄, Dahuang)

Dysmenorrhea: Nutgrass Galingale Rhizome (香附, Xiangfu) White Peony Root (白芍药, Baishaoyao) Chinese Angelica Root (当归, Danggui) Yanhusuo (延胡索, Yanhusuo) Hirsute Shiny Bugleweed Herb (泽兰, Zelan) Motherwort Herb (益母草, Yimucao) Hawthorn Fruit (山楂, Shanzha) Musk (麝香, Shexiang)

Hysteropsosis

Hysteropsosis: Sanchi Root (三七, Sanqi) Chinese Angelica Root (当归, Danggui) Motherwort Herb (益母草, Yimucao) Alumen (明矾, Mingfan) Snail (蜗牛, Woniu) Cherokee Rose Fruit (金樱子, Jinyingzi) Immature Bitter Orange (枳实, Zhishi) Tuber Fleeceflower Root (何首乌, Heshouwu) Chinese Thorowax Root (柴胡, Chaihu) Immature Bitter Orange (枳实, Zhishi) Shunk Bugbane Rhizome (升麻, Shengma) Membranous Milkvetch Root (黄芪, Huangqi)

Puerperal diseases

Postpartum hemorrhage: Sanchi Root (三七, Sanqi) Male Fern Rhizome (贯众, Guanzhong) Shepherdspurse Herb with Root (荠菜, Jicai) Purslane Herb (马齿苋, Machixian) Cattail Pollen (蒲黄, Puhuang)

Postpartum retention of urine: Shunk Bugbane Rhizome (升麻, Shengma) Magnetite (磁石, Cishi) Cicada Slough (蝉蜕, Chantui)

Postpartum abdominal pain: Hirsute Shiny Bugleweed Herb (泽兰, Zelan) Safflower (红花, Honghua) Hawthorn Fruit (山楂, Shanzha) Yanhusuo (延胡索, Yanhusuo) Cattail Pollen (蒲黄, Puhuang)

Postpartum perined edema: Pubescent Holly Root (毛冬青, Maodongqing)

Postpartum agalactosia: Cowherb Seed (王不留行, Wangbuliuxing) Uniflower Swisscentaury Root (漏芦, Loulu) Ant (蚂蚁, Mayi) Silkworm with Batrytis Larva (白僵蚕, Baijiangcan) Cushaw Seed (南瓜子, Nanguazi) Rice Bean (赤小豆, Chixiaodou) Ricepaperplant Pith (通草, Tongcao) Beautiful Sweetgum Fruit (路路通, Lulutong)

Lactifuge: Mirabilite (芒硝, Mangxiao) Malt (麦芽, Maiya) Dandelion (蒲公英, Pugongying) Sanchi Root (三七, Sanqi) Medicated Leaven (神曲, Shenqu)

Cracked nipple: Tendrilleaf Fritillary Bulb (贝母, Beimu) Borax (硼砂, Pengsha) Calamine (炉甘石, Luganshi) Frankincense (乳香, Ruxiang)

Infantile Emergency

Infantile high fever: Indigowoad Leaf (大青叶, Daqingye) Wild Mint (薄荷, Bohe) Cow-bezoar (牛黄, Niuhuang) Dwarf Lilyturf Root (麦门冬, Maimendong) Sweet Wormwood (青蒿, Qinghao) Cicada Slough (蝉蜕, Chantui) Chinese Thorowax Root (柴胡, Chaihu)

Infantile convulsion: Scorpion (全蝎, Quanxie) Croton Seed (巴豆, Badou) Cicada Slough (蝉蜕, Chantui) Snakegourd Root (瓜蒌根, Gualougen) Cow-bezoar (牛黄, Niuhuang) Earth Worm (地龙, Dilong) Tendrilleaf Fritillary Bulb (贝母, Beimu) Buffalo Horn (水牛角, Shuiniujiao) Gambirplant Hooked Stem and Branch (钩藤, Gouteng) Bamboo Shavings (竹茹, Zhuru)

Infantile infectious shock: Immature Bitter Orange (枳实, Zhishi)

Infantile respiratory system diseases

Infantile upper respiratory tract infection: Natural Indigo (青黛, Qingdai) Baikal Skullcap Root (黄芩, Huangqin) Franchet Groundcherry Calyx or Fruit (锦灯笼, Jindenglong) Silkworm with Batrytis Larva (白僵蚕, Baijiangcan) Hempleaf Negundo Chastetree (牡荆, Mujing) Honeysuckle Flower (金银花, Jinyinhua) Heartlaef Houttuynia Herb (鱼腥草, Yuxingcao) Dyers Woad Root (板蓝根, Banlangen)

Infantile bronchopneumonia: Cinnabar (朱砂, Zhusha) Kansui Root (甘遂, Gansui) Weeping Forsythia Capsule (连翘, Lianqiao) Honeysuckle Flower (金银花, Jinyinhua) Amur Barberry Root and Branchlet (小蘗, Xiaonie) Medicinal Evodia Root (吴茱萸, Wuzhuyu) Odorate Rosewood Root-wood (降香, Jiangxiang) White Mustard Seed (白芥子, Baijiezi) Heartlaef Houttuynia Herb (鱼腥草, Yuxingcao)

Infantile asthmatic bronchitis: Balloonflower Root (桔梗, Jiegeng) Gordon Euryale Seed (芡实, Qianshi) Medicinal Evodia Root (吴茱萸, Wuzhuyu) Ephedra (麻黄, Mahuang) Earth Worm (地龙, Dilong)

Infantile viral pneumonia: Shunk Bugbane Rhizome (升麻, Shengma) Honeysuckle Flower (金银花, Jinyinhua) Dyers Woad Root (板蓝根, Banlangen) Baikal Skullcap Root (黄芩, Huangqin) Coptis Rhizome (黄连, Huanglian)

Infantile night sweat: Figwortflower Picrorhiza Rhizome (胡黄连, Huhuanglian) Beardie (泥鳅鱼, Niqiuyu) Starwort Root (银柴胡, Yinchaihu) Chinese Wolfberry Root-bark (地骨皮, Digupi)

Infantile digestive system diseases

Infantile diarrhea: Whiteflower Patrinia Herb (败酱草, Baijiangcao) Spanishneedles Herb (鬼针草, Guizhengcao) Cinnabar (朱砂, Zhusha) Largehead Atractylodes Rhizome (白术, Baizhu) Wrinkled Gianthyssop Herb (藿香, Huoxiang) Stalactite (钟乳石, Zhongrushi) Swordlike Atractylodes Rhizome (苍术, Cangzhu) Tuckahoe (茯苓, Fuling) Cherokee Rose Fruit (金樱子, Jinyingzi) Honeysuckle Flower (金银花, Jinyinhua) Black Pepper Fruit (胡椒, Hujiao) Medicinal Evodia Root (吴茱萸, Wuzhuyu) Hyacinth Bean (扁豆, Biandou) Lotus Seed (莲子, Lianzi) Medicated Leaven (神曲, Shenqu) Smoked Plum (乌梅, Wumei) Cassia Bark (肉桂, Rougui) Dried Ginger (干姜, Ganjiang) India Mustard Leaf (芥菜, Jiecai) Malt (麦芽, Maiya) Flower of Chinese Trumpetcreeper (紫葳, Ziwei) Plantain Seed (车前子, Cheqianzi) Clove Flower-bud (丁香, Dingxiang) Garlic Bulb (蒜, Suan) Fistular Onion Stalk (葱白, Congbai) Common Yam Rhizome (山药, Shanyao)

Infantile dyspepsia: Plantain Seed (车前子, Cheqianzi) Mirabilite (芒硝, Mangxiao) Malt (麦芽, Maiya) Medicated Leaven (神曲, Shenqu) Largehead Atractylodes Rhizome (白术, Baizhu) Creeping Woodsorred Herb (酢浆草, Zuojiangcao) Common Yam Rhizome (山药, Shanyao) Villous Amomum Fruit (砂仁, Sharen) Swordlike Atractylodes Rhizome (苍术, Cangzhu) Black Pepper Fruit (胡椒, Hujiao) Hyacinth Bean (扁豆, Biandou) Clove Flower-bud (丁香, Dingxiang) Common Aucklandia Root (木香, Muxiang) Fig Receptacle (无花果, Wuhuaguo) Charred Hawthorn Fruit (焦山楂, Jiaoshanzha) Areca Seed (槟榔, Binlang) Chicken Gizzard Membrane (鸡内金, Jineijin)

Pyloric, spasm: Hematite (代赭石, Daizheshi)

Infantile retention of food: Charred Hawthorn Fruit (焦山楂, Jiaoshanzha) Areca Seed (槟榔, Binlang) Anhydrous Sodium Sulfate (玄明粉, Xuanmingfen) Aloes (芦荟, Luhui) Chinese Honeylocust Spine (皂角, Zaojiao) Immature Bitter Orange (枳实, Zhishi) Bitter Orange (枳壳, Zhiqiao) Officinal Magnolia Bark (厚朴, Houpo) Chicken Gizzard Membrane (鸡内金, Jineijin) Figwortflower Picrorhiza Rhizome (胡黄连, Huhuanglian) Chinese Wolfberry Root-bark (地骨皮, Digupi)

Infantile summer diarrhea: Talc (滑石, Huashi) Limonite(禹余粮, Yuyuliang) Plantain Seed (车前子, Cheqianzi) Wrinkled Gianthyssop Herb (藿香, Huoxiang)

Chalasia of candia: Fresh Ginger (生姜, Shengjiang)

Infantile bacterial dysentery: Common

Selfheal Spike（夏枯草，Xiakucao）Largeleaf Chinese Ash Bark（秦皮，Qinpi）Honeysuckle Flower（金银花，Jinyinhua）Chinese Pulsatilla Root（白头翁，Baitouweng）Common Aucklandia Root（木香，Muxiang）Coptis Rhizome（黄连，Huanglian）

Infantile acute icterohepatitis：Largeleaf Gentian Root（秦艽，Qinjiao）Christina Loosetrife Herb（金钱草，Jinqiancao）Capillary Wormwood Herb（茵陈蒿，Yinchenhao）Cape Jasmine Fruit（栀子，Zhizi）Rhubarb（大黄，Dahuang）Chinese Thorowax Root（柴胡，Chaihu）

Infantile urinary diseases

Infantile glomerular nephritis：Rrefers to "5．Vrological disease"

Infantile hyclrocele：Great-ventral Garden Spider（蜘蛛，Zhizhu）Chinese Gall（五倍子，Wubeizi）Chinese Clematis Root（威灵仙，Weilingxian）Kansui Root（甘遂，Gansui）

Infantile balanitis：Chinese Clematis Root（威灵仙，Weilingxian）Common Aucklandia Root（木香，Muxiang）Lightyellow Sophora Root（苦参，Kushen）

Incontinence of urine in children：Mantis Egg-case（桑螵蛸，Sangpiaoxiao）Vasps Nest（露蜂房，Lufengfang）Fistular Onion Stalk（葱白，Congbai）Fresh Ginger（生姜，Shengjiang）Malaytea Scurfpea Fruit（补骨脂，Buguzhi）Common Yam Rhizome（山药，Shanyao）Combined Spicebush Root（乌药，Wuyao）Sharpleaf Galangal Fruit（益智仁，Yizhiren）

Infantile nervous system diseases

Infantile epilepsy：Chlorite-schist（礞石，Mengshi）Chinese White Olive（青果，Qingguo）Arisaema with Bile（胆南星，Dannanxing）Pinellia Rhizome（半夏，Banxia）Cow-bezoar（牛黄，Niuhuang）Cicada Slough（蝉蜕，Chantui）Tall Gastrodia Rhizome（天麻，Tianma）

Disease of newborn

Neonatal jaundice：Giant Knotweed Rhizome（虎杖，Huzhang）Christina Loosetrife Herb（金钱草，Jinqiancao）Capillary Wormwood Herb（茵陈蒿，Yinchenhao）

Scleroderma neonatorum：Prepared Daughter Root of Common Monkshood（附子，Fuzi）Szechwan Lovage Rhizome（川芎，Chuanxiong）

Neonatal hemolytic disease：Licorice Root（甘草，Gancao）Motherwort Herb（益母草，Yimucao）Capillary Wormwood Herb（茵陈蒿，Yinchenhao）

Neonatal biliary atresia：Capillary Wormwood Herb（茵陈蒿，Yinchenhao）

Neonatal erysipelas：Cow-bezoar（牛黄，Niuhuang）

Infantile miscellaneous diseases

Morbid night crying of babies：Common Rush Stem Pith（灯芯，Dengxin）Chinese Gall（五倍子，Wubeizi）Pharbitis Seed（牵牛子，Qianniuzi）Cicada Slough（蝉蜕，Chantui）Bamboo leaf（竹叶，Zhuye）

Infantile salivation：Talc（滑石，Huashi）Vinegar（醋，Cu）Medicinal Evodia Root（吴茱萸，Wuzhuyu）Cassia Bark（肉桂，Rougui）Sharpleaf Galangal Fruit（益智仁，Yizhiren）Wrinkled Gianthyssop Herb（藿香，Huoxiang）Foutune Eupatorium Herb（佩兰，Peilan）

Infantile candidemia: Garlic Bulb（蒜，Suan）

Infantile frequent sighing: Inula Flower（旋覆花，Xuanfuhua）

Rubella: Herb of Siberian Cocklebur（苍耳草，Cangercao）Fineleaf Schizomepeta Herb（荆芥，Jingjie）Cicada Slough（蝉蜕，Chantui）Great Burdock Achene（牛蒡子，Niubangzi）Divaricate Saposhnikovia Root（防风，Fangfeng）Wild Mint（薄荷，Bohe）

Infantile stomatocace: Common Lophatherum Herb（淡竹叶，Danzhuye）Vinegar（醋，Cu）Gypsum（石膏，Shigao）Cinnabar（朱砂，Zhusha）Coastal Glehnia Root，and Fourleaf Ladybell Root（沙参，Shashen）Borax（硼砂，Pengsha）Great-ventral Garden Spider（蜘蛛，Zhizhu）Croton Seed（巴豆，Badou）Radish Seed（莱菔子，Laifuzi）Medicinal Evodia Root（吴茱萸，Wuzhuyu）Wheat Fruit（小麦，Xiaomai）Natural Indigo（青黛，Qingdai）

Infantile eczema: Rice Bean（赤小豆，Chixiaodou）Lightyellow Sophora Root（苦参，Kushen）Belvedere Fruit（地肤子，Difuzi）Calamine（炉甘石，Luganshi）

Infantile tinea capitis: Tuber Fleeceflower Root（何首乌，Heshouwu）

Infantile diaper rash: Root of Sinkiang Arnebia（紫草，Zicao）Stalactite（钟乳石，Zhongrushi）Globefish Muscle（绛香，Hetun）Honey（蜂蜜，Fengmi）Talc（滑石，Huashi）

Virus dermitis

Herpes zoster: Cowherb Seed（王不留行，Wangbuliuxing）Indian Chrysanthemum Flower（野菊花，Yejuhua）Red-kness Herb（水蓼，Shuiliao）Vinegar（醋，Cu）Nut-vomitive Poisonnut Seed（马钱子，Maqianzi）Chinese Lobelia Herb（半边莲，Banbianlian）Japanese Climbing Fern Spores（海金沙，Haijinsha）Giant Knotweed Rhizome（虎杖，Huzhang）Natural Indigo（青黛，Qingdai）Chinese Angelica Root（当归，Danggui）Shunk Bugbane Rhizome（升麻，Shengma）Chinese Gentian Root（龙胆草，Longdancao）Mantis Egg-case（桑螵蛸，Sangpiaoxiao）Earthworm（蚯蚓，Qiuyin）Chinese Gall（五倍子，Wubeizi）Scorpion（全蝎，Quanxie）Cow-bezoar（牛黄，Niuhuang）Fig Leaf（无花果叶，Wuhuaguoye）Purslane Herb（马齿苋，Machixian）Tuber Onion Leaf（韭菜，Jiucao）Realgar（雄黄，Xionghuang）Tuber Fleeceflower Root（何首乌，Heshouwu）

Flat want: Nutgrass Galingale Rhizome（香附，Xiangfu）Common Scouring Rush Herb（木贼，Muzei）Belvedere Fruit（地肤子，Difuzi）Vinegar（醋，Cu）Anhydrous Sodium Sulfate（玄明粉，Xuanmingfen）Pinellia Rhizome（半夏，Banxia）Root of Sinkiang Arnebia（紫草，Zicao）Manchurian Wildginger Herb（细辛，Xixin）Coix Seed（薏苡仁，Yiyiren）Cochinchinese Asparagus Root（天门冬，Tianmendong）White Mustard Seed（白芥子，Baijiezi）Purslane Herb（马齿苋，Machixian）Java Brucea Fruit（鸦胆子，Yadanzi）

Verruca vulgaris: Soyben（黄大豆，Huangdadou）Puncturevine Caltrop Fruit（刺蒺藜，Cijili）Sanchi Root（三七，Sanqi）Salammoniac（硇砂，Naosha）Arabic Cowry Shell（紫贝齿，Zibeichi）Nacre（珍珠母，Zhenzhumu）Toad（蟾蜍，Chanchu）Large Blister Beetle（斑蝥，Banmao）Garlic Bulb（大蒜，Dasuan）Java Brucea Fruit（鸦胆子，Yadanzi）

Infectious soft want: Yerbadetajo Herb（墨旱莲，Mohanlian）Chinese Gall（五倍子，Wubeizi）Coix Seed（薏苡仁，Yiyiren）

Suppurative dermatosics

Pustuar eruption: Talc（滑石，Huashi）Anhydrous Sodium Sulfate（玄明粉，Xuanmingfen）Coptis Rhizome（黄连，Huanglian）Acacia Catechu（孩儿茶，Haiercha）Common Selfheal Spike（夏枯草，Xiakucao）Pharbitis Seed（牵牛子，Qianniuzi）Heartlaef Houttuynia Herb（鱼腥草，Yuxingcao）Mirabilite Crystal（寒水石，Hanshuishi）Natural Indigo（青黛，Qingdai）Sulfur（硫黄，Liuhuang）Borax（硼砂，Pengsha）Vasps Nest（露蜂房，Lufengfang）Chinese Gall（五倍子，Wubeizi）Chinese Corktree Bark（黄柏，Huangbai）Walnut（胡桃仁，Hutaoren）Medicinal Evodia Root（吴茱萸，Wuzhuyu）Purslane Herb（马齿苋，Machixian）Green Gram Seed（绿豆，Lvdou）

Folliculitis: Belvedere Fruit（地肤子，Difuzi）Chalcanthnium（胆矾，Danfan）Vinegar（醋，Cu）Manyleaf Paris Rhizome（蚤休，Zaoxiu）Common Anemarrhea Rhizome（知母，Zhimu）Snake Slough（蛇蜕，Shetui）Chinese Gall（五倍子，Wubeizi）

Skin ulcer: Pig Nail（猪蹄甲，Zhutijia）Chinese Gall（五倍子，Wubeizi）Musk（麝香，Shexiang）Honey（蜂蜜，Fengmi）Soot（百草霜，Baicaoshuang）Natural Indigo（青黛，Qingdai）Coptis Rhizome（黄连，Huanglian）Fistular Onion Stalk（葱白，Congbai）Cow-bezoar（牛黄，Niuhuang）Dandelion（蒲公英，Pugongying）

Fungal dermitis

Head white ringworm: Croton Seed（巴豆，Badou）Aloes（芦荟，Luhui）Japanese Pagodatree Flower（槐花，Huaihua）Dasheen Tuber（芋头，Yutou）Lilac Daphne Flower-bud（芫花，Yuanhua）Sessile Stemona Root（百部，Baibu）Garlic Bulb（蒜，Suan）

Hand white ringworm: Large Blister Beetle（斑蝥，Banmao）Chinese Corktree Bark（黄柏，Huangbai）Oriental Variegated Coralbean Bark（海桐皮，Haitongpi）Sessile Stemona Root（百部，Baibu）

Vitiligo: Sulfur（硫黄，Liuhuang）Lithargyrum（密陀僧，Mituoseng）Borax（硼砂，Pengsha）Malaytea Scurfpea Fruit（补骨脂，Buguzhi）Cuttle Bone（乌贼骨，Wuzeigu）

Femoral white ringworm: Vinegar（醋，Cu）

Foot white ringworm: Diverse Wormwood Herb（刘寄奴，Liujinu）Vinegar（醋，Cu）Nut-Vomitive Poisonnut Seed（马钱子，Maqianzi）Yerbadetajo Herb（墨旱莲，Mohanlian）Green Tangerine Peel（青皮，Qingpi）Calamine（炉甘石，Luganshi）Flaccid Knotweed Herb（辣蓼草，Laliaocao）Siberian Solomonseal Rhizome（黄精，Huangjing）Cuttle Bone（海螵蛸，Haipiaoxiao）Snake Slough（蛇蜕，Shetui）Chinese Gall（五倍子，Wubeizi）Camphor（樟脑，Zhangnao）Mud Eel（鳝鱼，Shanyu）Common Floweringquince Fruit（木瓜，Mugua）Belvedere Fruit（地肤子，Difuzi）Gambirplant Hooked Stem and Branch（钩藤，Gouteng）Lobed Kudzuvine Root（葛根，Gegen）Tuber Fleeceflower Root（何首乌，Heshouwu）Common Cnidium Fruit（蛇床子，Shechuangzi）Alumen（白矾，Baifan）

Eczema dermatitis

Eczema: Belvedere Fruit（地肤子，Difuzi）Safflower（红花，Honghua）Talc（滑石，Huashi）Medicine Terminalia Fruit（诃子，Hezi）Chinese Lobelia Herb（半边莲，Banbianlian）Tree Peony Bark（牡丹皮，Mudanpi) Natural Indigo (青黛, Qingdai) European Verbena Herb (马鞭草, Mabiancao) Garden Burnet Root (地榆, Diyu) Coptis Rhizome (黄连, Huanglian) Calamine (炉甘石, Luganshi) Swordlike Atractylodes Rhizome (苍术, Cangzhu) Alumen (白矾, Baifan) Earth Worm (地龙, Dilong) Common Ducksmeat Herb (浮萍, Fuping) Garter Snake (乌蛇, Wushe) Chinese Corktree Bark (黄柏, Huangbai) Medicinal Evodia Root (吴茱萸, Wuzhuyu) Colophony (松香, Songxiang) Fistular Onion Stalk (葱白, Congbai) Common Yam Rhizome (山药, Shanyao) Cattail Pollen (蒲黄, Puhuang) Realgar (雄黄, Xionghuang) Chinese Angelica Root (当归, Danggui) Walnut (胡桃仁, Hutaoren) Common Cnidium Fruit (蛇床子, Shechuangzi)

Eczema of scrotum: Natural Indigo (青黛, Qingdai) Sulfur (硫黄, Liuhuang) Chinese Gentian Root (龙胆草, Longdancao) Babylon Weeping Willow Leaf (柳树叶, Liushuye) Sessile Stemona Root (百部, Baibu) Lightyellow Sophora Root (苦参, Kushen)

Contact dermatitis: Yerbadetajo Herb (墨旱莲, Mohanlian) Chinese Corktree Bark (黄柏, Huangbai) Chinese Fir Leaf (杉叶, Shanye) Herb of Bittesweet (白英, Baiying) Asiatic Rhinoceros Horn (犀角, Xijiao) Chinese Wolfberry Root-bark (地骨皮, Digupi) Ephedra (麻黄, Mahuang) Licorice Root (甘草, Gancao) Honey (蜂蜜, Fengmi)

Drug rash

Drug rash: Earthworm (蚯蚓, Qiuyin)

Urticaria

Urticaria: Belvedere Fruit (地肤子, Difuzi) Japanese Thistle Herb or Root (大蓟, Daji) Capillary Wormwood Herb (茵陈蒿, Yinchenhao) Talc (滑石, Huashi) Salt (食盐, Shiyan) Shunk Bugbane Rhizome (升麻, Shengma) Densefruit Pittany Root-bark (白鲜皮, Baixianpi) Motherwort Herb (益母草, Yimucao) Lightyellow Sophora Root (苦参, Kushen) Manchurian Wildginger Herb (细辛, Xixin) Silkworm Feculae (蚕砂, Cansha) Earthworm (蚯蚓, Qiuyin) Common Ducksmeat Herb (浮萍, Fuping) Cicada Slough (蝉蜕, Chantui) Honeysuckle Flower (金银花, Jinyinhua) Scorpion (全蝎, Quanxie) Chaulmoogratree Seed (大风子, Dafengzi) Fistular Onion Stalk (葱白, Congbai) Oriental Sesame Seed (黑芝麻, Heizhima) Clove Flower-bud (丁香, Dingxiang) Ephedra (麻黄, Mahuang) Divaricate Saposhnikovia Root (防风, Fangfeng) Fineleaf Schizomepeta Herb (荆芥, Jingjie) Puncturevine Caltrap Fruit (白蒺藜, Baijili) Tuber Fleeceflower Root (何首乌, Heshouwu)

Erythroderma desquamativum

Chronic eczema: Hindu Datura Flower (曼陀罗花, Mantuoluohua) Nut-vomitive Poisonnut Seed (马钱子, Maqianzi) Chinese Stellera Root (狼毒, Langdu) Pokeberry Root (商陆, Shanglu) Giant Knotweed Rhizome (虎杖, Huzhang) Natural Indigo (青黛, Qingdai) Root of Sinkiang Arnebia (紫草, Zicao) Membranous Milkvetch Root (黄芪, Huangqi) Chinese Angelica Root (当归, Danggui) Paniculate Swallowwort Root (徐长卿, Xuchangqing) Szechwan Lovage Rhizome (川芎, Chuanxiong) Malaytea Scurfpea Fruit (补骨脂, Buguzhi) Centipede (蜈蚣, Wugong) Umbellate Pore Fungus (猪苓, Zhuling) Ground Beetle (䗪虫, Zhechong) Garter Snake (乌蛇, Wushe) Black Pepper Fruit (胡

椒, Hujiao) Japanese Pagodatree Flower (槐花, Huaihua) Tonkin Sophora Root (山豆根, Shandougen) Glabrous Greenbrier Rhizome (土茯苓, Tufuling) Ephedra (麻黄, Mahuang) Dahurian Angelica Root (白芷, Baizhi)

Roseola: Weeping Forsythia Capsule (连翘, Lianqiao) Root of Sinkiang Arnebia (紫草, Zicao)

Neurodermatitis

Neurodermatitis: Safflower (红花, Honghua) Siberian Cocklebur Fruit (苍耳子, Cangerzi) Talc (滑石, Huashi) Vinegar (醋, Cu) Nut-vomitive Poisonnut Seed (马钱子, Maqianzi) Arsenolite Ore (砒霜, Pishuang) Chinese Stellera Root (狼毒, Langdu) Soyben (黄大豆, Huangdadou) Sulfur (硫黄, Liuhuang) Chinese Ligusticum Rhizome (藁本, Gaoben) Shrubalthea Bark (木槿皮, Mujinpi) Large Blister Beetle (斑蝥, Banmao) Croton Seed (巴豆, Badou) Walnut (胡桃仁, Hutaoren) Cochinchina Momordica Seed (木鳖子, Mubiezi) Iunate Peltate Sundew Herb (茅膏菜, Maogaocai) Chinaroot Greenbrier Rhizome (菝葜, Baqia) Realgar (雄黄, Xionghuang) Chinese Clematis Root (威灵仙, Weilingxian)

Cutaneous pruritus: Safflower (红花, Honghua) Mirabilite (朴硝, Piaoxiao) Puncturevine Caltrap Fruit (白蒺藜, Baijili) Root of Sinkiang Arnebia (紫草, Zicao) Garter Snake (乌蛇, Wushe) Tuber Fleeceflower Root (何首乌, Heshouwu)

Collagen disease

Erythema multiforme: Safflower (红花, Honghua) Kansui Root (甘遂, Gansui) Coptis Rhizome (黄连, Huanglian) Belvedere Fruit (地肤子, Difuzi)

Dermatasclerosis: Dan-shen Root (丹参, Danshen)

Sweat gland, sebaceous glands

Acne: Aloes (芦荟, Luhui) Loquat Leaf (枇杷叶, Pipaye) Ginkgo Seed (白果, Baiguo)

Brandy nose: Gypsum (石膏, Shigao) Pink Plumepoppy Herb with Root (博落回, Boluohui) Clam Shell (海蛤壳, Haigeqiao) Giant Gecko (蛤蚧, Gejie) Chaulmoogratree Seed (大风子, Dafengzi) Green Gram Seed (绿豆, Lvdou) Sessile Stemona Root (百部, Baibu) Coptis Rhizome (黄连, Huanglian)

Dermatitis

Chloasma hepaticum: Wild Mint (薄荷, Bohe)

White patch (leukoplakia): Lithargyrum (密陀僧, Mituoseng) Puncturevine Caltrap Fruit (白蒺藜, Baijili) Doubleteeth Pulbescent Angelica Root (独活, Duhuo) Sulfur (硫黄, Liuhuang) Malaytea Scurfpea Fruit (补骨脂, Buguzhi) Fig Receptacle (无花果, Wuhuaguo) Dodder Seed (菟丝子, Tusizi) Purslane Herb (马齿苋, Machixian) Safflower (红花, Honghua) Dahurian Angelica Root (白芷, Baizhi)

Hair diseases

Alopecia araeta: Rehmannia Dried Root (生地黄, Shengdihuang) Vinegar (醋, Cu) Yerbadetajo Herb (墨旱莲, Mohanlian) Malaytea Scurfpea Fruit (补骨脂, Buguzhi) Tuckahoe (茯苓, Fuling) Large Blister Beetle

(斑蝥，Banmao) Szechwan chinaberry Fruit (川楝子，Chuanlianzi) Fresh Ginger (生姜，Shengjiang) Chinese Arborvitae Leafy Twig (侧柏叶，Cebaiye) Hematite (代赭石，Daizheshi) Pinellia Rhizome (半夏，Banxia) Sulfur (硫黄，Liuhuang) Chinese Corktree Bark (黄柏，Huangbai) Babylon Weeping Willow Branchlet (柳枝，Liuzhi) Safflower (红花，Honghua) Tuber Fleeceflower Root (何首乌，Heshouwu)

Seborheic dermatitis: Tree Peony Bark (牡丹皮，Mudanpi) Chinese Gall (五倍子，Wubeizi) Dragon's Bone (龙骨，Longgu) Chinese Arborvitae Leafy Twig (侧柏叶，Cebaiye)

Hoary hair: Tuber Fleeceflower Root (何首乌，Heshouwu) English Walnut Seed (核桃仁，Hetaoren) Chinese Arborvitae Leafy Twig (侧柏叶，Cebaiye) Oriental Sesame Seed (黑芝麻，Heizhima)

Physicial skin disease

Chilblain: Safflower (红花，Honghua) Mirabilite Crystal (寒水石，Hanshuishi) Licorice Root (甘草，Gancao) Calamine (炉甘石，Luganshi) Mantis Egg-case (桑螵蛸，Sangpiaoxiao) Barbary Wolfberry Fruit (枸杞子，Gouqizi) Chinese Taxillus Twig (桑寄生，Sangjisheng) Chinese Corktree Bark (黄柏，Huangbai) Chinese Gall (五倍子，Wubeizi) Black Pepper Fruit (胡椒，Hujiao) Camphor (樟脑，Zhangnao) Tangerine Peel (橘皮，Jupi) Cassia Twig (桂枝，Guizhi) Cassia Bark (肉桂，Rougui) Colophony (松香，Songxiang) Fresh Ginger (生姜，Shengjiang) Oriental Sesame Seed (黑芝麻，Heizhima) Honey (蜂蜜，Fengmi) Garlic Bulb (大蒜，Dasuan)

Clavus: Safflower (红花，Honghua) Vinegar (醋，Cu) Pinellia Rhizome (半夏，Banxia) Sal-ammoniac (硇砂，Naosha) Malaytea Scurfpea Fruit (补骨脂，Buguzhi) Centipede (蜈蚣，Wugong) Chinese Wolfberry Rootbark (地骨皮，Digupi) Bunge Pricklyash (花椒，Huajiao) Small Centipeda Herb (鹅不食草，Ebushicao) Java Brucea Fruit (鸦胆子，Yadanzi) Licorice Root (甘草，Gancao) Snakegourd Fruit (瓜蒌，Gualou) Japanese Ampelopsis Root (白蔹，Bailian) Honey (蜂蜜，Fengmi) Bletilla Rhizome (白及，Baiji) Tuber Fleeceflower Root (何首乌，Heshouwu) Chinese Fir Leaf (杉叶，Shanye) Green Gram Seed (绿豆，Lvdou)

Insect dermatitis

Snake-bite: Realgar (雄黄，Xionghuang) Wrinkled Gianthyssop Herb (藿香，Huoxiang) Tokyo Violet Herb (紫花地丁，Zihuadiding) Mulberry Leaf (桑叶，Sangye) Common Dayflower Herb (鸭跖草，Yazhicao) Herb of Siberian Cocklebur (苍耳草，Cangercao) Indigowoad Leaf (大青叶，Daqingye) Vinegar (醋，Cu) Chinese Lobelia Herb (半边莲，Banbianlian) Mirabilite Crystal (寒水石，Hanshuishi) Pokeberry Root (商陆，Shanglu) Common Cruculigo (仙茅，Xianmao) Swordlike Atractylodes Rhizome (苍术，Cangzhu) Great-ventral Garden Spider (蜘蛛，Zhizhu) Brevicaude Pit Viper (蝮蛇，Fushe) Pepper Fruit (胡椒，Hujiao) Scabrous Doellingeria Herb (东风菜，Dongfengcai) Realgar (雄黄，Xionghuang)

Sarcoptidosis: Croton Seed (巴豆，Badou) Chaulmoogratree Seed (大风子，Dafengzi) Medicinal Evodia Root (吴茱萸，Wuzhuyu) Camphor (樟脑，Zhangnao) Realgar (雄黄，Xionghuang) Sessile Stemona Root (百部，Baibu) Vinegar (醋，Cu) Sulfur (硫黄，Liuhuang)

Surgical diseases

External humernal epicondylitis: Large Blister Beetle (斑蝥, Banmao) Japanese Buttercup Herb (毛莨, Maogen)

Arthritis in ankle joint: Bunge Pricklyash (花椒, Huajiao) Combined Spicebush Root (乌药, Wuyao)

Cervical spondylopathy: Vinegar (醋, Cu) Snake Slough (蛇蜕, Shetui) Agkistrodon Acutus (白花蛇, Baihuashe) Lobed Kudzuvine Root (葛根, Gegen)

Scapulohumeral periarthritis: Salt (食盐, Shiyan) Minium (铅丹, Qiandan) Dan-shen Root (丹参, Danshen) Asiatic Comelian Cherry Fruit (山茱萸, Shanzhuyu) Garlic Bulb (蒜, Suan) Rhizome or Root of Forbes Notopterygium (Incised Notopterygium Rhizome and Root (羌活, Qianghuo) Qianghuo) Mulberry Twig (桑枝, Sangzhi) Turmeric Rhizome (姜黄, Jianghuang) Cassia Twig (桂枝, Guizhi)

Stenosing tenovaginitis: Pangolin Scales (穿山甲, Chuanshanjia) Cassia Bark (肉桂, Rougui) Medicated Leaven (神曲, Shenqu)

Ischemic necrosis of femoral head: Chinese Eaglewood Wood (沉香, Chenxiang)

Lumber muscular.torsion: Rhubarb (大黄, Dahuang) Fresh Ginger (生姜, Shengjiang) Musk (麝香, Shexiang) Frankincense (乳香, Ruxiang) Myrrh (没药, Moyao) Sanchi Root (三七, Sanqi) Himalayan Teasel Root (续断, Xuduan) Fortune's Drynaria Rhizome, Baron's Drynaria Rhizome (骨碎补, Gusuibu) Chinese Clematis Root (威灵仙, Weilingxian) East Asian Tree Fern Rhizome (狗脊, Gouji)

Pain in the waist and lower extremities: Twotooth Achyranthes Root (牛膝, Niuxi) Siberian Cocklebur Fruit (苍耳子, Cangerzi) Nut-vomitive Poisonnut Seed (马钱子, Maqianzi) Tree Peony Bark (牡丹皮, Mudanpi) European Verbena Herb (马鞭草, Mabiancao) Licorice Root (甘草, Gancao) Largehead Atractylodes Rhizome (白术, Baizhu) Ground Beetle (䗪虫, Zhechong) Eucommia Bark (杜仲, Duzhong) Luffa Fruit (丝瓜, Sigua) Aspongopus (九香虫, Jiuxiangchong) Cassia Bark (肉桂, Rougui) Fresh Ginger (生姜, Shengjiang) Chinese Pine Node (松节, Songjie) Tuber Fleeceflower Root (何首乌, Heshouwu) Green Gram Seed (绿豆, Lvdou) Chinese Taxillus Twig (桑寄生, Sangjisheng) Doubleteeth Pulbescent Angelica Root (独活, Duhuo)

Sciatica: Nutgrass Galingale Rhizome (香附, Xiangfu) Nut-vomitive Poisonnut Seed (马钱子, Maqianzi) Chinese Stellera Root (狼毒, Langdu) Prepared Daughter Root of Common Monkshood (附子, Fuzi) Pangolin Scales (穿山甲, Chuanshanjia) Scorpion (全蝎, Quanxie) Coix Seed (薏苡仁, Yiyiren) Manchurian Wildginger Herb (细辛, Xixin) Doubleteeth Pulbescent Angelica Root (独活, Duhuo) Paniculate Swallowwort Root (徐长卿, Xuchangqing)

Hypertroplic spondylitis: Chinese Clematis Root (威灵仙, Weilingxian)

Systremma: White Peony Root (白芍药, Baishaoyao) Licorice Root (甘草, Gancao) Common Floweringquince Fruit (木瓜, Mugua)

Senile osteoarthritis: Ground Beetle (䗪虫, Zhechong) Glabrous Greenbrier Rhizome (土茯苓, Tufuling)

Painful heels: Twotooth Achyranthes Root (牛膝, Niuxi) Hairy Antler (鹿茸, Lurong) Chinese Clematis Root (威灵仙, Weilingxian) Chinese Taxillus Twig (桑寄生, Sangjisheng) Eucommia Bark (杜仲, Duzhong)

Osteopetrosis: Safflower (红花, Honghua) Nut-vomitive Poisonnut Seed (马钱子, Maqianzi) White Peony Root (白芍药, Baishaoyao) Szechwan Lovage Rhizome (川芎, Chuanxiong) Agkistrodon Acutus (白花蛇, Baihuashe)

Chronic osteomyelitis: Common Coltsfoot Flower (款冬花, Kuandonghua) Salt (食盐, Shiyan) Gypsum (石膏, Shigao) Calamine (炉甘石, Luganshi) Centipede (蜈蚣, Wugong) Pubescent Holly Root (毛冬青, Maodongqing) Garter Snake (乌蛇, Wushe) Large Blister Beetle (斑蝥, Banmao) Chinese Corktree Bark (黄柏, Huangbai) Croton Seed (巴豆, Badou) Cushaw Fruit Pedicel (南瓜蒂, Nanguadi) Frankincense (乳香, Ruxiang) Myrrh (没药, Moyao)

Traumatic injury: Common Aucklandia Root (木香, Muxiang) Safflower (红花, Honghua) Hindu Datura Flower (曼陀罗花, Mantuoluohua) Gypsum (石膏, Shigao) Iron Scales (生铁落, Shengtieluo) Dahurian Angelica Root (白芷, Baizhi) Udo Rhizome and Root (土当归, Tudanggui) Creeping Woodsorred Herb (酢浆草, Zuojiangcao) Balloonflower Root (桔梗, Jiegeng) Borax (硼砂, Pengsha) Ground Beetle (䗪虫, Zhechong) Chinese Corktree Bark (黄柏, Huangbai) Odorate Rosewood Root-wood (降香, Jiangxiang) India Madder Root (茜草, Qiancao) White Mustard Seed (白芥子, Baijiezi) Japanese Buttercup Herb (毛茛, Maogen) Lobed Kudzuvine Root (葛根, Gegen) Japanese Ampelopsis Root (白蔹, Bailian) Mirabilite (朴硝, Piaoxiao) Dragon's Blood (血竭, Xuejie) Himalayan Teasel Root (续断, Xuduan) Hirsute Shiny Bugleweed Herb (泽兰, Zelan) Small Centipeda Herb (鹅不食草, Ebushicao) Camphor (樟脑, Zhangnao) Snakegourd Fruit (瓜蒌, Gualou) Tuber Onion Leaf (韭菜, Jiucao) Rhubarb (大黄, Dahuang) Chinese Pyrola Herb (鹿衔草, Luxiancao)

Ankylosing spondylitis: Datura Flower (洋金花, Yangjinhua)

Bone fluoridation: Rehmannia Dried Root (生地黄, Shengdihuang) Borax (硼砂, Pengsha)

Joint tuberculosis: Coptis Rhizome (黄连, Huanglian) Turtle (鳖, Bie) Centipede (蜈蚣, Wugong) Giant Typhonium Rhizome (白附子, Baifuzi) Deglued Antler Powder (鹿角霜, Lujiaoshuang) Membranous Milkvetch Root (黄芪, Huangqi)

Fracture: Pyrite (自然铜, Zirantong) Earthworm (蚯蚓, Qiuyin) Manyprickle Acanthopanax Root (刺五加, Ciwujia) Williams Elder (接骨木, Jiegumu) Vinegar (醋, Cu) Mulberry Twig (桑枝, Sangzhi) Fortune's Drynaria Rhizome, Baron's Drynaria Rhizome (骨碎补, Gusuibu) Ground Beetle (䗪虫, Zhechong) Himalayan Teasel Root (续断, Xuduan) Frankincense (乳香, Ruxiang) Myrrh (没药, Moyao)

Bone tuberculosis: Large Blister Beetle (斑蝥, Banmao) Scorpion (全蝎, Quanxie) Myrrh (没药, Moyao) Frankincense (乳香, Ruxiang)

Ophthalmic disease

Hordeolum: Common Dayflower Herb (鸭跖草, Yazhicao) Common Lophatherum Herb (淡竹叶, Danzhuye) Swordlike Atractylodes Rhizome (苍术, Cangzhu) Human Milk (人乳汁, Renruzhi) Chinese Clematis Root (威

灵仙, Weilingxian)

Blear-eye: Mirabilite (芒硝, Mangxiao) Calamine (炉甘石, Luganshi) Climbing Groundsel Herb(千里光, Qianliguang) Honey (蜂蜜, Fengmi)

Dacryocystitis: Calamine (炉甘石, Luganshi)

Epidemic hemorrhagic conjunctivitis: Asiatic Plantain Herb (车前草, Cheqiancao) Feather Cockscomb Seed (青葙子, Qingxiangzi) Largeleaf Chinese Ash Bark (秦皮, Qinpi) Figwortflower Picrorhiza Rhizome (胡黄连, Huhuanglian)

Acute conjunctivitis: Common Scouring Rush Herb (木贼, Muzei) Mirabilite (芒硝, Mangxiao) Coptis Rhizome (黄连, Huanglian) Chinese Gentian Root (龙胆草, Longdancao) Peruvian Groundcherry Herb (灯笼草, Denglongcao) Wrinkled Gianthyssop Herb (藿香, Huoxiang) Honeysuckle Flower (金银花, Jinyinhua) Chinese Corktree Bark (黄柏, Huangbai) Leech (水蛭, Shuizhi) Dandelion (蒲公英, Pugongying) Climbing Groundsel Herb(千里光, Qianliguang)

Trachoma: Chalcanthnium (胆矾, Danfan) Watermelon Pulp (西瓜, Xigua) Garlic Bulb (蒜, Suan)

Pterygium: Chalcanthnium (胆矾, Danfan) Realgar (雄黄, Xionghuang) Cicada Slough (蝉蜕, Chantui) Pearl (珍珠, Zhenzhu)

Keratitis: Giant Knotweed Rhizome (虎杖, Huzhang) Licorice Root (甘草, Gancao) Calamine (炉甘石, Luganshi) Cicada Slough (蝉蜕, Chantui) Climbing Groundsel Herb (千里光, Qianliguang) Honey (蜂蜜, Fengmi)

Senile cataract: Desertliving Cistanche (肉苁蓉, Roucongrong) Magnetite (磁石, Cishi) Barbary Wolfberry Fruit (枸杞子, Gouqizi) Abalone Shell (石决明, Shijueming)

Glaucoma: Clove Flower-bud (丁香, Dingxiang) Areca Seed (槟榔, Binlang)

Obstruction of retinal artery: Lobed Kudzuvine Root (葛根, Gegen)

Central serous retinopsthy: Membranous Milkvetch Root (黄芪, Huangqi) Magnetite (磁石, Cishi) Motherwort Herb (益母草, Yimucao) Swordlike Atractylodes Rhizome (苍术, Cangzhu) Climbing Groundsel Herb (千里光, Qianliguang)

Myopia: Safflower (红花, Honghua) Szechwan Lovage Rhizome (川芎, Chuanxiong) Siberian Solomonseal Rhizome (黄精, Huangjing) White Mustard Seed (白芥子, Baijiezi)

Trichiasis: Chinese Gall (五倍子, Wubeizi)

Idiopathic tearing: Swordlike Atractylodes Rhizome (苍术, Cangzhu)

Night blindness: Swordlike Atractylodes Rhizome (苍术, Cangzhu) Alfalfa Root (苜蓿根, Muxugen) Goat Liver (羊肝, Yanggan)

Otopathy

Otitis externa: Chinese Corktree Bark (黄柏, Huangbai) Coptis Rhizome (黄连, Huanglian)

Obstruction of earwax: Chinese Honeylocust Spine (皂角刺, Zaojiaoci) Grassleaf Sweetflag Rhizome (石菖蒲, Shichangpu)

Otitis media suppurativa: Turmeric Roottuber (郁金, Yujin) Rangooncreeper Fruit (使君子, Shijunzi) Coptis Rhizome (黄连, Huanglian) Borax (硼砂, Pengsha) Calamine (炉甘石, Luganshi) Alumen (明矾, Mingfan) Snake Slough (蛇蜕, Shetui) Earthworm (蚯蚓, Qiuyin) Chinese Gall (五倍子,

Wubeizi) Honeysuckle Flower (金银花, Jinyinhua) Chinese Corktree Bark (黄柏, Huangbai) Scorpion (全蝎, Quanxie) Borneol (冰片, Bingpian) Bear Gall (熊胆, Xiongdan) Heartlaef Houttuynia Herb (鱼腥草, Yuxingcao) Garlic Bulb (蒜, Suan) Musk (麝香, Shexiang)

Sudden deafness: Safflower (红花, Honghua) Lobed Kudzuvine Root (葛根, Gegen) Magnetite (磁石, Cishi) Grassleaf Sweetflag Rhizome (石菖蒲, Shichangpu)

Meniere's disease: Pinellia Rhizome (半夏, Banxia) Ginkgo Seed (白果, Baiguo) Largehead Atractylodes Rhizome (白术, Baizhu) Tuckahoe (茯苓, Fuling) Hematite (代赭石, Daizheshi)

Drug-induced deafness: Siberian Solomonseal Rhizome (黄精, Huangjing)

Rhinopathy

Acute rhinitis: Small Centipeda Herb (鹅不食草, Ebushicao) Biond Magnolia Flower-bud (辛夷, Xinyi) Garlic Bulb (大蒜, Dasuan) Dahurian Angelica Root (白芷, Baizhi) Chinese Ligusticum Rhizome (藁本, Gaoben) Siberian Cocklebur Fruit (苍耳子, Cangerzi)

Chronic rhinitis: Wild Mint (薄荷, Bohe) Red Peony Root (赤芍药, Chishaoyao) Danshen Root (丹参, Danshen) Sal-ammoniac (硇砂, Naosha) Vasps Nest (露蜂房, Lufengfang) Small Centipeda Herb (鹅不食草, Ebushicao) Biond Magnolia Flower-bud (辛夷, Xinyi) Honey (蜂蜜, Fengmi)

Hypertrophic rhinitis: Biond Magnolia Flower-bud (辛夷, Xinyi)

Atrophic rhinitis: Coptis Rhizome (黄连, Huanglian) Aloes (芦荟, Luhui) Luffa Fruit (丝瓜, Sigua) Heartlaef Houttuynia Herb (鱼腥草, Yuxingcao) Honey (蜂蜜, Fengmi) Garlic Bulb (蒜, Suan)

Sinusitis: Siberian Cocklebur Fruit (苍耳子, Cangerzi) Licorice Root (甘草, Gancao) Chinese Angelica Root (当归, Danggui) Wrinkled Gianthyssop Herb (藿香, Huoxiang) Common Ducksmeat Herb (浮萍, Fuping) Acacia Catechu (孩儿茶, Haiercha) Croton Seed (巴豆, Badou) Watermelon Pulp (西瓜, Xigua) Blackberrylily Rhizome (射干, Shegan) Cow-bezoar (牛黄, Niuhuang) Heartlaef Houttuynia Herb (鱼腥草, Yuxingcao) Coptis Rhizome (黄连, Huanglian) Chinese Corktree Bark (黄柏, Huangbai) Dahurian Angelica Root (白芷, Baizhi) Biond Magnolia Flower-bud (辛夷, Xinyi)

Allergic rhinitis: Membranous Milkvetch Root (黄芪, Huangqi) Common Selfheal Spike (夏枯草, Xiakucao) Small Centipeda Herb (鹅不食草, Ebushicao) Large Blister Beetle (斑蝥, Banmao) Biond Magnolia Flower-bud (辛夷, Xinyi) Tree Peony Bark (牡丹皮, Mudanpi)

Nasal polyp: Sal-ammoniac (硇砂, Naosha) Swordlike Atractylodes Rhizome (苍术, Cangzhu) Great-ventral Garden Spider (蜘蛛, Zhizhu) Diplopod (马陆, Malu) Hindu Lotus Rhizome-node (藕节, Oujie) Realgar (雄黄, Xionghuang) Clove Flower-bud (丁香, Dingxiang)

Nasal hemorrhage: Common Rush Stem Pith (灯芯, Dengxin) Vinegar (醋, Cu) Rhubarb (大黄, Dahuang) Salt (食盐, Shiyan) Yerbadetajo Herb (墨旱莲, Mohanlian) Natural Indigo (青黛, Qingdai) Bletilla Rhizome (白及, Baiji) Cuttle Bone (乌贼骨, Wuzeigu) Aloes (芦荟, Luhui) Dragon's Blood (血竭, Xuejie) Garlic Bulb (蒜, Suan) Twotooth Achyranthes Root (牛膝, Niuxi) Cape Jasmine Fruit (栀子, Zhizi)

Guttural diseases

Laryngitis: Wild Mint (薄荷, Bohe) Vinegar (醋, Cu) Indian Mockstrawberry Herb (蛇莓, Shemei) Coptis Rhizome (黄连, Huanglian) Licorice Root (甘草, Gancao) Creeping Woodsorred Herb (酢浆草, Zuojiangcao) Honeysuckle Flower (金银花, Jinyinhua) Chinese Corktree Bark (黄柏, Huangbai) Figwort Root (玄参, Xuanshen) Blackberrylily Rhizome (射干, Shegan) Cow-bezoar (牛黄, Niuhuang)

Hoarse voice: Wild Mint (薄荷, Bohe) Coastal Glehnia Root, and Fourleaf Ladybell Root (沙参, Shashen) Cicada Slough (蝉蜕, Chantui) Balloonflower Root (桔梗, Jiegeng)

Aphonia: Ass-hide Glue (阿胶, Ejiao) Coastal Glehnia Root, and Fourleaf Ladybell Root (沙参, Shashen) Puff-ball (马勃, Mabo) Medicine Terminalia Fruit (诃子, Hezi) Cicada Slough (蝉蜕, Chantui)

Inflammation of the throat: Mirabilite (朴硝, Piaoxiao) Croton Seed (巴豆, Badou)

Acute tonsillitis: Asiatic Plantain Herb (车前草, Cheqiancao) Whiteflower Patrinia Herb (败酱草, Baijiangcao) Rehmannia Dried Root (生地黄, Shengdihuang) Vinegar (醋, Cu) Rhubarb (大黄, Dahuang) Giant Knotweed Rhizome (虎杖, Huzhang) Coptis Rhizome (黄连, Huanglian) Franchet Groundcherry Calyx or Fruit (锦灯笼, Jindenglong) Acacia Catechu (孩儿茶, Haiercha) Vasps Nest (露蜂房, Lufengfang) Cicada Slough (蝉蜕, Chantui) Honeysuckle Flower (金银花, Jinyinhua) Scorpion (全蝎, Quanxie) Watermelon Pulp (西瓜, Xigua) Tonkin Sophora Root (山豆根, Shandougen) Chinese Clematis Root (威灵仙, Weilingxian) Musk (麝香, Shexiang) Blackberrylily Rhizome (射干, Shegan) Dyers Woad Root (板蓝根, Banlangen) Ningpo Figwort Root (玄参, Xuanshen)

Polyp of vocal cors: Charred Hawthorn Fruit (焦山楂, Jiaoshanzha)

Globus hystericus: Borax (硼砂, Pengsha) Large Blister Beetle (斑蝥, Banmao) Dutchmanspipe Fruit (马兜铃, Madouling) Pinellia Rhizome (半夏, Banxia) Officinal Magnolia Bark (厚朴, Houpo) Common Perilla Leaf (苏叶, Suye)

Foreign body in esophagus and throat: Borax (硼砂, Pengsha) Hawthorn Fruit (山楂, Shanzha) Chinese Clematis Root (威灵仙, Weilingxian) Perilla Leaf (紫苏, Zisu)

Stomatosis

Periodontitis: Talc Powder (滑石粉, Huashifen) Shunk Bugbane Rhizome (升麻, Shengma) Dandelion (蒲公英, Pugongying) Garlic Bulb (蒜, Suan)

Periapical inflammation: Indian Mockstrawberry Herb (蛇莓, Shemei)

Angular stomatitis: Indian Mockstrawberry Herb (蛇莓, Shemei)

Toothache: Siberian Cocklebur Fruit (苍耳子, Cangerzi) Dahurian Angelica Root (白芷, Baizhi) Long Pepper Fruit (荜茇, Biba) Salt (食盐, Shiyan) Pinellia Rhizome (半夏, Banxia) Common Knotgrass Herb (萹蓄, Bianxu) Magnetite (磁石, Cishi) Smoked Plum (乌梅, Wumei) Szechwan Lovage Rhizome (川芎, Chuanxiong) Manchurian Wildginger Herb (细辛, Xixin) Vasps Nest (露蜂房, Lufengfang) Toad (蟾蜍, Chanchu) Chinese Gall (五倍子, Wubeizi) Bunge Pricklyash (花椒, Huajiao) Black Pepper Fruit (胡椒, Hujiao) Camphor (樟脑, Zhangnao) Lilac Daphne Flower-bud (芫花, Yuanhua) Japanese Buttercup Herb (毛茛,

Maogen) Chinese Clematis Root (威灵仙, Weilingxian) Realgar (雄黄, Xionghuang)

Recurrent stomatitis: Common Rush Stem Pith (灯芯, Dengxin) Talc (滑石, Huashi) Rhubarb (大黄, Dahuang) Dan-shen Root (丹参, Danshen) Anhydrous Sodium Sulfate (玄明粉, Xuanmingfen) Largeleaf Gentian Root (秦艽, Qinjiao) Sanchi Root (三七, Sanqi) Cow-bezoar (牛黄, Niuhuang)

Recurrent ulcer of mouth: Borax (硼砂, Pengsha) Manchurian Wildginger Herb (细辛, Xixin) Vasps Nest (露蜂房, Lufengfang) Ass-hide Glue (阿胶, Ejiao) Chinese Corktree Bark (黄柏, Huangbai) Medicinal Evodia Root (吴茱萸, Wuzhuyu) Watermelon Frost (西瓜霜, Xiguashuang) Akebia Stem (木通, Mutong) Green Gram Seed (绿豆, Lvdou) Clove Flower-bud (丁香, Dingxiang) Natural Indigo (青黛, Qingdai)

Oral lichen planus: Sweet Wormwood (青蒿, Qinghao)

Xerostomia: Dwarf Lilyturf Root (麦门冬, Maimendong) Barbary Wolfberry Fruit (枸杞子, Gouqizi) Coastal Glehnia Root, and Fourleaf Ladybell Root (沙参, Shashen)

Gingival bleeding: White Peony Root (白芍药, Baishaoyao) Ass-hide Glue (阿胶, Ejiao) Natural Indigo (青黛, Qingdai) Cow-bezoar (牛黄, Niuhuang)

Postextraction hemorrhage: Salt (食盐, Shiyan) Cuttle Bone (乌贼骨, Wuzeigu) Chinese Gall (五倍子, Wubeizi) India Madder Root (茜草, Qiancao)

Disfunction of mandibular articulation: Plantain Seed (车前子, Cheqianzi) Sanchi Root (三七, Sanqi) Chinese Angelica Root (当归, Danggui) Lightyellow Sophora Root (苦参, Kushen) Chinese Gall (五倍子, Wubeizi)

Tumor

Nasopharyngeal carcinoma: Dan-shen Root (丹参, Danshen) Stalactite (钟乳石, Zhongrushi) Sal-ammoniac (硇砂, Naosha) Tuckahoe (茯苓, Fuling)

Tyroid cancer: Pink Plumepoppy Herb with Root (博落回, Boluohui) Croton Seed (巴豆, Badou) Airpotato Yam Tuber (黄药子, Huangyaozi)

Lung cancer: Zedoray (莪术, Ezhu) Chinese Stellera Root (狼毒, Langdu) Bistort Rhizome (拳参, Quanshen) Common Selfheal Fruit-spike(Common Selfheal Spike (夏枯草, Xiakucao) Xiakucao) Umbellate Pore Fungus (猪苓, Zhuling) Largeleaf Chinese Ash Bark (秦皮, Qinpi) Fourstamen Stephania Root (防己, Fangji)

Mastoncus: Kansui Root (甘遂, Gansui) Cochinchinese Asparagus Root (天门冬, Tianmendong) Scorpion (全蝎, Quanxie)

Mammary cancer: Appendiculate Cremastra Pseudobulb (山慈姑, Shancigu) Vasps Nest (露蜂房, Lufengfang) Realgar (雄黄, Xionghuang)

Digestive tract cancer: Inula Flower (旋覆花, Xuanfuhua) Rehmannia Dried Root (生地黄, Shengdihuang) Hematite (代赭石, Daizheshi) Vinegar (醋, Cu) Manyleaf Paris Rhizome (蚤休, Zaoxiu) Chinese Stellera Root (狼毒, Langdu) Chlorite-schist (礞石, Mengshi) Largehead Atractylodes Rhizome (白术, Baizhu) Sal-ammoniac (硇砂, Naosha) Ginseng (人参, Renshen) Tuckahoe (茯苓, Fuling) Centipede (蜈蚣, Wugong) Toad (蟾蜍, Chanchu) Large Blister Beetle (斑蝥, Banmao) Croton Seed (巴豆, Badou) Gecko (守宫, Shougong) Cow-bezoar (牛黄,

Niuhuang) Tuber Onion (韭, Jiu) Chinaroot Greenbrier Rhizome (菝葜, Baqia) Airpotato Yam Tuber (黄药子, Huangyaozi) Chinese Clematis Root (威灵仙, Weilingxian) Musk (麝香, Shexiang)

Primary carcinoma of liver: Chinese Lobelia Herb (半边莲, Banbianlian) Common Selfheal Fruit-spike (Common Selfheal Spike (夏枯草, Xiakucao) Xiakucao) Large Blister Beetle (斑蝥, Banmao) Realgar (雄黄, Xionghuang) Clove Flower-bud (丁香, Dingxiang)

Cancinoma of kidney: Jackinthepulpit Tuber (天南星, Tiannanxing)

Tumor of bladder: Tonkin Sophora Root (山豆根, Shandougen)

Cancinoma of uterine cervix: Zedoray (莪术, Ezhu) Jackinthepulpit Tuber (天南星, Tiannanxing) Pinellia Rhizome (半夏, Banxia) Tendrilleaf Fritillary Bulb (贝母, Beimu) Sal-ammoniac (硇砂, Naosha) River-snail (田螺, Tianluo)

Oophoroma: Croton Seed (巴豆, Badou) Musk (麝香, Shexiang)

Chotioadenoma: Tonkin Sophora Root (山豆根, Shandougen)

Chorioepithelioma (chorionic epithelioma): Root of Sinkiang Arnebia (紫草, Zicao) Vasps Nest (露蜂房, Lufengfang)

Skin cancinoma: Nut-vomitive Poisonnut Seed (马钱子, Maqianzi) Alumen (白矾, Baifan)

Angiomyoma: Sinkiang Giantfennal Resin (阿魏, Awei) Aspongopus (九香虫, Jiuxiangchong) Herb of Bittesweet (白英, Baiying)

Angiosarcoma: Cochinchinese Asparagus Root (天门冬, Tianmendong)

Lymphoma: Toad (蟾蜍, Chanchu) Dwarf Lilyturf Root (麦门冬, Maimendong)

Side effect of large intestine: Chinese Clematis Root (威灵仙, Weilingxian) Dutchmanspipe Fruit (马兜铃, Madouling) Zedoray (莪术, Ezhu) Toad (蟾蜍, Chanchu) Large Blister Beetle (斑蝥, Banmao)

Anal disease

Anal fissure: Coptis Rhizome (黄连, Huanglian) Bletilla Rhizome (白及, Baiji) Sulfur (硫黄, Liuhuang) Rice Bean (赤小豆, Chixiaodou) Dried Ginger (干姜, Ganjiang) Myrrh (没药, Moyao)

Hemorhoid: Talc (滑石, Huashi) Hindu Datura Seed or Fruit (曼陀罗子, Mantuoluozi) Salt (食盐, Shiyan) Pinellia Rhizome (半夏, Banxia) White Peony Root (白芍药, Baishaoyao) Figwortflower Picrorhiza Rhizome (胡黄连, Huhuanglian) Shunk Bugbane Rhizome (升麻, Shengma) Hirsute Shiny Bugleweed Herb (泽兰, Zelan) Acacia Catechu (孩儿茶, Haiercha) Calamine (炉甘石, Luganshi) Lightyellow Sophora Root (苦参, Kushen) Alumen (明矾, Mingfan) Silkworm with Batrytis Larva (白僵蚕, Baijiangcan) Snake Slough (蛇蜕, Shetui) Cicada Slough (蝉蜕, Chantui) Chinese Gall (五倍子, Wubeizi) Honeysuckle Flower (金银花, Jinyinhua) Fig Receptacle (无花果, Wuhuaguo) Dragon's Blood (血竭, Xuejie) Tonkin Sophora Root (山豆根, Shandougen) Chinese Arborvitae Leafy Twig (侧柏叶, Cebaiye)

Pruritus ani: Calamine (炉甘石, Luganshi) Areca Seed (槟榔, Binlang)

Eczema ani: Camphor (樟脑, Zhangnao) Belvedere Fruit (地肤子, Difuzi) Lightyellow Sophora Root (苦参, Kushen)

Proctophosis: Manyleaf Paris Rhizome (蚤休, Zaoxiu) Limonite (禹余粮, Yuyuliang) Rangooncreeper Fruit (使君子, Shijunzi)

Shunk Bugbane Rhizome（升麻，Shengma）Chinese Gall（五倍子，Wubeizi）Cochinchina Momordica Seed（木鳖子，Mubiezi）Membranous Milkvetch Root（黄芪，Huangqi）Chinese Thorowax Root（柴胡，Chaihu）

Proctoptoma: Alumen（明矾，Mingfan）Chinaroot Greenbrier Rhizome（菝葜，Baqia）Shunk Bugbane Rhizome（升麻，Shengma）Immature Bitter Orange（枳实，Zhishi）Chinese Thorowax Root（柴胡，Chaihu）

Anusitis: Scorpion（全蝎，Quanxie）Heartlaef Houttuynia Herb（鱼腥草，Yuxingcao）

英文药名索引

C

D

E

F

G

M

N

O

S

T

U

汉语拼音药名索引

A

B

C

D

E

F

G

Q

R

S

E

T

天南星,Tiannanxing ………………… (319)

W

X

Y

月季花,Yuejihua …………………… (254)

Z

CURRICULUM VITAE OF LIU GONGWANG

DATE OF BIRTH: Nov. 20, 1943

SEX: Male

EDUCATION: BA of Traditional Chinese Medicine, Tianjin College of TCM, 1962～1968

WORKING EXPERIENCES: I have been working and teaching on TCM for more than 30 years. Doctor in chief, Hebei hospital, 1979. Director and associate professor, international training department of TCM, Tianjin College of TCM, (Tianjin, China), 1987. Director and Professor, Department of Acupuncture and Moxibustion, Tianjin College of TCM, (Tianjin, China), 1992～09, 2000. Director and Professor, Department of Chinese Medicine, Tianjin College of TCM, (Tianjin, China).

MEMBERSHIPS: General secretary of Foreign Medicinal Exchange Association, Tianjin, P. R. China.

PUBLICATIONS: *Fundamentals of Acupuncture and Moxibustion* (in English and Japanese), Editor in chief, May 1994.

Acupoints and Meridians (in English), Editor in Chief, 1997.

Techniques of Acupuncture & Moxibustion (in English), Editor in chief, 1998.

A Complement work of Present Acupuncture and Moxibustion (in Chinese), Editor in chief, 1998.

Chinese herbal Medicine (in Chinese and English), editor in chief, 2000.

The Prescriptions of TCM on Pain Syndrome, *Study of TCM Prescriptions*, 7, 1990.

Explanation on the Eight TCM therapeutic principles, *Study of TCM Prescriptions*, 5, 1990.

Explanation of TCM prescriptions, *Study of TCM Prescriptions*, 5.1999.

Discussion on the Four Elements of Ease the pain by Acupuncture, *Acupuncture research*, 4.1998.

The Treatment on Osteoporosis By TCM, 9.2000.

The treatment on The Syndrome Menopouse By TCM, 6.1999.

CLINICAL EXPERIENCE: Treatment of intractable pain and diseases related to nerve system, such as cerebral apoplexy, epilepsy and depression with acupuncture and Chinese herbs. Treatment of cancer of late stage with traditional and modern medicine.

MAILING ADDRESS:

Tianjin College Traditional Chinese Medicine

No.88, Yuquan road, Nankai District, Tianjin 300193, P.R.China

Tel.: 86-22-27491547

86-22-27486658 extend 83042 or 83044

Fax: 86-22-27374931

图书在版编目(CIP)数据

中药学:英文版/刘公望主编．-北京:华夏出版社,2001.1
(现代中医临床备要丛书)
ISBN 7-5080-2282-3

Ⅰ.中… Ⅱ.刘… Ⅲ.中药学-英文 Ⅳ.R28

中国版本图书馆 CIP 数据核字(2000)第 82297 号

华 夏 出 版 社 出 版 发 行
(北京东直门外香河园北里 4 号 邮编:100028)
新 华 书 店 经 销
北 京 建 筑 工 业 印 刷 厂 印 刷
787×1092 1/16 开本 35.75 印张 883 千字
2001 年 1 月北京第 1 版 2001 年 1 月北京第 1 次印刷
定价:150.00 元